Clinical Adult Neurology

Third Edition

Edited by

Jody Corey-Bloom, MD, PhD
Professor of Neurosciences
Department of Neurosciences
University of California, San Diego
La Jolla, California

with

Ronald B. David, MD
Attending Physician
Department of Pediatrics
St. Mary's Hospital
Associate Clinical Professor
Department of Pediatrics
Virginia Commonwealth University School of Medicine
Richmond, Virginia

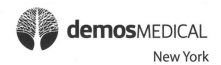

New York

Acquisitions Editor: R. Craig Percy
Cover Design: Amy Nordin
Copyeditor: Joann Woy
Compositor: Patricia Wallenburg
Printer: Bang Printing

Visit our website at www.demosmedpub.com

© 2009 Demos Medical Publishing, LLC. All rights reserved. This book is protected by copyright. No part of it may be reproduced, stored in a retrieval system, or transmitted in any form or by any means, electronic, mechanical, photocopying, recording, or otherwise, without the prior written permission of the publisher.

Medicine is an ever-changing science. Research and clinical experience are continually expanding our knowledge, in particular our understanding of proper treatment and drug therapy. The authors, editors, and publisher have made every effort to ensure that all information in this book is in accordance with the state of knowledge at the time of production of the book. Nevertheless, the authors, editors, and publisher are not responsible for errors or omissions or for any consequences from application of the information in this book and make no warranty, express or implied, with respect to the contents of the publication. Every reader should examine carefully the package inserts accompanying each drug and should carefully check whether the dosage schedules mentioned therein or the contraindications stated by the manufacturer differ from the statements made in this book. Such examination is particularly important with drugs that are either rarely used or have been newly released on the market.

Library of Congress Cataloging-in-Publication Data

Clinical adult neurology / edited by Jody Corey-Bloom, with Ronald B. David. — 3rd ed.
   p. ; cm.
  Rev. ed. of: Adult neurology / edited by Jody Corey-Bloom. 2nd ed. 2005.
  Includes bibliographical references and index.
  ISBN-13: 978-1-933864-35-8 (hardcover : alk. paper)
  ISBN-10: 1-933864-35-4 (hardcover : alk. paper)
  1. Neurology. 2. Nervous system—Diseases. I. Corey-Bloom, Jody. II. David, Ronald B. III. Adult neurology.
  [DNLM: 1. Nervous System Diseases—diagnosis. 2. Nervous System Diseases—therapy. 3. Neurologic Manifestations. WL 140 C6395 2009]
  RC346.A327 2009
  616.8—dc22

                     2008040667

Special discounts on bulk quantities of Demos Medical Publishing books are available to corporations, professional associations, pharmaceutical companies, health care organizations, and other qualifying groups. For details, please contact:

Special Sales Department
Demos Medical Publishing
386 Park Avenue South, Suite 301
New York, NY 10016
Phone: 800–532–8663 or 212–683–0072
Fax: 212–683–0118
Email: orderdept@demosmedpub.com

Made in the United States of America
08 09 10 11   5 4 3 2 1

Contents

▶ **III Neurologic Diseases and Disorders**

Foreword

Traditional textbooks convey knowledge. It is the goal of this text to convey not only essential knowledge, but also the collected wisdom of its many highly regarded contributors. This volume is divided into three sections:

▶ Adult Neurologic Examination
▶ Common Problems in Adult Neurology
▶ Neurologic Diseases and Disorders

Also included to facilitate a physician's use of this book are:

▶ Nosologic diagnosis tables
▶ "Pearls and Perils" boxes
▶ "Consider Consultation When . . ." boxes
▶ "Key Clinical Questions" boxes
▶ Selected annotated bibliographies
▶ A complete bibliography

The nosologic diagnosis tables are based on a discriminator model to promote clearer understanding and are superior to a criterion-based model and others that lack similar specificity.

> Whoever having undertaken to speak or write hath first laid for themselves some [basis] to their argument such as hot or cold or moist or dry or whatever else they choose, thus reducing their subject within a narrow compass.
> —*Hippocrates*

As Hippocrates has suggested, structure is the key to learning. Unless there is a structure onto which knowledge can be built, confusion and disorganization are the inevitable consequences.

Classification systems induce orderliness in thinking and enhance our ability to communicate effectively.

A review of the most enduring hierarchical classification systems, particularly that of Linnaeus (that is, phyla, genera, species), makes clear the value of grouping according to discriminating features, as well as the value of simplicity, expandability, and dynamism.

The goal, whatever the classification system, is to seek the most powerful discriminating features that will produce the greatest diagnostic clarity. Discriminating features should avoid crossing domains. Much of the confusion that arises in diagnosis may be the result of the clinician who unwittingly crosses the anatomic, pathologic, pathophysiologic, phenomenologic, and etiologic classification domains used in medicine (for example, the inclusion of anatomically-oriented "temporal lobe seizures" in a phenomenologically based classification system that includes complex partial seizures). Some conditions, such as brain tumors, are classified according to their histopathology and lend themselves well to this classification system. Others, such as headaches and movement disorders, are classified phenomenologically and are therefore much less easily classified. In other cases, discriminators must encompass inclusionary as well as exclusionary features. At times, we can only use a criterion-based system or construct tables to compare features.

Arbitrarily, we label as consistent features those which occur more than 75% of the time; features are considered variable when they occur less than 75% of the time. The diagnostic tables should be viewed, therefore, only as a beginning in the extremely difficult effort to make diagnosis more precise and biologically based. How well this book accomplishes the goals of identifying the most powerful discrimination features for maximum diagnostic clarity is limited by the current state of the art. In some areas, several features, when clustered together, serve to discriminate.

This text is designed to be pithy, not exhaustive, as there are already many available of this ilk.

This text is therefore in no way a singular effort and reflects the expertise of all who contributed in so many different ways and it is my hope that this is reflected in the quality of the effort. It is therefore my fondest wish that this text reside on your desk, rather than your bookshelf.

Ronald B. David, MD

Preface

Many of the contributors to this book are recognized authorities in their fields but were asked to participate because of their ability to meld their knowledge of a discipline with practical clinical experience. I would be highly remiss if I did not acknowledge their extraordinary contributions to this effort.

Section I of this book offers an organized discussion of the adult neurological evaluation including the history and examination, electrophysiological studies and neuroradiology. Section II covers common clinical problems in neurology and ways of evaluating, managing, and treating them. Section III illustrates the spectrum of specific neurologic diseases and disorders.

One of my motivations for editing this book was the opportunity to provide physicians involved in the primary care of patients with a methodical yet succinct guide to neurologic disease. Clearly, these are times that require a well-rationed, yet efficient, approach to the diagnosis of medical problems. Some instruments to aid in this endeavor were first pioneered by Dr. Ronald David, the Series Editor, in his volume on Pediatric Neurology. They include the "Features Table" which attempts to capture the discriminating, consistent and variable features of a disease. Likewise, the "Pearls and Perils" box emphasizes essences of a diagnosis in addition to some of the possible covert traps. "Consider Consultation When" should provide physicians with helpful guidelines for referral; "Key Clinical Questions" steers the clinician in his thinking and history taking.

It is my hope that you find the chapters in this book both comprehensive and practical and that *Clinical Adult Neurology* quickly becomes indispensable reference in your bedside and office decision-making.

Jody Corey-Bloom

Contributors

Joseph R. Berger, MD
Ruth L. Works Professor and Chairman
Department of Neurology
University of Kentucky
Lexington, Kentucky

Dennis N. Bourdette, MD
Chair and Roy and Eulalia Swank Family Research
    Professor
Department of Neurology
Oregon Health and Science University
Portland, Oregon

Marc C. Chamberlain, MD
Director and Professor
Departments of Neuro-Oncology and Neurology
Seattle Cancer Care Alliance
Seattle, Washington

Thomas C. Chelimsky, MD
Professor of Neurology, Anesthesia and Pediatrics
Department of Neurology
Case Western Reserve University and Medical Center
Cleveland, Ohio

Jody Corey-Bloom, MD, PhD
Professor of Neurosciences
Department of Neurosciences
University of California, San Diego
La Jolla, California

Nayan P. Desai, MD
Neurologist
Department of Neurology
Palo Alto Medical Foundation
Fremont, California

Joseph Drazkowski, MD
Director, EEG Lab
Department of Neurology
Mayo Clinic Arizona
Phoenix, Arizona

Ronald J. Ellis, MD, PhD
Associate Professor
Department of Neurosciences
University of California, San Diego
San Diego, California

Eva L. Feldman, MD, PhD
Russell N. DeJong Professor
Director, JDRF Center for the Study of Complications
    in Diabetes
Director, ALS Clinic
Department of Neurology
University of Michigan
Ann Arbor, Michigan

Douglas Galasko, MB, BCh
Professor
Department of Neurosciences
University of California, San Diego
San Diego, California

Steven G. Imbesi, MD
Professor
Radiology and Neurosurgery
Department of Radiology
University of California, San Diego
San Diego, California

Cheryl A. Jay, MD
Clinical Professor
Department of Neurology
University of California, San Francisco
San Francisco, California

Edward Kim, MD
Instructor
Department of Neurology
Oregon Health and Science University
Portland, Oregon

Anita A. Koshy, MD
Postdoctoral Fellow
Departments of Microbiology and Immunology, and
     Medicine
Stanford University School of Medicine
Stanford, California

Ruzica Kovacevic-Ristanovic, MD
Associate Professor
Northwestern University Feinberg School of Medicine
Department of Neurology
Evanston Northwestern Healthcare
Evanston, Illinois

Tomasz J. Kuzniar, MD, PhD
Assistant Professor
Northwestern University Feinberg School of Medicine
Division of Pulmonary and Critical Care Medicine
Evanston Northwestern Healthcare
Evanston, Illinois

Douglas J. Lanska, MD, MS, MSPH
Neurologist
Department of Medicine Service
Veterans Administration Medical Center
Tomah, Wisconsin
Professor of Neurology
Department of Neurology
University of Wisconsin School of Medicine and Public
     Health
Madison, Wisconsin

Stephanie Lessig, MD
Assistant Clinical Professor
Department of Neurosciences
University of California, San Diego
San Diego, California

Lawrence F. Marshall, MD
Professor and Chief of Neurosurgical Services
University of California, San Diego
San Diego, California

Michele K. Mass, MD
Associate Professor
Department of Neurology
Oregon Health and Science University
Portland, Oregon

Andrew D. Massey, MD
Associate Professor
Department of Internal Medicine
Kansas University School of Medicine, Wichita
Wichita, Kansas

Eli S. Neiman, DO
Department of Neurology
New Jersey Neurological Institute
Edison, New Jersey

Richard K. Olney, MD
Professor
Department of Neurology
University of California, San Francisco
San Francisco, California

Michael S. Rafii, MD, PhD
Assistant Professor
Department of Neurosciences
University of California, San Diego
La Jolla, California

John F. Rothrock, MD
Professor and Vice Chair
Department of Neurology
University of Alabama at Birmingham
Birmingham, Alabama

James W. Russell, MD, MS, FRCP
Associate Professor
Department of Neurology
University of Maryland School of Medicine
Baltimore, Maryland

Melody Ryan, Pharm D, MPH
Associate Professor
Departments of Pharmacy Practice and Science, and
     Neurology
University of Kentucky
Lexington, Kentucky

Stephen J. Ryan, MD, MA
Associate Professor
Department of Neurology
University of Kentucky
Lexington, Kentucky

Sith Sathornsumetee, MD
Instructor
Department of Medicine (Neurology)
Faculty of Medicine Siriraj Hospital
Mahidol University
Bangkok, Thailand

J. Robinson Singleton, MD
Associate Professor
Department of Neurology
University of Utah
Salt Lake City, Utah

John T. Slevin, MD, MBA
Professor
Departments of Neurology, and Molecular Biomedical
    Pharmacology
Veterans Administration Medical Center
University of Kentucky Medical Center
Lexington, Kentucky

Mark A. Stacy, MD
Associate Professor
Department of Medicine (Neurology)
Duke University Medical Center
Durham, North Carolina

Evelyn S. Tecoma, MD, PhD
Professor
Department of Neurosciences
University of California, San Diego
La Jolla, California
San Diego Veterans Administration Healthcare System
San Diego, California

Ruth H. Whitham, MD
Chief
Department of Neurology
Portland Veterans Affairs Medical Center
Professor
Department of Neurology
Oregon Health and Science University
Portland, Oregon

Richard M. Zweifler, MD
Chief
Department of Neurology
Sentara Healthcare
Adjunct Professor
Department of Neurology
Eastern Virginia Medical School
Norfolk, Virgina

SECTION 1

ADULT NEUROLOGIC EXAMINATION

CHAPTER 1

The Neurologic History and Examination of the Adult

Douglas Galasko

Outline

► Overall goals
► The neurologic history
► Neurologic examination

Overall Goals

The traditional approach of using the history and examination to guide diagnostic decision-making reaches a peak in patients with neurologic problems. Even in an age of technology and high resolution neuroimaging tests, the "old-fashioned" clinical approach to neurology remains relevant. Imaging and other laboratory studies are powerful tools, which complement but do not replace a meticulous history and examination. For example, neuroimaging procedures are not routinely helpful in the evaluation of common clinical problems, such as headache and lower back pain, where clinical evaluation remains the mainstay. Similarly, the history is critical in deciding whether—and how—to evaluate a patient for the common symptoms of headache, vertigo, pain, or episodic loss of consciousness. For non-neurologists, the brain and its offshoots often seem intimidating and difficult to assess thoroughly and efficiently. This chapter highlights important principles of the neurologic history and examination of adults, emphasizing how the examination can be tailored to fit specific clinical situations (Box 1.1). In addition to a single comprehensive approach, selected components of the history and examination can be used for screening the nervous system, evaluating elderly individuals, and testing cognitive abilities.

Integrating symptoms and signs into a diagnosis is part of the art of medicine. The utility of specific parts of the neurologic history or examination can be rigorously evaluated, using evidence-based approaches, to help determine the most useful elements that provide positive ("rule-in") or negative ("rule-out") evidence of specific disorders. For example, when distinguishing syncope from seizures, a loss of consciousness with prolonged sitting or standing and preceding feelings of diaphoresis or light-headedness are the symptoms that best ruled out a seizure, whereas waking up with a sore tongue, having a sense of déjà vu or other unusual feelings before spells, or having repeated muscle jerking for a minute or two during spells is indicative of a seizure. For carpal tunnel syndrome, features that best predict electrodiagnostic evidence of median nerve compression include sensory symptoms in a plausible distribution, decreased sensitivity to pain in the median nerve territory, and weak thumb abduction. Nocturnal paresthesiae, Phalen's and Tinel's signs, and thenar atrophy have much less diagnostic value.

The Neurologic History

General Principles

A *screening* neurologic history should center on common problems relevant to a patient's age, gender, or medical history. For example, in an elderly patient, questions should cover stroke, memory ability, gait and falls, and the special senses of vision and hearing. In patients with hypertension or ischemic coronary disease, inquiry about transient ischemic attacks or stroke is important, while in insulin-dependent diabetics, symptoms of cerebral ischemia and cranial and peripheral neuropathy should be sought.

When a patient's *major complaint* consists of or includes neurologic dysfunction, the history should be focused and detailed. The onset, course, and tempo of symptoms, and whether they are intermittent, relapsing

> ▼
>
> **Box 1.1** Overall goals in neurologic assessment
>
> **History**
> ▶ Identify and characterize neurologic symptoms; try to map onto syndromes or classes of disease.
> ▶ Localize the site(s) of origin of the symptoms.
> ▶ Determine etiologic or risk factors.
> ▶ Define the degree of disability due to the neurologic problem: e.g., mobility, social or occupational function.
>
> **Examination**
> ▶ Localize the site(s) of origin of neurologic symptoms.
> ▶ Rule out serious neurologic causes of common symptoms such as headaches.
> ▶ Assess the extent of impairment of function.
>
> **Integrated goal**
> ▶ Establish a diagnosis in terms of anatomic localization, likely etiology, and the extent of impairment of daily function that results.

with normal function between episodes, or constant should be clarified. Many neurologic symptoms are difficult to describe, and patients should be encouraged to provide a detailed account of their nature, using lay language rather than technical or jargon terms that may be misunderstood—a clear description can guide the physician to decide that the symptoms represent specific syndromes such as vertigo, migraine, seizure, or stroke. For intermittent or episodic symptoms that recover completely, such as headaches, seizures, vertigo, or transient ischemic attacks, clinical judgment depends on the history alone. If the nature of the symptoms renders the patient an inadequate historian—as may occur for strokes, seizures with loss of consciousness, and memory disorders—an informant is essential. This may require a phone call or an additional clinic visit. A goal of history-taking is to group symptoms into a syndrome diagnosis if possible. For example, the description of a throbbing headache may be insufficient to characterize it as migraine. If nausea and photophobia accompany the headache, and visual phenomena such as scintillations sometimes precede it, then the migraine syndrome is obvious.

The *onset* of neurologic symptoms often helps narrow the differential diagnosis. For example, the sudden or rapid onset of focal loss of neurologic function is typical of an ischemic or hemorrhagic stroke. The subacute onset of a similar focal deficit suggests a mass lesion. On the other hand, many disorders that involve degeneration of the central or peripheral nervous system begin insidiously and show steady progression, with a course measured in months or years. The clinician should ask whether any unusual events or exposures preceded the onset of

symptoms, including headache, infections, medications, and trauma. In patients with focal weakness or sensory symptoms suggesting injury or entrapment of a peripheral nerve, the history should include a search for predisposing factors such as sleeping or sitting in an unusual position, previous injuries or fractures, and repetitive limb motion at work or during hobbies.

The *clinical course* of neurologic conditions helps to narrow the diagnosis. Episodic conditions that produce transient neurologic symptoms that then revert to normal include migraine and other headaches, vertigo, seizures, and transient cerebral ischemia. Acute attacks of multiple sclerosis are characterized by neurologic deficits with rapid onset, over hours or more commonly a day or two, followed by a gradual but often incomplete recovery over days to weeks. After a stroke or trauma, the brain usually shows some degree of recovery, which may continue for many months after the original insult. Fluctuation of deficits occurs in many neurologic conditions and is commonly reported as fatigue. This is especially true of disorders affecting structures that enable rapid conduction of nerve impulses, such as myelin and the neuromuscular junction. Multiple sclerosis and myasthenia gravis are prime examples of conditions with weakness that fluctuates from day to day, and patients with these disorders may report tiring after the increased effort needed to complete formerly routine activities. A chronic, steadily progressive course, measured over years, is typical of inflammatory or degenerative disorders.

It is important to inquire about risk factors for neurologic conditions. Because almost any type of neurologic condition can be inherited, including degenerative conditions, dementia, movement disorders, seizures, muscle diseases, and peripheral neuropathies, the *family history* should be noted. If one strongly suspects an inherited disorder, a comprehensive assessment may include obtaining medical records on other family members, interviewing relatives of the patient, and examining family members who may have the disorder of interest. For many inherited neurologic disorders, it is possible to test for pathogenic DNA mutations and to use the information for prognosis and, in some instances, for genetic counseling.

Environmental (or nongenetic) risk factors for neurologic conditions form an enormous list. Only a few examples will be mentioned here. If symptoms suggest a stroke or transient ischemic attack, then the history should focus on the heart (including valvular conditions or arrhythmias such as atrial fibrillation that may predispose to embolism, symptoms of coronary atherosclerosis, and cardiac surgery) and on hypertension, diabetes, and smoking. Many systemic diseases can affect the nervous system, for example, diabetes mellitus, cancer and its treatment, chronic renal failure, systemic lupus erythematosus, and collagen vascular disorders. Among infectious disorders, human immunodeficiency virus (HIV) infection may result in symptoms affecting the entire nervous system, especially cognitive impairment, focal weakness, seizures, weakness, and sensory symptoms due to spinal cord or peripheral nerve involvement.

Occupations or hobbies may predispose to neurologic problems. Repetitive movements may lead to pain and weakness among workers on assembly lines or checkout stands, people typing at computer terminals, professional musicians, and workers who use vibrating tools. These symptoms do not automatically imply nerve damage, because damage or inflammation to muscles, tendons, and joints may explain the clinical picture. A meticulous examination and ancillary tests such as electromyography (EMG) or X-ray studies may be needed to clarify the diagnosis.

It is also important to inquire about *medications* and *abuse of alcohol and drugs*. These substances can damage the central nervous system, producing cognitive and behavioral symptoms and contributing to vascular disorders. They may also affect the peripheral nerves. Some common scenarios include elderly patients whose confusion, lethargy, or cognitive changes can be explained by polypharmacy; patients receiving cancer chemotherapy, who develop neuropathy or cerebellar ataxia; and patients receiving psychotropic medications, who become delirious or develop movement disorders such as tremor, parkinsonism, or tardive dyskinesia.

The neurologic history should cover *psychiatric symptoms*. In some cases, the psychiatric history may reveal factors that contribute to patients' perception of their neurologic symptoms. For example, conversion reactions may manifest as pseudoseizures, unusual movement disorders, blindness, sensory loss, or paralysis. Although the bizarre and nonphysiologic nature of symptoms or signs helps to clarify many of these diagnoses, patients may sometimes have combined neurologic and psychiatric disorders, such as mixed pseudoseizures and genuine seizures. Diagnostic acumen often needs to be supported by physiologic testing (electromyography or electroencephalogram) or neuroimaging studies to define the etiology of the symptoms. In patients with chronic pain, including chronic daily headaches, factors such as anxiety and depression may exacerbate or amplify the symptoms. Patients with neurologic disorders often develop psychiatric symptoms, which may be amenable to treatment. Sometimes these symptoms result from patients' awareness of their disability (e.g., reactive depression in patients with paralysis), or they may be part of the disease, for example, agitation and delusions in patients with Alzheimer's disease, or emotional lability in patients with frontal lobe lesions. By identifying and assessing the importance of these symptoms, the clinician can determine their impact on the patient's functional ability and the need for specific treatment.

Because neurologic conditions may cause disability, it is critical to assess the impact of symptoms on the patient's daily life, whether this is temporary or permanent, and whether rehabilitation, assistive devices, or help from other people may be needed. This judgment will include the findings on physical examination. For most patients with chronic neurologic diseases, it is important to ask about the patient's level of independence in carrying out basic activities of daily living (walking, dressing, grooming, eating, bathing, and toileting) and more complicated "instrumental" activities such as driving, shopping, managing finances, and carrying out hobbies. If a neurologic condition may interfere with a patient's occupation, the history should include a description of the nature of the job and its demands.

Specific Syndromes

A single chapter cannot cover important elements of history-taking related to every neurologic symptom and condition likely to be encountered. Much of this task will fall to later chapters that describe the diagnostic approach to specific disorders. Instead, a few conditions will be selected either because of their relatively high frequency or the clinical difficulty that they tend to cause. These are highlighted in Table 1.1.

The Neurologic Examination

General Principles

Screening Examination

The full neurologic examination is not efficient in a screening situation, and a "bare essentials" examination should retain elements that cover the nervous system from head to toe, emphasize those components that can be assessed more objectively, and focus on findings that may indicate disorders related to a patient's age or medical history.

In younger adults, usually enough information is gleaned about cognitive function from taking a history to decide whether a formal mental status examination is needed or not. A basic screening examination should include selected cranial nerves (especially II, eye movements [III, IV and VI], and VII), gait, muscle strength, coordination, and tendon reflexes (including plantars). Testing shoulder abduction, wrist extension, and finger spreading is a good screen for strength in the arms. Gait testing, including having patients rise from a chair or from a squat without using their arms, walk on tiptoes, heels, and tandem is generally an adequate screen of muscle strength in the legs. In the absence of symptoms or of other findings, little is to be gained from systematically testing sensation.

In elderly patients, in addition to the just mentioned screens, it is important to test the special senses of vision and hearing, memory (e.g., by testing delayed recall of a list of words), and gait, including rising from a chair and climbing stairs. A series of functional tests described by

Table 1.1 Key historical features of neurologic conditions

Condition	Key features
Seizure vs. pseudoseizure or syncope	Generalized seizures (grand mal) should include loss of consciousness, and may include injury, tongue-biting, and incontinence.
	Complex partial seizures may include unusual behavior and bizarre emotional states, and usually last seconds to minutes, followed by a longer period of mental clouding.
	Most seizures produce postictal depression lasting longer than postsyncopal.
	Syncope is often preceded by lightheadedness, and occurs after prolonged sitting or standing.
Migraine headache	Severe headache, often unilateral. Associated symptoms include visual aura, nausea, photophobia, and phonophobia.
	Positive response to treatment with triptan or ergot medications, or after sleep in a dark room.
	Distinguish from tension or muscle-contraction headache which is more often described as band-like, squeezing, jabbing, or pressure, and is bilateral.
Dizziness	Vertigo is a feeling of rotating or being tilted relative to surroundings, usually worsened by changing head position and often accompanied by nausea. It should be distinguished from presyncope or lightheadedness, whereas "dizziness" often includes faintness and graying of vision.
Dysarthria vs. aphasia	Both may make speech difficult to understand. After a transient ischemic attack, patients who are aphasic often report difficulty thinking what to say, finding words. or understanding other people.
	Dysarthria often includes feelings that the tongue or mouth feels heavy, and speech is thick or slurred.
Forgetfulness	Amnestic and dementing conditions cause difficulty in retaining new or recent information, while older memories are preserved.
	Patients with memory lapses due to impaired attention or concentration often describe these lapses in great detail. Patients with impaired recent memory often deny problems or are vague on details.
	History from an informant is important.
Numbness, tingling and pain in peripheral nerve territory	Numbness is a negative symptom; the affected area may feel dead or lame. Paresthesia is a positive symptom, suggesting both nerve damage and regeneration. It is often described as tingling, pins and needles, or burning and tends to follow the territory of a root or nerve.
	Radicular pain often produces brief, severe, lancinating pain.
	Pain may not precisely follow a nerve or root distribution, e.g., carpal tunnel syndrome may produce pain in the forearm or higher.
Backache	It may be difficult to distinguish nerve root compression or sciatica from musculoskeletal pain.
	Radiation of pain to the thighs or lower extremity is more likely to be neurogenic.
	Back pain in a patient with known or suspected cancer may indicate metastatic spread, especially to the epidural space.

Tinetti and Ginter (1988) may help to identify the risk of physical dependence and falls.

Comprehensive neurologic examination

To elicit findings accurately and consistently, and to integrate the findings to suggest a locus of abnormality, a sound knowledge of the basic anatomy and organizing principles of the brain and peripheral nervous system is essential. Many textbooks deal with this, and several are listed among the references. A number of areas are sources of confusion for non-neurologists, and will be covered here and emphasized in the other chapters on specific syndromes.

By carrying out the clinical ritual of the neurologic examination in a structured manner, one is least likely to make errors of omission or commission. A key skill is to be able to discard findings as unphysiologic, inconsistent with the suspected diagnosis, or artifacts due to the patient's lack of complete effort or cooperation. Dividing the examination into modules that test fairly discrete brain areas or functional systems works well. When presenting or writing up the neurologic examination, the customary approach is "top down," that is, starting with mental status, then proceeding through cranial nerves, motor function, coordination, sensation, reflexes, balance, and gait. One can deviate from this order in the clinical examination, and it is often useful to test integrative functions such as gait and balance earlier. However, the traditional sequence has merits: it is methodical and comprehensive, divides the nervous system into anatomic and physiologic modules, and tests more objective parts of the examination (such as cranial nerves and motor function) before more subjective elements (such as sensation).

Many neurologic findings can be dichotomized as present or absent. For others, the examiner needs to describe a gradation of abnormalities. It is difficult even for experienced clinicians to rate the severity of signs consistently. Aids such as numerical grading of findings can be

Table 1.2 Grading systems for muscle strength and tendon reflexes

Medical Research Council scale

Strength

5	Movement against full resistance of examiner
4	Movement against some resistance
3	Movement against gravity, not resistance
2	Movement only with gravity eliminated
1	A flicker or trace of voluntary movement
0	No voluntary movement

Tendon reflexes

4+	Pathologically increased, e.g., spreads to other sites, or clonus is evident
3+	Increased; may be a variant of normal or associated with anxiety
2+	Normal
1+	Barely present or present only with facilitation
0	Absent

helpful, provided that the examiner can define each grading level. Two examples for which numbers have a standard clinical definition are the assessment of muscle strength from 0 to 5 and the recording of tendon reflexes (Table 1.2).

The terms "intermittent" or "equivocal" tend to be applied to neurologic findings in inverse relationship to the examiner's clinical expertise. With a few exceptions (such as cutaneous reflexes and frontal release signs that may fatigue), a positive neurologic finding should be repeatedly and consistently detectable. Some of the more fickle signs include the plantar response, tendon reflexes, and the testing of pain and light touch. When findings behave erratically—for example, a plantar response that sometimes is flexor and sometimes extensor—the examiner's inconsistency is more often at fault than the patient's nervous system. Similarly, asymmetrical tendon reflexes that do not fit the distribution of a nerve root, plexus, or pathway should be retested and found to be reproducible before they are accepted as definite findings. Careful technique when performing the examination is the best way to prevent these problems. Several elements of the neurologic examination that require special care are highlighted in later sections.

Another problem is the extent of effort and cooperation provided by the patient. For tests of muscle strength and speed of movements, the patient must be motivated to make as good an effort as possible, whereas for testing tendon reflexes and muscle tone, relaxation is important. In the presence of pain, a patient may not make a complete effort to contract a muscle group. Recording strength as "decreased but limited by pain" is appropriate. Testing sensation is the most subjective part of the neurologic examination, and abnormal findings should be interpreted based on their anatomic and physiologic consistency. For example, a spatial gradient is typical of impaired cutaneous sensation, with less severe impairment as the zone of normal sensation is approached. Sharp demarcation of normal and maximally impaired sensation is less plausible (but can occur in a severe or complete nerve injury). Asymmetry is a key indicator of a focal neurologic finding. It is important to compare the patient's left and right side, bearing in mind that people who are strongly left- or right-handed may show a minor degree of asymmetry of muscle strength or bulk.

A number of "normal" changes are found in many otherwise healthy elderly people. Small pupils that react poorly to light, impaired upward gaze, wasting of the first dorsal interosseous muscle, slight stooping of posture, impaired position and vibration sense in the feet, decreased (or sometimes absent) ankle reflex, and frontal release signs such as the glabella and snout reflexes are interesting findings that lack clinical or localizing significance.

To gain the most from the neurologic examination, it should be regarded as more than a checklist of tests carried out independently of each other or of the history. It is helpful to consider the examination as a way to test hypotheses and identify patterns of dysfunction that can be integrated into systems, syndromes, or levels of the nervous system. For example, if an elderly patient complains of the sudden onset of weakness of the right arm, a stroke is a likely cause. The examination should pay special attention to testing for weakness and upper motor neuron findings in the right arm, and also in the right face and leg, which would indicate a left-sided brain lesion. If left facial weakness is found ("crossed paralysis"), the localization shifts to the brainstem, in which case other cranial nerve findings should be carefully sought. If a right hemiparesis is apparent, the examiner should test carefully for aphasia, which would help to localize the lesion to the cortex rather than to a subcortical site such as the internal capsule.

Mental Status Examination

When a patient provides a coherent history rich in details, cognitive abilities are usually intact. If neurologic symptoms do not point to a disease process likely to affect cognition, then this intuitive impression of cognitive function is usually accurate. However, subtle abnormalities or circumscribed areas of cognitive loss can be overlooked without formal testing. In elderly patients, because of the increased prevalence of dementing disorders, it is important to screen for the presence of cognitive dysfunction, notably memory impairment.

Many clinicians develop their own approach to assess mental status. This can be successful, particularly if it covers major areas of cognitive function. Structure and order are important in conducting a mental status examination, to help interpret apparent deficits correctly. Memory, language, and attention should be assessed before testing other areas, because impairment in these major cognitive abilities often result in poor performance on other tasks. For example, aphasia may result in difficulty following verbal instructions or making verbal or written responses, rendering tests of construction or calculation difficult to interpret. Patients with attention deficits or delirium may have difficulty following complex verbal instructions or registering all of the elements to be learned in a memory task. Elderly patients may take a little longer than younger adults to perform certain tests, but if allowed sufficient time, they perform normally. These and other principles to provide a brief but accurate test of mental status are detailed in Table 1.3.

Brief screening tests, such as the Mini-Mental State Examination (MMSE) (Folstein 1975) or the Blessed Information-Memory-Concentration Test (Blessed et al., 1968), are concise, structured, and yield standardized and interpretable total scores. They can detect dementia, especially Alzheimer's disease, and can track progression over time. However, they do not assess language, visuospatial abilities, or abstraction well. Highly educated patients can score normally on the MMSE even in the presence of mild dementia. The examiner should be aware of how the patient's age, education, or native language may influence mental status test scores. Patients with low levels of education may perform suboptimally on tests of drawing, language, and abstraction. If clinician and patient do not speak the same language, then testing must be done using an interpreter. Validated translations of tests such as the MMSE can be extremely helpful in this challenging situation.

Cranial Nerves

The clinical usefulness of testing each cranial nerve varies, and selective emphasis is best for a typical clinical neurologic examination. Because olfaction and taste are difficult to test sensitively and are unlikely to be the sole features of significant neurologic illness, these are usually omitted. For the other cranial nerves, this section assumes that the reader knows the basic sequence of the examination. Rather than presenting a complete guide to the examination, it will focus on details that enhance the accuracy of the examination.

Table 1.3 Key elements of the mental status examination

Condition	Key features
Attention	Refers to sustained effort. Tests include counting backwards from 20, serial subtraction (e.g., serial 3s from 50), reciting months backwards.
Recent or short-term memory	Recall of a list after a delay, e.g., three or four unrelated words, or a name and address (e.g., John Brown, 42 Market Street, Chicago). Present the list or address to the patient several times to ensure that they register the information. The delay before testing recall should last at least 5 minutes and is filled with other testing to distract the patient. Can also ask the patient to describe details of recent news events.
Remote memory	Less important to test than recent memory. Should be preserved even in severe anterograde amnesia. Ask for names of former U.S. presidents; dates of important historical events.
Orientation	Test knowledge of time and place; orientation for person is not useful clinically since it is impaired only in severe disorders. May need to make allowances, e.g., retired or unemployed patients may not track the date.
Language	Aphasia is unlikely if naming is normal, therefore test naming in detail by showing the patient familiar objects and their parts, e.g., watch, stem or winder, band or strap, clasp or buckle. Is output fluent (many words, not necessarily highly meaningful) or nonfluent (telegraphic speech)? Can the patient follow a two-step verbal command? Can the patient repeat a sentence, e.g., "no ifs, ands, or buts," or "the lawyer's closing argument convinced him?" Can the patient write a dictated sentence?
Visuospatial and constructional ability	A good bedside screening test is to ask the patient to draw the face of a clock, fill in the numbers, then set the time, e.g., to 11:20 or 3:30. Copying intersecting pentagons (from the Mini-Mental State Exam) can be used.
Abstraction	Explaining proverbs tests memory and schooling rather than problem-solving. Instead, ask a patient to explain similarities between word pairs, e.g., table-chair, ship-horse, poem-statue.
Calculation	Dyscalculia is rarely an isolated or localizing finding, therefore a lower priority to test routinely. Abilities depend on education. Ask the patient to calculate change, e.g., how many quarters in $3.75, and to subtract numbers.
Hemineglect, praxis, visual agnosia	These are not worth testing as part of a routine mental state examination. Hemineglect is important chiefly in patients with left hemiparesis; the patient should be asked to identify where they perceive bilateral sensory stimuli.

Brief examination of the visual fields is much less sensitive than formal measurement by perimetry, but attention to detail can improve the yield of clinical testing. It is unlikely that a clinician will reliably detect a slightly enlarged blind spot or a small field deficit, and more reasonable goals are to be able to detect larger deficits, such as those affecting a quadrant or hemifield of vision. Each eye should be tested individually, using a small visual stimulus; a colored pen cap or preferably a red-topped pin are better than fingers. All four quadrants of each visual field should be examined, since quadrantic field deficits can occur. While the patient fixes gaze on the examiner's nose, the stimulus is brought in slowly (to avoid testing motion perception, a sensitive visual ability) from outside the visual field until the patient notices it. This is more sensitive than asking the patient to count fingers (large targets are much easier stimuli than smaller ones) or to identify moving fingers. Visual acuity is not commonly affected by neurologic conditions, with rare exceptions such as optic neuritis and retinal ischemia. Decreased acuity usually results from refractive problems of cornea, lens disorders such as cataracts, or macular degeneration. Acuity is best tested with correction, that is, while the patient wears glasses or contact lenses, or looks through a pinhole.

Testing pupillary reactions is more sensitive when carried out in a darkened room, because it is easier to see constriction of the baseline dilated pupils. A strong flashlight or ophthalmoscope light should be used. This makes it easier to detect unreactive pupils, "sluggish" reactions to light, or the small pupil characteristic of Horner's syndrome.

Eye movements inform greatly about the function of the ocular muscles; cranial nerves III, IV, and VI; the brainstem, cerebellum and vestibular apparatus; and the cortex. Smooth pursuit, or tracking of a steadily and slowly moving target such as the examiner's index finger, may be assessed while examining the range of eye movements. Nystagmus may only be apparent on extremes of lateral or vertical gaze. It should be described according to its nature (for example, rotary or linear), and according to the direction of the rapid phase. *Saccades* are rapid voluntary eye movements, tested by having a patient quickly change gaze from straight ahead to full left and right, then up and down. Slow saccades can occur in neurodegenerative conditions, while overshoot or undershoot suggest cerebellar dysfunction.

Important details of examining and interpreting cranial nerves V to XII are presented in Table 1.4. One area

Table 1.4 Elements of the cranial nerve examination

Condition	Key features
II: Visual fields	Small visual field defects are easily missed. To enhance their detection, test each eye individually. Use a small visual stimulus, e.g., a colored pen cap or better still a red-topped pin. Test all four quadrants of each visual field. While the patient fixes gaze on your nose, bring the target in slowly from beyond the limit of the field.
II, III: Pupil reaction	Best tested in a darkened room. Use a strong flashlight or ophthalmoscope.
III, IV, VI: Eye	Test the full horizontal and vertical range; ask about double vision and look for nystagmus. Check smooth movements pursuit and rapid eye movements (saccades).
V: Sensory	There are three divisions of the trigeminal nerve; test each division by examining the forehead, cheek, and mandible. The corneal reflex depends on both V and VII.
VII: Motor	Central or upper motor neuron facial weakness almost always spares the forehead and often eyelid closure. Lower motor neuron or true nerve VII lesions cause weakness of the entire hemiface. Test forehead wrinkling, strong closure of the eyelids, symmetry of smiling, puffing out cheeks.
VIII: Hearing	First screen for diminution of overall hearing ability; if hearing is normal, then the Weber or Rinne tests will not be useful.
VIII: Vestibular	Nystagmus may originate from vestibular, brainstem, or cerebellar dysfunction. Vestibular (peripheral) nystagmus may only be seen by abolishing visual fixation, or using postural tests such as head shaking or the Hallpike maneuver.
IX: Sensory	The gag reflex does not need to be tested routinely in all patients. It is of value when other lower cranial nerves are affected, to help localize dysarthria, or to help assess a patient's ability to protect their airway if they aspirate.
X: Motor	Symmetrical and strong elevation of the palate on saying "aaah" is the basic test. Uvula position is less helpful, since it may deviate slightly from center as a normal variant.
	To test for dysarthria, have a patient say "la-la-la; mi-mi-mi; gaa-gaa-gaa" (tests lingual [XII], labial [VII], and palatal [X] consonants, respectively). Have edentulous patients wear their dentures for accurate testing.
XI	Sternocleidomastoid (SCM) and trapezius muscles are very strong. In addition to testing head turning to the left (the action of the right SCM) and the right (the action of the left SCM), also test forward flexion of the head against resistance.
XII	Slight deviation of the tongue on protrusion is usually of no consequence. Test for weakness, e.g., patient pushes tongue into cheek against the resistance of the examiner's index finger

to highlight is the testing of hearing. The Weber (tuning fork placed on the center of the forehead) and Rinne (air and bone conduction are compared in each ear) tests are useful to help classify the cause of hearing loss, but are unnecessary if hearing is clinically normal. Hearing is intact for clinical purposes if the patient can perceive the sound of a vibrating 256-Hz tuning fork held a few inches away from either ear, a whispered question in each ear, or the rustling of the patient's hair just above each ear.

Muscle Strength and the Motor System

Attention to technique can enhance the accuracy of testing muscle strength. It is best to expose and visualize limb muscles, and avoid testing patients who are wearing several layers of clothing. Exposure also allows inspection of muscle bulk and a search for abnormalities such as fasciculations. To grade muscle strength, examiners compare themselves against patients, and should try to use muscles of similar strength to those being tested. Thus, when testing shoulder abduction (deltoid), hip flexion, knee extension, or other movements by powerful muscles, the examiner should use upper body strength, pressing with both arms if needed. Conversely, to test abduction of the little finger or thumb, much less effort is required, and the examiner can use his own little finger or thumb. When searching for subtle weakness, it is helpful to start testing with the patient's muscle groups in a position that places them under a mechanical disadvantage. This applies especially to joints that can be locked: instead of trying to

overcome a hyperextended elbow joint, the examiner should make the patient start with a flexed elbow and try to straighten it against resistance. Another trick is to use leverage when testing strength. For example, when testing the strength of a patient's extended arms, pushing down at the wrist is more effective and sensitive than doing so at the elbow. Many of the muscle groups of the legs are very large and difficult to overcome. To demonstrate minor degrees of weakness, functional tests may be used to pit a patient's own body weight against these muscles, for example, having a patient walk on tiptoes or heels, or rise from a chair with arms folded across the chest (Table 1.5).

As with other parts of the neurologic examination, it is important to compare left and right as well as proximal and distal. The examiner should try to integrate findings into consistent patterns of disease; for example, upper motor neuron versus lower motor neuron, antigravity muscle weakness in stroke, distal muscle weakness in polyneuropathy, and weakness maximal at proximal muscles (shoulders, hips) in myopathy (Table 1.6). If the history suggests the possibility of focal weakness due to pathology affecting a peripheral nerve, root, or plexus, then a more detailed examination of all of the muscles in that region may be needed. Many books describe the testing of muscles innervated by branches of peripheral nerves in great detail, as listed in the references. Peripheral nerve injury or entrapment is common, and patterns seen in common disorders such as carpal tunnel syndrome, ulnar neuropathy, peroneal neuropathy, and

Table 1.5 Patterns of muscle weakness

	Discriminating features	Consistent features	Variable features
Upper motor neuron (UMN)	Increased ("spastic") tone Increased tendon reflexes, often spread Pathological reflexes, e.g., extensor plantar	Weakness especially of antigravity muscle groups	Muscle bulk relatively preserved Impaired fine motor skills
Lower motor neuron (LMN)	Weakness is worst distally Tendon reflexes focally decreased or absent	Weakness in territory of affected nerve(s)	Wasting, especially in more severe lesions Fasciculations
Stroke (or other lesion) in cortex or internal capsule	Hemiparesis, affecting at least two out of face, arm and leg Sudden onset if stroke	Antigravity pattern of weakness, mainly extensor muscles, best appreciated in the arms UMN signs	Associated findings: aphasia, visual field deficits, hemisensory loss
Stroke (or other lesion): brainstem	Crossed paralysis: facial weakness on opposite side to limb weakness	Weakness, UMN signs	Other cranial nerve, cerebellar or sensory abnormalities
Polyneuropathy	Symmetrical weakness, worst distally	LMN signs	Sensory impairment in similar pattern
Myopathy, myositis, dystrophy	Weakness usually is proximal and symmetrical	Slow progression	Loss of reflexes Muscle tenderness Wasting

Table 1.6 Actions and innervation of selected muscles

Action	Main muscle	Nerve	Main root
Arm abduction	Deltoid	Axillary	C5
Elbow flexion, palm upward	Biceps	Musculocutaneous	C5,6
Elbow flexion, hand vertical	Brachioradialis	Radial	C5,6
Elbow extension	Triceps	Radial	C7,8
Wrist extension	Extensor carpi radialis	Radial	C6,7
Wrist flexion	Flexor carpi ulnaris	Ulnar	C8
Finger extension	Extensor digitorum	Radial	C7
Spreading fingers apart	Interossei	Ulnar	C8,T1
Thumb abduction	Abductor pollicis brevis	Median	T1
Hip flexion	Quadriceps femoris	Femoral	L2,3,4
Thigh adduction	Adductors	Obturator	L2,3,4
Knee flexion	Hamstrings	Sciatic	L5,S1
Foot dorsiflexion	Tibialis anterior	Peroneal	L4,5
Foot plantar flexion	Gastrocnemius and soleus	Tibial	S1,2
Foot eversion	Peronei	Peroneal	L5,S1
Foot inversion	Tibialis posterior	Tibial	L4,5

lumbosacral root lesions should be learned in detail and are described in another chapter of this book. In addition to performing strong movements, muscles are also called upon to carry out fine motor skills. Dexterity may be tested by having the patient rapidly tap the index finger to the thumb, open and close the fist, and tap each foot on the floor. These movements may be slowed after a stroke or in Parkinson's disease and may be irregular in rate and rhythm in cerebellar disorders. Marked slowing or difficulty in performing bimanual movements may be an early sign of Parkinson's disease.

Extrapyramidal Motor System

Movement disorders involve the extrapyramidal motor system, consisting of the basal ganglia and their connections. Physical findings may be characterized as positive (abnormal movements such as tremors, myoclonus, or chorea), or negative (such as slowing of movement or increased muscle tone). Specific disorders are discussed in later chapters. Aspects of tremor and tone will be discussed here, because they are often misinterpreted. First, when assessing tremor, the rate and amplitude are helpful, because the resting tremor of Parkinson's disease is slower than an action or postural tremor. The relationship of the tremor to movement should be tested. A resting tremor, characteristic of Parkinson's disease, occurs when a limb is relaxed, and often increases with nervousness or activity such as walking. Although this tremor usually does not affect fine motor skills, associated findings of bradykinesia and rigidity may do so. A postural tremor is faster, and best seen when the hands are held outstretched. It may be accompanied by an action tremor, a rapid tremor

that is maximal while carrying out fine motor tasks such as pointing or writing. This tremor is sometimes mistakenly called *cerebellar tremor* because it may appear while a patient carries out the finger-to-nose test. Cerebellar "intention tremor" is not a genuine oscillation or tremor, but is due to overshooting or undershooting the target.

Muscle tone is most readily tested in the upper extremities. The patient should be relaxed, through distraction if necessary, and the examiner should provide enough support to the limb being moved to ensure that it is relaxed. Movements should include elbow flexion–extension, wrist flexion–extension, and forearm pronation–supination. The limb should be moved relatively slowly, to assess whether a sustained increase in tone is present throughout the range of movement, which indicates rigidity. Mild rigidity can be elicited by retesting tone while the patient makes fine movements with the opposite arm (called *facilitation*)—for instance, opening and closing the fist.

Coordination

Coordination is easy to test, but may be tricky to interpret, since abnormal performance of "cerebellar" tasks may be due to causes other than cerebellar lesions. Slowness on finger-to-nose or rapid alternating movement is nonspecific: it can occur after a stroke or in Parkinson's disease. An irregular rate or rhythm of movement and difficulty making rapid movements to a precise target are hallmarks of cerebellar hemisphere problems, whereas gait ataxia indicates midline cerebellar involvement. To detect a mild cerebellar problem, the clinical tests should be demanding. Thus, on finger-to-nose pointing, the patient should have to extend the arm fully in order to touch the

Table 1.7 Tendon reflexes and their nerve and root innervation

Reflex	Peripheral nerve	Root
Triceps	Radial	C6–8
Biceps	Musculocutaneous	C5,6
Brachioradialis	Radial	C5,6
Quadriceps (knee)	Femoral	L2–4
Gastrocnemius-soleus (ankle)	Sciatic/tibial	S1,2

examiner's finger. Similarly, the patient should be encouraged to perform rapidly alternating movements, such as pronating and supinating the hands, as quickly as possible. The key part of the heel-to-shin test is the patient's ability to slide the heel of one foot accurately along the shin of the opposite leg, rather than the speed of movement.

Reflexes

Attention to technique can enhance the reliability of eliciting the tendon reflexes. It is important to optimize the patient's positioning to elicit these reflexes, so that muscles are relaxed and the tendon to be tested is at a slight stretch. For upper extremity reflexes, the patient should relax the limb completely (letting forearms rest in her lap) or the examiner should support the relaxed limb. To elicit the triceps reflexes, a good position can be achieved by the examiner supporting the patient's abducted arm by holding it at the elbow crease, with the elbow passively hanging down at 90 degrees. To test the ankle reflex, the ankle should be passively dorsiflexed to place the Achilles tendon on a slight stretch. The type of reflex hammer makes a difference: hammers with heavier heads, especially the queen's square type, make better contact over the tendon than the smaller tomahawk hammers. Tendon reflexes should not show dramatic fatigue or variability, and if a reflex is increased, decreased, or absent, that sign should be reproducible on repeated testing. A standard system for grading the strength of tendon reflexes is shown in Table 1.2. The nerve and root innervation of the commonly tested deep tendon reflexes is shown in Table 1.7.

Much folklore surrounds the plantar response, and the neurologic literature is replete with eponyms in addition to that of Babinski, describing a variety of locations within the S1 dermatome where this reflex can be elicited. The basic method requires the examiner to scratch the outer edge of the sole (rather than a more medial zone, which may trigger a plantar grasp or flexion response), curving toward the ball of the foot. Although the stimulus should be slightly noxious, it is often useful to start with a gentle scratch, and then repeat with increasing firmness until a reflex is seen. Too strong a stimulus will trigger a withdrawal response that includes dorsiflexion of the entire foot and pulling away of the big toe and resembles a "positive Babinski sign." A true extensor plantar response includes extension of the big toe, often accompanied by fanning of the rest of the toes. Although an extensor plantar response may fatigue over many repeated tests, it should be a finding that can be reproducibly identified more than once.

Frontal release signs are also known as primitive reflexes, and include the glabellar, snout, pout, suck, and grasp reflexes. These are normally present in infants and absent in normal adults. They reappear in a percentage of clinically normal elderly individuals, and in frontal lobe lesions, Alzheimer's disease, and Parkinson's disease. Although interesting as phenomena, these signs are not frequent or reliable enough to add specific diagnostic or localizing information to practice. The superficial reflexes refer to the abdominal, cremasteric, and anal reflexes. Although they may be absent in spinal cord or nerve root disease, they are often difficult to interpret reliably, and their value is supportive. Other signs should be given greater weight in assessing spinal cord or sacral nerve root function.

Sensation

Because it is one of the most subjective parts of the examination, sensation is best tested after muscle strength, coordination, and reflexes. Several types of sensation ("modalities") should be tested, since there are distinct sensory pathways for these different stimuli. Sensory deficits usually are incomplete; however, total loss of sensation may occur in large strokes, spinal cord lesions, peripheral nerve trauma, or severe peripheral neuropathy. Usually, sensory deficits show a pattern of gradual transition from decreased sensation to normal, from distal to proximal. Sensory deficits in the territory of roots or peripheral nerves may be less extensive than maps of sensory dermatomes would predict, due to overlap between adjacent sensory nerves. The sensory examination is most likely to yield helpful information if one approaches it with hypotheses in mind, searching for corroborative evidence for the history or examination findings. It is common for patients to report some degree of variation from one stimulus to the next, and it is difficult to provide exactly the same pin-prick or light touch as sensory testing proceeds from one area to the next.

Pin-prick is the easiest modality to test reliably over the whole body. A safety pin or toothpick makes a convenient testing tool, but a new one must be used for each patient to avoid the risk of spreading infectious diseases such as hepatitis or HIV. As a screen, it is sufficient to compare the left and right arms and legs, and to sample proximal and distal areas of each limb. If the history in-

Table 1.8 Impaired sensation

	Discriminating features	Consistent features	Variable features
Polyneuropathy: large fiber	Selective decrease of position, vibration, touch discrimination	Maximal distally, glove–stocking configuration, symmetrical Decreased reflexes	Distal muscle weakness with or without wasting Other sensory modalities impaired
Polyneuropathy: small fiber	Selective decrease of pain and temperature sensation	Maximal distally, symmetrical Reflexes preserved	Burning pain. Dysautonomia: color and sweating changes
Multifocal neuropathy (mononeuritis multiplex)	Patchy, asymmetrical, spares some branches of nerves	Weakness and reflex loss in distribution of affected nerves Sensory loss less apparent	Usually rapid or subacute onset; accompanied by pain
Spinal cord compression (subacute or chronic)	Sensory level Upper motor neuron signs below level of lesion	Bilateral sensory loss and weakness	Pain Impairment of bowel and bladder control.
Peripheral nerve or root lesion	Findings confined to territory of one nerve or root	Weakness and/or numbness, tingling and sensory loss	May be acute (e.g., trauma) or chronic (e.g., entrapment)

dicates sensory symptoms or other neurologic findings are present, then a more detailed examination must be carried out to try to map the sensory deficit. Temperature is conducted by the same small-caliber nerve fibers as is pain. Because it is much harder to test reliably, temperature sensation is not tested as a routine, but may be used to corroborate findings on pin-prick testing. A tube of cold water or a cool metallic object such as a tuning fork may be used as a stimulus. Vibration sense is not a unitary sensation, because it is conveyed through large-caliber and other sensory nerves. Joint position sense is a more pure test of large-caliber sensory nerve fibers. This modality is extremely sensitive, allowing the perception of small movements. Position sense is best tested by grasping the thumb, finger, or toe at its side and moving the digit through a short range of a few degrees.

Sensory deficits have several hallmark patterns. Polyneuropathy produces symmetrical stocking–glove impairment of joint position sense and fine touch (large fiber), pinprick and temperature (small fiber), or all of these modalities. Lesions of nerve roots or peripheral nerves may result in signature areas of impaired sensation, usually easiest to show by testing pin-prick. These areas are detailed in *Aids to the Examination of the Peripheral Nervous System* (Medical Research Council 1975). Spinal cord lesions produce a sensory level, which should be carefully sought by testing pin-prick. Lesions affecting the sacral sensory nerve roots or the most caudal part of the spinal cord may produce sensory deficits restricted to the perianal region: so-called "saddle anesthesia" (Table 1.8).

Gait and Balance

As mentioned earlier, it can be useful to test gait before most of the neurologic examination, because it is a key in-

tegrative movement. If a patient can rise from a chair, walk on heels and toes, and tandem walk, then leg muscle strength is most likely normal. Abnormalities of gait should be interpreted by using information from the overall neurologic examination to decide which systems or pathways, and thus what types of pathologic processes, are responsible. Patients with a variety of balance or gait problems attempt to compensate by standing and walking with their feet further apart and by taking smaller steps. Therefore, these two findings are nonspecific. Similarly, difficulty with tandem walking may occur in a variety of gait disorders, and is universal in patients aged 80 or older.

Some gait disorders produce characteristic patterns. Cerebellar disorders of gait are marked by irregularity in the rate and rhythm of leg movements, with inaccurate foot placement and unsteadiness, leading to a lurching, drunk-looking gait. It is important to remember that midline lesions affecting the vermis of the cerebellum may produce truncal ataxia, in which gait unsteadiness is not accompanied by dysmetria or abnormalities of rapid alternating movement. Other classic examples of gait disorders include the high-stepping, foot-slapping gait of peripheral neuropathy; the stooped, shuffling gait with decreased arm swing typical of Parkinson's disease; the waddling gait of proximal weakness as seen in myopathy or muscular dystrophy; and the dragging and circumduction of the affected leg seen in hemiparetic stroke. In addition to the gait abnormalities, these disorders typically advertise their presence by a pattern of characteristic findings on the systematic neurologic examination.

Balance is difficult to assess clinically, since it is a complex ability that depends on visual, vestibular, and position sense input, which are integrated into appropriate and timely postural and other motor responses. Romberg's test is a standard clinical approach to test static balance, in which the patient stands with feet next to each other and eyes closed. The presence of sway while the patient stands in this position is often normal, whereas the need to open their eyes or take a corrective step is not. Because visual input is removed with the eyes closed, the Romberg maneuver tests position sense and, to a lesser extent, vestibular input to balance. Dynamic balance (i.e., the response to maintain balance after a perturbation) is difficult to test clinically. One test for postural instability involves standing behind the patient (whose feet are placed slightly apart), requesting that they try to stay on balance, and pulling sharply on their shoulders. The normal response is for the patient to sway backward briefly, then make corrective leg muscle contractions or take a step and regain balance. Patients with Parkinson's disease and impaired postural reflexes tend to topple, therefore, the examiner must be prepared to catch and support the patient.

Annotated Bibliography

De Myer WE. *Technique of the neurological examination*, 4th ed. New York: McGraw-Hill, 1993.
   A well-illustrated guide to the neurologic examination, supplemented with self-test material to assist learning.
Medical Research Council. *Aids to the examination of the peripheral nervous system*. London: Author, 1975.
   This brief guide has excellent photographs showing how to examine muscles supplied by every major peripheral nerve of clinical relevance.
Patten J. *Neurological differential diagnosis*, 2nd ed. London: Springer-Verlag, 1996.
   This book uses excellent schematic drawings to integrate elements of the neurologic history and examination with neuroanatomy.
Strub RL, Black FW. *The mental status examination in neurology*, 4th ed. Philadelphia: FA Davis, 1999.
   A thorough introductory text that clearly explains the elements of mental status testing.

CHAPTER 2

Electroencephalography and Evoked Potential Studies

Joseph Drazkowski and Eli S. Neiman

Outline

▶ Basic mechanisms
▶ Recording technology
▶ Normal EEG
▶ Abnormal patterns
▶ EEG in the differential diagnosis of epilepsy
▶ Epilepsy surgery
▶ Computer EEG
▶ Evoked potentials
▶ Summary

The nervous system functions through the conduction of electrical impulses. The field of clinical neurophysiology comprises the recording and measurement of this electrical activity. Commonly used clinical neurophysiology tests include routine electroencephalography (EEG) and evoked potentials (EP), EEG telemetry, and intraoperative monitoring of EEG and EPs.

Electroencephalography is a recording of the spontaneous electrical activity of the cerebral cortex. The EEG was first recorded in the late 19th century by Caton, in dogs. In the early 20th century, Hans Berger recorded an EEG in humans and soon recognized the importance of the procedure for the practice of neurology. Prior to the advent of computed tomography (CT) and magnetic resonance imaging (MRI), EEG was the only noninvasive test for detection and localization of various cerebral lesions. Today, EEG is essential in the care of persons with epilepsy and remains important in evaluation of persons with encephalopathy, dementia, specific infections, altered consciousness, and coma (Table 2.1).

Evoked potentials are the time-locked electrical responses of the nervous system to a specific stimulus, such as a flash of light, a sound, or an electrical stimulus to a peripheral nerve. The minute electrical signals evoked by such a stimulus can be recorded only by sophisticated electronic computer averaging techniques. This was first accomplished by Dawson in 1951. The recording of EPs was once the most sensitive and specific test for multiple sclerosis (MS), but this application has been replaced by MRI. Evoked potential recordings are now used in the outpatient setting when a person is suspected of having MS on the basis of neuroimaging. Evoked potential use has also moved into the operating room and intensive care unit as an aid to monitoring the integrity of the nervous system in special situations.

Basic Mechanisms

Each neuron in the central nervous system (CNS) actively maintains a state of disequilibrium by pumping out sodium and pumping in potassium, in a 3:2 ratio (more sodium goes out than potassium goes in). The inside of the neuron is maintained at an electrically negative potential by this pump, and by the intrinsic negative charge on cytosolic proteins. The voltage difference across the cell membrane is determined by the ion concentrations and can be calculated using the *Nernst equation*; it averages –140 mV. Electrical signaling in the nervous system occurs when the transmembrane potential is changed via the opening or closing of ion channels. As ion channels open and ions rush across the membrane down their electrochemical gradients, the transmembrane potential changes. In dendrites (the receptive or input portion of the neuron), shifts in membrane potential occur as a response to inputs from other cells. These membrane potentials are summated and, when they reach a threshold, cause the neuron to "fire" (depolarize) and send an action potential (electrical impulse) down the axon (output

Table 2.1 Electroencephalogram in various neurological conditions

Condition	Discriminating features	Consistent features	Variable features
Encephalopathy		Generalized slow rhythms	FIRDA, triphasic waves
Focal brain lesion	Persistent focal delta activity	Normal activity elsewhere	Focal loss of fast (β) activity
Focal epilepsy, interictal	Focal spike discharge	Normal activity elsewhere	Focal slowing (θ and δ)
Focal epilepsy, ictal recording	Focal rhythmic evolving spike or rhythmic ictal discharges	Normal activity elsewhere	Scalp recording may be completely normal in some frontal lobe epilepsy
Primary generalized epilepsy	Generalized high-amplitude spike-and-wave, 3 Hz or higher frequency	Normal background rhythms	Interictal recording may be completely normal.
Secondary generalized epilepsy	Slow spike-and-wave (1.5–2.5 Hz)	Background slowing	

portion of the neuron). At the end of the axon, the electrical impulse induces release of neurotransmitters that act on another dendrite, thus completing the cycle of interneuron communication and transmission.

The action potential is the most dramatic aspect of neuronal function, but is not the source of EEG signals. Lasting only a millisecond, the action potential is too short to be recorded easily. The EEG signal represents the variations in transmembrane potential in the dendritic portion of the neuron. These changes occur over the course of tens to hundreds of milliseconds. The electrical field generated by each neuron is minute, and is undetectable in routine situations. Only when millions of neurons act in synchrony does the electrical activity sum to a large enough voltage to be recordable on the scalp EEG. Using standard technology, a single EEG channel detects the summated electrical activity of a 6-cm^2 region of cortex. Scalp EEG signals are measured in microvolts, and are a thousand times smaller than electromyogram (EMG) and electrocardiogram (ECG) signals. Large groups of neurons discharge synchronously owing to coordinated input to the dendritic tree from subcortical afferents, typically from the thalamus. Thalamocortical connections are thought to form a reverberant circuit, and these oscillations are felt to give rise to the familiar α-rhythm (see later discussion). In disease states, abnormal activity produces patterns such as rhythmic slowing and spike-and-wave discharges that replace normal activity.

Recording Technology

Recording the EEG requires highly specialized and sensitive equipment owing to the small voltage of the signals. By convention, EEG electrodes are placed at standard locations separated by either 10% or 20% of the head circumference. This is known as the *international 10-20 system*. In a standard EEG, 21 or more scalp electrodes are applied. Electrode positions on the left side of the scalp are designated by odd numbers; on the right by even numbers. Those applied in the midline are give the subscript "z" for zero. Frontal electrodes are named "F," ("Fp" is the frontal polar head region), temporal electrodes are named "T," occipital electrodes are named "O," and so on. A map of standard electrode locations is shown in Figure 2.1. In general, the numbers assigned to the electrode site are larger in positions on the more posterior temporal aspects of the head and are larger the farther they are away from the midline in the coronal orientation.

Many of the obvious patterns seen on a typical EEG recording are *artifacts*; that is, EEG activity of noncerebral origin. The eyes are powerful generators of electrical fields, and eye movements are often the most prominent feature of a recording in the frontal head region. Scalp muscles also generate high-amplitude potentials that can easily obscure the lower-amplitude EEG. One of the most common errors in recording technology is failure to obtain good electrical contact when the electrode is applied to the scalp (high impedance). Poorly applied electrodes may act like an antenna and introduce stray electrical signals to the recording (noise). Head or body movement may also create artifact on the EEG and, if rhythmic, may be mistaken for an abnormal EEG, thereby possibly leading to misdiagnosis. The high gains used in EEG amplifiers make the recording susceptible to even tiny amounts of stray electrical noise. The responsibility of identifying and correcting sources of noise during the recording falls to the technologist performing the test.

Normal α-wave background rhythms have an average amplitude of about 50–70 μV, with other physiologic potentials ranging from 2 to 300 μV. The typical EEG instrument amplifies physiologic signals approximately one million times. The final output of the EEG is a tracing with a "sensitivity" expressed in microvolts per millimeter. Typical sensitivity values are 5–30 μV/mm. The EEG amplifier is a differential amplifier; that is, it amplifies the difference between two inputs (usually adjacent elec-

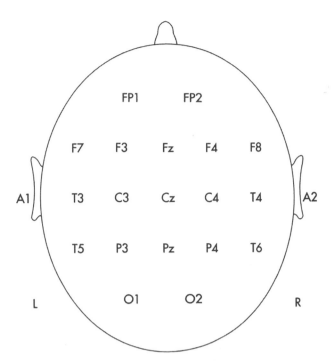

Figure 2.1 The 10–20 electrode system, showing names and placements of standard electrodes.

trodes) and rejects signals that are the same in each of the two inputs (common mode rejection). This amplifier can be configured in two ways, using either unipolar (referential) or bipolar montages.

In a referential (unipolar) montage, each channel displays the activity of a single active electrode subtracted from an inactive (or relatively inactive) reference electrode that is common to all channels in the recording (Figure 2.2). Referential recordings have both advantages and disadvantages. It is fairly easy to determine the point of maximum amplitude of an event, just by finding the chan-

nel with the highest amplitude output. Polarity is also easily determined as long as the reference is not contaminated. When the common reference channel is active with EEG or artifact, this unwanted activity contaminates the signal in all channels. Similarly, amplitudes may be distorted slightly because of the physical distance from the reference: more distant electrodes may display higher amplitudes only because of their distance from the reference (longer inter-electrode distance).

In bipolar montage recordings, channels are arranged in chains, with each channel representing the difference usually between adjacent electrodes. Bipolar montages therefore display EEG gradients rather than true amplitudes. This form of recording also has advantages and disadvantages. Bipolar recordings are immune to common reference effects. Focal activity can usually be localized by looking for a *phase reversal*, which is usually negative in polarity (surface negative discharge). This distinction can be difficult when the maximum amplitude is at the end of an electrode chain where no phase reversal occurs. Occasionally, high-amplitude activity with widespread fields and low gradients may not be well seen because of the small potential difference between electrodes.

The appearance of the EEG is partly determined by the choice of filters used during the recording. The electrical field of the human brain oscillates at frequencies ranging from below 1 Hz to well above 100 Hz. However, routine EEG analysis centers on a band of activity from 1 Hz to 25 Hz. By convention, different frequencies are referred to by different names. Activity of 3 Hz or slower is called *delta* (δ), from greater than 3 Hz to less than 8 Hz *theta* (θ), from 8 Hz to 12 Hz *alpha* (α), and faster frequencies are called *beta* (β). Frequency components above 20 may distort normal sinusoidal waveforms, making them look sharper than they really are. Filters that reduce the amplitude of high-frequency activity (also

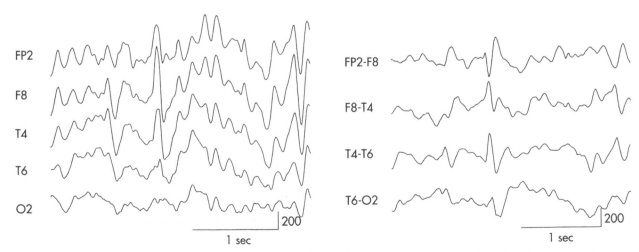

Figure 2.2 The figure on the left illustrates a sharp wave on a referential montage with a common inactive reference. The figure on the right shows the same EEG segment using a bipolar montage relative to its neighboring electrode.

called *low-pass filters*) are useful when muscle artifact obscures the EEG activity. Muscle activity typically is composed of high-amplitude signals much faster than 25 Hz. Changing the high-frequency filter may reduce unwanted muscle artifact and allow viewing of the otherwise artifact-ridden EEG. Typical high-frequency filter (low-pass filter) settings range from 35 Hz to 70 Hz, with 15-Hz filters used for excessively noisy recordings. Low-frequency filters (*high-pass filters*) affect slow signals. *Excessive filtering* can mask or distort important EEG signals. Equally significant, excessive filtering can alter the appearance of artifacts and make them appear as EEG abnormalities when they are not. The practice of running an entire EEG with filters set at the narrowest bandpass, practiced in some laboratories, leads both to missing important findings and over-interpretation of artifacts.

A standard EEG is recorded in an electrically isolated room or at the hospital bedside. Recording sessions for an awake-only EEG last at least 20 minutes, and for an awake and asleep recording at least 30 minutes. For 50 years, the recording was traditionally made on a wide, folded paper, but this has been supplanted in most labs by digital technology. Computerized digital EEG allows easier handling and storage of the large amounts of data generated. With digital EEG, after the record is acquired, one can change the filter settings, montages, and paper speed, and quickly move to points of interest in the

recording with out having to turn pages. Recordings are made by technologists, who should preferably be certified by the American Board of Registered EEG Technologists. Interpretation of the EEG is performed by a neurologist with training in EEG diagnostics. In recent years, the growth of EEG fellowships and explosion of technological innovations and clinical applications (especially in epilepsy) has led the American Board of Psychiatry and Neurology to offer certification of special competency in clinical neurophysiology.

Normal EEG

The normal EEG of an adult appears different in the waking and sleeping states. In the waking state, the most prominent EEG activity is the posterior dominant rhythm, also known as the α-rhythm (8–13 Hz), which is seen maximally in the occipital region. α-rhythm is present when the patient is awake and the eyes are closed, and is usually "blocked" (attenuated) by eye opening. The posterior dominant rhythm is often a mixture of several closely related frequencies, giving it a modulated or waxing-and-waning appearance. Low-amplitude widespread β-rhythm (13 Hz+) may also be seen as a normal inherited variant or due to sedative and other medications. Figure 2.3 shows normal features of the waking EEG.

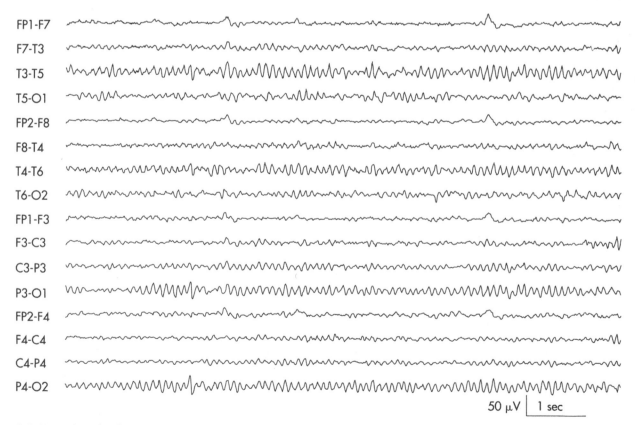

Figure 2.3 Normal awake electroencephalogram in a young adult.

In the transition to drowsiness, the α-rhythm gradually reduces in amplitude and slows slightly in frequency. In some cases, the α-rhythm in early drowsiness may transition to higher-amplitude, monotonous, generalized rhythmic activity. Low-amplitude θ-rhythm may be seen as an early feature of drowsiness. Such θ activity in the fully awake state would be abnormal (see later discussion on generalized slowing), but is normal as the patient becomes drowsy. Interpretation of slowing requires consideration of the context in which it appears. Technologist comments on the recording, change to slow rolling eye movements, and eventually disappearance of movement artifact provide important clues about the state of the patient. Deeper in drowsiness, the EEG shows low-amplitude generalized θ- and β-wave activity. Some specific patterns may be seen during drowsiness. Positive occipital sharp transients of sleep (POSTS) are of positive polarity, located in the occipital region, sharply contoured, and transient (occur briefly). Positive occipital sharp transients of sleep sometimes form briefly sustained rhythmic runs mimicking sharp waves. Vertex waves (V-waves) are seen in stage I sleep and persist into deeper sleep stages. These surface negative waves are often very sharply contoured, and are located at the vertex (Cz electrode). An uncommon finding in the normal drowsing EEG is the small sharp spike (SSS), also sometimes called a *benign epileptiform transient of sleep* (BETS). These are discussed in more detail in the section on spike discharges. The EEG of drowsiness is shown in Figure 2.4.

In stage II sleep, stage I patterns persist, but the background becomes more active, with higher amplitudes and the appearance of minor amounts of δ-wave activity. The defining characteristics of stage II sleep are *sleep spindles* and *K complexes*. A sleep spindle is a brief (1–3 second duration) discharge of 12–14 rhythms, moderate in amplitude (30–60 µV typically), enclosed in a spindle-shaped envelope. These are usually distributed symmetrically about the midline in the fronto-central head regions. The K complex is located in the same regions as the spindle, and may appear as a combination of vertex wave with an after-coming slow wave, with superimposed spindle-like components. The K complex is often triggered by external stimuli.

Stage III and stage IV sleep may be encountered but are not usually recorded during daytime routine EEG. The transition from stage II to stage III occurs when the background is comprised of more than 20% δ-wave activity (a definition that is less exact than might appear). Stage IV sleep has greater than 50% δ-wave activity. Deeper sleep stages usually show no spindles, K complexes, vertex waves, or POSTS.

Most vertebrates dream during a stage of sleep characterized by rapid eye movements (REM sleep). During REM sleep in humans, there is near-complete paralysis of skeletal muscles, sparing the extraocular muscles. The EEG of REM sleep shows low-amplitude diffuse slowing with occasional α-like rhythms. Rapid eye movements ap-

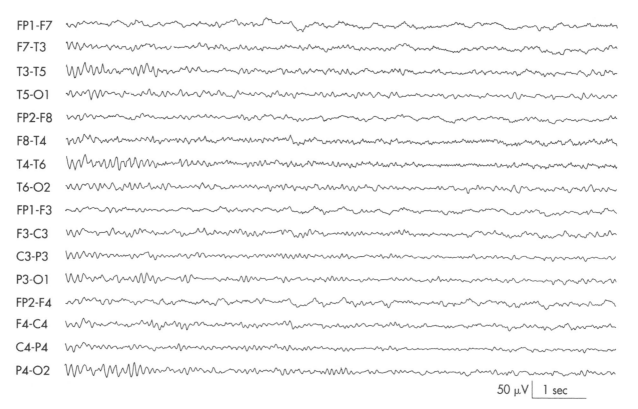

Figure 2.4 Electroencephalogram showing normal drowsiness.

pear as rhythmic saw-tooth-shaped θ-wave activity in the frontal and fronto-polar regions. In a normal adult, the nocturnal cycle of light sleep to deep sleep followed by the initial REM period takes about 90 minutes.

Above the age of 60, certain distinct changes in the EEG are considered normal for age. As one gets older, temporal θrhythms become more prominent during the waking state. Normal elderly individuals may also have a slightly slower posterior dominant rhythm in contrast to young adults. In drowsiness, diffuse slowing (usually θ) is common, and at times may appear paroxysmal. Some normal elderly adults may exhibit bifrontal rhythmic δ activity during drowsiness.

"Normal Variant" Patterns

Many rare, but normal, patterns occur in EEG. Most of these patterns occur in less than 1–2% of the population, but there are enough distinct normal variants so that one or two of them will be seen per week in a typical EEG laboratory. Unfortunately, many of these normal variants are both rhythmic and sharply contoured, thus mimicking abnormal activity, since rhythmicity and sharp contour are hallmarks of the epileptic EEG. These normal variant patterns, to the uninitiated, may appear distinctly abnormal. The subject has been reviewed by Klass and Westmoreland.

Rhythmic temporal θ of drowsiness (RTD) is seen in 1–2% of normal adolescents. The discharge is often sharply contoured, sometimes taking on a triangular or saw-tooth appearance. The sharp component is surface negative. Amplitudes are 30–60 μV, and the discharge has a wide field centered on the mid temporal to anterior temporal regions. The discharge may persist in rhythmic form, with frequencies of 4–7 Hz, for more than 10–20 seconds or, more commonly, may appear briefly for 2–5 second runs. On some occasions, just a single wave, sharply contoured, may be seen. Unlike a temporal lobe seizure (which is a rhythmic, temporal, sharply contoured triangular discharge lasting 5–30 seconds), the RTD maintains a single frequency (i.e., is monorhythmic) throughout its course and does not evolve or change to progressively slower frequencies. In distinction to seizure activity, which induces postictal slowing or suppression, normal variants such as RTD produce no disturbance of the background rhythm. When Gibbs first described this pattern, it was felt to indicate epilepsy or psychopathology and was called *psychomotor variant* (discouraged term), although population studies have since shown it to be a benign pattern.

Persons older than age 40 may also show bursts of θ activity, usually either widespread or posterior, in the transitions from waking to stage I sleeping states. *Wicket spikes* are rhythmic, sharply contoured θ waves, sometimes with a spike component, that are seen in the mid

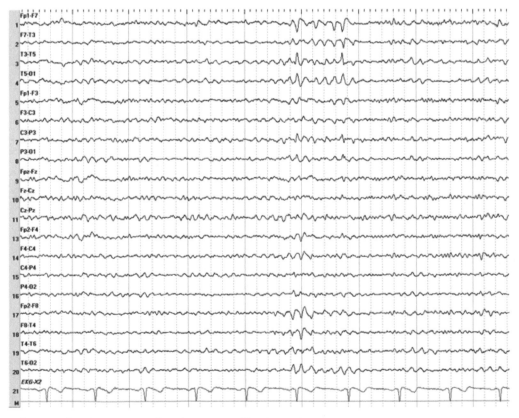

Figure 2.5 Bilateral temporal wicket waves, a sharply contoured benign variant.

temporal regions of many elderly. The sharp component is surface negative. Again, like RTD, the wicket spike is distinguished as nonepileptiform because it is strictly monorhythmic, within the background rhythm, with no clear after-going slow wave and without evolution (Figure 2.5). The distinction may be difficult when only a single spike component, rather than a train of waves, is present.

Mu (μ) rhythm is a sharply contoured, comb-shaped rhythmic wave associated with motor cortex. The sharp component is surface negative. Usually of low to moderate amplitude, it is seen in the central regions (electrodes C3 and C4), overlying motor cortex. The discharge is seen in the waking and drowsing states in bursts lasting 1–5 seconds, sometimes longer. The frequency is usually slightly faster than the posterior dominant rhythm. Actual movement, or even the mere thought of movement of the contralateral hand, blocks the rhythm. An alert technologist can confirm the nature of the pattern by having the patient move the contralateral hand and commenting on the recording. In some individuals, especially children, the posterior dominant rhythm may exhibit the peculiar property of merging adjacent waves, dropping its apparent frequency content in half. The *slow α variant* is a harmonic of the normal rhythm. It usually has a higher amplitude than the regular posterior rhythm, and can be unilateral (one side slow, the other fast). These harmonics are usually seen in early drowsiness.

Perhaps the most controversial of the normal rhythmic variants is *subclinical rhythmic epileptiform discharge of adults* (SREDA). SREDA is usually seen in older adults. It may be focal to any head region, although it is most often seen in the temporal regions. Unlike most of the normal rhythmic variants, it is not a monorhythmic discharge.

Breach rhythm is a unique pattern that by itself is not indicative of brain dysfunction. Breach rhythms result from bony skull defects and are most often seen in postsurgical patients. The skull defect leads to reduced electrical impedance and less filtering of high frequencies, thus allowing for higher amplitude waveforms and faster frequencies over the scalp/skull defect. Increased penetration of faster frequencies leads to an apparent sharpening of the EEG rhythms, so that waveforms that are actually normal may look like sharp waves. In addition, special attention must be paid, so that a sharp wave or spike in the area of the breach rhythm is not overlooked as mere breach artifact (Figure 2.6).

Abnormal Patterns

The multitude of abnormal EEG patterns can be categorized into those that are slow versus those that are sharp; and those that are focal versus those that are generalized. An additional modifier of *rhythmic*, *periodic*, or *sporadic*

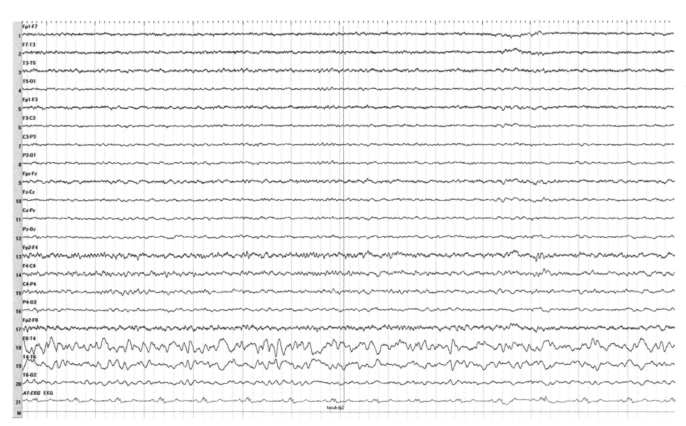

Figure 2.6 Breach rhythm. This patient has a burr hole or skull defect underlying the T4 recording electrode.

(the terms occasional or irregular may also be used) completes the basic classification schema of abnormal EEG patterns.

Slowing

Generalized slowing of the EEG is the hallmark of encephalopathy or generalized disturbances of global brain function. In the hospital setting, diffuse slowing is most often found with toxic or metabolic etiologies, and may also be seen in posthypoxic comas, degenerative diseases such as Alzheimer's dementia, postictal states, and similar generalized processes. The severity of the condition causing the encephalopathy is usually correlated with the degree and amplitude of the slowing. In adults, slowing in the θ range is usually associated with mild to moderate encephalopathies that usually correlate clinically with lethargy or slight confusion. In contrast, δ slowing is usually seen in stupor or coma states. Sequential EEG may provide a quantitative and sensitive measure of a patient's clinical improvement or decline, and is sometimes the most accurate way to assess the success of treatment before clinical changes become evident. A diffusely slow EEG is shown in Figure 2.7.

Certain forms of slowing may have special meaning and deserve special mention. *Frontal intermittent rhyth-mic delta activity* (FIRDA) is a monorhythmic, sinusoidally shaped, high-amplitude δ activity that is intermittent and typically appears for runs of 1–5 seconds during light drowsiness. FIRDA can be seen in any generalized encephalopathy, but it is often indicative of a transition in the patient's condition, as opposed to a stable clinical state. Originally, FIRDA was associated with deep midline lesions and was felt to reflect altered thalamo-cortical synchronization (Figure 2.8).

Triphasic waves are high-amplitude, rhythmic 1–2 waves, with a characteristic three-phase appearance (small positive–large negative–small positive deflection). These waves are usually located maximally in the fronto-central region and may exhibit the unique property of an *antero-posterior lag*, with the activity appearing in the anterior head region 40–100 msec earlier than in the posterior head region. Triphasic waves are classically associated with hepatic encephalopathy, but may occasionally be seen with renal failure, hypercarbic encephalopathy, and other conditions (Figure 2.9). Triphasic waves are called "atypical" when they exhibit posterior maxima, lack or show reversed anteroposterior phase lag, or exhibit variable morphology. Unfortunately, there can be a blurring of distinguishing features among FIRDA, triphasic waves, and even atypical spike-and-wave patterns, emphasizing the point that EEG findings must be interpreted in the clinical context.

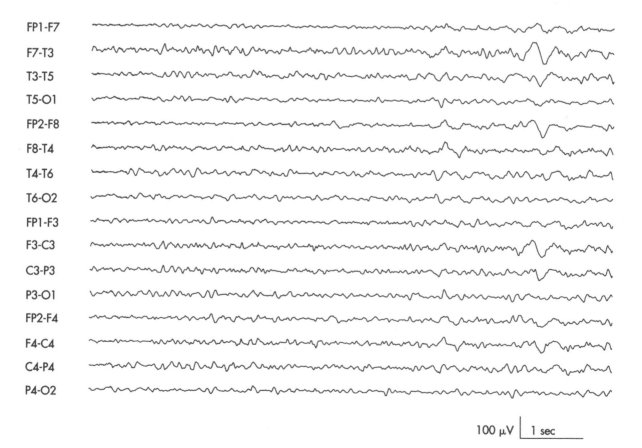

100 μV | 1 sec

Figure 2.7 Generalized slowing of electroencephalogram is the hallmark of encephalopathy.

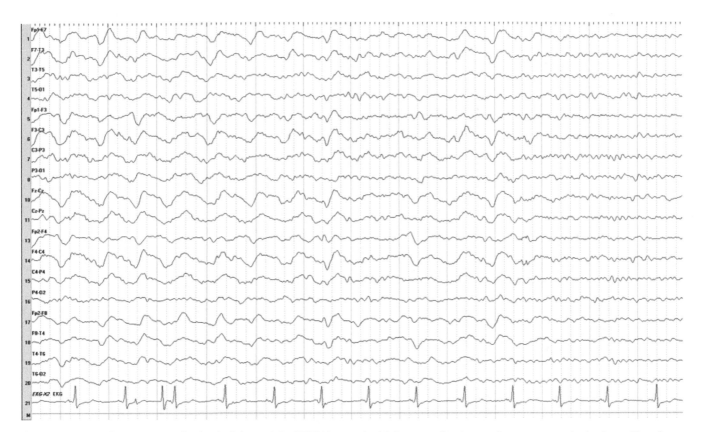

Figure 2.8 Frontal intermittent rhythmic delta activity (FIRDA); note the highest amplitude waveforms are seen in the frontal head regions.

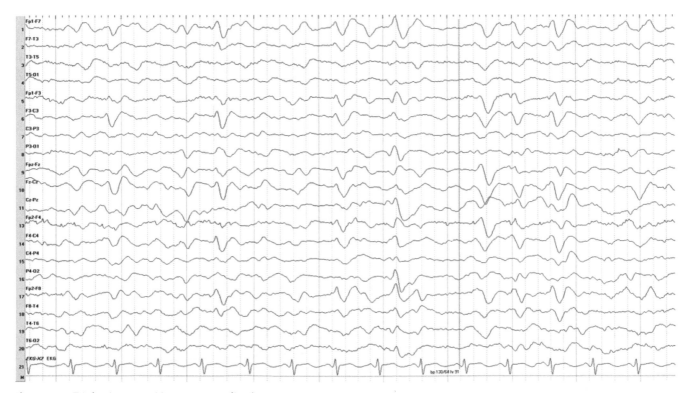

Figure 2.9 Triphasic waves. Maximum amplitudes are seen in the fronto-central head regions.

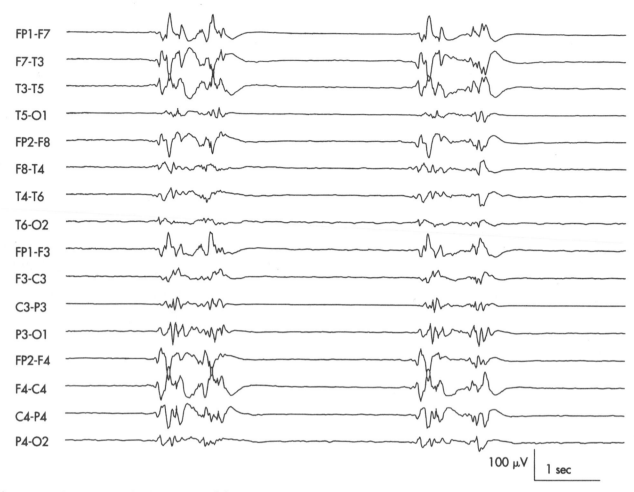

Figure 2.10 Burst suppression is a pattern of alternating high-amplitude bursts and very low-amplitude suppressed intervals.

Specific EEG patterns seen in stupor and coma patients may help with prognosis. *Burst suppression* is a pattern of alternating suppressed EEG intervals (at least 2 seconds of <20 mV) and paroxysmal bursts of mixed sharp and slow activity of higher amplitude (Figure 2.10). The burst suppression pattern is nonspecific with regard to etiology and can be seen in end-stage/ongoing seizure activity, hypothermia, anoxic–ischemic encephalopathy, and even iatrogenic situations such as medically induced coma. So-called "rhythmic" patterns may also be seen in coma. These include spindle coma, θ-coma, and α-coma patterns, which consist of diffuse unvarying appearance of their respective EEG components. The diffuse distribution of activity, lack of variability, and little or no response to stimuli differentiate these patterns from normal EEG. Care should be taken not to confuse these patterns with normal EEG, as the prognosis for the rhythmic patterns is usually quite poor. Rhythmic and burst suppression patterns are also seen with severe diffuse cerebral damage and medication overdoses. Burst suppression may be iatrogenic, deliberately induced with barbiturates or other medications to treat status epilepticus, provide neuroprotective levels of

anesthesia during neurosurgery, or induced in the management of increased intracranial pressure. When not iatrogenic, both burst suppression and rhythmic coma patterns are associated with poor outcomes, especially when the etiology is anoxic–ischemic injury.

Clinical brain death is usually accompanied by electrocerebral silence (ECS). Electrocerebral silence is defined as no detectable brain activity greater than 2 μV. Guidelines suggest that ECS can be determined only when the EEG is performed according to specific protocols and interpreted by knowledgeable readers. An ECS recording is not necessary to determine clinical brain death. Recording the EEG at maximal sensitivity settings makes it susceptible to recording and misinterpreting artifact as cerebral activity. The EEG should be used as a complementary tool in the clinical determination of brain death, and should be reserved for cases when one of the clinical features of brain death is not available or reliable.

Focal slowing is the hallmark of focal brain lesions, and can take several forms. Persistent polymorphic δ activity is most strongly associated with lesions undercutting the cortical–white matter connections. Destructive

▼▼

Pearls and Perils

EEG slowing

▶ Generalized slowing can be seen in many conditions, including encephalopathies (renal, hepatic, other metabolic), toxic states (lithium, sedatives, anticonvulsants), and degenerative conditions (Alzheimer's disease, others).

▶ Generalized slowing is not usually seen in psychiatric disease.

▶ Focal slowing usually suggests a static lesion (stroke, tumor, other) but may have a transient cause (postictal state, migraine, transient ischemic attack).

lesions of cortex often produce suppression of the EEG, first appearing as loss of faster-frequency components (β) in the area of the lesion and progressing to dropout of all activity. Intermittent focal slowing, interspersed in a normal appearing background, may also be seen with focal lesions. The significance of intermittent slowing versus persistent slowing remains uncertain. In known epilepsy patients, intermittent slowing may be the scalp recording expression of deeper subclinical epileptic activity. Conversely, not all intermittent slowing signifies epilepsy and, more commonly, it is a relatively nonspecific finding. Prior to the days of neuroimaging, focal EEG slowing or suppression was one of the few methods of finding lesions such as subdural hematomas or tumors (Figure 2.11). Today, EEG is clearly inferior to either CT or MRI when looking for focal structural lesions.

Periodic

Periodic patterns on EEG arise in a small number of special situations that, although relatively rare, are important to recognize. Periodic patterns are composed of high-amplitude complexes, often with sharp components, that repeat in an essentially rhythmic manner. These recordings may be focal or generalized, and are classified according to repetition rate, relationship to the EEG background, and wave morphology.

Periodic lateralized epileptiform discharges (PLEDS) are focal sharp waves that recur with a nearly periodic repetition rate ranging from 0.2 to 2 seconds (Figure 2.12). There is marked slowing of the background rhythms in the region of the PLEDS. This pattern is seen in patients with acute structural lesions, often in the setting of a generalized encephalopathy. PLEDS may also represent an end-stage pattern in status epilepticus, as seizure discharges occur in an "exhausted" brain.

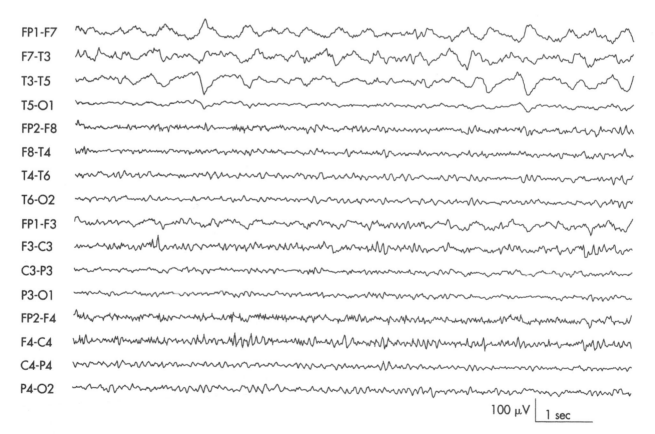

$100 \, \mu V$ | 1 sec

Figure 2.11 Focal slowing in a patient with a brain tumor.

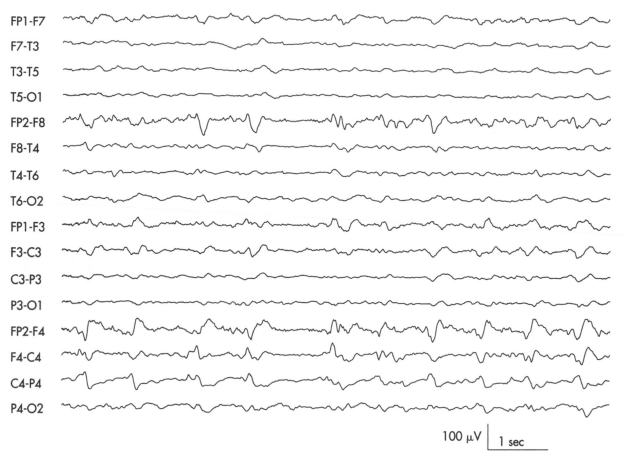

Figure 2.12 Periodic lateralized epileptiform discharges (PLEDS), due to embolic stroke.

Several infectious diseases are associated with periodic EEG patterns. For example, herpes encephalitis is often accompanied by a temporal (PLED) or bitemporal (BIPED) periodic pattern with high-amplitude sharp waves repeated every 2–6 seconds. The periodic pattern usually emerges during the first 2–3 days of the illness, making EEG one of the earliest diagnostic tests for this treatable disorder. Subacute sclerosing panencephalitis, a rare disorder associated with atypical measles infection, shows an EEG pattern of generalized, paroxysmal, periodic bursts every 5–20 seconds against a flat background. The EEG in Creutzfeldt-Jakob disease initially shows nonspecific diffuse or focal slowing. However, within a month or two of onset, periodic sharp waves recurring every 0.5–2 seconds begin to appear. The EEG is presently the only specific noninvasive test for Creutzfeldt-Jakob disease; 14-3-3 protein in the cerebrospinal fluid is suggestive (14-3-3 may be also positive in many neurodegenerative disorders) and brain biopsy is confirmatory. Periodic EEG patterns may also be seen in posthypoxic/anoxic coma, may suggest a poor prognosis.

In status epilepticus, the EEG shows an evolution from discrete seizures through a continuous seizure pattern, with suppression intervals gradually appearing in the late stages. In untreated status epilepticus, the suppression intervals become frequent, prolonged, and rhythmic. Prognosis declines as the EEG pattern advances through these stages. In these and other causes of coma, periodic sharp discharges are associated with poor prognosis. *Stimulus-induced rhythmic, periodic ictal discharges* (SIRPIDs) was first described by Hirsch and colleagues in 2004, in the critically ill. These rhythmic and periodic discharges can be induced by touch stimulation or even an abrupt noise in the patient's room. These periodic discharges often end after the stimulus has stopped. The pathophysiology of SIRPIDs is still unknown, as is the prognosis and treatment of patients with this stimulus-induced periodic EEG pattern (Figure 2.13).

Epileptiform

The EEG signature of the epilepsies is the interictal spike discharge. Identification of interictal spikes is perhaps the most common and significant reason for performing routine EEG. The spike is a brief discharge, lasting between 20 and 70 msec, and is both high enough in amplitude and sharp enough in waveform to clearly stand out from the ongoing background. Often, the spike discharge is

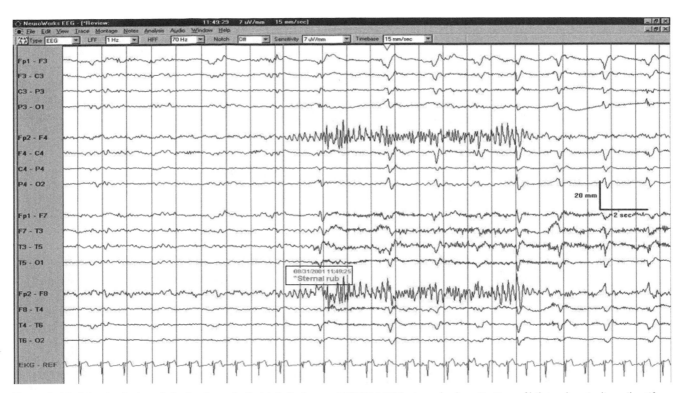

Figure 2.13 Stimulus-induced rhythmic periodic ictal discharges (SIRPIDs). With sternal rub, activation of bilateral periodic epileptiform discharges occurs. (Courtesy of Dr. Lawrence Hirsch)

closely followed by an after-coming slow wave, typically lasting 200–600 msec. Sharp waves share morphology with spike waves, but are longer in duration, lasting between 70 and 200 msec. Spikes and sharp waves (epileptiform activity) are classified by their distribution (whether generalized or focal); location (temporal, frontal, central, and so on); amplitude, rhythmicity, and state dependence (waking or sleeping); prominence of after-coming slow wave; how frequently they occur; and associated clinical signs.

Accurate interpretation of epileptiform discharges is essential to determining their clinical significance. The presence of spike discharges has a false-positive rate (patients with spikes but no seizures), and the absence of spikes has a false-negative rate (patients with seizures but no spikes). The false-positive rate depends strongly on the type of spike discharge. Anterior temporal spikes, characteristic of temporal lobe epilepsy (TLE), are a very reliable finding, and over 90% of patients with anterior temporal spikes have epilepsy. Spikes in other locations are less reliable. Generalized spike-and-wave may often be seen in persons without seizures (see later discussion), and the specificity varies even among subtypes of a given discharge. In patients with proven epilepsy, the EEG may be negative (that is, show no spikes, or only a normal or nonspecific pattern) owing to undersampling issues. Spikes may occur infrequently and, since the EEG is recorded for only 20–30 minutes, this may not be long enough to record abnormalities. A single EEG is abnormal in only about 30% of patients with epilepsy. Repeating the EEG, with sleep deprivation, increases the diagnostic yield. Two and three serial EEGs yield abnormalities in 46% and 59% of cases, respectively. However, since more than 20% of epilepsy patients have persistently normal EEGs despite multiple recording sessions, epilepsy remains a clinical diagnosis. A normal routine EEG cannot rule out a seizure disorder. Conversely, an abnormal EEG can make epilepsy a more likely diagnosis but is not, by itself, diagnostic of epilepsy.

The use of EEG to search for spikes is important not only to confirm and classify epilepsies, but also to aid in the prognosis for seizure recurrence in special circumstances. In patients presenting with a single seizure, the risk of having a second seizure is twice as great for patients when epileptiform abnormalities are present. The use of EEG to assess the risk of seizure relapse in a well-controlled patient who wishes to stop medications is more controversial. In a large meta-analysis, abnormal EEG was associated with a relative risk of 1.45 for relapse over a 1- to 2-year follow-up interval. Others have suggested that the emergence of epileptiform abnormalities on serial EEGs during medication taper is more predictive of relapse.

When spikes are not seen in a routine EEG, so-called activation procedures may be useful to help provoke abnormal discharges. Hyperventilation, which produces a mild hypocapnia, can lead to slowing on the

> ### Pearls and Perils
>
> #### EEG and epilepsy
>
> ▶ A normal EEG may be found in 20–70% of cases with epilepsy, and repeated tracings should be ordered if suspicion is high.
>
> ▶ "Spike discharges" on EEG may actually be normal variants such as benign epileptiform transients of sleep (BETS), vertex waves, RTDs, and wicket spikes.
>
> ▶ Seizures that persist despite adequate medication may be misclassified or may not be epilepsy.

EEG, especially in young patients, or trigger spike-and-wave discharges that are usually generalized. Repetitive flashes of a strobe light at frequencies ranging from 2 to 20/sec usually trigger a normal occipital response voltage called *photic driving*. In some, the photic response may be markedly asymmetric, suggesting dysfunction of the underlying occipital brain region. Others, however, may be photosensitive, and the flash triggers diagnostic spike-

and-wave discharges. Sleep deprivation prior to recording the EEG may also activate spike discharges. Capturing sleep during an EEG recording may be the most important activating procedure in bringing to the surface and provoking focal and generalized epileptiform abnormalities. In fact, all of these activation procedures are routinely used in suspected epilepsy patients to increase the diagnostic yield of EEG.

Generalized Spike-and-Wave

The generalized spike-and-wave discharge is characteristic of generalized epilepsies. The classic form is the 3-per-second spike-and-wave, shown in Figure 2.14. The spike is high-amplitude and narrow, and often contains two or more phases. The after-coming slow wave is also high-amplitude, of uniform morphology, and lasts about 300 msec, terminating immediately as another spike-and-wave complex arises. The first discharges in a burst repeat slightly faster than 3-per-second, up to 3.5–4 per second, and, as the burst progresses, these discharges gradually slow to slightly below 3-per-second. In prolonged discharges, a blunting of consciousness, known as

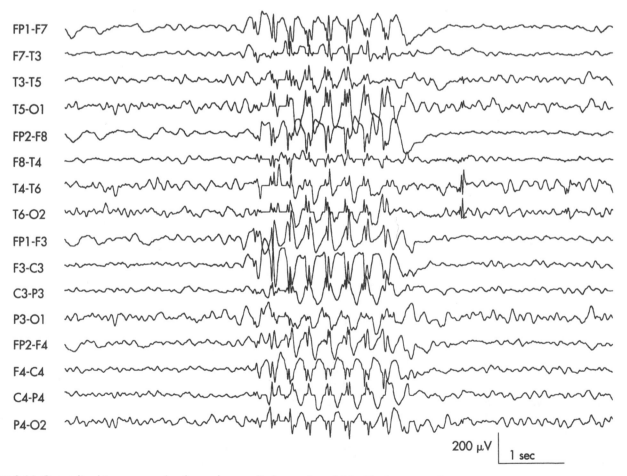

200 µV | 1 sec

Figure 2.14 Generalized 3-per-second spike-and-wave discharges in a child with absence epilepsy.

an *absence seizure*, may occur. Children of 5–10 years of age with this condition usually come to attention because someone noted "staring spells." Many will outgrow their seizures, although some will eventually develop generalized tonic–clonic seizures. Medications such as phenytoin and carbamazepine are unlikely to be effective, and may provoke worsening of discharges in these patients. This type of epilepsy is often inherited as an autosomal dominant trait with variable penetrance. Siblings of these patients may exhibit the EEG trait and yet never have a clinical seizure, reinforcing the notion that the presence of spike-and-wave on EEG, by itself, is not diagnostic of epilepsy, but must be correlated with clinical history.

Spike repetition rates other than 3-per-second are associated with other seizure types. Discharges consistently faster than 3-per-second are more likely to be seen in primary generalized epilepsies. *Rapid spike-and-wave* at 4–5 per second is seen in juvenile myoclonic epilepsy (JME). This is a syndrome of three distinct seizure types: absence, myoclonic, and generalized tonic–clonic. Onset is usually in early adolescence, and patients rarely outgrow their epilepsy. Although the rapid spike-and-wave discharge is strongly associated with JME, these patients may also display other spike types in their EEG. The EEG in JME is often normal interictally, and the diagnosis is sometimes strictly made on clinical evaluation. Patients with JME frequently have absence seizures, with typical 3-per-second spike-and-wave. Another spike discharge seen in JME is a run of very rapid, low-amplitude spike discharges above 15–20 per second, with or without associated slow wave. The polyspike in JME is sometimes time-locked to a myoclonic jerk.

Even faster repetition rates of generalized spike-and-wave are seen in the family of 6-per-second spike-and-wave discharges. Hughes has proposed a classification of these 6-per-second spike-and-wave discharges as WHAM or FOLD variant discharges. *WHAM variant discharges* are seen in the *w*aking state, with *h*igh amplitude, *a*nterior scalp predominance, and in *m*ale patients. WHAM variants of the 6-per-second spike-and-wave have a relatively high association with generalized tonic-clonic seizures. *FOLD variant discharges*, on the other hand, are seen in *f*emales, in the *o*ccipital region, with *l*ower amplitude (less than 50 μV for the spike component), and in *d*rowsiness only, and are associated with a lower risk of epilepsy. Less than 30% of patients with FOLD discharges have seizures.

The *phantom spike* is a very-low-amplitude, 6-per-second spike-and-wave discharge that is generally located in the posterior head regions and is regarded as a normal variant. Another discharge with the same general repetition rate is the 14-and-6-per-second positive spike-and-wave. This discharge, best seen on referential montages, has a distinctive characteristic of positive surface polarity of the spike component, is most often seen in young people, and is considered a normal variant.

Generalized spike-and-wave discharges, by definition, are seen in all head regions. They may display a phenomenon called *fractionation* or minor shifting asymmetries. Patients with generalized epilepsy may have discharges that are seen in focal regions of the scalp, although the regions will shift from one side to the other in the course of a single recording or on serial recordings. An important consideration in the differential diagnosis is *secondary bilateral synchrony*, which is seen when a focal discharge spreads rapidly and appears to be a generalized discharge. The distinction is an important one, as therapy (medication or surgery) is often guided by the type of EEG abnormality/epilepsy that is ultimately diagnosed. Resective surgery is possible in partial but not generalized epilepsy.

Focal Spike and Sharp Wave Discharges

The localization-related epilepsies are the most common adult epilepsies. They differ from the generalized epilepsies in that partial seizures arise in a specific epileptic focus. When the focus is related to a known pathologic process, such as a tumor, vascular malformation, post-traumatic lesion, or stroke, the epilepsy is termed *symptomatic*. *Cryptogenic* seizures have no known cause. Some genetic epilepsy may also be of partial or focal onset.

Recently, progress has been made in understanding the cryptogenic epilepsies. Accurate diagnosis with the assistance of EEG is important in the successful management of these patients. The diagnostic finding on EEG that suggests a partial seizure disorder is the focal spike or sharp wave that is restricted to a particular scalp distribution. Focal epileptiform activity is usually less uniform in appearance, less repetitive, often less rhythmic, and has a lower-amplitude slow component, compared to generalized spike-and-wave discharges. Spikes and sharp waves are felt to carry equal diagnostic significance, although some have suggested that spike sharpness may be predictive of seizure control.

The anterior temporal spike discharge is seen in patients with temporal lobe, and sometimes frontal lobe, seizures (Figure 2.15). The discharge is variable in its amplitude and morphology. The field is widespread, often extending into frontal, mid, and posterior temporal regions. The anterior temporal spike is seen most frequently in drowsiness, unilaterally, and ipsilateral to the seizure focus. Many patients with temporal lobe seizures will display spike discharges independently from both temporal regions. Bilateral independent spike discharges may signify independent epileptic foci in both temporal lobes, but may often be seen as secondary phenomena in patients with purely unilateral disease. The distinction is important when planning surgical treatment. The anterior temporal spike has a high specificity for epilepsy, with about

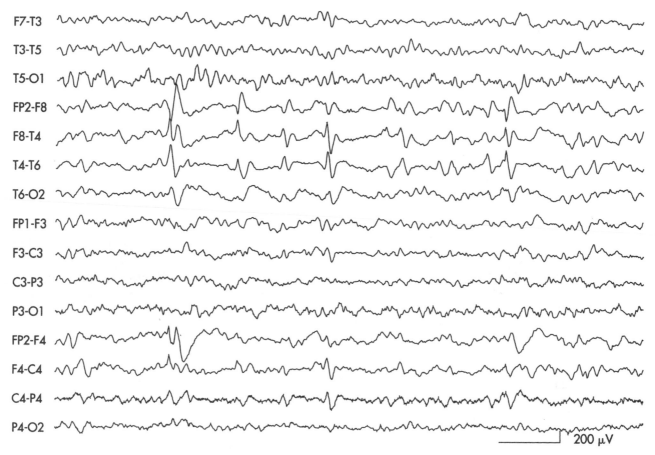

Figure 2.15 Right anterior temporal spike discharge in a patient with complex partial seizures and mesial temporal sclerosis. Phase reversal seen at the common electrode F8.

90% of patients with this discharge having clinical seizures. People with occipital, central, or frontal spikes are less likely (40–60%) to have epilepsy.

Several specific types of focal spikes deserve special attention. A rare EEG finding is the midline spike appearing near the scalp vertex in patients with epilepsies arising from frontal midline brain structures. Associated seizures may involve rhythmic leg movements (arising from the leg primary motor cortex), unusual body posturing (fencer's posture arising from the supplementary motor area), or peculiar movements such as bicycling leg movements, pelvic thrusting, and other features that do not look like common seizures. The pathologic midline spike may be difficult to distinguished from the normal vertex sharp wave of sleep, especially in children, in whom the normal V-waves often appear quite sharp.

Several forms of focal spike discharge are best regarded as normal variants. The most important of these is the BETS. This is a low- to moderate-amplitude discharge (<50µV), with a widespread field centered in the mid temporal regions. The morphology is usually a single or diphasic form with low-amplitude after-coming slow wave. The discharge is seen exclusively in early sleep

stages, and is not associated with focal slowing. Population studies have shown that this discharge is equally common in persons with and without epilepsy.

Persons blind from infancy may have occipital *needle spikes*, which are named for their very sharp morphology, very brief duration of 10–35 msec, and characteristic occipital localization. Persons with cerebral palsy (CP) will sometimes demonstrate so-called CP spikes in the central (sensorimotor) head region. Needle spikes and CP spikes are not associated with epilepsy.

EEG in the Differential Diagnosis of Epilepsy

A clinician will often order an EEG when a patient has spells that may be seizures. The clinical spectrum of seizure-like events is great, and includes a number of nonepileptic events that can mimic seizures. Important imitators of epilepsy include spells of psychiatric conditions such as conversion disorders, anxiety or panic attacks, and dissociative state syndromes. These are known as nonepileptic seizures (NES) or pseudoseizures. Epilepsy may also be misdiagnosed in NES of nonpsychiatric origin, including variant forms of migraine, transient ischemic attacks, movement disorders, cardiogenic syncope, and episodic endocrine spells such as hypoglycemia.

Furthermore, some seizures do not look like "typical" seizures. Frontal lobe seizures, for example, may have a bizarre clinical appearance. Patients with frontal lobe epilepsy (FLE) will often have a normal EEG, occasionally even during a definite epileptic seizure, making the diagnosis difficult. Because of the large size of the frontal lobe, the epileptiform activity may not be reflected on the surface EEG, especially if the seizure discharge remains localized. Patients with TLE may present clinically with confusional spells, episodes of bizarre behavior, or panic attacks.

Some patients with epileptic spikes on EEG may turn out to have pseudoseizures. Studies of patients diagnosed by neurologists as having epilepsy, referred to specialty centers for tertiary care, have reported a misdiagnosis rate of 20%. An even higher rate of misdiagnosis occurred in the opposite direction, however, when seizures were of a peculiar enough type that physicians dismissed the spells as psychiatric. Approximately 25% of cases diagnosed by neurologists as having NES turn out to have epilepsy when monitored in an EEG telemetry unit (EMU). The coexistence of epilepsy and NES was estimated to be about 10–15%. As an example, outcomes of telemetry monitoring in 394 patients at the Barrow Neurological Institute are compared to preadmission diagnosis in Figure 2.16. Recording one or multiple typical events in an EMU affords the best chance of arriving at the proper diagnosis. Every attempt to record all typical events should be made, owing to the possibility of having both NES and epilepsy in the same patient. Since patients consistently under-report seizures, clinicians should have a low threshold for admission to an EMU, even if the patient describes only "rare events."

Electroencephalographic telemetry units are inpatient wards of a hospital, equipped with specialized EEG instruments capable of recording, storing, and analyzing EEG and video data continuously. These digital video EEG recordings allow detailed analysis of any recorded spells. During an EMU admission, patients are often either weaned off their anticonvulsant medications or have their anticonvulsant doses reduced to encourage recording and analysis of typical events. Having the patient or family members confirm that the observed episodes are indeed typical of the attacks prompting medical attention, combined with analysis of the EEG during the attack, greatly improves the chances for correct diagnosis. In people with suspected epilepsy who have not responded adequately to medications, EMU admission often confirms the diagnosis and type of epilepsy. Diagnosis of events as NES during an EMU admission can often allow for cessation of potentially toxic antiepileptic drugs (Table 2.2).

Epilepsy Surgery

Medications fail to provide complete control of seizures in 30–60% of cases. For patients with partial epilepsy, surgery is an important therapeutic option. Typical "cure

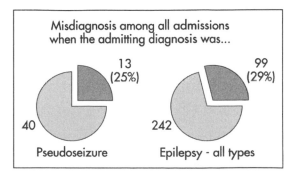

Figure 2.16 Misdiagnosis in a population of patients with poorly controlled epilepsy. Data from 394 referrals to the epilepsy clinic at the Barrow Neurological Institute, comparing the diagnosis at time of referral to the diagnosis obtained after video electroencephalographic telemetry.

Table 2.2 Major indications for electroencephalography

Situation	Reason for EEG
New-onset seizure	Evaluate risk of recurrence
	Classify seizure type if abnormality found
Selecting drug therapy	Classify seizure type
Uncertain if spells are really seizures	Finding of spike discharges helps support diagnosis
	Video EEG telemetry offers definitive diagnosis
Seizures continue despite drugs	Video EEG telemetry to evaluate for epilepsy treatment and confirm epilepsy diagnosis
Prolonged seizure-free interval	Assess risk of relapse when drug discontinued
Stupor and coma	Degree of slowing is sensitive indicator of progress
	Certain patterns portend poor prognosis
	Rule out subtle status epilepticus
Encephalitis	Periodic pattern or temporal slowing and sharp waves is early indicator of herpes infection
Dementias	Normal EEG raises suspicion of depression
	Periodic pattern suggests Creutzfeldt-Jakob disease
	Abnormal EEG suggests possible "organic" process

rates" for TLE at established epilepsy surgery centers range from 60 to 70%, with an additional 20% of patients showing a marked reduction in seizure frequency. Frontal lobe epilepsies and epilepsies arising at other localizations are less common, and have slightly lower success rates with surgery. Current evidence shows that surgery is far more likely to lead to a seizure-free outcome than medical treatment. A recent Canadian study has shown clear effectiveness of early surgery compared to medical therapy in refractory epilepsy patients. Seizure-free rates from all of the new antiseizure drugs either recently released or under development are all below 10%, averaging a disappointing 1–2%.

Presurgical evaluation of epilepsy patients should be undertaken as soon as a patient with partial epilepsy fails to gain freedom from seizures despite adequate trials of two or three medications. The cornerstone in the diagnostic workup for epilepsy surgery is the EEG. Recording

of seizures in an inpatient EMU allows for confirmation of the diagnosis of epilepsy and often localization of the seizure focus. A focal seizure onset is shown in Figure 2.17. Certain EEG patterns at the time of seizure onset are highly predictive of focus localization. The "initial focal" and "delayed focal" patterns correctly identify lobe and lateralization in over 90% of cases. Accurate seizure onset data, when combined with neuroimaging, are often accurate enough to allow a resective surgery to be completed without invasive diagnostic testing. Tremendous advances have been made in neuroimaging for epilepsy surgery, although video EEG telemetry remains a vital component of the evaluation. An important aspect of the presurgical evaluation involves ruling out multifocal epilepsy. Typically, recording five consecutive concordant seizures is required to achieve a high confidence that the vast majority come from the same side. The recording of seizures on video EEG typically requires a 5–7 day hos-

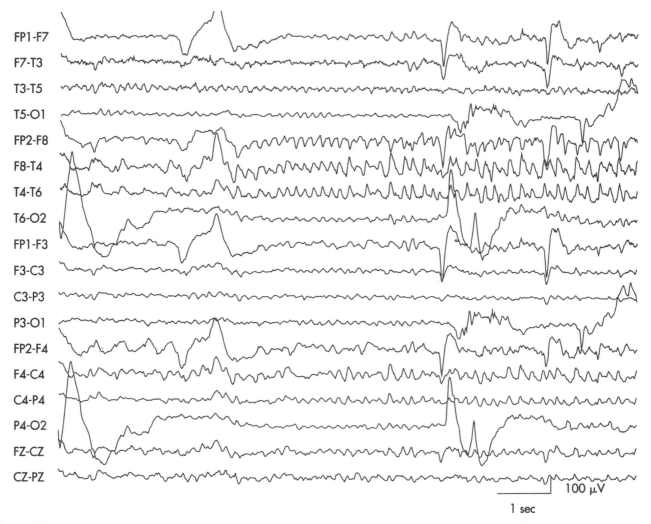

Figure 2.17 Electroencephalogram showing a temporal lobe seizure onset in a 28-year-old with a 15-year history of complex partial seizures that were uncontrolled despite maximal medical therapy. The patient has been seizure-free following removal of the right amygdala and hippocampus.

pitalization. The volume of data generated during a prolonged stay in the EMU is great, and it is not feasible for an electroencephalographer to review every minute of the recorded EEG. Computer techniques have done much to ease this burden, as current recording systems are usually equipped with computer-driven automatic detection of spikes and seizures.

In about a quarter to a third of potential surgical candidates, the information obtained by noninvasive diagnostic tests (including neuroimaging and surface electrode recordings) is ambiguous, thereby necessitating surgical implantation of electrodes inside the skull. Invasive EEG electrodes may be thin strips or two-dimensional grids placed in the subdural space or thin multicontact wires implanted into the brain substance. Depth wire recordings typically target the hippocampus and other deep limbic structures. The target sites for depth wires are selected with the assistance of MRI guidance technology. Each technique has advantages that make it appropriate for specific cases. Subdural grid electrodes allow for a seizure focus to be localized to a narrow region. They can also be used in "mapping" the functions of the cortex that underlies them, thus improving surgical planning to avoid *eloquent* (language, motor function) cortex. Recent advances in functional MRI techniques may be complementary and, in the future, may replace the need to perform grid mapping to localize eloquent cortex. Depth electrodes can record from brain structures that are not recordable with subdural or scalp electrodes. Since the vast majority of medically refractory partial epilepsy arises from deep limbic structures, depth electrodes provide the most unambiguous localization. Permanent complication rates from either technique are in the range of 1–2%.

Ambulatory telemetry may occasionally serve as a lower-cost substitute for inpatient video EEG telemetry. Electrodes are applied, and a recording device is worn and carried around for 24–72 (or more) hours, with the patient returning the device and a seizure diary for analysis. The modern recording apparatus records continuously to digital storage for later review. The patient or family can mark typical events on the device to alert the reviewer to an appropriate event location on the record. Ambulatory EEG is particularly useful to quantify 3-per-second spike-and-wave discharges most often occurring during sleep, and often not captured during routine outpatient EEG recording. When clear-cut seizures are recorded, the ambulatory EEG can "rule in" a seizure disorder. A normal recording is often seen during ambulatory recordings and, unfortunately, cannot be used to rule out certain (e.g., frontal lobe) types of epilepsy. Ambulatory EEG can sometimes provide lateralizing data, but is probably not adequate for surgical localization.

When medications do not control seizures adequately, and the patient is not a surgical candidate, another option is the vagal nerve stimulator (VNS). This device is approved by the U.S. Food and Drug Administration (FDA) and has been on the market for a number of years. The device is easily implanted in outpatient surgery, with the output electrode attached to the left vagus nerve. The VNS is not effective in all who receive it and, at best, may reduce the number and severity of seizures. Unlike medications, the therapeutic effectiveness of VNS often improves with time, without exposing the patient to the potential side effects of antiseizure medications. The device is "dumb" in that the stimulation consists of simple cycling between on and off modes. Stimulation parameters may be adjusted quickly and easily using a handheld programmer. Seizure reduction with the VNS rivals many of the newer antiseizure drugs. The battery is replaceable and has a life expectancy of several years, depending on the stimulation parameters.

New devices that are not yet FDA approved include an indwelling "smart" device that may be implanted over epileptogenic cortex. When a focal resection cannot be completed, this device may be considered. This device is trained to detect abnormal electrocorticography identified to be associated with the patient's clinical seizures. In response to the detection of abnormal signal, the device delivers a small electrical stimulation to the underlying cortex in an attempt to abort the abnormal discharge. Seizure prediction devices are also in development, with the hope of providing seizure prediction minutes to hours before seizure onset.

Computer EEG

The computer has taken over the EEG laboratory. As a tool for recording, storing, and displaying data, digital EEG is superior, and also cheaper, than older paper-based technologies. Computer recording allows mathematical analysis of the EEG using methods such as power spectrum computation, dipole analysis, and coherence analysis. The computer can reformat the EEG from a difficult-to-interpret acquistion to a visually appealing and impressive full-colored "topographic map." There are a number of sources of error in these procedures, however, and they cannot yet be recommended for routine clinical use, except in some special cases of epilepsy and, potentially, in the evaluation of dementia. No current computer system can account for the many normal variant patterns seen on EEG. Likewise, computer analysis of the EEG is particularly susceptible to minor errors in technique, and can produce erroneous results in particular settings, such as mild drowsiness, medication effects, and artifacts. For the most part, these applications remain research tools. However, compressed spectral analysis (CSA) can be a useful clinical tool, especially in monitoring depth of anesthesia and the presence of a burst-suppression pattern, either in the operating room or intensive care unit. The CSA can also be a sensitive tool in noting changes during neurovascular procedures, such as carotid endarterectomy.

Evoked Potentials

Following stimulation of sensory nerves, an afferent impulse goes through specific pathways and synapses in relay nuclei to reach the brain, where it is processed by neurons in primary sensory areas. As the signal passes through each step of the way, it produces a minute electrical impulse. These impulses are too small to be recorded without averaging techniques, as the raw signal is smaller than ongoing EEG activity. Repetitive stimulation leads to repeated identical responses along the pathway in question. Recording these evoked responses on the computer leads to cancellation of the random EEG signals, and reinforcement of the time-locked EP, when the appropriate number of responses are averaged. The signal-to-noise ratio improves with the square root of the number of repetitions. Measuring the time and amplitude of the EP peaks provides an accurate, quantitative assessment of sensory function along the pathway in question.

Evoked potentials can be recorded in many ways, but three modes are commonly used in clinical medicine. *Visual EPs* (VEPs) are recorded by repetitive visual stimulation, usually with an alternating black and white checkerboard pattern displayed on a screen in front of the patient at a predetermined visual angle and stimulus intensity. A positive cortical peak representing arrival of the nerve impulses at the occipital lobe is seen between 95 and 105 msec after the stimulus. Pattern-reversal VEP requires the attention and cooperation of the patient; without it, inconsistent and nonreproducible results will be obtained. In uncooperative patients, flash stimulation can be used but is less precise. Flash stimulation produces a more variable response than pattern reversal VEP but may be sufficient to demonstrate gross integrity of the anterior visual pathways to the cortex.

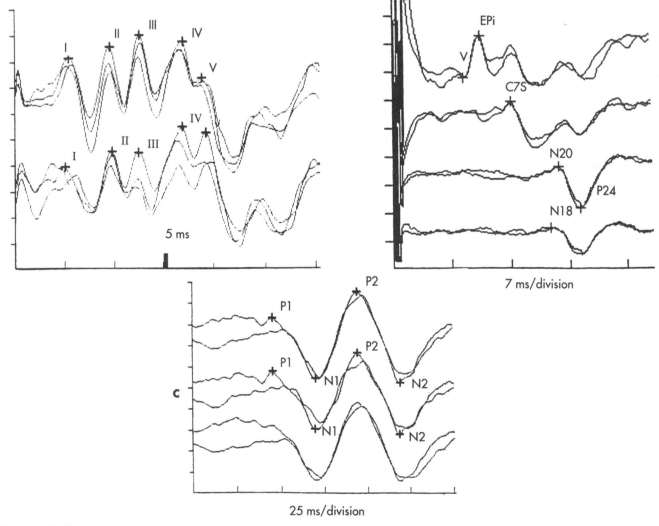

Figure 2.18 Normal evoked potential studies in typical clinically used modalities.

Somatosensory EPs are recorded following electrical stimulation of a peripheral nerve. Commonly used nerves include the median, peroneal, and posterior tibial nerves. For example, median nerve stimulation produces peaks recorded at the neck and scalp, representing transmission through the brachial plexus (typically 9–11 msec), nucleus cuneatus in the brainstem (13–14 msec), and primary sensory cortex (18–20 msec). Similar waveforms can be recorded in the other commonly tested nerves as the impulse passes along the specific pathway.

Brainstem EPs (BAEPs) are obtained following delivery of a loud click to the ear, usually at 60 dB above threshold. A series of five consistently reproducible peaks come from each of five structures along the auditory pathway: acoustic nerve (1.5–2.5 msec), cochlear nucleus (2–3 msec), superior olivary nucleus (3–4 msec), lateral lemniscus (4.5–5.5 msec), and medial geniculate bodies of the thalamus (5.5–6.5 msec).

Exact latencies for all EPs depend on the technique used in the lab where the study is obtained. Each lab should establish its own normal ranges from a series of normal controls. Examples of EPs are seen in Figure 2.18. Evoked potentials were once important in confirming conduction defects in suspected multiple sclerosis. The superior sensitivity of MRI, as well as the broader amount of information provided, has largely supplanted EPs for this use. VEPs are still useful to confirm either active or remote optic neuritis, however. BAEPs provide proof that an auditory stimulus reaches the CNS and so are objective evidence of hearing function. BAEPs are presently the best method of evaluating hearing threshold in neonates, infants with meningitis, and other children at risk for hearing loss. BAEPs are very sensitive to acoustic nerve dysfunction from schwannomas, meningiomas, and other tumors of the cerebellopontine angle. Conduction hearing loss produces elevation of the hearing threshold without change in central interpeak latencies. Sensorineural hearing loss produces increased interpeak latencies as the stimulus intensity is reduced, so that changes in the latency–intensity relationship can differentiate conduction deficits from neurologic causes of hearing loss. An important use of EP is to provide continuous monitoring of nerve, spinal cord, brainstem, and cortical function in anesthetized or comatose patients. Tibial somatosensory EPs, for example, are used to monitor spinal cord integrity during lumbar and thoracic spine surgery, whereas median EPs are used for upper cervical surgical procedures. BAEPs, on the other hand, can help preserve hearing in resections of schwannomas, and are a good monitor of brainstem integrity during posterior fossa surgery.

Summary

Electroencephalographic and EP studies allow a unique view of the function of the brain and provide information that is complementary to other investigations. EEG is of fundamental importance in the outpatient management of epilepsy. It provides supporting evidence for its diagnosis, aids in the classification of seizure type and/or epilepsy syndrome, assists with prognosis and, in some cases, monitors adequacy of therapy. For patients who do not respond to anticonvulsant medications, EEG telemetry is essential in the evaluation for epilepsy surgery. EEG is a useful adjunct for evaluating prognosis in dementias, encephalopathies, and coma. Evoked potential studies have more limited utility but remain important in optic neuritis, hearing loss, acoustic neuroma, and intraoperative monitoring, where their use may lower neurosurgical complication rates.

Acknowledgments

This chapter is dedicated to the memory of John Archibald R.EEG T. and Dorothea Brittenham R.EEG. T. Mr. Archibald was the chief technologist of the Barrow Neurological Institute Epilepsy Monitoring Unit from 1992 through 1996. Ms. Brittenham was instrumental in establishing technical standards for EEG still used today and teaching numerous physicians and technicians alike to perform and interpret EEGs and EPs. Also a debt of gratitude to Mr. and Mrs. Drazkowski and Dr. and Mrs. Neiman for their love and support.

Annotated Bibliography

Daly DD, Pedley TA. *Current practice of clinical electroencephalography*, 2nd ed. New York: Raven Press, 1990.
An excellent and practical manual for illustrations of normal variants, technical matters, and major classes of waveforms and their clinical correlations.

Daube JR. *Clinical neurophysiology*, 3rd ed. 2008 [Contemporary neurology series.] New York: Oxford University Press, 2008.
A concise review of the essential areas of all clinical neurophysiology including basic neurophysiology and the practical applications of EEG, EMG, EPs, and evaluation for epilepsy surgery.

Luders H, Lesser RP. *Epilepsy: Electroclinical syndromes*. London: Springer-Verlag, 1987.
An overview of various epilepsy syndromes with emphasis on their respective EEG manifestations. Very useful guide to the value of EEG in managing patients with epilepsy.

Niedermeyer E, Lopes da Silva F. *Electroencephalography: Basic principles, clinical applications, and related fields*, 5th ed. Baltimore: Williams & Wilkins, 2005.
The electroencephalographer's bible, containing exhaustive reference information about EEG, EP, and related information.

CHAPTER 3

Electrodiagnosis of Neuromuscular Disease

J. Robinson Singleton, James W. Russell, and Eva L. Feldman

Outline

- ▶ Principles of nerve conduction studies
- ▶ Principles of electromyography
- ▶ Electromyographic assessement of denervation
- ▶ Electrodiagnosis of specific disorders
- ▶ Neuromuscular junction disorders
- ▶ Summary

Electrodiagnostic medicine is defined by the American Association of Electromyography and Electrodiagnosis as the "clinical and electrophysiological evaluation of the function of nerve roots, peripheral nerves, neuromuscular junctions, muscles, spinal reflexes, and evoked potentials arising from the spinal cord and brain." This chapter focuses on the two most common electrodiagnostic techniques: nerve conduction studies (NCS) and electromyography (EMG). Collectively, these techniques are commonly referred to as EMG, although, strictly speaking, this designation should be reserved for electromyography only. Clinical EMG is an extremely useful tool and is best employed as an extension of the neurologic history and examination. In our laboratories, an electrodiagnostic consultation consists of a neurologic history, focused examination, and appropriate EMG studies. This allows for the most accurate diagnosis of peripheral nervous system disease before designing an appropriate treatment program.

This chapter will first discuss principles of nerve conduction studies and EMG, and then address the use of EMG in confirming or refuting a neurologic diagnosis.

Principles of Nerve Conduction Studies

After obtaining a neurologic history and completing a focused examination, the electrodiagnostician usually begins the evaluation with NCS. Common NCS include those of sensory nerves, motor nerves, and the neuromuscular junction. In each case, the nerve of interest is stimulated and the response recorded.

Stimulation

The stimulator is a hand-held device with two silver-plated service electrodes or wetted felt pads 0.5–0.1 cm in diameter; these are applied to the skin, and current passes through them to stimulate the nerve of interest below. With bipolar stimulation, both electrodes (the cathode and anode) are placed over the nerve. The cathode, or negative pole, attracts cations and is closest to the recording site. The anode, or positive pole, attracts anions and is farthest from the recording site. Current flows from anode to cathode and negative charges accumulate under the cathode and depolarize the nerve. In a routine stimulator, the cathode and anode are usually 2–3 cm apart. Alternatively, electroencephalogram (EEG) or monopolar needles can be used.

The stimulator is designed to deliver a square-wave pulse of electrical energy to the skin. Both intensity and duration of the stimulation can be controlled. There are two types of stimulation: constant-voltage or constant-current. In constant-voltage stimulation, the current varies with the skin and electrode impedance. In contrast, in constant-current stimulation, the current adjusts to the electrode impedance. Constant current is better for serial assessment of the level of shock intensity as a measure of nerve excitability and is routinely employed in our laboratories. The stimulus intensity varies between 150 and 300 V (20–40 mA) for a healthy nerve. Durations are from 0.05 to 1 msec. The stimulation threshold is defined as the level required to achieve a response, and at maximal threshold all axons are activated.

Recording

Electrical impulses are recorded either directly from depolarization of nerve fibers or from depolarization of muscle fibers. The sensory nerve action potential (SNAP) represents the sum of electrical depolarizations passing along the sensory nerve of interest beneath a recording electrode after electrical stimulation of the nerve. The compound muscle action potential (CMAP) represents the electrical sum of muscle depolarizations recorded at the muscle end plate, the site where peripheral nerve meets muscle. There are two types of recording electrodes: needle and surface. When recording from sensory nerves, needle electrodes will both increase the amplitude and decrease the noise, but are rarely used because they are invasive and technically more demanding. In motor nerves, the advantage of needle electrodes is that there is less interference from other muscles, so there is better definition of the initial deflection (also known as *takeoff*) of the CMAP. This can be advantageous when recording from proximal muscles that are difficult to isolate. The disadvantage of using needle electrodes for motor recording is that it records only a small portion of the CMAP.

More commonly, surface electrodes are used for both sensory and motor recordings. Electrodes, with conduction paste to reduce impedance, are taped to the skin. A larger disc ground electrode is also placed on the skin a few centimeters distant from the recording electrodes. Signal from the ground is subtracted (in the preamplifier) from the waveform signal to eliminate environmental noise such as 60-cycle electrical interference. Although there is a smaller amplitude and less favorable signal-to-noise ratio when using surface electrodes for sensory nerve recordings, they are more easily employed and less painful for the patient than needle electrodes. Sensory recordings require a 100,000-fold amplification, which also magnifies the noise in the system. Averaging of sensory responses can remove this noise and allow a clearer definition of the sensory signal. The degree of enhancement of the signal is proportional to the square root of the number of trials. For example, averaging four sensory trials will decrease the noise-to-signal ratio by two.

Surface electrodes offer a definite advantage when recording from motor nerves. Surface electrodes record the CMAP from all fibers innervated by a nerve. The onset in this instance will reflect the conduction of the fastest fibers, whereas the amplitude will reflect the number of muscle fibers activated and the timing of their activation. It is important that surface electrodes are placed over the motor nerve end plate. During a motor recording, a commonly encountered error is an initial positive deflection in the CMAP. This indicates the recording electrode is not over the end plate. With both sensory and motor recordings, it is important to decrease the skin impedance by cleaning off oils, trimming calluses, and avoiding smeared electrode paste. If excessive noise is still encountered, it could indicate an error in either the gain or filter settings, or that the ground requires moistening.

Electrical potentials recorded from surface electrodes pass through a preamplifier, which subtracts the signal common to both the G1 and G2 electrodes (common mode rejection) and then passes the net signal on to the EMG machine. In all contemporary machines, this analogue signal is then digitized, allowing both storage and manipulation of the digital waveform (e.g. altered sensitivity) prior to display. Most contemporary EMG machines have automatic instrument settings that manipulate this digital signal. Filter settings for sensory recordings should eliminate signal components with waveforms slower than 20 KHz and more frequent than 2 KHz. The gain is set between 10 and 20 µV per division. In contrast, for motor recordings, filters are set between 2 and 10 KHz, while the gain is between 1 and 2 mV.

▼

Pearls and Perils

Nerve stimulation

▶ Clearly label the anode and cathode and, if necessary, rotate the anode off the nerve.

▶ Avoid measurement from the anode rather than the cathode for distance measurements.

▶ Avoid high skin impedance by removing grease and callous and, if the patient is edematous, stimulate with needle electrodes.

▶ Record results only after supramaximal stimulation.

▶ Avoid NCS in patients with central lines and Swan-Ganz lines inserted directly into the heart.

▶ Avoid stimulator artifact, which can occur if the stimulator and recording electrodes are placed too closely together or the recording electrodes are placed too far apart.

▶ Always place a ground between the stimulating and recording electrodes.

▶ Adequately warm skin and underlying tissue prior to NCS (>32°C in upper extremities, >31°C in lower extremities). Nerve conduction studies from cool nerves yield a distinctive pattern of prolonged distal latency, reduced conduction velocity, and increased response amplitude.

Motor Nerve Conduction

During motor nerve conduction studies, the active or recording electrode is designated as G1 and is placed over the muscle end plate; G2 is the reference electrode and is placed on tendon or bone. Supramaximal stimulation (sufficient to obtain the largest CMAP amplitude) is used for this and all other nerve conduction recordings.

Calculation of a correct motor conduction velocity depends on three components: (a) the terminal or distal latency, (b) an accurate measurement of the CMAP, and (c) a correct distance calculation. The terminal or distal latency represents the integrity of the nerve from the point of stimulation to the axon terminals. It is dependent upon the length of the axon terminals, the time required for neuromuscular junction transmission, and the time for generation of the CMAP. The latency of the CMAP is measured at the takeoff and corresponds to the fastest conducting nerve fibers. Compound muscle action potential amplitude measurements are from baseline to negative peak and correspond to the number of muscle fibers activated. For a correct calculation of conduction velocity, a motor nerve is stimulated at both a distal and proximal point along the main nerve trunk. The distance between the cathodes is measured. Conduction velocity represents the distance in meters between the cathodes divided by the proximal latency minus the distal latency in seconds. A common source of error in motor recordings is the use of submaximal stimulation, which can lead to inaccurate takeoffs and variable CMAPs. A small initial negative CMAP peak may occur if a high gain is used. This deflection can arise from the nerve and is usually ignored. In contrast, a small positive CMAP dip indicates that G1 is not over the end plate and must be repositioned. Frequently, volume conduction can occur from other muscles. This can be due to overzealous stimulation of more than one nerve. Alternatively, anomalous innervation may exist, and volume conduction could reflect a true anatomic variation.

Sensory Nerve Conduction Studies

There are two common types of sensory recordings: orthodromic and antidromic. In an orthodromic recording, stimulation of the digital sensory nerves elicits a response at a more proximal site along the nerve trunk. Alternatively, stimulation of a proximal site along the nerve results in an *antidromic recording* from digital nerves. Sensory amplitudes can be measured baseline to negative peak, our method of preference. Sensory amplitudes are a reflection of the density of innervation.

Sensory conduction velocities can be calculated directly, based on the distal latency alone, since there is no need to factor out the time delay incurred by motor nerves in neurochemical transmission across the neuro-

muscular junction. In this instance, the distance between the cathode and the recording G1 electrode is divided by the initial distal latency. More proximal sensory conduction velocities are calculated identically to motor nerves, as described earlier.

Measurement Variability

Several factors can contribute to variability in nerve conduction studies. For both sensory and motor nerves, conduction velocity increases 0.7–2.4 m/s (or about 5%) per degree between 29–48°C. Thus, temperature control is crucial to performing accurate, reproducible nerve conduction studies. In the authors' laboratories, we require the hand warmed to 32°C and the foot to 31°C, and use thermal packs. Heating lamps are also employed for limb warming. If the skin is 34°C, the muscle is approximately 37°C. If a limb is inadequately warmed, artificial increases in distal latencies, with corresponding slowed conduction velocities are observed, together with an *increase* in the response amplitude, especially for sensory responses.

Age is another important variable in nerve conduction studies. Conduction velocities for full-term infants are 50% that of adults. Between the ages of 3 and 5 years, childhood velocities reach adult values. After the age of 60, motor conduction velocities are on average 10% slower than before the age of 60 and, by 70, are 15% slower. By the age of 70, median sensory amplitudes are decreased by one-third when compared with responses measured between the ages of 18 and 25 years.

Anatomic variation in nerves also contributes to variability. Both proximal and distal conduction velocities are slower in the legs when compared to the arms. An inverse relationship is also present between height and conduction velocity, so that the taller the individual, the slower the conduction velocity. Conductions velocities are greater proximally than distally, because of decreased distal axon diameters, shorter internodal distances, and the temperature gradient of distal arms and legs.

Principles of Electromyography

Electromyography is the study of motor unit potentials, defined as the summated electrical potentials of all muscle fibers in one motor unit firing in response to activation of a single lower motor neuron. Most commonly, a concentric needle electrode is passed through muscle fibers, where it detects both the intracellular and extracellular potentials. The three major parts of the needle examination include evaluations of (a) insertional activity, (b) abnormal spontaneous activity, and (c) motor unit action potentials (MUAPs). Careful attention to each component will improve the diagnostic capacity of the examination.

Insertional Activity

Insertional activity is examined at an amplifier gain of 20–100 µV per division. As the needle passes through muscle, irritation of muscle fiber membranes produces potential changes, which deflect the trace on the screen. This normal insertional activity indicates to the examiner that he is recording from muscle, and should stop within 20–100 msec after needle movement is stopped. A marked decrease in insertional activity implies either that the needle is not in muscle or that the muscle has undergone severe chronic fibrosis or replacement by fat. Severe, acute ischemia of muscle due to vascular occlusion or compartment syndromes may also produce decreased or absent insertional activity. Conversely, prolonged insertional activity suggests abnormal muscle membrane irritability.

Abnormal Spontaneous Activity

When the needle is no longer being moved, normal muscle is electrically silent. Spontaneous electrical activity with the needle at rest is generally pathologic. Abnormal spontaneous activity arises when a muscle fiber loses its innervation. Clinical entities associated with abnormal spontaneous activity include denervation due to axonal injury to motor nerve fibers, and muscle fiber necrosis (because portions of individual muscle fibers separated by necrosis from their motor end plate become denervated). Motor axonal injury occurs with many neuropathies. Myofiber injury occurs in inflammatory myopathy, dystrophies, and metabolic disorders of muscle, such as hyperkalemic periodic paralysis. These same myopathic disorders often produce abnormal prolongation of insertional activity, as described earlier.

The most commons forms of abnormal spontaneous activity are *positive waves* and *fibrillation* potentials. Positive waves are potentials generated from injured single muscle fibers and represent the repolarization phase of the muscle action potential. Fibrillation potentials are bi- or triphasic potentials with an initial positive component and are thought to represent distant recording spontaneous discharge from a single denervated muscle fiber. Fibrillation potentials are of variable amplitude (20–200 µV) with a rhythmic discharge pattern (0.5–20 Hz). Fibrillation potential amplitude depends upon fiber size. Chronically denervated, atrophied muscle has small-amplitude fibrillation potentials, whereas recent denervation of a hypertrophied fiber yields a large-amplitude potential. Various rating scales exist for quantifying fibrillation potentials. We employ the following empiric scale: 1+ indicates sustained fibrillation potentials in two areas of muscle; 2+, fibrillations in half of insertion sites; 3+, activity found in all areas examined, and 4+, abnormal potentials fill the baseline in all areas and make interpretation of voluntary response difficult.

Other forms of abnormal spontaneous activity include fasciculation potentials, complex repetitive discharges, myokymia, myotonia, neuromyotonia, and cramp potentials. *Fasciculations* represent the spontaneous contraction and accompanying electrical discharge of one entire motor unit. Although frequently associated with denervated motor units in amyotrophic lateral sclerosis (ALS), fasciculations may also be noted in other chronic denervating conditions, or as a normal variant, especially following exercise.

Several high-frequency discharges can be distinguished and have distinctive clinical significance. These discharges often are provoked by needle insertion, indicating increased biochemical irritability of muscle fibers, although they also frequently occur spontaneously. *Complex repetitive discharges* are sustained, high-frequency, rhythmic bursts with a distinctive "machine noise" sound that typically signals very chronic denervating injury. By contrast, *myokymic discharges* are trains of brief, high-amplitude, high-frequency discharges, classically seen following ionizing radiation injury or therapy. Clinical *myotonia*, transient muscle stiffness following brief isometric exercise, is associated with repetitive discharge featuring a continuously changing frequency and amplitude yielding a distinctive "dive-bomber" quality. Myotonic discharges or related "neuromyotonia" may be encountered in myotonic dystrophy or in metabolic derangements of muscle membrane ion channels (referred to as "channelopathies"), such as hyper- or hypokalemic periodic paralysis. Finally, continuous, rhythmic high-frequency discharges of simple morphology, "cramp potentials," may signal hyper-irritability of injured muscle but is usually a normal variant.

Motor Unit Action Potentials

Motor unit action potentials represent the summation of individual muscle fiber action potentials from one motor unit. Motor unit action potentials are described based on their activation pattern, or recruitment, as well as their amplitude, duration, and configuration. *Recruitment pattern* describes the preprogrammed, orderly, and invariant order in which motor units are activated in response to increasing voluntary effort. Small MUAPs are recruited first, typically firing in semirhythmic bursts of seven to eight and, with increased effort, increase their firing rate to 15–20. Incremental effort recruits additional motor units of increased size, each firing initially at seven to eight and quickening their firing rate as effort is increased. Figure 3.1 shows a schematic representation of motor unit recruitment in normal muscle.

Three other characteristics distinguish the MUAP waveform: *amplitude*, arbitrarily determined as the height (in microvolts) from greatest positive to greatest negative deflection; *duration*, during which the oscilloscope trac-

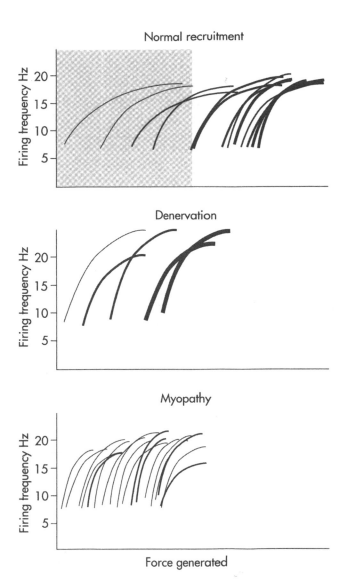

Figure 3.1 Schematic motor unit recruitment patterns demonstrated on needle examination of patients with normal muscle, denervation, or myopathy. Each curve represents an individual motor unit, with frequency of depolarization measured as a function of total force generated. Line thickness gives a measure of relative motor unit size. As described in the text, during normal recruitment (*top panel*), small motor units are recruited first, increasing their firing rate to 10–15 before recruitment of subsequent, larger units. During the electromyographic evaluation, the greatest information can be obtained by evaluating the first three to five motor unit action potentials, the area demarcated by shading in the top panel. Either denervation or myopathy decreases maximum power generated. In denervation, loss of some motor units results in increased firing rate of remaining units, whose size is often increased. In myopathy, power generated by each individual muscle fiber and motor unit is decreased, so recruitment occurs more rapidly. Due to fiber splitting, motor units are often smaller in size.

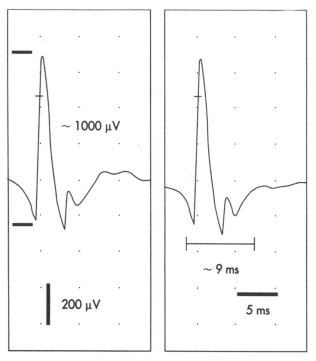

Figure 3.2 Two sequential recordings of a typical normal motor unit action potential (MUAP). Waveform is unchanged from one firing to the next. As indicated by the scales, this MUAP is about 1,000 μV in amplitude, and 9 msec in duration. This MUAP has two phases and five turns.

ing is deflected from the baseline (in msec); and *turns* and *phases*, that is, the number of times within a MUAP that the tracing changes polarity or crosses the baseline, respectively. A typical MUAP is shown in Figure 3.2. Proximity of the needle to the MUAP of interest dramatically alters these characteristics. For adequate recording, the rise time of the first negative deflection should be less than 0.5 msec, indicating close proximity of MUAP and needle. A typical MUAP will have a duration of less than 10 msec, fewer than five phases, and a stereotyped morphology with each firing. Amplitude varies from one MUAP to the next, but is typically less than 2,000 μV for each of the first four MUAPs recruited.

Electromyographic Assessment of Denervation

By examining the recruitment pattern for the first three to five MUAPs in several sites for each muscle, the electromyographer may recognize decreased recruitment due to neurogenic injury. Two criteria are commonly used in the authors' lab:

- *Increased MUAP amplitude.* In normal muscle, the first three to four MUAPs all have an amplitude of less than 2,000 μV. Discovery of high-amplitude (>2,000 μV) motor units among the first three or four on the screen in more than 20% of the sites examined suggests neurogenic loss of relatively smaller motor units, necessitating early recruitment of larger motor units.

- *Fast firing MUAPs.* Ordinarily, recruitment of a subsequent MUAP occurs before the previous motor unit reaches a firing rate of 15. Discovery of individual motor units firing at more than 20, regardless of their amplitude, suggests neurogenic loss of other motor units that would normally be recruited in support as effort is increased.

Recruitment changes are the first recognizable EMG signs of functional disconnection between motor neuron and muscle, present immediately upon injury, before the appearance of spontaneous activity (2–3 weeks) or alterations in MUAP morphology observed with reinnervation (>6 weeks). Subtle or early changes may be difficult to detect in the absence of other signs. Moreover, discovery of decreased recruitment, in itself, does not provide information about the duration of the injury, its cause (e.g., axonal injury versus demyelination), or its location (e.g., damage to motor neuron, root, plexus, or axon).

Attention to the morphology of the motor units in a muscle with decreased recruitment offers information about both chronicity of injury and associated reinnervation. In partially denervated muscle, surviving motor axons send out terminal sprouts that reinnervate denervated muscle fibers. Recently reinnervated fibers lack proper synchronization with the rest of the adopted motor unit, and may not respond to every axonal signal. Thus, motor units containing recently reinnervated fibers are of long duration and often have a ragged, polyphasic morphology that can alter from one firing to the next because of dropout of individual fibers. When extreme, so-called "satellite potentials" may represent fibers firing so late that they are time-locked with, but not within the waveform of the primary motor unit. As reinnervated connections mature, polyphasic behavior gives way to well-consolidated units of increased amplitude. Cyclic denervation and reinnervation may lead to consolidation of surviving muscle fibers into a few gargantuan motor units (amplitudes of 5,000–15,000 μV) in ALS and chronic radiculopathies.

Following traumatic nerve crush, transection, localized ischemia, or other complete axonal denervation, regenerating axons must extend from the point of injury down the remnant nerve sheath, usually at a rate of 2–3 cm per month. Distinctive low-amplitude, complex, and long-duration *nascent motor units* herald reinnervation of the denervated muscle, and may be observed as early as 6 weeks following injury in paraspinal and other very proximal muscles. The electrodiagnostic presence of such nascent motor units may portend a comparably good prognosis for recovery of strength before any voluntary muscle activity can be observed clinically.

Electromyographic Assessment of Myopathy

Activation of muscle acetylcholine receptors generates a wave of depolarization that is carried away from the motor end plate into the depth of the muscle fiber through the T-tubule system, assuring a synchronized contraction of the entire fiber, a condition that optimizes the force generated by the muscle. Myopathy, whether due to metabolic injury, ion channel dysfunction, or inflammatory necrosis of muscle fibers, decreases the efficiency and power of muscular contraction, often by desynchronizing one portion of a motor unit or myofiber from another. As a result, the unifying electrodiagnostic abnormality in myopathy is increased recruitment: a greater than expected number of motor units must be recruited to generate a given power of muscular contraction. Schematic representations of recruitment in normal muscle, following denervation, or in myopathy are compared in Figure 3.1.

In mild disease, this subtle effect can be very difficult to recognize or quantify. In profound myopathy, voluntary effort may rapidly fill the screen with motor units, yet generate no perceptible movement of the examined limb, indicating essentially complete electromechanical dissociation. One simple rule of thumb is that in larger muscles (e.g., biceps, deltoid), the patient should be able to generate force recognizable by the examiner while only a single motor unit is firing near the inserted EMG needle. If initial voluntary effort always produces multiple motor units near the needle, a myopathy should be considered.

Changes in MUAP morphology may also distinguish myopathy, although this is not invariable. Myopathic motor units are often of low amplitude, short duration, and very polyphasic, reflecting desynchronization of firing both within individual fibers and between fibers in a given motor unit. Often, in more severe myopathy, no motor unit has an amplitude greater than 1,000 μV. Although in isolation, myopathic motor units may closely resemble the nascent units observed in reinnervation, these two may be distinguished in the context of dramatically different recruitment patterns.

Finally, fibrillation potentials may be observed in inflammatory myopathies and some dystrophies, reflecting functional denervation of portions of individual muscle fibers by necrosis. Other distinctive repetitive discharges associated with myopathies have been discussed earlier. Complex combinations of abnormal spontaneous activity, decreased recruitment, and myopathic motor units should make the examiner think of injury due to toxins, severe chronic illness, or inclusion body myositis. A comparison of EMG findings in denervation and myopathy is presented in Table 3.1.

Table 3.1 Electrodiagnostic comparison of denervation and myopathy

	Denervation	Myopathy
Motor symptoms	Weakness often distal	Weakness often proximal
Sensory symptoms/signs	Depends on process	No
SNAP	Depends on process	Normal
CMAP	Reduced amplitude	Often normal
EMG	Decreased recruitment: (loss of some motor units requires remaining motor units to provide more effort; reinnervation leads to large motor units)	Increased recruitment: (because all motor units inefficient, more motor units necessary to generate same level of power)
Electrodiagnostic criteria	1 Any of first three MUAPs is >2000µV (in >20% of sites) 2 Any of first three MUAPs fires >20Hz before recruitment of additional motor units	1 Impossible to voluntarily generate just one MUAP on screen 2 No large MUAPs. MUAPs are of short duration, low amplitude, and polyphasic
Abnormal spontaneous activity	Often	Often

Electrodiagnosis of Specific Disorders

Nerve Conduction Studies/ Electromyography as a Diagnostic Tool

In a number of specific diseases, EMG and NCS can be of benefit in rendering a diagnosis. In general, electrodiagnostic studies excel in localizing the site of a peripheral nerve lesion (e.g., motor neuron, nerve root, plexus, distal nerve axon), distinguishing denervating from demyelinating injury, and quantifying the contributions of sensory and motor axonal injury in neuropathy. Nerve conduction studies and EMG are the most sensitive methods for diagnosing abnormalities of neuromuscular junction transmission, such as myasthenia gravis. As described earlier, EMG recognizes myopathy and may distinguish inflammatory myopathy (which may respond to immunosuppressive therapy) from metabolic myopathy (which is unresponsive to immunosuppressive therapy). Nerve conduction studies offer a quantitative and reproducible assessment of current nerve function, allowing objective measurement of disease progression and response to treatment.

Diagnostic limitations of electrodiagnosis must be considered. Nerve conduction studies and EMG are relatively insensitive measures of subtle axonal or muscle injury (as compared to microscopic analysis of biopsy specimens, for instance), and may find no abnormalities in early disease or conditions in which irritation of nerve fibers lead to pain but no permanent injury. They cannot substitute for clinical judgment, and normal results should not be used to dismiss complaints of localized pain, myalgias, or exercise intolerance. Biopsy of nerve or muscle, imaging in search of soft tissue or bony compression, or repeat evaluation after an interval of watchful waiting may be necessary to demonstrate subtle abnormalities.

Large myelinated sensory fibers carry vibration and proprioceptive information, whereas pain and temperature sensibility are mediated by small, unmyelinated, or thinly myelinated axons. Sensory NCS assess only large myelinated sensory fibers, and will be normal in cases of small-fiber neuropathy, which may be seen in diabetes or prediabetes, amyloidosis, leprosy, or as a hereditary condition. These neuropathies frequently present with pain, paresthesias, and occasionally with autonomic dysfunction. Quantitative sensory testing, recording of sympathetic skin responses, quantitative sudomotor axon reflex testing (QSART), R-R interval evaluation, and skin biopsy for intraepidermal nerve fiber counting may complement NCS in determining the extent of injury to small unmyelinated fibers and autonomic involvement. Finally, EMG and NCS provide information exclusively about lower motor neurons and peripheral sensory fibers. Weakness, sensory loss, or autonomic dysfunction due to spinal cord or brain lesions will produce only subtle recruitment changes, and no alterations in motor or sensory conductions, unless concurrent peripheral nerve injury is present.

Entrapment and Compression Neuropathies: Upper Extremity

Nerve injuries due to entrapment or compression are readily recognized by NCS. In general, the diagnostic approach combines conduction measurements across accessible sites of entrapment with needle EMG to confirm localization and determine the extent of denervation. Entrapment frequently causes localized demyelination before frank axonal injury. Thus, demonstration of drop in conduction velocity or conduction block across an entrapped nerve segment is the most sensitive measure of early injury. Knowledge of motor innervation allows localization by examining successive muscles innervated by the nerve of interest for evidence of denervation.

Compression of the median nerve at the wrist—carpal tunnel syndrome—is the most common upper extremity nerve entrapment. Risk factors include repetitive hand or forearm motion, especially under load, and weight gain. Wrist and hand pain; paresthesias radiating into hand, forearm, or shoulder; and ultimately sensory loss, thumb and finger weakness, and thenar atrophy occur as a result of compression of the median nerve between wrist bones and the transverse carpal ligament. Electrodiagnosis takes advantage of the accessibility of both the median and ulnar nerves at the wrist. Specific criteria for sensory latencies have been established. In our laboratories, a median sensory distal latency of more than 3.7 msec, or a difference side to side of more than 0.5 msec is sufficient to suggest the diagnosis of median entrapment at the wrist. In equivocal cases, orthodromic sensory recording of conduction across the short midpalmar to wrist segment is more sensitive.

Proximal entrapment of the median nerve is rare. Compression of the pure motor anterior interosseus branch (usually by fibrous bands attached to the flexor digitorum superficialis) can be established by showing denervation of pronator quadratus and flexor pollicis longus, but not distal muscles of the main median nerve (e.g., adductor pollicis brevis). Compression of the median nerve between two heads of the pronator teres (pronator syndrome) causes decreased conduction in the forearm segment, and denervation of distal median muscles, sparing the pronator teres.

Ulnar entrapment occurs most commonly at the elbow, as the nerve passes through the cubital tunnel and retrocondylar groove. Compression against the proximal ulna is a common chronic injury due to resting elbows on tables, car windows, or chair rests. Electrodiagnosis depends on demonstrating ulnar slowing or conduction block across the elbow. Because of variable innervation, proximal ulnar forearm muscles (flexor carpi ulnaris) may or may not show denervation. Sparing of abductor pollicis brevis helps to distinguish ulnar neuropathy from lower trunk plexopathy. Compression of the ulnar nerve at the wrist in Guyon's canal (between pisiform and hook of the hamate) spares the dorsal cutaneous branch but causes denervation of finger intrinsics and prolonged distal sensory latencies in the typically measured palmar branches.

Radial nerve injury at the axilla ("crutch palsy)" can be distinguished from spiral groove compression (humerus fracture, "Saturday night palsy") by sparing of the triceps in the latter case. Because the proximal radial nerve cannot be approached directly, demonstration of focal conduction block is difficult, and care must be taken to exclude a middle trunk plexopathy (rare) or C7 radiculopathy. Brachioradialis (a C5–C6 innervated muscle) is often spared in both conditions, and radial sensory responses should be normal in C7 radiculopathy. Uncommonly, the posterior interosseus branch may be compressed by fracture, rheumatoid arthritis, or soft tissue swelling, typically causing denervation of extensor carpi ulnaris, but often sparing the supinator.

Entrapment Neuropathies: Lower Extremity

Peroneal nerve compression as it swings beneath the head of the fibula is the most common focal neuropathy of the lower extremity and one of the most accessible to electrodiagnosis. Entrapment often occurs beneath the peroneus longus, which is typically spared from denervation. Peroneal conduction across the fibular head is slowed, and denervation of the anterior tibialis and extensor digitorum brevis is common. Peroneal and tibial nerves are both branches of the sciatic nerve, which may be entrapped at the sciatic notch on its exit from the pelvis, or less commonly by fibers of the piriformis muscle, through which the sciatic nerve frequently passes. Severe sciatic neuropathy may be distinguished from L5–S1 radiculopathy by sparing of gluteal and paraspinous muscles. Partial sciatic injury often preferentially affects peroneally innervated muscles, and should be distinguished from peroneal neuropathy by assessing involvement of the short head of the biceps femoris, a muscle that receives innervation exclusively from peroneal fibers proximal to the popliteal fossa. The distal tibial nerve may be entrapped in the tarsal tunnel between the laciniate ligament and the inferior aspect of the medial malleolus, producing low-amplitude motor responses and prolonged distal motor latency at the adductor hallices.

Femoral nerve entrapment occasionally follows trauma, psoas hematoma, or vigorous surgical positioning, with proximal thigh pain and knee extensor weakness. Nerve conduction studies are often of limited value. Sparing of obturator-innervated adductors excludes lumbar plexopathy. Imaging for pelvic mass or hematoma is often warranted. Meralgia paresthetica, focal entrapment of the lateral femoral cutaneous nerve beneath the inguinal ligament, produces paresthesias and sensory loss across the proximal lateral thigh, most commonly in the setting of recent weight gain. In thin individuals, direct side-to-side comparison of sensory nerve conduction can confirm the diagnosis.

Rheumatoid or osteoarthritis, autoimmune or connective tissue diseases, or prolonged physical labor can predispose to multifocal entrapment mononeuropathies, but the clinician should also consider metabolic disease (diabetes) or vitamin deficiencies that may render peripheral nerves more vulnerable to compressive injury. Hereditary predisposition to pressure palsy (HNPP) should be suspected if the patient relates a series of recurrent, prolonged palsies, often following trivial injury.

Table 3.2 Motor weakness

Neuromuscular disorder	Discriminating features	Consistent features	Variable features
Anterior horn cell disease	1 Normal sensory studies	1 Low amplitude or absent CMAP 2 Extremity and paraspinal denervation 3 Diffuse muscle fasciculations	1 Mild decrement in CMAP amplitude with 2-Hz repetitive stimulation
Polyradiculopathy	1 Normal sensory studies	1 Extremity and paraspinal denervation	1 Prolonged F-wave latencies or absent F-waves
Plexopathy	1 Focal low or absent SNAP amplitudes in the distribution of a plexus, e.g. brachial, lumbar 2 No paraspinal denervation	1 Low or absent CMAP amplitudes in a plexus distribution 2 Extremity denervation	1 Prolonged F-wave latencies or absent F-waves in the affected limb(s)
Myasthenia gravis	1 Reparable decrement in CMAP amplitude (≥10%) in two nerves with 2-Hz repetitive stimulation	1 Normal CMAP amplitude 2 Increased jitter ± blocking with SFEMG	
Myopathy	1 Short duration, small amplitude MUAPs 2 Normal sensory study	1 Increased recruitment of MUAPs	1 CMAP amplitude normal or reduced depending on degree of atrophy
Demyelinating polyneuropathy	1 Widespread reduction in conduction velocities (<70% normal) and increase in distal latencies (>125% normal) 2 Preserved distal CMAP amplitudes	1 Absent or prolonged F-wave latencies 2 Abnormal sensory studies depending on the type of demyelinating neuropathy	1 Temporal dispersion 2 Partial conduction block
Axonal polyneuropathy	1 Widespread reduction in conduction velocities (<70% normal) and mildly prolonged distal latencies 2 Reduced CMAP and SNAP amplitudes	1 Large, long duration polyphasic MUAPs	1 Absent or mildly prolonged F-wave latencies
Mononeuritis multiplex	1 Multifocal reduction in CMAP and SNAP amplitudes 2 Multifocal mild reduction in conduction velocities	1 Large, long duration polyphasic MUAPs	1 Absent or mildly prolonged F-wave latencies

Nerve conduction studies of HNPP patients frequently demonstrate a mild demyelinating neuropathy featuring conduction slowing more than conduction block, even in nerves not reported to have been previously affected.

Motor Neuronopathies

Injury to peripheral motor neurons in specific sites along their course (from the anterior horn of the spinal cord, through ventral spinal roots, to recombination in brachial or lumbosacral plexus and distally) produces distinctive electrodiagnostic features that aid in diagnosis (Table 3.2). Focal injury to motor neuron cell bodies may occur with infection (e.g., poliomyelitis or HIV), intramedullary spinal cord mass lesions, or syrinx. More commonly, motor neuron disease is degenerative; either sporadically, as in ALS; hereditarily, as in the spinal muscular atro-

phies; or through autoimmune activities, as in multifocal motor neuropathy with conduction block.

Amyotrophic lateral sclerosis may be considered the electrodiagnostic prototype of motor neuron degeneration: sensory responses are normal, and motor responses show decreased amplitudes reflecting muscle atrophy, but essentially preserved distal latencies and conduction velocities. In contrast to typical radiculopathies, F-responses are often easily elicitable, frequently of normal latency, and may produce unusually large-amplitude waveforms reflecting chronic consolidation of motor units. Chronic denervation and subsequent reinnervation lead to dramatically enlarged motor units, as denervated fibers are reinnervated by the terminal sprouts of surviving motor neurons. This leads to a characteristic EMG pattern of decreased recruitment of very large (2,000–10,000 μV) motor units in the presence of abnormal spontaneous activity (often of large amplitude) and, characteristically, fasciculations.

To meet formal criteria for ALS, denervation must be observed in muscles of multiple myotomes of at least three of the four body segments (head, upper extremities, thoracic paraspinal muscles, lower extremities). Denervation in thoracic paraspinal muscles rarely occurs with trauma, and strongly suggests ALS in the appropriate clinical setting (also common in patients with diabetes). Proximal motor conductions should be performed on every patient evaluated for ALS in hopes of finding multifocal conduction block, evidence for multifocal motor neuropathy. These patients often have high titers of circulating anti-GM1 ganglioside antibodies, indicating autoimmune neuronal injury, and may respond to immunosuppression with intravenous gammaglobulin or cyclophosphamide.

Electrodiagnostic Approach to Peripheral Polyneuropathy

Electrodiagnostic characterization of peripheral neuropathy follows a clear framework to subdivide neuropathies into manageable diagnostic groups. The fundamental questions to be answered are: (a) Does the neuropathy involve sensory fibers, motor fibers, or both? (b) Is it primarily axonal or demyelinating? (c) Is the process acute, subacute, or chronic? and (d) What is the extent of axonal injury? As described in the following sections, NCS play a critical role in answering the first two questions, while needle EMG offers information about the severity and chronicity of axonal injury. Most polyneuropathies begin distally, involving distal fibers of multiple nerves equally. If only selected distal nerves are affected, multiple mononeuropathies due to compression, vasculitis, or infiltration should be considered. Frequently, in more severe neuropathies, distal motor and sensory responses will be absent, offering little information about the character of the neuropathy. The electrodiagnostician should proceed proximally (e.g., radial sensory, peroneal motor responses recorded from the anterior tibialis) until a nerve with a recordable distal latency and amplitude is discovered, to document the extent of the neuropathy. A protocol for the initial assessment of polyneuropathy is summarized in Box 3.1.

Sensory Neuropathy

Nerve conduction studies readily distinguish sensory and motor nerve involvement in peripheral neuropathy. Distal sensory responses are a specific measure of large myelinated axonal loss. Sensory potentials with amplitudes less than 50% of the lower limit of normal indicate clear axonal injury. Note that older individuals frequently experience decreased sensory amplitudes,

---

Box 3.1 Protocol for the initial assessment of polyneuropathy

Conduction studies

▶ Test most symptomatic site when symptoms/signs are mild or moderate, least involved if severe.

▶ Record motor amplitude, distal latency, conduction velocity, and F-response for the peroneal motor (extensor digitorum brevis).

▶ If abnormal, repeat sequence for tibial motor (abductor hallucis).

▶ If no responses, repeat protocol and peroneal motor recording at the:
  – Anterior tibialis muscle
  – Ulnar motor (hypothenar)
  – Median motor (thenar)

▶ Record sensory amplitude, distal latency, and conduction velocity for the sural sensory (ankle). If not clearly normal, consider averaging.

▶ Median sensory (index finger). If antidromic response is absent or a focal entrapment is suspected, record from the wrist stimulating the palm.

▶ Abnormalities should result in evaluation of opposite extremity and/or evaluation of additional peripheral nerves.

Needle examination

▶ Examine anterior tibial, medial gastrocnemius, first dorsal interosseous (hand), and lumbar paraspinal muscles.

▶ If they are normal, intrinsic foot muscles should be examined.

▶ Confirm abnormalities by examining at least one contralateral muscle.

---

and that absent sural responses should not be considered pathologic in patients over 75 years of age. Small, thinly myelinated, and unmyelinated fibers do not contribute to the sensory potential, so painful small-fiber sensory neuropathies may produce normal sensory conductions. Because sensory responses are all recorded distally, and more proximal stimulation of sensory nerves is impractical, conduction block and slowing due to demyelination cannot be easily recorded from sensory nerves. Pure sensory axonal neuropathies cannot be reliably distinguished electrically from sensory neuronopathies. In each, there is a loss of sensory potentials with preservation of motor amplitudes and conductions. Although rare, pure sensory neuropathies and/or neuronopathies are most commonly seen in paraneoplastic syndromes, autoimmune disorders (especially Sjögren's syndrome), vitamin E deficiency, cis-platinum or pyridoxine toxicity, elderly women (idiopathic sensory neuropathy), and inherited disor-

> ### Box 3.2 Pure sensory neuropathies
>
> ▸ Paraneoplastic syndromes
> ▸ Autoimmune disorders (Sjögren's syndrome)
> ▸ Vitamin E deficiency
> ▸ Vitamin B$_{12}$ deficiency
> ▸ *Cis*-platinum neuropathy
> ▸ Pyridoxine toxicity
> ▸ Idiopathic sensory neuropathy
> ▸ Hereditary sensory neuropathy
> ▸ Friedreich's ataxia
> ▸ Bassen–Kornzweig disease

ders, including hereditary sensory neuropathy types I–IV, Friedreich's ataxia, and Bassen–Kornzweig disease. Box 3.2 lists sensory neuropathies.

Motor Neuropathy: Demyelinating versus Axonal

Distal motor responses and proximal conduction along motor nerves offer robust diagnostic tools for assessing axonal and demyelinating injuries. Primary demyelination is typically the result of autoimmune attack of myelin in distal nerves, as in acute inflammatory demyelinating polyneuropathy (AIDP, also known as Guillain–Barré syndrome), chronic inflammatory demyelinating polyneuropathy (CIDP), or a consequence of hereditary defects in myelin deposition. An understanding of the physiology of nerve conduction is important for appreciating the various nerve conduction findings indicative of demyelination. Peripheral axons are insulated along their entire length by segments of myelin elaborated by Schwann cells, and they are broken between each Schwann cell by a short *node of Ranvier*. Conduction of an action potential proceeds down the axon in a *saltatory* fashion, regenerating at each node, at a velocity 5–20 times faster than that achievable by demyelinated axons. Primary demyelination occurs at random nodes of Ranvier along the entire length of the axon in a *segmental* pattern, preserving the physical continuity of the axon except in the most severe cases. Mild segmental demyelination disrupts normal saltatory conduction along some axons within the nerve, slowing the conduction velocity of these axons. As demyelination becomes more profound, conduction through some axons is blocked entirely, functionally disconnecting the motor neuron from the innervated muscle and resulting in weakness. Demyelinating effects summate distally, reflecting the greater burden of segmental injury in longer nerves.

Three distinctive motor response features (temporal dispersion, diminished conduction velocity, and conduction block) suggest primary demyelination. In mild dis-

ease, distal latencies are prolonged, but amplitude may be essentially normal, indicating preservation of distal axons. Temporal dispersion is a normal characteristic of the motor action potential and reflects the difference in conduction time between the slowest and fastest fibers within a nerve. With demyelination, the difference in time necessary to transmit a signal along the most severely affected axons is increased, prolonging the CMAP duration. By stimulating the motor nerve more proximally, a longer portion of axon is observed, and the effects of segmental demyelination summate: proximal CMAP duration of more than 125% of distal CMAP duration indicates pathologic temporal dispersion and suggests demyelinating injury. Proximal stimulation also allows recording of conduction velocity along the proximal nerve segment, which will be slowed in demyelination.

With more severe demyelination, some fibers will not transmit signals along their entire length, resulting in conduction block. A drop in proximal CMAP amplitude of more than 50% compared with the distal response indicates conduction block. In general, conduction block is a more prominent feature of acquired demyelinating injury in AIDP or trauma, whereas heroic temporal dispersion and uniformly slowed conduction velocities, out of proportion to the decrease in CMAP amplitude, are characteristic features of hypertrophic hereditary demyelinating neuropathies like hereditary motor sensory neuropathy type I (HMSN I, also known as Charcot–Marie–Tooth disease) and hereditary motor sensory neuropathy type III (HMSIII, also known as Dejerine–Sottas disease). Even though weakness is profound and decreased recruitment is noted, abnormal spontaneous activity is typically absent from the needle exam, indicating structural continuity of peripheral axons. Severe or advanced forms of both hereditary and acquired demyelinating diseases can be accompanied by true axonal loss, indicated by the appearance of abnormal spontaneous activity on needle exam. A list of the common causes of demyelinating neuropathy is presented in Box 3.3.

Mixed Motor and Sensory Neuropathy

Metabolic stress and microvascular ischemia (as seen in diabetes), in addition to toxic injury and nutritional deficiencies, affect both sensory and motor neurons with the longest distal axons, leading to distal axonal degeneration and focal loss of myelin. This type of neuropathy, classified as a sensorimotor "mixed" (i.e., components of both axon loss and demyelination) polyneuropathy is exceedingly common. Electrically, these neuropathies present as absent or low-amplitude sural sensory potentials with mild reduction in motor amplitudes and conduction velocities. Recorded sensory potentials and CMAPs reflect the dropout of axons with decreased amplitude of the response. Because the surviving axons conduct essentially

Box 3.3 Common causes of demyelinating neuropathies

Segmental demyelinating, motor > sensory polyneuropathy
▶ Acute inflammatory demyelinating polyneuropathy
▶ Chronic inflammatory demyelinating polyneuropathy
▶ Monoclonal gammopathy of undetermined significance
▶ Pharmaceuticals
  – Amiodarone
  – Perhexiline
  – High-dose Ara-C
▶ AIDS
▶ Hereditary neuropathy with susceptibility to pressure palsies (HNPP)

Uniform demyelinating mixed sensorimotor polyneuropathy
▶ Hereditary motor sensory neuropathy
▶ Metachromatic leukodystrophy
▶ Adrenomyeloneuropathy

Box 3.4 Etiologies of sensorimotor mixed polyneuropathy

Mixed axon loss, demyelinating sensorimotor polyneuropathy
▶ Diabetes mellitus, impaired glucose tolerance
▶ Uremia

Axon loss, motor > sensory polyneuropathy
▶ Axonal Guillain–Barré syndrome
▶ Porphyria
▶ Hereditary motor sensory neuropathy
▶ Lead neuropathy
▶ Dapsone neuropathy
▶ Vincristine neuropathy

Axon loss, mixed sensorimotor polyneuropathy
▶ Amyloidosis
▶ Chronic liver disease
▶ Nutritional diseases
  – Vitamin B deficiency
  – Folate deficiency
▶ Alcoholism
▶ Sarcoidosis
▶ Connective tissue diseases
  – Rheumatoid arthritis
  – Periarteritis nodosa
  – Systemic lupus erythematosus
  – Churg–Strauss vasculitis
  – Hypereosinophilia syndrome
▶ Toxic neuropathy
  – Acrylamide
  – Ethylene oxide
  – Hexacarbons
  – Organophosphorus esters
  – Glue sniffing
▶ Metal neuropathy
  – Chronic arsenic intoxication
  – Mercury
▶ Drug-induced
  – Colchicine
  – Ethambutol
  – Metronidazole
  – Misonidazole
  – Nitrofurantoin
  – Chloroquine
  – Disulfiram
  – Nitrous oxide
▶ Neuropathy of chronic illness
▶ AIDS

normally, distal latency is not markedly prolonged. The mild slowing of conduction velocities is attributed to two phenomena: early focal demyelination and axonal loss of the fastest conducting myelinated fibers. No conduction block is observed unless focal injury is present across the recorded segment. Box 3.4 presents a list of the common etiologies of sensorimotor mixed polyneuropathy.

Radiculopathies and Plexopathies

Injury to nerve roots is common in both the cervical and lumbar spine due to degenerative spondylosis, herniated disk, trauma or, more rarely, impingement of mass lesions, metastatic or intrinsic extradural tumors, vascular anomalies, or abscess. In the cervical region, electrodiagnosis helps distinguish radiculopathy from brachial plexopathy through careful anatomic localization. Injury to the exiting nerve root by compression in the ventral root exit zone does not impinge on sensory nerve cell bodies, which are positioned outside the neural foramen in the dorsal root ganglia (DRG). Even though proximal connections between the DRG and spinal cord may be injured, resulting in characteristic pain, dermatomal sensory loss, and paresthesias, continuity is preserved between the sensory nerve cell body and the distal afferent axon. Thus, a critical general principle regarding electrodiagnosis of radiculopathy is that clinical sensation is impaired, but distal action potentials of sensory nerves are preserved. In contrast, compression or stretch injury beyond the level of the DRG leads to prominent decreased sensory response amplitudes in plexopathy.

Table 3.3 Electrodiagnostic comparison of motor neuronopathy, radiculopathy, and plexopathy

	Motor neuronopathy	**Polyradiculopathy**	**Plexopathy**
Motor signs/symptoms	Weakness involving multiple myotones and peripheral nerve distribution		
Sensory loss	No	Often	Yes
SNAP	Normal	Normal	Low amplitude
CMAP	Low amplitude or absent	Low amplitude	Low amplitude
F-responses	Often present. Normal latency	Sometimes absent	Often absent
		Mild prolongation	Conduction block or severe prolongation
Paraspinous denervation	Yes	Usually	No

Needle examination of specific muscles may further aid in localization to cervical roots or brachial plexus. Denervation in paraspinous muscles indicates injury to very proximal dorsal root rami. The dorsal scapular nerve to the rhomboids, and long thoracic nerve to the serratus anterior muscle, leave the C5 root and C5, C6, and C7 roots, respectively, prior to incorporation into the upper trunk. Sparing of these muscles localizes the lesion to the upper trunk of the brachial plexus. Differentiating between C8–T1 radiculopathy and lower trunk plexopathy can be difficult, since peripheral muscles served are essentially identical. Sensory nerve action potential of the median cutaneous nerve of the forearm will be reduced in lower trunk plexopathy, but not in C8 radiculopathy. Low cervical paraspinous muscles are spared in plexopathy.

A similar conundrum confronts the electromyographer attempting to distinguish lumbosacral plexopathy from L5–S1 radiculopathy, since the sciatic trunk carries most fibers from each proximal distribution. L5–S1 radiculopathy is more common. Sural sensory responses should be spared in this disorder, but in fact are often absent or reduced due to age or local trauma. Nerves to the gluteal muscles depart the lumbosacral plexus early, and are often spared in plexopathy, but often show denervation in significant L5–S1 radiculopathy. Generalized clinical and electrodiagnostic features of motor neuronopathy, radiculopathy, and plexopathy are compared in Table 3.3.

Neuromuscular Junction Disorders

Neuromuscular junction (NMJ) disorders share a common theme: toxic or autoimmune injury to components of the NMJ reduces the fidelity of transmission, resulting in weakness that is often variable with effort or over time. A brief review of the physiology of the NMJ aids in understanding electrodiagnosis of these disorders (Figure 3.3). Depolarization of the axon terminal opens membrane calcium (Ca^{2+}) channels, and Ca^{2+} influx triggers release of acetylcholine (ACh) molecules from vesicles at the axon terminal. Acetylcholine diffuses across the neuro-

muscular synaptic junction to bind to ACh receptors on the muscle end plate. Binding to a sufficient number of receptors triggers membrane depolarization and synchronized contraction of the muscle fiber. Unbound ACh is rapidly degraded by acetylcholinesterase in the synaptic cleft. With each subsequent stimulation, the store of immediately available ACh is reduced, and a smaller number of ACh quanta are released. Fortunately, a large surplus of both ACh and ACh receptor provides a "safety margin" that allows threshold depolarization across every stimulated NMJ under normal circumstances. Recruitment of additional ACh from stores in the presynaptic axon terminal ensure that this safety margin is maintained, even with prolonged exercise or repeated stimulation.

Some common NMJ diseases and toxins are listed by their site of action in Figure 3.3. Myasthenia gravis

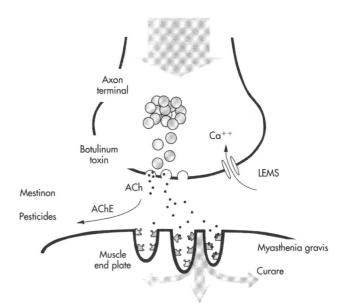

Figure 3.3 Steps in neuromuscular junction (NMJ) transmission are represented here and described in the text. Diseases and toxins affecting the NMJ are shown at their sites of action. ACh, acetylcholine; AChE, acetylcholinesterase; LEMS, Lambert–Eaton myasthenic syndrome.

Table 3.4 Diagnostic comparison of neuromuscular junction disorders

	Myasthenia gravis (MG)	Lambert–Eaton myasthenic syndrome (LEMS)
Symptoms	Normal baseline strength, with fatigable weakness	Baseline weakness, improves with exercise
Common sites	Bulbar/ocular muscles	Limb muscles; associated autonomic dysfunction
Pathophysiology	Postsynaptic	Presynaptic
Autoimmune attack of:	ACh receptors	Ca^{2+} channels
Electrodiagnosis		
CMAP amplitude	Often normal	Often decreased
Repetitive stimulation	6–30% decrement	Little or no decrement
Postexercise CMAP amplitude	Little or no facilitation	50–300% facilitation

(MG) and Lambert–Eaton myasthenic syndrome (LEMS) serve as prototypes of postsynaptic and presynaptic damage, respectively. Myasthenia gravis, the most common NMJ disorder, results from autoimmune destruction of postsynaptic ACh receptors. The defining symptom of MG is rapidly progressive weakness with exercise. In essence, the safety margin of NMJ transmission is decreased, so that even slight depletion of ACh results in failure of postsynaptic depolarization for many muscle fibers. Pyridostigmine (Mestinon) helps by inhibiting acetylcholinesterase, thus making more ACh available at the postsynaptic end plate. By comparison, in LEMS, autoimmune destruction of the presynaptic Ca^{2+} channels results in radically decreased ACh release at all times. Patients with LEMS are chronically weak but, paradoxically, brief exercise increases their strength. These disorders can be distinguished by NCS techniques. Contrasting findings reflect their different sites of injury to the NMJ and underline their pathophysiology, as outlined in Table 3.4.

Repetitive nerve stimulation of a target muscle is a simple (but relatively insensitive) NCS method for evaluation of NMJ abnormalities. Repetitive stimulation typically follows evaluation of the CMAP and can be performed at any site where a clearly defined CMAP from just one muscle can be obtained. Stimulation sufficient to generate a maximal CMAP amplitude is determined to assure that all innervated motor units are being excited. Patients with LEMS usually have low-amplitude CMAPs, reflecting ACh depletion, whereas the CMAPs of MG patients are often normal. The patient is then given a train of electrical stimuli at 0.5-second intervals, usually a total of four, to deplete released ACh quanta with each stimulation. Amplitudes of successive generated CMAPs are compared. Normal individuals will show no change in CMAP amplitude, since the large safety margin of ACh and ACh receptor excess allows for NMJ transmission even with partial depletion of released ACh. However, patients with MG will show a decrement or decrease in CMAP amplitude, reflecting the failure of NMJ trans-

mission for some muscle fibers with damaged ACh receptors. A CMAP amplitude drop of 6–10% is considered significant if technical errors can be excluded. In

▼

Box 3.5 Electrodiagnostic approach to the weak patient

Conduction studies
▶ Record sensory amplitude, distal latency, and conduction velocity for the sural sensory (ankle).
▶ If sural equivocal or technically difficult:
  – Opposite sural
  – Ulnar sensory
▶ Record motor amplitude, distal latency, and conduction velocity for the ulnar motor (hypothenar). Repetitive supramaximal stimulation at wrist (2 × 4 stimuli) before and immediately after 5 seconds of maximal voluntary exercise (fingers should be restrained or taped together).
▶ If proximal weakness predominates:
  – Record motor amplitude, distal latency, and conduction velocity for the spinal accessory motor (trapezius). Repetitive supramaximal stimulation at wrist (2 × 4 stimuli) before and immediately after 5 seconds of maximal voluntary exercise.
▶ If legs weaker:
  – Record sensory amplitude, distal latency, and conduction velocity for the peroneal nerve (EDB).
▶ Abnormality in any of the above requires further evaluation of suspected disorder (e.g., polyradiculopathy, myopathy, neuromuscular transmission abnormality

Needle examination
▶ Examine selected distal and proximal muscles, in upper and lower limbs, including paraspinal. For example, biceps brachii, first dorsal interosseous (hand), vastus lateralis, anterior tibialis, medial gastrocnemius, lumbar paraspinal muscles.

symptomatic patients with MG, a decrement of 10–30% is common. Evaluation of fatigable muscles is more likely to demonstrate a decrement. Lambert–Eaton myasthenic syndrome and NMJ toxins feature a less dramatic decrement to repetitive stimulation at electrode 2.

A second maneuver distinguishes LEMS from MG. Increasing the rate of repetitive stimulation to 20 (or having the patient forcefully activate the muscle of interest for 10 seconds) floods the neuromuscular junction with ACh. Increased synaptic ACh temporarily allows greater fidelity of NMJ transmission for LEMS patients. This is reflected in facilitation of the CMAP to 150% or even 300% of its pre-exercise amplitude, often close to normal. By comparison, in MG patients, postexercise stimulation will yield a CMAP that is essentially unchanged in amplitude from initial recordings, indicating "repair" of their decrement.

Accurate interpretation of repetitive stimulation depends on achievement of a maximal CMAP as a baseline. If stimulation is submaximal, a spurious facilitation may be observed following exercise in normal subjects. Similarly, cooling can reproduce a decrement in the absence of disease. A generalized protocol for the electrodiagnostic approach to the weak patient is shown in Box 3.5.

Repetitive stimulation may evoke no decrement in myasthenics with weakness confined to bulbar or ocular muscles. If ACh receptor antibody titers are negative or equivocal, but MG is suspected on clinical grounds, the patient should be referred to an experienced electromyographer who can perform *single-fiber EMG* evaluation. Single-fiber EMG detects asynchrony of NMJ transmission between different muscle fibers served by the same motor neuron (i.e., in the same motor unit), a condition that precedes NMJ block in MG. Single-fiber EMG is more sensitive than other methods discussed for detection of a NMJ disorder, and it can also detect NMJ asynchrony associated with recent reinnervation.

Myopathy

Nerve conduction studies typically play a modest role in evaluation of myopathy. Typically, strength is decreased out of proportion to reduction in CMAP amplitude, reflecting electromechanical dissociation rather than axonal loss as the pathophysiology. The CMAPs may be either normal or mildly reduced if muscle has been replaced by fat or connective tissue in longstanding disorders. Sensory responses should be normal.

Electrodiagnostic features of myopathy have been discussed in some detail under the earlier EMG technique section. A basic electrodiagnostic algorithm combining EMG features and duration of weakness is presented in Figure 3.4. A careful search for abnormal spontaneous

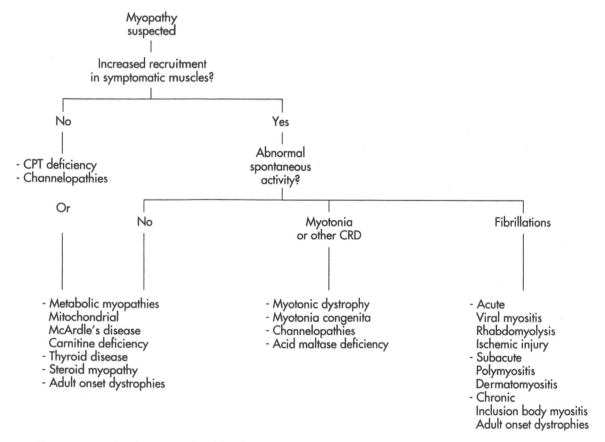

Figure 3.4 Electromyographic diagnostic algorithm for myopathy and dystrophy.

activity is important, since inflammatory myopathies are often amenable to treatment. Experience allows detection of muscle areas that have been replaced by fat or connective tissue (decreased insertional activity, spongy "feel" at the tip of the needle), suggesting chronic injury in many dystrophies. Repetitive discharges (myotonia, neuromyotonia) in the setting of myopathic motor units should suggest myotonic dystrophy, or channelopathies such as myotonia congenita and paramyotonia.

Summary

Nerve conduction studies and needle EMG serve as a quantitative extension of the neurologic examination. Nerve conduction studies localize compressive lesions, determine the extent of sensory and motor nerve contributions to neuropathy, assess NMJ integrity, and distinguish between demyelination and axonal denervation. Electromyography distinguishes traumatic injury and degeneration due to motor neuronopathies, radiculopathies, or peripheral neuropathy. Needle evaluation provides information about chronicity of disease and plays a critical role in diagnosis of myopathies. Specialized NCS and EMG techniques are the most sensitive measures of neuromuscular junction injury. Coupling a patient's history, clinical examination, and electrodiagnostic studies frequently yields an informative diagnosis, allowing for effective therapeutic intervention.

Acknowledgments

This work was supported in part by NIH RO1 NS40458 (JRS), NIH NS42056, the Juvenile Diabetes Research Foundation Center for the Study of Complications in Diabetes (JDRF), the Office of Research Development (Medical Research Service), Department of Veterans Affairs (JWR), NIH RO1 NS38849, the Juvenile Diabetes Research Foundation Center for the Study of Complications in Diabetes, and the Program for Understanding Neurological Diseases (PFUND) (ELF).

Annotated Bibliography

American Association of Electrodiagnostic Medicine. Guidelines in electrodiagnostic medicine. *Muscle Nerve* 1992;15:229–253.
Mini-monograph provides procedures for nerve conduction studies and needle EMG in general classes of neuromuscular diseases.

Daube JR. Electrodiagnostic studies in amyotrophic lateral sclerosis and other motor neuron disorders. *Muscle Nerve* 2000;23:1488–1502.
Focused review describes specific EMG features of denervation in detail and explains typical EMG findings in a variety of motor neuronopathies.

Feldman EL, Grisold W, Russell JW, Zifko UA. *Atlas of neuromuscular diseases.* Wien, Austria: Springer-Verlag, 2005.
Summarizes the nerve conduction and EMG findings in a broad spectrum of neuromuscular diseases. The organization of diseases is particularly helpful.

Kimura J. *Electrodiagnosis in diseases of nerve and muscle: Principles and practice.* New York: Oxford University Press, 2001.
Serves as the classic electrodiagnostician's guide. All topics relevant to EMG are covered in sufficient detail to allow understanding. A brief but well-written anatomy section is very useful to the beginning electromyographer.

Oh S. *Clinical electromyography: Nerve conduction studies.* Philadelphia: Lippincott Williams & Wilkins, 2002.
Extensive textbook describes all aspects of nerve conduction studies with careful attention to technical issues.

CHAPTER 4

Neuroradiology: Diagnostic Imaging Strategies

Steven G. Imbesi

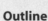

Outline

▶ Imaging modalities
▶ Problem-solving approache
▶ On the horizon

Imaging Modalities

Many imaging modalities exist today in neuroradiology, and the optimal use of each technique depends on a good understanding of its advantages and disadvantages.

Plain Films

Plain x-ray films were the mainstay of neuroradiology before the advent of computed tomography (CT) and magnetic resonance imaging (MRI), which show much greater anatomic detail. Nevertheless, plain films still give a good general overview of anatomy by providing excellent pictures of the bony structures. This can be useful in cases of head trauma, congenital abnormalities such as craniosynostosis (early suture closure resulting in deformities of the skull) or cephaloceles, osseous dysplasias, bone abnormalities due to Paget's disease and multiple myeloma, degenerative changes and deformities of the spine, and facial abnormalities. Plain films are also helpful to establish anatomic relationships for presurgical or radiation planning, and to screen for the presence of foreign bodies (in particular to identify potentially hazardous metal prior to MRI).

Plain film radiography involves exposure to ionizing radiation and thus should be avoided or limited in pregnant women since fetuses are particularly vulnerable, especially in the first trimester. Plain films offer almost no information about the brain or spinal cord, locations where other modalities such as CT or MRI should be used.

Computed Tomography

The development of CT was a breakthrough, allowing information to be obtained about the inner contents of the skull and the spine. Although CT is excellent for evaluation of cortical bone, it is also helpful in tissue differentiation between fat, fluid, soft tissue, bone, and air. Through the use of iodine contrast, the imaging capabilities of CT are expanded considerably. Changes in the blood–brain barrier lead to contrast enhancement, so that neoplasms, infarcts, and inflammatory processes are more readily detected. Computed tomography has become an extremely rapid imaging technique and therefore lends itself well to evaluating unstable patients, such as those with acute traumatic injuries. Computed tomography is often the modality of choice when biopsy guidance is needed.

Computed tomography employs ionizing radiation emitted from an x-ray tube, which moves in a circular fashion around a patient. As the radiation passes through the patient, it is attenuated by differences in tissue density, and this change is sensed by detectors also arranged in a circular gantry. The information from the detectors is then sent to a computer for reconstruction of an image, appearing as a "slice" of the imaged region of interest. The configuration of the CT scanner has evolved, the latest being a multi emitter, multidetector arrangement with a contiguous helical acquisition capable of extremely rapid scanning and exquisite reconstruction. This rapid image acquisition, in conjunction with the dynamic administration of iodinated contrast material, also allows the cerebral and neck vasculature to be reconstructed, thus creating computed tomographic angiography (CTA) images.

Computed tomography is not free of hazards. Of great concern is the relative risk of iodinated contrast material in people who are allergic to iodine or who have poor renal clearance of iodine as a result of renal failure or multiple myeloma. A history of contrast allergy is not an absolute contraindication to the administration of iodine, since nonionic iodine contrast agents can now be used, or patients can be premedicated with steroids or antihistamines. Prednisone is typically given as 50 mg, 12 and then 2 hours prior to administration of contrast, whereas diphenhydramine (Benadryl) may be given as 50 mg, 2 hours prior to iodine contrast in patients with a history of minor reactions. Iodine is excreted by the kidneys and should be used cautiously in patients with diminished renal function (that is, those with a creatinine level greater than 1.5). Liberal intravenous fluids should be administered and, in some cases, dialysis may be necessary.

As informative as CT may be, its images are fraught with artifacts from bone, metal, or patient motion. Owing to the adjacent dense petrous bone, the posterior fossa is often difficult to evaluate well, particularly when the image is degraded by motion. Metal from dental fillings or surgical clips can interfere with the image, causing beam-hardening artifacts. The girth of the patient may also be a limiting factor, producing image degradation.

The primary plane of scanning is axial. This may limit the ability to visualize certain structures, although coronal images can be obtained directly if the patient is able to extend their head and neck. Otherwise, the computer can use the axial images to reconstruct views in different planes (known as *image reformatting*), but the image detail is never as sharp as true acquisitions. For that reason, MRI has major advantages by presenting direct multiplanar anatomy in virtually any plane, as opposed to the limited planes of CT.

Magnetic Resonance Imaging

Magnetic resonance imaging is the most recent widely available advance in radiologic imaging. Its advantages over CT include direct multiplanar imaging, the lack of ionizing radiation, and increased soft tissue contrast resolution. Additional capabilities include magnetic resonance angiography (MRA), in which blood vessels are imaged without use of iodinated contrast, and magnetic resonance spectroscopy (MRS) that detects brain metabolites and provides biochemical physiologic information.

Magnetic resonance imaging is based on exciting nuclear spin states with a radio frequency generator in a strong magnetic field and measuring the induced current in receiver coils. The amplitude of the induced current is proportional to the number of excited nuclei exerting a net magnetic vector. The decay of the induced current can be used to calculate relaxation parameters specific for each tissue type. By varying the time interval between excitation pulses (*repetition time* or T_R), as well as the interval between excitation pulse and echo—or signal readout (*echo time* or T_E)—one can use the specific tissue relaxation properties to discriminate different tissue types. For example, fat gives a high (strong) signal intensity on studies with short T_R and short T_E, whereas water gives high signal intensity on studies with long T_R and long T_E. Magnetic resonance imaging scanners measure single-proton hydrogen nuclei in water and relatively short chain fats. The MRI signals in larger molecules decay too rapidly for current clinical imaging applications; however, hydrogen protons in these larger molecules are detected by MRS.

Contrast studies can highlight tissue appearance in regions of differential perfusion or breakdown of the blood–brain barrier. Furthermore, MRI uses chelated gadolinium as a contrast agent. Chelated gadolinium does not contain iodine and is only rarely associated with acute reactions, very few of which are serious. Recent reports, however, of nephrogenic systemic fibrosis (NSF) induced by gadolinium contrast have limited the use of this contrast agent in patients with reduced renal clearance capability; specifically, a glomerular filtration rate (GFR) of less than 60 is considered a relative contraindication, and a GFR of less than 30 an absolute contraindication, unless the information to be obtained with contrast enhancement is deemed critical to patient survival.

The increased tissue contrast resolution with MRI makes it the diagnostic study of choice for many soft-tissue applications. The direct multiplanar imaging capabilities and lack of distortion from adjacent osseous structures make MRI ideal for imaging most of the central nervous system (CNS), particularly the posterior fossa and spinal cord. Increased contrast resolution means greater sensitivity for the detection of subtle masses, meningitis, white matter tract disease (demyelinating or dysmyelinating), early infarction (particularly that of the brainstem and posterior fossa), and most inflammatory or infectious processes (Tables 4.1 and 4.2).

Magnetic resonance angiography is another application. The most commonly used MRA imaging method depends on the effect of flowing blood that places "fresh spins" of nonexcited blood hydrogen nuclei (which can produce a strong readout signal) into a slab of saturated tissue (purposefully previously suppressed by repeated excitations prior to obtaining the readout signal), resulting in an image of the vasculature. Ironically, by the same physiology of flowing blood, blood vessels in routine MRI show as regions of low signal or "flow void," since the excited blood hydrogen nuclei leave the imaged slice prior to acquisition of the readout signal. Magnetic resonance angiography is an excellent modality for evaluating vascular anomalies, aneurysms, and vessel stenosis/occlusion. However, angiography remains the gold standard for imaging complex vascular structures such as arteriovenous malformations (AVMs).

Table 4.1 Tissue signals on CT and MRI

Signals on CT		
Air	Very very dark	−1,000 to −100 HU
Fat	Very dark	−100 to −20 HU
Water	Dark	0 to +20 HU
Muscle	Gray	30 to 60 HU
Bone	Bright	over +200 HU

Signals on MRI	T1	T2
Air	Very dark	Very dark
Cortical bone, calcium	Very dark	Very dark
Fat	Bright	Gray
Water	Dark	Bright
Muscle	Gray	Gray

HU = Hounsfield units

Table 4.2 MRI vs. CT: what to use

Brain		
Supratentorial tumor	MR	CT
Infratentorial tumor	MR	
Demyelinating disease	MR	
Meninges	MR	
Infarcts		
Early	MR	
Subacute	MR	CT
Chronic	MR	CT
Trauma		
Acute hemorrhage	MR	CT
Subacute hemorrhage	MR	
Chronic hemorrhage	MR	
Calcification		CT
Aneurysm, AVM	MR	CT
Temporal bone		CT
Orbit (except retinoblastoma)	MR	
Skull base		
Bone erosion		CT
Fracture		CT
Marrow replacement	MR	
Meningioma	MR	
Paranasal sinuses		
Screen		CT
Fracture		CT
Mucous vs. tumor	MR	
Spine		
Degenerative changes		CT
Epidural abscess	MR	
Radiculopathy	MR	CT*
Myelopathy	MR	

*CT myelogram

Magnetic resonance spectroscopy has also now become a relatively routine additional sequence acquisition in the magnetic resonance neuroimaging armamentarium. Magnetic resonance spectroscopy exploits the small differences in nuclear spin rates (chemical shifts) of protons in different molecular moieties caused by the local electronic environment created by the surrounding electron cloud. Magnetic resonance spectroscopy analyzes the biochemical substances in the brain (such as cerebral cellular constituents, neuronal metabolites, and neurotransmitters) and provides physiologic information to complement the anatomic findings of MRI. When confronted with a lesion on MRI, MRS can help categorize the abnormality and differentiate between neoplastic, inflammatory/infectious, vascular (infarction), degenerative, and metabolic pathologic processes.

Unfortunately, like all modalities, MRI also has limitations. First, contraindications to MRI examinations exist, including pacemakers; metal in the brain, orbit, or on blood vessels not specifically cleared for MRI; most cochlear implants; surgically placed neurostimulator leads; many other types of metal in the body; body habitus; and weight. Relative contraindications include pregnancy, claustrophobia, and inability to hold still for relatively long periods (the last two factors may be alleviated with general anesthesia). Magnetic resonance imaging studies may be limited by artifacts caused by adjacent metal (for example, dental repairs and spinal metal hardware), motion, or vascular flow artifact.

Angiography

Angiography is an invasive technique used to study blood vessels in great detail. It uses x-rays with film or digital radiography to record a moving picture of the actual flow of blood. Iodine contrast is injected via catheters that are placed selectively or superselectively into specific blood vessels feeding the area of interest (Figure 4.1). Angiography shows blood vessels in the greatest detail and represents the gold standard in the evaluation of vascular disease in the brain and spine, including aneurysms, AVMs, and vasculitis. It may also be a precursor to recently developed neurointerventional procedures, which include thrombolysis, angioplasty/stenting, and embolization of AVMs, tumors, and aneurysms.

The drawback to angiography is that it is invasive and carries a risk of about 0.5% for complications such as bleeding at the puncture site (commonly causing a groin hematoma because the access point is usually the femoral artery), allergic reactions, infection, stroke, blindness, vascular damage, loss of limb, and even death. Therefore, in certain situations, such as screening for

Pearls and Perils

MR scanning

▶ The patient's body habitus and weight must be within the physical limits of the MRI.

▶ Patients cannot be claustrophobic and must be physically able to hold still for relatively long periods of time.

▶ Patients must be able to lie flat in a tight space—use in patients with congestive heart failure or nausea can be dangerous.

▶ If patients require sedation, qualified personnel must be available to monitor them.

▶ If there is a history of a possible orbital metallic foreign body such as from welding or metal grinding, patients should undergo screening radiographs of the orbit. Orbital metallic foreign bodies are an absolute contraindication.

▶ Prior surgery, in particular brain aneurysm surgery, with the placement of metallic vascular clips, requires specific clearance by the manufacturer (need lot and model number). A negative intraoperative magnet test is preferred.

▶ Cochlear, ocular, penile, and heart valve prostheses, in addition to vascular filters, require specific clearance. Most vascular stents are safe within 6 weeks of placement, but this factor should be confirmed.

▶ Use of MRI during pregnancy is controversial. Pregnancy should be considered a relative contraindication, particularly in the first trimester.

▶ Cervical halos should be nonferromagnetic for MRI use. Most orthopedic hardware is safe for MRI. Size, configuration, and orientation of axis are important. An examination should be discontinued if a patient experiences discomfort.

▶ Patients should wait at least 6–8 weeks after cardiac bypass or other surgeries, particularly if surgical clips are close to vital structures.

▶ BBs and shrapnel are ferromagnetic and dangerous. Bullets and shotgun pellets are generally nonferromagnetic and relatively safe if not located within or adjacent to vital structures such as the neural axis, orbital globe, heart, major blood vessels, etc. Each must be considered as contaminants since age may change these properties.

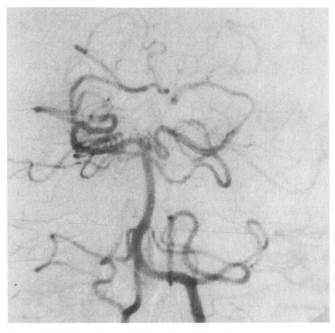

Figure 4.1 Normal vertebral artery angiogram.

carotid atherosclerotic disease in workups for transient ischemia, a less invasive test such as carotid ultrasound or MRI/MRA is preferred, reserving angiography for subsequent therapeutic intervention. Historically, angiography was used to diagnose intracranial masses by determining displacement of blood vessels by neoplasms or other intracranial lesions that also produce mass effect such as subdural hematomas. At present, CT and MRI provide much more specific and less invasive detection.

Ultrasound

Ultrasound is based on the production of mechanical vibrations by applying a current to a piezoelectric crystal in a transducer head, causing the crystal to oscillate at a set frequency. When the crystal is placed in contact with the skin, the vibrations are conducted through the body. Some of the vibrations are reflected at interfaces of different tissues and are measured by the transducer, which also functions as a receiver. The interval between the applied pulse and the reflected signal (echo) is proportional to the distance traveled, allowing the calculation of object depths. The echo display brightness is proportional to the reflected signal intensity. The amount of reflection at an interface of two tissues is proportional to the difference in acoustic properties of the tissue types. Therefore, interfaces with air, bone, or metal (each of which has extreme acoustic values relative to soft tissue) result in near complete reflections. On the other hand, transmission through water involves no interfaces and should generate no echoes (anechoic).

Another ultrasound application utilizes the change in frequency that occurs when an echo is produced by a moving object (Doppler effect). This allows the calculation of flow velocities in blood vessels, an important component of vascular evaluation. Transcranial Doppler directs ultrasound waves into the brain, enabling many intracranial blood vessels to be identified, as well as the direction of flow through them. Neuroradiologic applications of ultrasonography in adults include evaluation of carotid vessels for plaques, stenosis, dissection, or subclavian steal; evaluation of intracranial vasculature for spasm after hemorrhage or trauma; ultrasound-guided needle biopsies; and intraoperative localization of brain and spinal cord tumors.

Advantages of ultrasound include the lack of ionizing radiation, direct multiplanar imaging, portability, real-time imaging, and relatively low cost. Its disadvantages include relatively poorer tissue contrast resolution, operator dependence, and inability to view beyond air, bone, or metal.

Nuclear Medicine and Positron Emission Tomography

Nuclear medicine studies record γ-ray photoemissions resulting from the radioactive decay of unstable atomic isotopes. Emissions are measured by crystal detectors with electronically set energy ranges calibrated to the isotope of interest. These usually produce planar images, however, moving detectors can be scanned in multiple projections and analyzed with a computer to produce a cross-sectional image known as single-photon emission computed tomography (SPECT). Nuclear medicine studies use radioactive atoms attached to specific carrier molecules. Because these molecules are often biologically active, and because spatial resolution is poor, nuclear medicine studies provide information that is generally more physiologic than anatomic.

Neuroradiologic applications include cerebral blood flow studies to identify regions of decreased cerebral perfusion, confirm brain death, or evaluate regions of seizure activity; bone scans to evaluate metastatic lesions in the spine; and triple-phase bone scans or Indium white blood cell (WBC) scans to identify osteomyelitis. Indium cisternograms are used to evaluate suspected cerebrospinal fluid (CSF) leaks, extra-axial cysts, and ventricular shunt function, and to confirm the presence of normal pressure hydrocephalus. Functional brain scans with Technitium^{99m}-HMPAO and I^{123} spectamine can be used for early detection of cerebral infarction (within 1 hour) or to evaluate collateral blood flow in preparation for cerebral vascular surgery. Indium WBC scans and thallium studies may be used to evaluate cerebral abscesses or tumors, respectively. SPECT has been used to identify patterns of brain hypometabolism as a marker of Alzheimer's disease and other dementias, but its sensitivity is not optimal.

The advantages of nuclear medicine studies include specific physiologic information and very few contraindications. Disadvantages include poor spatial and anatomic resolution, radiation exposure, limited clinical applications, relatively long study times, and, in some cases, nonspecificity of findings.

Positron emission tomography (PET) is a very recent imaging development, and resembles SPECT, since both use a radioactive compound producing photons and result in cross-sectional imaging. Although in SPECT the measured photon is a direct product of the radioactive decay, in PET a parent compound undergoes β$^+$ decay, in which one of the daughter decay products is a positron—an entity that has the identical mass of an electron but is positively charged (also called *antimatter*). The emitted positron travels a short distance (usually less than 1 cm) and collides with an electron, resulting in an annihilation reaction producing two photons traveling in opposite directions. These photons are detected tomographically and analyzed using a computer to generate images. Most isotopes of carbon, nitrogen, and oxygen are positron emitters, as is fluorine18, and can be attached to a wide range of biologically active compounds. These compounds accumulate in regions of increased perfusion, oxygen consumption, or glucose utilization; regions of protein synthesis; or regions containing specific receptors.

Positron emission tomography may be used for evaluating brain masses for determining the rate of metabolic activity (higher rates generally imply a higher degree of malignancy), localizing seizure foci, distinguishing postsurgical change or radiation necrosis from tumor recurrence, diagnosing Alzheimer's dementia, and evaluating metabolic brain disorders and posttraumatic changes; PET has also been used to map brain activity during cognitive tasks. Positron emission tomographic imaging yields physiologic information with poor anatomic and spatial resolution. Other disadvantages include lack of availability due to rapid decay times (only available at a limited number of centers with a nearby cyclotron to produce the isotope), high expense, and the need for concurrent use of an anatomic imaging modality (usually MRI) to improve anatomic localization.

Myelography

Myelography is an invasive procedure requiring an intrathecal lumbar or cervical needle puncture to gain access to the CSF, where iodine contrast is injected. Formerly, an oil-based iodine contrast called *Pantopaque* was used, which needed to be removed. Now, excellent nonionic water-soluble intrathecal contrast agents are used. These agents are excreted by the kidneys, do not have to be removed, and have a rarer incidence of side effects and complications.

Myelography followed by CT is extremely informative in assessing spinal degenerative disease and its effects on the spinal cord and nerve roots. Although it has been superseded by MRI for many purposes, myelography is an option when MRI is contraindicated or cannot be obtained, such as when metallic orthopedic hardware causes excessive artifact. Myelography can effectively show extradural spinal disease due to disc extrusion or osteophytes. It is sensitive to the presence of intradural extramedullary lesions such as meningiomas or metastases, as well as arteriovenous (A–V) fistulas. However, myelography is less specific than MRI because it lacks good soft-tissue differentiation. Subsequently, MRI is clearly superior when the question of spinal intramedullary disease is raised.

If there is a possible complete block to the flow of the CSF in the spine, lumbar puncture should be avoided because of the risk of herniation, and C1–C2 puncture should be performed instead. Myelography may be extremely risky in the presence of epidural spinal infection because the needle may traverse an epidural abscess and seed the subarachnoid space. Therefore, in the workup of spinal infection, MRI is preferred on the grounds of greater safety and specificity.

Cisternography

As an extension of a myelographic procedure, intracranial cisternography following placement of intrathecal iodinated contrast agents can be performed and is useful in the diagnosis of arachnoid cysts within the cavarum or calvarium CSF leaks. Radionuclide cisternography can be performed for similar abnormalities and in cases of suspected normal pressure hydrocephalus.

Spinal Intervention

Under radiologic guidance, injection of contrast material into intervertebral discs (discography), the epidural space, or aimed at nerve roots or articular facets may be performed for diagnosis. Similarly, once location of the needle tip is confirmed, pharmacologic agents injected into these same regions can then provide therapeutic relief. Recently, widespread acceptance and performance of *vertebroplasty*, the placement of methylmethacrylate into vertebral body compression fractures (either osteoporotic or pathologic) via transcutaneous needle insertion with needle tip positioning into the vertebral body, usually by a transpedicular approach, has resulted in tremendous immediate pain relief and fracture stabilization for this otherwise relatively untreatable problem, allowing patients, usually previously bedridden, to resume normal activities of daily living.

Endovascular Neurointerventional Procedures

Via angiographic access, superselective vessel catheterization can be used for embolization of AVMs, vascular tumors, and aneurysms. Embolization may make use of polyvinyl alcohol (PVA) foam particles, cyanoacrylates, and in some cases alcohol, coils, and balloons. Detachable microcoils are also commonly used to treat intracranial aneurysms. Detachable balloons are effective in the treatment of cavernous carotid fistulas. Vascular tumors

such as meningiomas are often treated by flow-directed tiny PVA foam particles, whereas soft-tissue tumors can be treated with direct intra-arterial chemotherapy administration. Thrombolysis may be performed in cases of hyperacute strokes within less than 6 hours of onset. After superselective catheterization of arteries, tissue plasminogen activator (TPA) or urokinase may be infused to dissolve fresh thrombi directly. Angioplasty can be used to treat proximal cerebral artery vasospasm, a complication of subarachnoid hemorrhage. Additionally, intra-arterial infusion of papaverine can be helpful for more distal vascular spasm, although the agent is effective for only short periods of time and may need to be repeated. Finally, angioplasty with stenting for arthrosclerotic stenotic lesions of the carotid arteries is now an acceptable alternative to carotid endarterectomy surgery.

Problem-solving Approaches

Brain Disorders

Trauma

Computed tomography remains the most efficient and effective means of evaluating acute head trauma, and can readily detect hemorrhage and other effects. Epidural hematomas have a characteristic extra-axial biconvex or lenticular shape. In the acute phase, they are of high density and appear white. These are often associated with skull fractures that cross meningeal grooves or dural sinuses, resulting in subsequent rupture of the associated vessel, meningeal artery, or venous sinus, respectively (Figure 4.2). Patients may initially present with a lucent interval, making detection by imaging critical prior to the development of serious neurologic deterioration due to cerebral compression from the adjacent mass effect of the lesion. Although epidural hematoma is well known to be a medical emergency, the even more common subdural hematoma can be just as serious. Subdural hematomas have a typical extra-axial crescent shape and, in the acute, phase appear white, whereas a subacute or chronic subdural will be less dense, appearing gray or black, respectively. A subdural hematoma may occur in the absence of a skull fracture. These lesions are due to rupture of the traversing cortical veins where they join with the dural sinuses. Subdural hematomas are common manifestations of head trauma, can also be associated with significant mass effect on the adjacent brain parenchyma, and may be accompanied by other serious traumatic injury such as contusions and shears.

Cerebral contusions are intraparenchymal "brain bruises" caused by contact between the cortical surface and the adjacent calvarium. They can be either hemorrhagic or bland (edematous). The lesions may occur adjacent to the area of impact (coup) or opposite the site of impact (con-

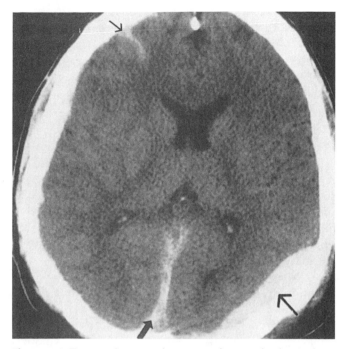

Figure 4.2 Trauma. Computed tomography reveals a lenticular high-density collection in the left occipital region indicating an acute epidural hematoma (*large arrow*). The high density and thickening along the posterior falx is consistent with an inter-hemispheric subdural hematoma (*broad medium-sized arrow*). The high density along a right frontal sulcus (*small arrow*) indicates subarachnoid hemorrhage.

trecoup). They do not always manifest immediately, reaching their maximum extent after a latency of 4–7 days; therefore, serial CT studies may be needed. Shear injuries—also known as diffuse axonal injury (DAI)—are also intra-parenchymal lesions, but occur deeper in the brain than cerebral contusions, at gray–white matter junctions, along major white matter tracts such as the corpus callosum, and in the brainstem. Like contusions, shear injuries may be hemorrhagic but are more commonly bland. These bland edematous changes are therefore more readily detected by MRI than CT (Tables 4.3 and 4.4).

Fractures of the skull and facial bones can be detected by plain films or more readily by CT. Fractures may be a marker of underlying intracranial injury. Although nondepressed skull fractures may be of less clinical importance, depressed skull fractures (more easily recognized by CT) can be very significant. Depression of at least 5 mm (the width of the skull) warrants neurosurgical attention because such fractures are often associated with open injuries and tears of the dura.

Skull base fractures may result in a CSF leak. Fine-cut CT, particularly in the coronal plane, is an effective way of determining the presence of basal skull fractures (Figure 4.3). Evaluation for CSF rhinorrhea may be initiated with radionuclide cisternography. This can be followed by fine-cut CT scanning in the area of suspicious

radionuclide concentration with iodine contrast cisternography, if necessary.

High-resolution CT is the optimal means of evaluating the temporal bone for possible fractures. Longitudinal fractures appear along the long axis of the temporal bone and are more common than transverse fractures. They usually result in ossicular dislocation and conductive hearing loss. Transverse fractures cross the axis of the petrous portion of the temporal bone and are usually more serious, damaging the VII and VIII cranial nerve complex, resulting in sensorineural hearing loss and facial paralysis.

Direct vascular trauma may result in frank lacerations of vessels, pseudoaneurysm formation, and fistulas.

Table 4.3 Hemorrhage on CT

Stage	Time	State
Acute	0–1 week	Bright
Subacute	1–3 weeks	Isodense
Chronic	>3 weeks	Dark

1 The signal of hemorrhage on computed tomography (CT) varies with time. The bright signal largely depends on the hemoglobin (protein) concentration, which eventually breaks down and is diluted. In anemia, the bright signal may not show with acute hemorrhage.
2 In some cases of hyperacute hemorrhage, the signal of actively extravasating blood may be isointense (gray) rather than bright due to its liquid (unclotted) state. A memory aid for the timing of isointense blood is the "rule of sevens," i.e., 7 seconds or 7 days.
3 The signal of chronic hemorrhage is dark (like cerebrospinal fluid) on CT, so that differentiation between a chronic subdural hematoma and a subdural hygroma may be difficult. Magnetic resonance imaging may be needed to distinguish between the two.
4 Subdural hematomas along the tentorium cerebelli can be very difficult to detect on CT.

Table 4.4 Hemorrhage on MRI

Stage	Time	State	T1	T2
Hyperacute	0–6 hours	OxyHgb	Iso	Iso
Acute	6 hours–3 days	DeoxyHgb	Iso	Dark
Subacute (early)	3–7 days	Intracell MET	Bright	Dark
Subacute (late)	1–3 weeks	Extracell MET	Bright	Bright
Chronic	3 weeks–forever	Hemosiderin	Dark	Dark

OxyHgb,= oxyhemoglobin; DeoxyHgb, deoxyhemoglobin; intracell MET, intracellular methemoglobin; Extracell MET, extracellular methemoglobin.

1 Hemorrhage changes in a different manner on magnetic resonance imaging (MRI) than on computed tomography (CT). In addition to protein breakdown, changes also occur in paramagnetic effects.
2 In the hyperacute stage, detection of subarachnoid hemorrhage can be very difficult because it may have the same signal as adjacent cerebrospinal fluid unless fluid-attenuating inversion recovery (FLAIR) imaging sequences are obtained.
3 Because none of the signals of hemorrhage on MRI are exactly the same as water on all pulse sequences, this can help differentiate a chronic subdural hematoma from a subdural hygroma.
4 Extracellular MET may also persist forever in the brain if the blood–brain barrier becomes intact prior to macrophage invasion, which is required for conversion to hemosiderin.

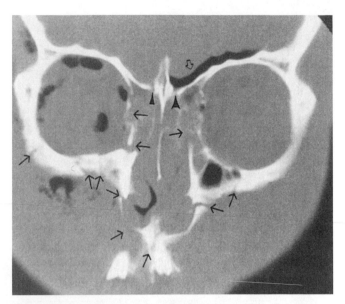

Figure 4.3 Trauma. Coronal computed tomography of the face demonstrating multiple complex facial fractures (*black arrows*). There are also fractures at the cribriform plate at the base of the skull (*arrowheads*), and pneumocephalus in the left subfrontal region (*open arrow*). Meningitis may be a potential complication.

Rapidly enlarging soft tissues, subarachnoid hemorrhage, or active wound bleeding may warrant urgent radiographic evaluation by angiography. Arteriovenous fistulae, most commonly a carotid artery–cavernous sinus fistula or vertebral artery–vertebral vein fistula, may develop as a result of vascular trauma, or a dural A–V fistulae can occur following thrombosis of a dural sinus. The carotid–cavernous fistula may manifest as proptosis and chemosis. Computed tomography may reveal a dilated superior ophthalmic vein. Angiography is necessary for definitive evaluation, and neurointerventional techniques such as balloon occlusion of the fistulae may be needed for final treatment. Arterial lacerations or pseudoaneurysms should be diagnosed acutely by angiography. In many cases, these can be treated by neurointerventional techniques using detachable balloons, or coils, or both.

Neoplasms

Evaluation of cerebral neoplasia can be performed effectively by CT or MRI. The use of contrast agents is very helpful in defining the extent and nature of the underlying neoplasm. For lesions above the tentorium cerebelli, noncontrast CT is an inadequate examination, since small lesions may be missed; however, the addition of contrast material results in satisfactory visualization of these lesions. For masses below the tentorium, where beam-hardening artifacts from adjacent temporal bones degrade the CT images, lesions may be missed even following contrast administration. Magnetic resonance imaging is superior

Table 4.5 Frequency of brain tumors

Metastasis	40%
Gliomas	25%
Meningiomas	15%
Pituitary adenomas	10%
Schwannomas	<10%
Other	1%

to CT in the detection of neoplastic lesions, in particular those in the posterior fossa, and should be performed in all patients especially those who have a contraindication to iodinated contrast material that precludes a contrast-enhanced CT scan (Table 4.5).

When evaluating metastatic disease, one should pay attention not only to the brain parenchyma but also to the bones, which may be affected by metastases, particularly those from lung, breast, and prostate, as well as lymphoma. On CT, one should scrutinize the bone windows in addition to the brain windows. When searching for metastatic disease with MRI, it is important to look carefully at the bone marrow signal on T1-weighted images,

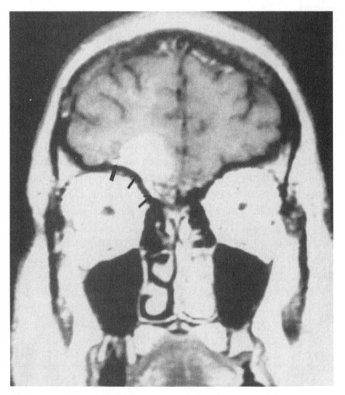

Figure 4.4 Extra-axial tumor. T1-weighted post-gadolinium magnetic resonance imaging showing an extra-axial enhancing mass arising from the right subfrontal region of the cranium, with a broad-based dural surface attachment (*arrows*). These features are characteristics of a meningioma.

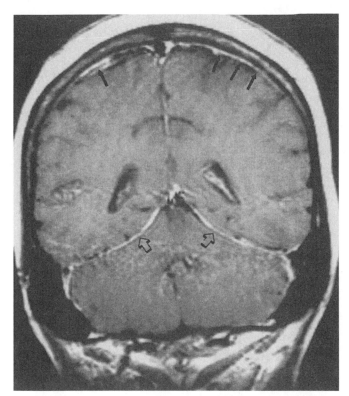

Figure 4.5 Meningeal tumor. T1-weighted post-gadolinium coronal magnetic resonance imaging of the brain demonstrating abnormal contiguous meningeal enhancement over the convexities (*solid arrows*), which may be seen in infections, neoplasia, and other conditions—in this case, lymphoma. There is also enhancement of the tentorium (*open arrows*).

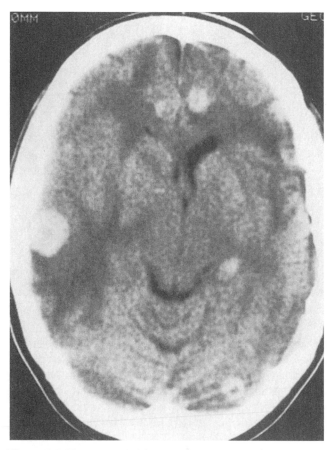

Figure 4.6 Metastases. Axial noncontrast computed tomography shows multiple scattered high-density nodules throughout the brain with surrounding vasogenic edema, suggestive of hemorrhagic metastases, or possibly septic emboli. Biopsy showed metastatic melanoma.

which normally has a homogeneous appearance in the skull and the clivus. The meninges must be examined carefully to detect extra-axial lesions such as meningioma (Figure 4.4) or metastatic disease, for example from the breast, lung, or melanoma, or from lymphoma. Meningeal involvement is best imaged by T1-weighted postgadolinium MRI scans taken in the coronal and axial planes (Figure 4.5).

Some tumors, such as oligodendrogliomas, craniopharyngiomas, astrocytomas, dermoids, and meningiomas, tend to calcify, whereas others may cause bone destruction. These changes are best seen on CT. On the other hand, the most sensitive indicator of early bone marrow involvement is MRI, in which the T1-weighted images demonstrate loss of bright bone marrow signal. Some tumors may be hemorrhagic, which assists in the differential diagnosis (Figure 4.6 and Table 4.6).

Tumors may present as ring-enhancing lesions and can mimic the appearance of inflammatory lesions such as abscesses. Glioblastoma multiforme (GBM) typically has a ring-enhancing configuration due to its necrotic center, often with eccentric thickening where blood vessels enter (Figure 4.7). Juvenile pilocytic astrocytomas may present

as an enhancing nodule with or without an adjacent rim-enhancing cyst. Metastatic lymphoma in immunosuppressed patients often presents as a periventricular

Pearls and Perils

Brain tumors

▶ The use of iodine or gadolinium contrast agents markedly increases the conspicuity of most brain tumors.

▶ Metastatic lesions are much more easily seen with contrast agents. They often appear as one or more nodules surrounded by extensive edema.

▶ A solitary lesion does not necessarily exclude a metastasis; 40–50% are single when found.

▶ Some brain neoplasms and other mass lesions typically do not enhance. These include lower-grade astrocytomas, lipomas, epidermoids, and arachnoid cysts.

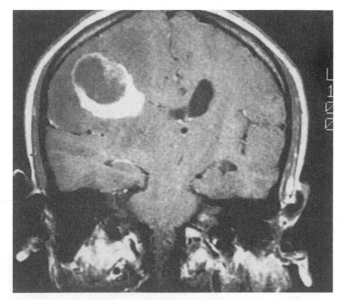

Figure 4.7 Intraparenchymal tumor. T1-weighted postgadolinium coronal magnetic resonance imaging demonstrates a ring-enhancing mass with surrounding edema in the right parietal lobe, causing midline shift and compressing the right lateral ventricle. The mass is eccentrically thickened along its medial inferior border. This appearance is typical of a glioblastoma multiforme, which was confirmed on biopsy.

ring-enhancing lesion. Sometimes it is difficult to determine if a ring-enhancing lesion is a neoplasm, an inflammatory process, or other lesion. Clinical history, characterization of imaging patterns, and MR spectroscopy (Figure 4.8) can be helpful, although biopsy may ultimately be necessary (Box 4.1).

When initially viewing an intracranial mass, it is important to determine whether it arises from within the brain (intra-axial) or from outside the brain (extra-axial), since this will significantly change the differential diagnostic possibilities. Magnetic resonance imaging has the distinct advantage of true multiplanar anatomic presentations, which facilitates this determination. Computed tomography may fail to demonstrate a dural attachment of an extra-axial lesion (Table 4.7).

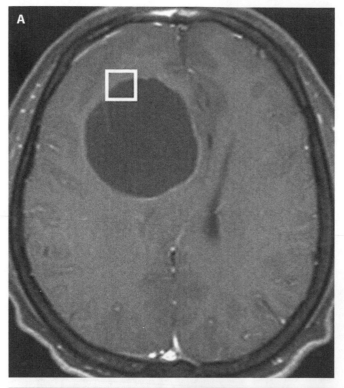

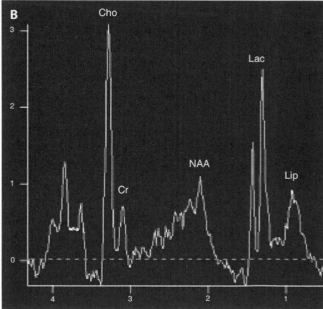

Figure 4.8 Glioblastoma multiforme. **A:** Axial T1-weighted magnetic resonance imaging (MRI) with gadolinium contrast and MR spectroscopy voxel shows a large right frontal intraparenchymal mass with peripheral enhancement, necrotic center, and right to left midline shift. **B:** Short T_E MR spectra demonstrates diminished N-acetylaspartate (NAA), decreased creatine (Cr), markedly elevated choline (Cho), elevated lactate (Lac), and elevated lipid (Lip), a pattern indicative of highly malignant neoplasm.

Table 4.6 Common hemorrhagic brain tumors

Primary	Metastatic
Glioblastoma multiforme	Melanoma
Ependymoma	Choriocarcinoma
Pituitary adenoma	Renal cell carcinoma
Oligodendroglioma	Thyroid carcinoma
	Adenocarcinoma

Table 4.7 Features of intra-axial and extra-axial masses

Imaging features: intra-axial mass
  Cortex pushed out
  Infiltrates brain
  Narrows cisterns
Typical intra-axial masses
  Glioma (includes astrocytoma, ependymoma, oligodendroglioma, GBM)
  Brain metastasis
  Primitive neural ectodermal tumor (PNET)
  Hemangioblastoma
  Primary cerebral lymphoma
Imaging features: extra-axial mass
  Cortex pushed in
  Dural base: flat, broad based, dural "tail"
  Bone changes
  Widens cisterns
Typical extra-axial masses
  Meningioma
  Schwannoma
  Pituitary adenoma
  Epidermoid, dermoid, lipoma
  Meningeal metastasis
  Secondary lymphoma
  Arachnoid cyst

Vascular disease

The term *stroke* encompasses a wide group of cerebral vascular disorders with differing clinical presentation, pathology, etiology, prognosis, and treatment.

Cerebral infarction. Ischemic cerebral vascular disease leading to cerebral infarction is the most common cause of stroke. The usual mechanisms include arterial stenosis/occlusion or embolism, or both, from atherosclerotic vascular narrowing/ulceration, arterial thrombosis, atherosclerotic embolic debris, or embolism from cardiac sources.

The acute phase of an infarct may become apparent on MRI within an hour of the stroke, particularly with diffusion-weighted imaging, and on CT in 6–24 hours, depending on lesion size. Earlier than this, CT is often completely normal. On CT, changes may be quite subtle, with evidence of mild mass effect manifested by sulcal effacement due to slight brain swelling, or the normal band of low-density medial to the insula (the insular ribbon) may be lost. On CT, there may be decreased density or, on T2-weighted MRI, increased signal intensity secondary to the increased water content in the neuronal cells (cytotoxic edema). Additionally, it is this cytotoxic edema that results in *restricted water diffusion in the cell*, allowing early identification of the lesion on diffusion-weighted MRI (Figure 4.9).

If contrast is given in the acute phase, blood vessels in the region of the infarct may enhance. This *intravascular enhancement sign* is seen more often on MRI than on CT. Later, one may visualize meningeal enhancement in the territory of the infarct, again more obvious on MRI. Early thrombosis of the feeding vessel leading to the area of infarction may show as loss of the vascular flow void on MRI or as a hyperdense artery on CT.

During the subacute phase, which may last from a few days to a few weeks, the likelihood of hemorrhage increases. Although an infarct may not be frankly hemorrhagic initially, it may develop petechial hemorrhage later, usually along the gyral surfaces. The petechial hemorrhage appears on CT or MRI as a wavy cortical pattern, and may progress to a denser, deeper intraparenchymal hemorrhagic pattern. During this phase, the pattern with contrast agent administration changes from predominantly meningeal to increasingly intraparenchymal enhancement, usually taking on a wedge-shaped appearance. Brain swelling progressively diminishes.

In the chronic phase of an infarct, encephalomalacia develops, with focal volume loss appearing as a dark area on CT or a bright area on T2-weighted MRI. Compensatory enlargement of the adjacent ventricle may occur. Congenital infarction may produce gross loss of brain, leaving a cyst lined by gliotic white matter communicating with the adjacent ventricle, referred to as *porencephaly*.

Vascular evaluation. When there is a history of transient ischemic attack, amaurosis fugax, or an infarct, a vascular workup should be performed. The most sensitive ultrasound assessment of the carotid arteries is obtained by duplex evaluation, combining an image of anatomic features (e.g., carotid plaques) with Doppler evaluation of carotid blood flow velocity. From the peaks of systolic velocity and waveforms, a percent stenosis of the diameter

Box 4.1 Common ring-enhancing lesions

Mnemonic: MAGIC DR
M: Metastases
A: Aneurysm
G: Glioma
I: Infections (abscess)
C: Clot (resolving hematoma)
D: Demyelinating process (e.g., active multiple sclerosis plaque)
R: Radiation change

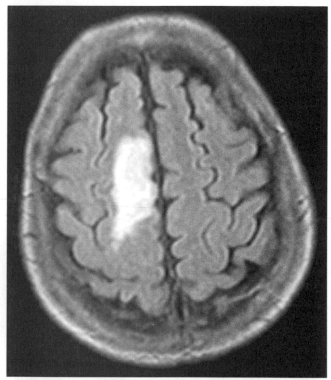

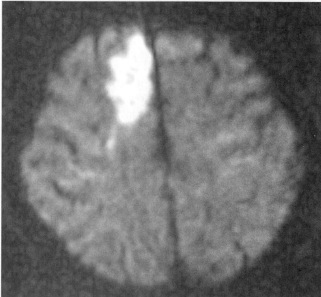

Figure 4.9 Acute infarct. **A:** Axial FLAIR magnetic resonance image (MRI) shows a region of increased signal intensity in the right medial frontal lobe involving the gray and adjacent white matter compatible with a right anterior cerebral artery infarct. **B:** Diffusion-weighted MRI confirms the lesion is an acute infarct.

cardiac embolic source), or both, further evaluation of the brain's vasculature can be obtained by angiography, using CT, MRI, or catheter contrast angiography. Both CTA and MRA are noninvasive and can be performed with considerable accuracy. On MRA, a two-dimensional *time-of-flight* technique is chosen to cover the entire neck from the thoracic inlet to the skull base. A three-dimensional time-of-flight technique, which gives greater detail but less area coverage than the two-dimensional type, can be chosen to display the circle of Willis. One should beware of flow and dephasing artifacts, particularly at the petrous bone and whenever there are sharp bends in vessels, because these may cause false-positive stenoses. Two-dimensional MRA may overestimate the degree of true carotid stenosis but is more dependable than ultrasound for detecting tandem stenoses. With the use of gadolinium contrast agent, a three-dimensional technique can now be acquired of the neck vessels, resulting in less saturation artifact and more accurate determination of the degree of vascular stenosis, as well as the detection of extremely slow flow such as that seen in a carotid "string sign." Computed tomography angiography also provides accurate information on the degree of vascular narrowing; however, high-density material such as calcification in atherosclerotic plaque or the normal skull base bone may lead to image artifact and possible misinterpretation of the examination.

Catheter angiography can also accurately measure the degree of vascular stenosis (Figure 4.10). However, being an invasive procedure and given the accuracy of CTA and MRA, it is usually reserved to answer a specific question regarding the patient's condition. Catheter angiography can better delineate collateral flow, vascular steal, vasculitis, and associated lesions such as tandem stenoses, intracerebral aneurysms, and AVMs, as well as tumor vascularity. Although MRA is an excellent screening test and can usually detect aneurysms as small as 3 mm, catheter angiography remains the gold standard to diagnose small vascular abnormalities. Catheter angiography is also necessary to fully evaluate the feeding arteries, vascular nidus, and draining veins of an AVM, and is, of course, mandatory prior to endovascular therapy such as embolization for AVMs, A–V fistulae, and aneurysms; angioplasty for stenoses or vasospasm (Figure 4.11); and superselective chemotherapy infusion for tumors.

Most recently, CT or MR perfusion examinations have become clinically available to further evaluate cerebrovascular physiology, and these have shown great promise to expand the time window for administration of thrombolytic agents in the presence of acute cerebral ischemic disease. This technique can produce cerebral blood flow (CBF), cerebral blood volume (CBV), and blood mean transit time (MTT) maps that demonstrate perfusion mismatches of infarcted versus ischemic—yet

of the internal carotid artery is estimated. Ultrasound evaluation of the carotid arteries is noninvasive compared to catheter carotid angiography, but its accuracy is extremely operator-dependent. Therefore, a skilled ultrasonographer should perform the evaluation.

Following initial screening by ultrasound of the carotid arteries or echocardiography (to locate a possible

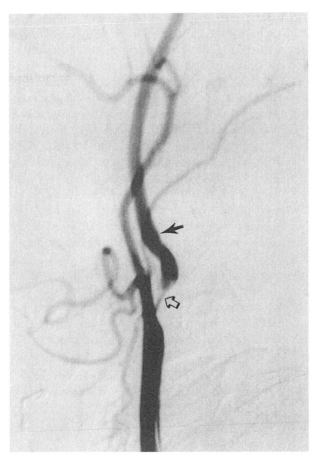

Figure 4.10 Vascular stenosis. Lateral view of a left common carotid angiogram demonstrating high-grade stenosis at the proximal left internal carotid artery. There is 83% diameter stenosis (*open arrow*) relative to the normal expected diameter of the left internal carotid artery (*solid arrow*).

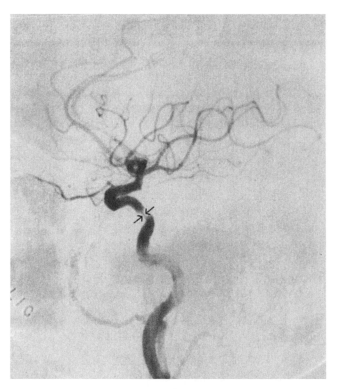

Figure 4.11 Vascular stenosis. Left common carotid angiogram demonstrating high-grade stenosis of the intracranial pericavernous left internal carotid artery (*arrows*). This lesion is not amenable to surgical repair, but could be treated with carotid angioplasty and stenting.

still viable—brain parenchyma (ischemic penumbra), which is potentially salvageable (Figure 4.12), while limiting the risk of hemorrhagic complications.

Unusual causes of ischemic cerebrovascular disease. One should consider other causes of ischemic cerebral vascular disease, particularly if the patient is young or lacks risk factors for arteriosclerosis. Arterial dissection is due to a tear within the vessel wall leading to either a false lumen (appearing as a double lumen on angiography) or subintimal hematoma (appearing as vessel narrowing). Arterial dissection most commonly affects the proximal internal carotid artery just distal to the carotid bifurcation or the vertebral artery from C1–C2 to the skull base. The most specific way of demonstrating dissection, particularly if a subacute thrombus is present in the vessel wall, is by MRI, because angiography may show only vessel narrowing (the effect of the lesion on the vascular lumen), whereas MRI depicts the actual hematoma in the vessel wall.

Vasculitis is most accurately diagnosed by catheter angiography, since the lesions are commonly located in the smaller vessels of the distal vasculature. Therefore, sharp focus and great detail are required to find these areas of subtle narrowing and luminal irregularity. The causes of vasculitis include collagen vascular disease (for example, systemic lupus erythematosus or scleroderma), necrotizing disorders (such as giant cell arteritis, Takayasu disease, or periarteritis nodosa), drug-related disease, or infections (tuberculosis, syphilis). Drugs of abuse, such as cocaine, amphetamines, or heroin may cause vascular spasm, vasculitis, thrombosis, or intraparenchymal hemorrhage leading to brain infarction in typical or atypical locations. Septic emboli with scattered brain abscesses may also occur.

The basal ganglia, particularly the putamen and globus pallidus, develop infarction (often bilateral and symmetric) in rare metabolic conditions such as Leigh's disease and propionic acidemia. Toxic causes of cerebral anoxia, including poisoning due to carbon monoxide or cyanide, also may affect the basal ganglia symmetrically.

Magnetic resonance imaging is an excellent modality to evaluate venous thrombosis, an often-overlooked cause of stroke. On spin echo, one may see the bright signal of subacute thrombus in a dural sinus, such as the superior sagittal sinus. Phase-contrast magnetic resonance venograms (MRV) can demonstrate the lack of flow in many venous structures, such as the major dural sinuses (the superior sagittal sinus, the straight sinus, or the trans-verse sinuses) or the smaller draining veins (the superficial cortical veins or the deep internal cerebral veins). On contrast-enhanced CT, one may encounter the delta (δ) sign, noted in the major dural sinuses but most commonly seen at the torcula (the triangular-shaped junction of the straight sinus, superior sagittal sinus, and transverse sinuses at the occiput). This is caused by the absence of signal in the center of the sinus due to the occluding thrombus but with bright enhancement at the periphery of the sinus secondary to the small, contrast-filled collateral venous channels in the sinus wall.

Intracranial hemorrhage. Primary intracranial hemorrhage in the absence of trauma accounts for 15% of strokes. The usual causes are hypertension (50%), amyloid angiopathy (20%), vascular malformations (15%), and other causes such as coagulopathy, drugs, infarction, neoplasia, or rarely, infectious processes.

Hypertensive hemorrhages are most commonly identified by their intraparenchymal location in the putamen (Figure 4.13) or thalamus, or less commonly in the pons, cerebellum, or subcortical regions. The risk of amyloid angiopathy increases with age. Deposition of amy-

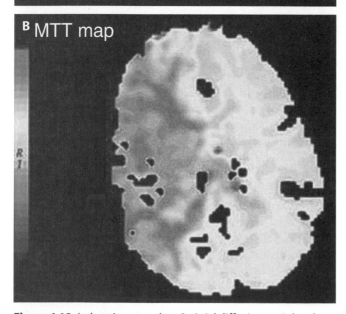

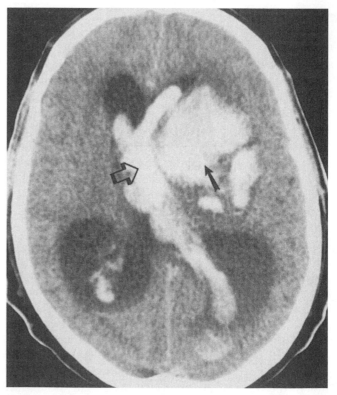

Figure 4.12 Ischemic penumbra. **A:** Axial diffusion-weighted magnetic resonance imaging (MRI) reveals foci of increased signal from acute infarction in the right frontal lobe deep white matter. **B:** Axial MR perfusion mean transit time map depicts a large region of delayed cerebral perfusion (diffusion–perfusion mismatch) throughout the entire right middle cerebral artery territory, compatible with ischemic but not yet infarcted brain parenchyma.

Figure 4.13 Hypertensive hemorrhage. Axial noncontrast computed tomography of the brain showing a large intraparenchymal hemorrhage arising from the left basal ganglia (*solid arrow*) and causing midline shift to the right, with leakage of blood into the lateral ventricles (*open arrow*) and subsequent development of hydrocephalus.

loid along vessel walls leads to loss of vessel integrity and subsequent hemorrhages, typically located in the peripheral lobar areas. Although imaging studies may be suggestive, the diagnosis is confirmed by demonstrating vascular amyloid on biopsy.

Coagulopathies can cause intracranial hemorrhage. Coagulopathies may be secondary to anticoagulation with Coumadin, heparin, and aspirin, or they may be due to primary disorders such as disseminated intravascular coagulopathy, thrombotic thrombocytopenic purpura, hemophilia, and hemolytic–uremic syndrome. Meningitis or encephalitis may be associated with peripheral (usually petechial) gyral hemorrhages and may mimic subarachnoid hemorrhage. Contrast usually shows gyral enhancement of the leptomeninges, dural enhancement of the pachymeninges, or both.

Neoplasms may undergo hemorrhage. The use of iodine or gadolinium as a contrast agent may reveal an enhancing nodule adjacent to a hematoma, suggesting a neoplasm. The primary brain neoplasm that tends to hemorrhage most often is glioblastoma multiforme, followed by ependymoma, oligodendroglioma, and pituitary adenoma. Metastatic lesions with a high likelihood of hemorrhage include melanoma, choriocarcinoma, renal cell carcinoma, thyroid carcinoma, and adenocarcinoma.

About 15% of cases of hemorrhage are due to vascular malformations. Arteriovenous malformations are the most common type, but hemorrhage may also result from cavernous malformations, rarely from capillary telangiectasia, and very uncommonly from developmental venous anomalies (DVAs). An AVM is a congenital shunt between the arterial and venous system, in which microfistulae are found instead of capillaries, causing the left-to-right shunt. Increased flow through AVMs may lead to the formation of arterial aneurysms or venous varices. Evaluation of an AVM may start with CT to demonstrate hemorrhage, with punctate or serpentine calcifications found in up to 25%. Magnetic resonance imaging shows numerous vascular flow voids at the region of the nidus, in addition to enlarged feeding arteries and draining veins. Magnetic resonance angiography may help to show the detail of the AVM, but the definitive diagnostic workup requires detailed catheter angiography, which may be combined with specific endovascular therapies (embolization) and followed by surgical removal. The radiologic angiographic hallmark of an AVM is early venous drainage during the arterial phase and the presence of a vascular tangle or nidus.

Cavernous malformations are very slow-flowing vascular malformations. Like other vascular malformations, they usually do not cause significant mass effect unless they bleed. They are best detected by MRI, which may reveal the footprints of prior hemorrhage (the presence of low-signal-intensity hemosiderin), particularly in gradient echo studies. Spin echo sequences may indicate subacute hemorrhage as high T1 signal extracellular methemoglobin (Figure 4.14). Phase-contrast MRA can be even more sensitive to slowly flowing blood and may demonstrate *cavernomas*, which can be invisible on catheter angiography due to the extremely slow flow.

A DVA (formerly known as *venous angioma*) is an unusual appearing collection of veins that actually drains normal brain parenchyma. On angiography, its appearance may be bizarre, taking on a medusa's head shape of tangled veins draining into a single venous channel, seen only in the venous phase on angiography. Developmental venous anomalies only rarely produce bleeding or mass effect. Capillary telangiectasias are tiny vascular malformations that may only very rarely undergo punctate hemorrhage. Again, the best way to detect their footprints is by MRI, using gradient echo sequences sensitive to hemosiderin (if prior bleeding has occurred) and to the inherent deoxyhemoglobin within these lesions; otherwise, this entity is more commonly recognized as showing a punctuate area of enhancement (usually in the pons) following contrast material administration.

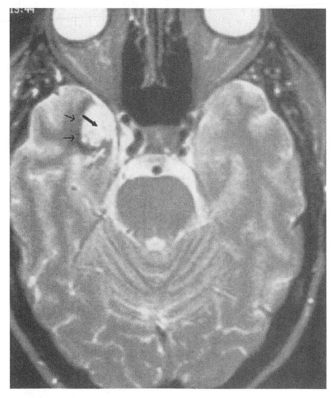

Figure 4.14 Hemorrhage in a patient with temporal lobe epilepsy due to cavernous hemangioma. Axial T2-weighted magnetic resonance imaging reveals an area of high signal (*solid arrow*) with surrounding low signal (*smaller paired arrows*), consistent with subacute hemorrhage with a rim of surrounding hemosiderin.

Subarachnoid hemorrhage Primary (nontraumatic) subarachnoid hemorrhage accounts for about 5% of strokes. The most common cause is aneurysm rupture (80%), followed by vascular malformations (15%), and rarely coagulopathy, drugs, or sepsis. Aneurysmal hemorrhage represents a neurosurgical emergency. About 2% of people harbor aneurysms, as shown by surveys of cerebral angiograms or of autopsy specimens. If an aneurysm bleeds, there is a 50% chance of rebleeding and a 50% chance of mortality if left untreated. The risk of a hemorrhage from an aneurysm is approximately 1–2% per year. Aneurysms are usually found at arterial bifurcations and are related to faster or disturbed blood flow. Most aneurysms are located around the circle of Willis (Table 4.8). Indeed, if an aneurysm is peripheral to the circle of Willis, one should consider the possibility of a mycotic aneurysm, AVM-induced aneurysm, or other lesion.

When acute subarachnoid hemorrhage is suspected, the initial evaluation should be CT to identify the site of maximal blood collection as a predictor of the site of the aneurysm. This should be followed by detailed catheter angiography to define the aneurysm, although CTA or MRA may also be helpful. Because there is a 20% chance of multiple aneurysms, a complete cerebral angiogram should be performed. A good-quality cerebral angiogram should define the aneurysm, its exact location, the direction that it is pointing, the nature of its neck, whether there is adjacent arterial spasm, and if other aneurysms are present. Additionally, at the same setting, the aneurysm could then be treated endovascularly with detachable coils following the diagnostic procedure, if appropriate criteria are met such as a narrow aneurysm neck, ability to access the aneurysm via catheter navigation, and no arterial branch incorporated into the aneurysm sac wall.

Infection

Neuroimaging studies may be helpful in the evaluation of certain types of brain infections, particularly encephalitis, abscesses, and meningeal and parameningeal abnormalities. The use of contrast with CT or MRI is extremely important to make the disease process much more conspicuous. For encephalitis and to detect meningeal and subependymal abnormalities, MRI is more sensitive than CT. For lesions that calcify (such as old cysticercosis or

Table 4.8 Common locations of aneurysms

Anterior communicating artery	35%
Posterior communicating artery	35%
Middle cerebral artery	20%
Basilar artery	5%
Posterior fossa and other sites	<5%

▼

Pearls and Perils

Aneurysms

▶ If several aneurysms are present on angiography, the decision as to which aneurysm has bled is usually based on aneurysm size (the largest being the most likely to have ruptured) as well as associated information obtained on the angiogram and clues from other neuroimaging studies:

  a Site of greatest blood collection:

    – Interhemispheric fissure: anterior communicating artery origin

    – Sylvian fissure: ipsilateral posterior communicating or middle cerebral artery origin

    – Prepontine cistern: basilar artery origin

    – Foramen magnum or fourth ventricle: posterior inferior cerebellar artery origin

  b Active extravasation of contrast from the aneurysm.

  c Adjacent vascular spasm.

  d Irregularity of the aneurysm (Murphy's teat).

▶ If an aneurysm is not found by cerebral angiography, a repeat study should be performed 1–2 weeks later; an aneurysm may go undetected because it has clotted or vasospasm is present at the time of initial angiography.

▶ In nonhemorrhagic situations (e.g., in a patient with family history of aneurysms), MRA is a reasonable noninvasive screen and can detect unruptured aneurysms as small as 3 mm.

granulomatous lesions) and for lesions arising from the skull (e.g., complications of sinusitis or mastoiditis), CT is more revealing than MRI, particularly in demonstrating areas of skull base erosion on scans taken in the coronal plane. However, MRI may be more helpful in demonstrating the extent of dural involvement or transdural penetration of a disease process. Communicating hydrocephalus may be a complication of meningitis and is detectable by either CT or MRI.

Magnetic resonance imaging is superior in detecting encephalitis because it shows white matter changes earlier than CT and is better at revealing areas of adjacent edema. Complications such as brain abscess can be detected readily by CT or MRI with contrast agents. Herpes simplex causes a devastating form of encephalitis and is a medical emergency because early treatment may be lifesaving. This virus has a predilection for the insula and temporal lobe, and is identified more readily by MRI than CT. In some cases it may mimic a tumor mass.

Human immunodeficiency virus (HIV) infection and a host of HIV-related diseases commonly affect the nervous system. In HIV infections of the brain, CT or MRI shows progressive central and peripheral volume loss and deep white matter changes, usually without enhancement. In patients with HIV, brain involvement due to toxoplasmosis or lymphoma may produce focal neurologic deficits, with lesions that are readily detected by either contrast CT or MRI. Toxoplasmosis appears as nodular, ring-like, or bull's-eye enhancing lesions with surrounding edema, usually 1–2 cm in size and located in the basal ganglia or gray–white matter junctions. Lymphoma lesions can appear to be almost identical to toxoplasmosis, but tend to cluster around the ventricles and may be somewhat larger, from about 2–3 cm. They also are more typically ring enhancing rather than nodular or bull's-eye in shape, and they may show hyperdensity on CT or low T2 signal intensity on MRI due to the high nuclear-to-cytoplasmic ratio of the small "blue" cells that comprise this lesion. Additionally, MRS is an excellent modality to differentiate these two, sometimes confusing, lesions rather than the usual initiation of empiric therapy or brain biopsy.

Cytomegalovirus (CMV) can cause ependymitis in patients with HIV. Ependymitis is readily detected as an area of periventricular high signal on T2-weighted MRI, which enhances with gadolinium. CMV retinitis is difficult to detect by CT or MRI unless, a secondary hemorrhage occurs. At the cauda equina or a peripheral nerve level, CMV polyradiculitis can readily be seen on MRI with gadolinium and fat suppression techniques (Figure 4.15).

Mycobacteria (usually *Mycobacterium tuberculosis* or *avium*), the most common HIV-related opportunistic infection worldwide, may present with thick meningeal enhancement (best seen on MRI) and scattered enhancing granulomas throughout the brain. Cryptococcus, another common HIV-related disease, tends to affect the Virchow-Robin perivascular spaces, which show dilatation and occasionally mild enhancement. The adjacent meninges may also enhance and thicken. Again, this is usually best seen on MRI with contrast.

Intravenous drug abuse may result in complications such as vasculitis, septic emboli, mycotic aneurysms, infarcts, and brain abscesses. Whereas brain abscesses and infarcts can be detected with CT or MRI, vasculitis and mycotic aneurysms may be subtle and are usually best evaluated by highly detailed cerebral catheter angiography.

Multiple sclerosis and white matter diseases

Multiple sclerosis is by far the most commonly acquired demyelinating disease, resulting in white matter changes that are most sensitively revealed by MRI (Figure 4.16). Numerous lesions are found, potentially anywhere in the white matter. Sites of predilection are periventricular re-

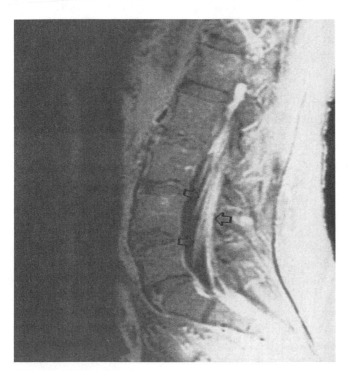

Figure 4.15 Cytomegalovirus (CMV) polyradiculitis in a patient with acquired immune deficiency syndrome. T1-weighted sagittal magnetic resonance imaging postgadolinium of the lumbar spine reveals multiple enhancing nerve roots in the cauda equina (*open arrows*).

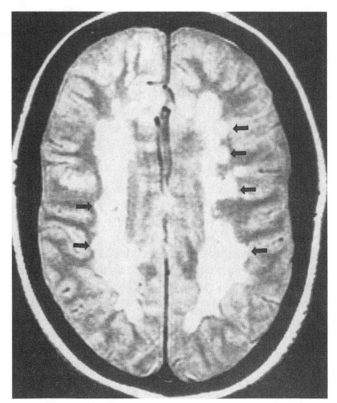

Figure 4.16 Multiple sclerosis. Axial proton density magnetic resonance imaging of the brain demonstrating focal and confluent areas of high signal intensity in the periventricular white matter. The configuration is nodular or knuckle-like, reminiscent of fingers curled around the ventricles (*arrows*)—the so-called Dawson's fingers.

gions (in particular around the atria), the corpus callosum, brainstem (especially at the root of the fifth cranial nerve), cerebellum, medulla, and cervical cord. Subtle lesions may be seen affecting the optic nerves. Active hyperacute lesions (usually <6 weeks old) may enhance with gadolinium. Occasionally, active lesions may result in tumefaction, with mass effect and surrounding edema. In chronic multiple sclerosis, one may see areas of volume loss.

The specific diagnosis of multiple sclerosis cannot be made by imaging alone because other disease processes, such as Lyme disease and even subacute arteriosclerotic encephalopathy, may closely mimic the pattern of white matter changes (Box 4.2). Use of sagittal fluid-attenuating inversion recovery (FLAIR) sequences can help differentiate demyelination from ischemia by demonstrating lesions at the callosal–septal interface (this location being common in demyelinating conditions but not in ischemia). However, multiple sclerosis is most accurately diagnosed by combining clinical and laboratory findings, including neuroimaging studies, CSF examination, and evoked potential studies.

Infectious diseases such as HIV tend to produce diffuse symmetric deep white matter changes primarily in the frontal regions, without significant mass effect or enhancement when contrast is given. Progressive multifocal leukoencephalopathy (PML) produces more focal, asymmetric, peripherally located white matter lesions primarily in the parieto-occipital lobes, without mass effect, that can rarely show mild enhancement.

Autoimmune causes of white matter abnormalities include acute disseminated encephalomyelitis (ADEM), which may follow a vaccination or viral illness, and subacute sclerosing panencephalitis (SSPE), a rare delayed complication after a measles infection. In these conditions, white matter changes may contain areas of contrast enhancement, sometimes showing slight mass effect, and may be scattered widely throughout the brain and spinal cord. Autoimmune diseases such as lupus erythematosus may also produce periventricular white matter changes.

Cyclosporine and methotrexate toxicity, as well as other chemotherapeutic agents, may lead to diffuse white matter changes; lesions that are potentially reversible if the etiology is identified early and cessation of the drug is prompt. Carbon monoxide and cyanide tend to affect the basal ganglia but may also involve areas of the deep white matter. Drugs such as heroin, cocaine, and amphetamines may produce white matter changes in a nonspecific diffuse periventricular pattern. Radiation change may be seen along the confines of the radiation ports and may also produce a tumor-like area of enhancement with surrounding edema (radiation necrosis).

Vascular causes of white matter changes on imaging include hypertension and arteriosclerosis. Binswanger's disease (subcortical arteriosclerotic encephalopathy) is a

---

> **Box 4.2** Deep white matter abnormalities on imaging
>
> **Demyelinating diseases:**
> Primary: Multiple sclerosis
> Secondary:
>   1 Infection: E.g., progressive multifocal leukoencephalopathy, HIV, Lyme disease
>   2 Autoimmune: Acute disseminated encephalomyelitis, SSPE
>   3 Metabolic: Osmotic (central pontine myelinolysis), Leigh's disease
>   4 Toxic: Methotrexate, cyclosporine, alcohol, carbon monoxide, cyanide, CNS irradiation
>   5 Vascular: Hypertension, arteriosclerosis, anoxia, migraine
>   6 Trauma: Shear injuries
> **Dysmyelinating diseases:**
>   1 Adrenoleukodystrophy, metachromatic leukodystrophy, Alexander's disease, and other rare disorders

---

rare cause of dementia in which diffuse periventricular deep white matter changes and scattered lacunar infarcts are seen. Anoxic encephalopathy may lead to diffuse white matter changes, as well as basal ganglia infarction, and migraine may rarely produce scattered, deep white matter T2 hyperintensities on MRI. In hypertensive encephalopathy, transient white matter changes may occur in the subcortical areas of the posterior circulation that revert to normal upon resolution of the hypertensive crisis.

Finally, dysmyelinating diseases are rare inherited disorders that lead to malformation of myelin and extensive breakdown of the white matter.

Congenital disorders

Many disorders of neural development manifest in children and are not within the scope of this chapter. A variety of congenital disorders may be found in adults and may be first suspected because of detection on neuroimaging. Computed tomography is often adequate to make the diagnosis, although the multiplanar presentation of MRI may be much more advantageous in determining the specific type of congenital defect.

Cephaloceles may manifest as defects in the skull with protrusions of brain or meninges, or both. These defects may be initially seen on plain films and may be further evaluated by CT scans to assess the relationship of the cephalocele to the skull. Cephaloceles may be related to other underlying disease processes such as Chiari malformations, holoprosencephaly, and aqueductal stenosis.

Corpus callosum agenesis may be suspected on CT scan by the flaring of the lateral ventricles in a "race car" configuration (with the anterior horns of the lateral ventricles widely separated as well as flared atria). Magnetic resonance imaging is the optimal way to image corpus callosal agenesis and also can show associated anomalies such as a callosal lipoma, Arnold-Chiari malformation, Dandy-Walker deformity, or schizencephaly.

Phakomatoses are neural crest disorders that lead to epidermal and neural abnormalities. In tuberous sclerosis, gray matter heterotopias, subependymal nodules, and giant-cell astrocytomas may develop. Other phakomatoses such as von Recklinghausen's disease (neurofibromatosis type I), neurofibromatosis type II, or von Hippel-Lindau disease may be associated with CNS tumors in adults.

Schizencephaly is considered to be a form of gray matter heterotopia that extends from the periphery of the brain to the ventricle. In "open-lipped" schizencephaly, there is a CSF cleft between the invaginations of gray matter, whereas "closed-lipped" schizencephaly lacks a CSF space between the gray matter lips. Magnetic resonance imaging can differentiate these abnormalities from a porencephalic cyst, which is lined by gliotic white matter and not gray matter.

Seizure disorders

Magnetic resonance imaging best evaluates seizures associated with a temporal lobe focus. Multiplanar volume acquisition with thin-section, high-resolution, T1-weighted images, as well as coronal inversion recovery (FLAIR) sequences, can yield highly detailed anatomic presentations of the temporal lobe and, in particular, the hippocampus to show mesial temporal sclerosis, vascular malformations, or neoplasms. Gradient echo MRI studies can be used to search for areas of small vascular malformations that may have bled periodically in the past, setting up a seizure focus. Positron emission tomography is used in some centers to help determine the site of origin of seizure foci in patients for whom seizure surgery is being considered. Magnetic resonance spectroscopy of the hippocampus can also show evidence of neural volume loss indicative of mesial temporal sclerosis prior to the development of anatomic imaging findings.

Skull Base Lesions

Anterior skull base

Paranasal sinuses and nasopharynx. Computed tomography is the simplest and most cost-effective way to screen for disease of the paranasal sinuses. Coronal images are usually obtained, because this technique most closely duplicates the anatomy as seen by the endoscopic sinus surgeon. The paranasal sinuses are most commonly affected by acute, allergic, or chronic inflammatory disease. Inflammatory changes may show on CT as areas of mucoperiosteal thickening, air fluid levels, or total

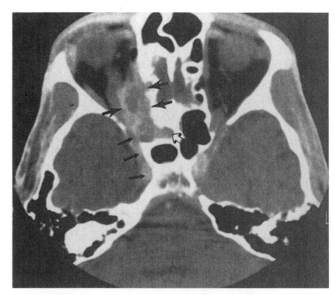

Figure 4.17 Infection. Axial computed tomography with contrast at the level of the orbits demonstrates intraorbital extension of sinusitis (open arrow) leading to an orbital abscess (*large arrows*) as a result of an Aspergillus infection. The intraorbital infectious process extends posteriorly into the cavernous sinus (*solid arrows*).

opacification. Sinusitis may be complicated by osteomyelitis, extension of infection to invade the orbit, cavernous sinus, anterior skull base, meninges, or brain (Figure 4.17), as well as vascular involvement possibly resulting in brain infarction.

The most common malignancy of the nasopharynx and paranasal sinuses is squamous cell carcinoma, whereas other tumors such as lymphoma and minor salivary gland tumors are less frequent. Computed tomography may demonstrate skull base invasion and subsequent spread to meninges or brain. Several benign neoplasms, including papillomas of the nasal cavity and juvenile nasopharyngeal angiofibroma of the pterygopalatine fossa may invade the anterior skull base. To help plan surgery for these types of lesions, MRI and CT may both be needed (Table 4.9).

The eye and orbit. Either CT or MRI can be used to evaluate the orbit. Ocular lesions, such as primary uveal melanoma or metastatic melanoma, are best imaged by MRI to search for paramagnetic effects of melanin (bright on T1-weighted images, dark on T2-weighted images). In evaluating a malignancy of the eye, MRI can also show extension along the optic nerve and involvement of meninges and cavernous sinus, which is best seen with contrast and fat suppression. Again, MRI is best for showing demyelination of the optic nerve in optic neuritis. To support the additional diagnosis of multiple sclerosis, demyelination may be sought in the brain. Abnormalities of the extraocular muscles, such as thyroid ophthalmopathy, metastasis, and orbital pseudotumor,

Table 4.9 Skull base lesions

Primary skull base lesions
   Infections
   Cephaloceles
   Meningioma
   Pituitary adenoma
   Craniopharyngioma
   Metastasis
   Osseous neoplasms
   Schwannoma
   Paraganglioma
   Epidermoid
   Arachnoid cyst
Extracranial to intracranial routes of skull base lesion extension
   Direct invasion through the bone
   Perineural spread (cranial nerve V, VII)
   Pterygopalatine fossa
   Orbital apex
   Eustachian tube to temporal bone
   Carotid canal
   Jugular foramen

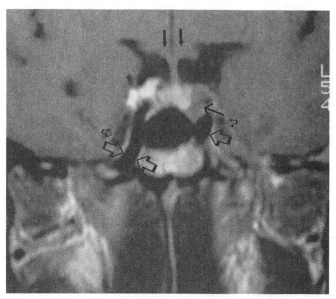

Figure 4.18 Pituitary adenoma. Coronal T1-weighted magnetic resonance imaging postgadolinium, through the sella turcica, shows lack of enhancement of the left lateral aspect of the pituitary gland (*solid arrow*). Magnetic resonance imaging is better than computed tomography since it reveals much more information about adjacent structures, including the optic chiasm (*paired solid arrows*), the carotid arteries passing through the cavernous sinuses (*large open arrows*), and Meckel's cave containing the trigeminal nerve ganglion (*small open arrows*).

can be evaluated by either MRI or CT, as can masses or inflammation involving the lacrimal gland or periosteum.

Mid skull base

In evaluating the sella turcica and parasellar regions, MRI has advantages over CT because it can clearly demonstrate structures adjacent to the pituitary gland, such as the carotid arteries and the cavernous sinus, the optic chiasm, and the meningeal surface from which a meningioma may arise. A wide variety of lesions may produce radiologic abnormalities in this region (Box 4.3). On either MRI or CT, a pituitary microadenoma typically appears as a relatively hypointense area of the gland when contrast is given (Figure 4.18), owing to the slow uptake

of contrast by the tumor relative to the normal gland, which lacks a blood–brain barrier. On the other hand, a macroadenoma (defined as a pituitary tumor larger than 1 cm) tends to enhance with contrast as brightly as the rest of the gland. To diagnose microscopic adrenocorticotropic hormone (ACTH)-secreting pituitary adenomas, superselective petrosal vein sampling may be necessary.

Posterior skull base

High-resolution CT scanning in the coronal and axial planes is the optimal way of obtaining detailed imaging of the temporal bone, which may be involved in mastoiditis and secondary cholesteatoma. If diagnosed late, these conditions may lead to destruction of the middle ear ossicles, invasion of the inner ear structures, cranial nerve VII palsy, venous thrombosis, meningitis, or brain abscess.

Magnetic resonance imaging is best for evaluating the cerebellopontine angle (CPA). Neoplasms of the temporal bone or CPA cistern include a vestibular schwannoma arising from the sheath of cranial nerve VIII (75%) (Figure 4.19), meningioma (10%), epidermoid tumors (5%), arachnoid cysts (5%), paragangliomas (glomus tympanicum and glomus jugulare), schwannomas arising from other cranial nerves, and, rarely metastasis.

Common lesions of the clivus include chordomas, chondrosarcomas, and metastases. Loss of bone marrow

Box 4.3 Differential diagnosis of sellar and suprasellar masses

Mnemonic: SATCHMOE

S: Sellar/suprasellar pituitary adenoma
A: Aneurysm
T: Tuberculosis and other granulomatous disease
C: Craniopharyngioma and Rathke's cleft cyst
H: Histiocytosis X, hamartoma
M: Meningioma, metastasis
O: Optic nerve glioma
E: Epidermoid/dermoid/teratoma

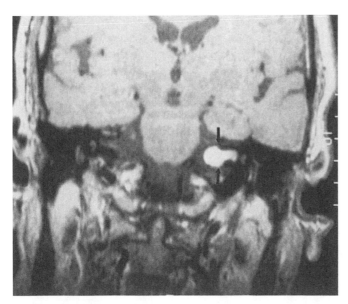

Figure 4.19 Vestibular nerve schwannoma. Coronal T1-weighted magnetic resonance imaging postgadolinium, demonstrating an enhancing ice cream cone–shaped mass involving the left internal auditory canal. The extracanalicular part of the mass is rounded like a scoop of ice-cream (*double arrows*) and is centered directly at the internal auditory canal. There is also slight widening of the internal auditory canal opening, the porous acusticus.

signal on MRI is often the earliest sign. Further evaluation of the bone matrix may be accomplished by CT. The foramen magnum may be involved by neoplasms (particularly meningiomas) and is the site of congenital abnormalities (Chiari malformations with tonsillar ectopia), as well as vascular abnormalities. In the case of meningiomas, MRI is the best modality to demonstrate dural relationships of the tumor. For vascular abnormalities (tortuous vertebral and basilar arteries or aneurysms), MRI with MRA or direct catheter angiography may be needed. Areas such as the jugular foramen may be evaluated by MRI or CT in search of neoplasms such as paragangliomas, schwannomas, or metastatic tumors.

Spine abnormalities

Trauma

Evaluation of acute spinal trauma usually begins with plain films to obtain a general overview and to search for fractures, subluxations, malalignment, and soft-tissue injuries. Further osseous detail can be obtained by CT. For spinal ligamentous injury or intraspinal abnormalities—for example, epidural hematoma, nerve root avulsion, and spinal cord contusion—and delayed complications such as myelomalacia or syrinx formation, MRI is best. To evaluate acute spinal vascular injuries, CTA or MRA may be adequate. However, angiography may be neces-

sary, allowing neurointerventional procedures to be used to treat active hemorrhage.

Neoplasia

Radiographically, the spaces of the spinal canal are described as extradural, intradural-extramedullary, and intradural-intramedullary. In addition, one should be alert for extraspinal processes that can invade the spine from adjacent soft tissues (Figure 4.20). When extradural disease is caused by neoplasia, metastatic cancer is by far the most common cause. Spinal metastasis often invades the bone marrow. This can be seen very early on MRI as signal dropout on T1-weighted images (loss of the normal fat signal). Magnetic resonance imaging may identify spinal metastasis earlier than radionuclide bone scans and provides much greater anatomic detail. Metastases to the spine commonly arise from primary tumors of the lung, breast, prostate, melanoma, and lymphoma. Myeloma may also affect the spine, resulting in compression fractures and possible extension into the spinal canal. Benign tumors of the spine are rare, and include giant-cell tumor in the vertebral body and aneurysmal bone cyst, osteoid osteomas, and osteoblastoma when located in the posterior elements. A common benign entity of the vertebral body is the hemangioma. Correlation with CT and plain films is often helpful to evaluate the cortical bony aspects of the tumor and to characterize the bone matrix.

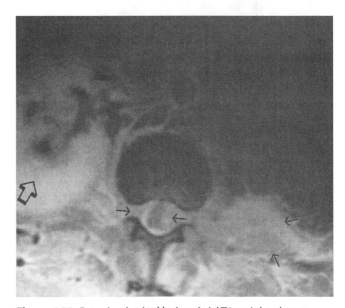

Figure 4.20 Extradural spinal lesion. Axial T1-weighted postgadolinium magnetic resonance imaging of the lumbar spine with fat saturation reveals abnormal meningeal enhancement entering the neural foramen, causing compression of the thecal sac (*linear arrows*) and extending into the paravertebral soft tissues bilaterally. A functioning right kidney (*open arrow*) is seen, but the left kidney is not visualized due to nonfunction because of obstruction. The inferior vena cava is thrombosed (*large solid arrow*).

Intradural-extramedullary tumors may be primary or metastatic. Meningiomas arise mainly in the thoracic spinal canal (80%), with the remainder (20%) being cervical, and, very rarely, lumbar. They tend to have a broad-based dural surface attachment and enhance very brightly with gadolinium. Schwannomas arise from nerve sheaths, whereas neurofibromas invade both the sheaths and the nerves. A variety of neoplasms can seed the meninges, for example, via CSF spread from primary neural tumors such as glioblastoma, ependymoma, neuroblastoma, and primitive neuroectodermal tumors, or from hematogenous metastatic tumor, such as from the lung or the breast, and melanoma. Leukemia and lymphoma may also be seen and can be either primary or metastatic.

Intradural-intramedullary neoplasms include ependymomas, astrocytomas, hemangioblastomas, lipomas, dermoids (Figure 4.21), and rarely, metastasis. Ependymomas are the most common primary intraspinal neoplasm and occur primarily at the conus and the filum terminale but can affect any part of the spinal cord. On MRI, they appear as either a solid enhancing or a partially enhancing (necrotic) mass with or without a cystic

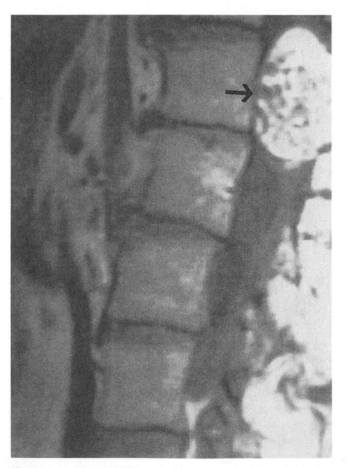

Figure 4.21 Intramedullary spinal lesion. Sagittal T1-weighted magnetic resonance imaging demonstrates an intramedullary mass with mottled high-intensity signal suggesting the presence of fat. The mass was found to be a fat-containing dermoid.

component or hemorrhage, or both. Astrocytomas can have a similar appearance. However, they are usually located in the cervical and upper thoracic cord. Spinal hemangioblastoma is less common, appearing as a cyst with an eccentric enhancing mural nodule or as an enhancing nodule alone. Intramedullary lipomas and dermoids can be distinguished by their high fat content.

Magnetic resonance imaging has become the most important tool for imaging intraspinal neoplasms. Computed tomography myelography may be sensitive to neoplasms in an extradural or even an intradural location, but is less specific when compared with MRI. Also, if suspicion exists of complete block within the spinal canal, myelography requires a C1–C2 puncture to avoid reducing pressure below the level of the block, to prevent potential herniation of the brain.

Degenerative disease

Many components of the spine can produce symptoms due to compression of the spinal cord or nerve roots. Degenerative disc disease may be due to frank herniation, bulges, or disc and osteophyte complexes. Herniation of the disc may be focal—localized at the disc interspace level; extruded—discs migrate out from the disc interspace level either upward or downward while remaining attached to the parent disc; or sequestered—a disc fragment that becomes detached from its parent disc and migrates away from the disc interspace. Whether symptoms occur depends on the location of disc herniation. Discs that are central (midline) may result in cord compression and myelopathy, whereas those that herniate into a neural foramen or into a subarticular or lateral recess may impinge on the adjacent nerve roots, resulting in a radiculopathy (Figure 4.22).

Osteophytes may contribute to stenotic changes depending on their location. Those at the edges of disc interspaces may protrude into the central canal and carry the adjacent disc back with them. This forms a disc–osteophyte complex, or hard disc, and may require surgical removal. Osteophytes may cause stenosis at the central canal, the subarticular or lateral recess, or at the neural foramen (Figure 4.23). Degeneration of the articular facet joints may result in hypertrophy of the superior articular facet, which not uncommonly causes stenosis at the neural foramen. A disc that bulges laterally may also cause foraminal stenosis. Hypertrophy of the adjacent pedicle or congenital short pedicles may lead to stenosis of the central canal or lateral recess. Degenerative changes to facet joints can also lead to synovitis and the development of synovial cysts that can subsequently compress an adjacent nerve root.

Computed tomography myelography is an excellent means of evaluating degenerative spinal disease due to bony hypertrophy. It has been replaced to a large extent by MRI, which is less invasive and gives additional in-

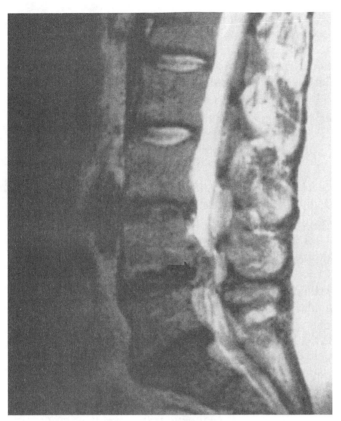

Figure 4.22 Disc herniation. Sagittal T2-weighted magnetic resonance imaging shows narrowing of the thecal sac at the L4–L5 level due to a mass corresponding to disc signal (*arrow*). This is an extruded herniated disc that has migrated cephalad from the disc space.

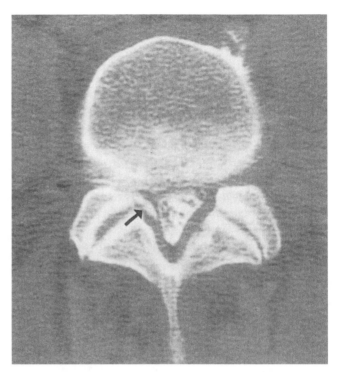

Figure 4.23 Osteophyte. Computed tomography myelogram shows a large osteophyte narrowing the thecal sac and right lateral recess (*arrow*).

formation about the adjacent spinal cord, nerve roots, and bone marrow changes in the adjacent vertebra. For example, early vertebral end plate changes (type I) may be seen on MRI as areas of edema or granulation tissue and therefore may enhance. Later changes may include fatty end plate changes (type 2) and sclerosis at the end plates (type 3). Clinical judgment is often needed to determine the significance of these abnormal imaging findings.

Recurrent back pain after spinal surgery is referred to as the "failed back." This syndrome has numerous causes, with recurrent disc prolapse at the operative site and development of scar tissue high on the list. Imaging with contrast helps distinguish these problems because scar tissue enhances, whereas the disc tends not to do so. In either case, MRI is the optimal means of evaluation, provided that surgery did not introduce a substantial amount of metal into the individual's body, resulting in significant imaging artifact that may preclude satisfactory evaluation (Box 4.4).

Infection

The most common cause of spinal infection is *Staphylococcus*, which is usually the result of seeding from the chest, kidneys, or a cardiac valvular source, as well as iatrogenically, either following surgery or from intravenous drug use. Other pyogenic spinal infections may be due to *Streptococcus* or *Escherichia coli*. Vertebral osteomyelitis and discitis may progress to an epidural or paravertebral abscess. Epidural abscess may compress the thecal sac, leading to spinal cord compromise, cauda equina syndrome, or both. Tuberculosis, brucellosis, and fungal infections such as coccidiomycosis and cryptococcus also may affect the spine. Tuberculosis most commonly affects the lower thoracic spine and produces bony changes that may be complicated by an epidural abscess. The discs are affected late, in contrast to pyogenic bacterial infections that affect the discs early.

Box 4.4 Causes of failed back surgery

▶ Residual or recurrent disc herniation
▶ Disc herniation elsewhere
▶ Scar formation
▶ Facet arthrosis
▶ Discitis, osteomyelitis, arachnoiditis, neuritis
▶ Epidural hematoma
▶ Failed instrumentation or bone fusion

Imaging for a spinal infection often starts with plain films of the spine, which may show early signs such as loss of disc interspace height or irregularity of the subchondral aspects of the vertebral end plates. For more definitive diagnosis, MRI is the technique of choice because it is very sensitive to the changes of osteomyelitis and discitis, and can detect an epidural abscess (Figure 4.24). Computed tomography myelography can demonstrate an epidural abscess, but it is not specific. Other extradural defects including epidural hematoma, epidural neoplasm, and herniated discs, can have a similar appearance. Also, when performing a spinal puncture, there is a danger of traversing an abscess with the needle and seeding the subarachnoid space. Therefore, especially if MRI is available, CT myelography should be avoided in this situation.

It is sometimes unclear whether an abnormal enhancing area in the spine represents postsurgical scar, epidural neoplasm, or infection. An infectious cause may be sought by radionuclide scanning with Indium[111]-labeled leukocytes, or gallium, or using a three-phase bone scan with technetium. The most specific way to diagnose spinal infection and determine the causative organism is by needle biopsy under CT or fluoroscopic guidance.

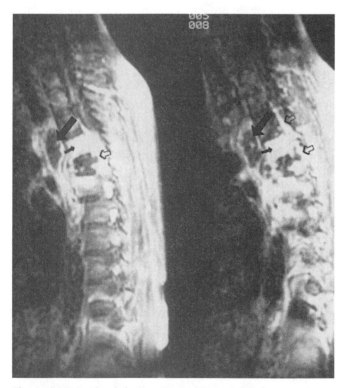

Figure 4.24 Epidural abscess. Sagittal T1-weighted magnetic resonance imaging postgadolinium in a patient with acute myelopathy shows abnormal enhancement of upper thoracic vertebral body (*small solid arrow*) and in the epidural space (*open arrows*), consistent with osteomyelitis and an epidural abscess causing severe central canal stenosis. There is also a prevertebral fluid collection indicating an abscess (*large solid arrow*) adjacent to the thoracic aorta and posing a major vascular threat.

Inflammation of the intradural nerve roots (polyradiculitis) with abnormal enhancement (Figure 4.15) may occur with HIV-related CMV. Similar enhancement can occur in other viral illnesses, Guillain-Barré syndrome, and arachnoiditis. Sarcoidosis, tuberculosis, metastatic meningeal carcinomatosis, and lymphoma are also potential considerations, although the enhancement pattern is usually more nodular with these entities. Magnetic resonance T1-weighted imaging with gadolinium using fat saturation is the best way to visualize these lesions.

Demyelinating disease

Multiple sclerosis is the most common demyelinating disease to affect the spinal cord. Magnetic resonance imaging may show hyperintensities in the white matter on T2-weighted imaging, and active plaques may enhance when contrast is given. Transverse myelitis may lead to a similar appearance of the spinal cord.

Congenital abnormalities

Congenital spinal defects are often initially noticed on plain films, which may show scoliosis, or defects such as spina bifida, hemivertebrae, or block vertebrae. Computed tomography and MRI are valuable if further workup is needed. Magnetic resonance imaging may be useful in demonstrating associated defects, such as a tethered cord (held in an abnormally low position by lesions such as lipomas) or diastematomyelia (a defect with a bony bar or a fibrous band that splits the cord). The Chiari I malformation, with unusually low cerebellar tonsils that may have an associated syrinx (usually cervical), is best evaluated by MRI, as are myelomeningoceles (seen in association with spinal dysraphism or Arnold-Chiari [Chiari II] malformation).

On the Horizon

The field of radiology is subject to profound influences by cutting-edge technologies. Several advances are mentioned briefly.

Digital radiography allows lower radiation exposure, electronic manipulation of images, and digital transfer and storage of images. Multidetector spiral CT has allowed faster acquisition of images, and now spiral CTA is being used as a noninvasive screen or confirmatory study for carotid disease (stenosis or dissection), aneurysm workup, and other vascular disorders. Sonographic resolution continues to improve, and new sonographic contrast agents—some in current use for vascular sonography—may extend the role of neurosonography. Intraoperative neurosonography is becoming widely used to aid in surgical resection of lesions. In addition, high-intensity, focused ultrasound itself can be used therapeutically, such as in thermal tumor ablation or vascular thrombolysis. In nuclear medicine, a host of new carrier compounds are being tested and may yield important information about brain physiology. These compounds can also be linked to therapeutic agents to act as a "magic bullet," once reaching their intended target receptor. New research with supercomputers may obviate the need for collimators, decrease the dose of radiopharmaceutical needed, and greatly increase the spatial resolution of nuclear medicine studies.

In no area of radiology do changing technologies hold more promise than MRI. New ultra-fast MRI systems allow image acquisition times rapid enough to prevent movement artifact. Real-time MRI is being tested and now occasionally used for image-guided interventional procedures at academic centers. Magnetic resonance spectroscopy continues to improve, and now three-dimensional "whole-brain" acquisition is possible, which holds promise for physiologic brain studies via individual metabolite brain mapping. Functional MRI is defined as any MRI technique that is sensitive to the activation of neuronal tissue. The technique most used is based on cerebral perfusion, and has the ability to image the inherent hemoglobin oxygenation state without exogenous contrast material—known as blood oxygenation level dependent (BOLD) contrast—since there is a disproportionate increase in regional cerebral blood flow and hemoglobin oxygenation level after brain activation, relative to the local surrounding metabolic rate. This technique allows mapping of brain activation with different tasks, and is being used at present to map eloquent regions of the brain and enhance our understanding of how the brain functions. Other newer sequences, such as arterial-spin labeling, are being investigated, and may provide greater sensitivity and spatial localization of brain activation mapping as well as less patient motion artifact and precise measurements of cerebral blood flow. The role of diffusion-weighted imaging, now in common clinical practice for the early detection of cerebral ischemia, has been further expanded by exploiting the inherent anisotropy (limited movement) of water molecules within neuronal axon bundles to generate diffusion tensor images of the white matter tracts throughout the brain. This type of imaging can show whether a neoplasm has invaded an eloquent tract such as the corticospinal tract (precluding complete resection) or if the tract is merely displaced (allowing safe removal of the entirety of the lesion). Additionally, white matter fractional anisotropy mapping holds promise for detecting white matter abnormalities, such as multiple sclerosis, earlier than conventional T2-weighted or FLAIR sequences. With the use of state-of-the-art super-high-field strength magnets (3 Tesla and above), the resolution of MRI will be greatly increased, leading to superb images, such that MRA will rival digital subtraction catheter angiography and obviate the need for invasive diagnostic vascular examinations. Finally, there are exciting possibilities involving MRI using atoms other than hydrogen, for example ^{13}C, ^{23}Na, and ^{31}P, particularly in conjunction with MR spectroscopy.

Annotated Bibliography

Edelman RR, Hesselink JR, Zlatkin MB, Crues JV, eds. *Clinical magnetic resonance imaging*, 3rd ed. Philadelphia: WB Saunders Elsevier, 2006.
A comprehensive review of the use of MRI in clinical practice.
Grossman RL, Yousem DM. *Neuroradiology: The requisites*, 2nd ed. Philadelphia: Mosby Elsevier, 2003.
An excellent, easy-to-understand overview of the basics of neuroradiology.
Harnsberger HR. *Diagnostic imaging: head and Neck*. Salt Lake City: Amirsys, 2004.
An extensive and well-illustrated survey of head and neck imaging.
Osborne AG. *Diagnostic imaging: Brain*. Salt Lake City: Amirsys, 2004.
An extensive and well-illustrated survey of brain imaging.
Ross, JS. *Diagnostic imaging: Spine*. Salt Lake City: Amirsys, 2004.
An extensive and well-illustrated survey of spine imaging.

COMMON PROBLEMS IN ADULT NEUROLOGY

Syncope and Seizures

Andrew D. Massey

The task of evaluating a patient who comes to the office or emergency room complaining of a momentary loss of consciousness, but who appears otherwise well at the time of the visit, makes many physicians uncomfortable. When no diagnosis is immediately reached, the physician must decide if a potentially serious disorder is present and the patient should be admitted for observation and a series of tests, or if the patient can safely be discharged home and assessed as an outpatient. In addition, there is the question of what tests are necessary to arrive at the correct diagnosis, in what order they should be performed so as to minimize the time and expense of an evaluation, or when might it be appropriate and safe to simply observe the patient without subjecting them to a laundry-list of investigations.

Not uncommonly, a firm diagnosis of the problem is not arrived at with the initial encounter, or the wrong diagnosis is mistakenly assumed, sometimes with unfavorable life-long consequences (for example, incorrectly labeling a patient as having epileptic seizures). The goals of this chapter are to review the basic pathophysiologic concepts involved with transient interruption of consciousness, apply these concepts to several common disorders, understand when laboratory tests may be helpful in reaching a diagnosis, and recognize when the patient's symptoms may be due to a potentially serious disorder requiring immediate attention.

Definitions

Syncope is a term used to describe a sudden, brief, and reversible loss of consciousness usually accompanied by flaccid muscle tone that is often, but not uniformly, due to acute impairment in cerebral blood flow. Terms sometimes used by patients to describe syncope include: *blackout*, *faint*, or even *seizure*. Syncope should be differentiated from symptoms of feeling *dizzy*, *light-headed*, or *woozy*, which the patient may use to describe a near loss, but not complete loss, of consciousness. These latter terms often are meant to describe symptoms of impending loss of consciousness or *near-syncope*. Although some authors use the term *seizure* to describe any sudden behavioral change, and reserve the term *epileptic seizure* when this behavior is brought about by a paroxysmal discharge of cortical neurons, in this chapter the term *seizure* will be synonymous with *epileptic seizure*.

Syncope

Epidemiology

Approximately 3% of all emergency room visits in the United States are for syncope. In the younger patient, the most common cause is neurally mediated syncope, whereas in the elderly orthostatic hypotension or cardiovascular causes are more frequent (Table 5.1). In the past, nearly one-half of all incidents remained undiagnosed even after prolonged observation and diagnostic studies. However, more recently, newer diagnostic tests utilizing prolonged outpatient cardiac monitoring, electrophysiologic laboratory studies of the heart, tilt table testing to reproduce orthostatic stress, video-EEG recording, and the

---

Table 5.1 Common causes of transient loss of consciousness

Neurally mediated syncope
Situational syncope
　Micturition syncope
　Tussive syncope
　Deglutination syncope
　Defecation syncope
　Glossopharyngeal neuralgia
　Carotid sinus hypersensitivity
Orthostatic syncope
Cardiac syncope
　Arrhythmia
　Valvular heart disease
　Cardiomyopathy
　Atrial myxoma
　Cardiac tamponade
　Pulmonary embolus
Cerebrovascular disease
　Vertebrobasilar insufficiency
　Subclavian steal
　Vertebrobasilar migraine
Brainstem compression
　Arnold-Chiari malformation
　Hydrocephalic attacks
　Epileptic seizure
Psychiatric disorders
　Panic attacks
　Somatization disorder
　Psychogenic unresponsiveness
　Malingering

---

wider application of the psychiatric interview, have enabled a reliable diagnosis in nearly 85%.

Syncope may underscore a severe condition such as a cardiac arrhythmia and the risk for sudden death if left untreated. However, in spite of the forewarning, it seems that if the cause for the syncopal episode remains undiagnosed, and no indication of heart disease is evidenced from the patient's initial examination, history, or electrocardiogram (ECG), the risk of serious morbidity or mortality is low. The greatest danger for serious consequences comes with the diagnosis of cardiac syncope; so consequently, initial investigations should focus on discovering or excluding a cardiovascular source.

Pathogenesis

Consciousness is the awareness of oneself and one's surroundings, whereas, *unconsciousness* is the inability to have subjective experiences and respond to sensory stimuli. The cerebral cortex and brainstem reticular activating system normally function to maintain consciousness, and diseases that produce dysfunction of either, or both, lead to an unconscious state. Consciousness may be interrupted by one of four basic mechanisms: decreased cerebral blood flow (which happens with asystole of 5–8 seconds, or with an absolute drop in blood pressure to ,≤60 mm Hg), impaired delivery to the brain of necessary nutrients such as oxygen or glucose, interruption of the brain's normal neuronal function by neurotoxins, or disruption of the brain's neuronal electrical activity such as occurs during a seizure.

Initial Approach

The critical step in attaining a correct diagnosis is an accurate and sufficient history. Obtaining details of the circumstances leading up to the event, the behavior and subjective sensations witnessed or experienced during the event, and the condition and activities of the patient upon regaining consciousness are most important. Because the patient, due to his unconscious state, is often unable to provide all of this information, it is crucial that a reliable witness be interviewed.

It must first be established that consciousness was in fact lost. Alternatively, was the incident due to some other condition besides syncope? Were the symptoms due to a spinning sensation or true vertigo, disequilibrium, temporary weakness, or a brief confusional state during which time the patient appeared awake but disoriented? These symptoms would suggest alternative diagnoses different from those producing syncope.

Knowing the patient's position when consciousness was lost is essential. If syncope occurred during a postural change toward a more upright position, orthostatic syncope must be considered (especially in a patient with a history of multiple events, all occurring soon after making postural changes). Syncope that occurs after standing for a prolonged period of time is consistent with either orthostatic hypotension or neurally mediated syncope. Cardiac arrhythmia, an epileptic seizure, or a transient ischemic attack (TIA) will occur independent of the position of the patient.

If syncope occurs with physical exertion, a cardiac cause should be seriously considered. Severe valvular heart disease (e.g., aortic stenosis), obstructive cardiomyopathy, acute coronary ischemia, or pulmonary hypertension may all cause syncope brought on by exertion, and a thorough evaluation to confirm or exclude these diagnoses must be initiated. If headache accompanies the exertionally induced syncope, a posterior fossa mass or congenital abnormality such as an Arnold-Chiari malformation might be present. Other clues to a cardiac source are symptoms of palpitations, dyspnea, chest pain, a personal history of heart disease, or a family history of sudden death occurring at a young age (e.g., prolonged QT interval, or hypertrophic cardiomyopathy). Following a syncopal event, if the patient complains of "the worst headache" of his life, it is essential to exclude a subarachnoid hemorrhage.

Syncope occurring only in relation to specific activities such as micturition, coughing, swallowing, or defecating suggests a *situational syncope*. A seizure or migraine attack may be ushered in by an aura. Syncope during exercise of the arm, sometimes preceded by an aching pain involving the arm, could be the result of a subclavian steal syndrome. Dysarthria, diplopia, vertigo, disequilibrium, and/or focal weakness and sensory changes preceding or following the syncopal event signals vertebrobasilar ischemia, or if followed by a headache (especially in a young female patient) may be due to vertebrobasilar migraine.

If the duration of unconsciousness is more than 5 minutes, the disorder is less likely to be neurally mediated syncope or orthostatic hypotension. In these conditions, unconsciousness is rarely longer than a few minutes, and often lasts less than 1 minute unless the patient suffers a traumatic head injury as a result of the fall or is prevented from falling to the ground (e.g., in a phone booth). Cardiovascular, cerebrovascular, or metabolic conditions (or a seizure that is confused with syncope) may result in a prolonged period of unconsciousness. Urinary incontinence can occur with either neurally mediated syncope or a seizure, but a deeply bitten tongue strongly argues for a recent generalized tonic–clonic seizure, especially if the tongue is laterally bitten (the tip of the tongue may sometimes be bitten when the patient falls from other causes).

The physical examination must include a complete general and neurologic examination, and should be performed as soon after the syncopal event as possible. Diagnostic signs may vanish as the time between the event and the examination increases. Unfortunately, many patients are examined well after the event has occurred, when they are conscious and asymptomatic. With recurring episodes, it can be helpful diagnostically to teach family or friends of the patient to measure pulse rate, blood pressure, respirations, and response to noxious or other stimuli. With the prevalence of personal home video recorders, recurring episodes of syncope might be captured on tape, so that the behavior during and immediately following the event can be reviewed for clues as to the diagnosis.

The blood pressure and pulse should at least be measured with the patient lying and then standing. It is best if the supine pressure is obtained after the patient has rested on his back for 10 minutes. After standing, the pulse and blood pressure are measured immediately and again at 1 and 2 minutes. If there is a trend for the blood pressure to slide downward, the recording in the upright position should be continued until the lowest point is reached or syncope comes about. Criteria for the diagnosis of orthostatic hypotension are given later in this chapter in the section on orthostatic hypotension.

With subclavian steal, the blood pressure will show a significant difference when measured in the normal arm compared to the affected arm. The heart examination may reveal either an irregular, fast, or slow pulse suggesting an arrhythmia. Presence of a murmur could identify valvular heart disease as the basis for syncope. Findings of congestive heart failure put the patient at a higher risk for serious morbidity or mortality following a syncopal event. Recognition of asymmetrical weakness or reflexes, a Babinski response, visual field deficit, or language error should lead to a more extensive neurologic evaluation, with the possible findings of cerebrovascular disease or other intracranial lesion.

Laboratory Tests

When a cause for the syncopal event is reliably determined, the diagnosis is often made from the history and physical examination. The role of laboratory tests is usually to confirm what is already suspected. However, certain tests are sometimes helpful as screening tools and, in the case of an ECG, could help the physician decide if the patient is at higher risk for significant morbidity or sudden death, and may influence a decision to admit to the hospital or dismiss from the emergency room. Nonselective cardiac testing is rarely rewarding, not economically justified, and can sometimes be associated with unnecessary risk.

General metabolic profiles or hemograms are uncommonly helpful in detecting a diagnosis that is not already suspected. A hemogram can be used to confirm a significant anemia in a patient with a recent gastroin-

Pearls and Perils

Evaluation of patients with syncope

▶ The patient's description of the event should always be confirmed by a reliable witness whenever possible.

▶ The correct diagnosis can often be established or suspected at the time of the initial examination. Laboratory studies are often helpful only in confirming a suspected diagnosis.

▶ Cardiovascular and orthostatic syncope are more common in the elderly, whereas neurally mediated syncope is more common in the young.

▶ The elderly patient may have multiple reasons for syncope, including heart disease, arrhythmia, medication effect, and orthostatic hypotension.

▶ It is helpful to examine the patient as close in time to the event as possible.

▶ A supine blood pressure and pulse after the patient has remained prone for at least 10 minutes, and then after standing for at least 2 minutes should be performed in nearly every evaluation for syncope.

▶ The ECG is important in the initial evaluation not only for diagnostic purposes, but to help stratify the patient into either a high- or low-risk group for serious morbidity or mortality.

▶ Prolonged ECG monitoring is indicated when a history of heart disease is present, and when the cause of syncope remains unknown after the initial assessment.

testinal hemorrhage and orthostatic hypotension, but may not be as sensitive as testing stool for occult blood when the hemorrhage is too fresh to result in a measurable change in the hematocrit. A metabolic profile may confirm a prerenal azotemia when congestive heart failure or depleted intravascular volume is presumed. A recent generalized tonic–clonic seizure may produce all of the following: high anion gap metabolic acidosis due to unmeasured lactic acid, elevation of the creatine phosphokinase (CPK) because of rhabdomyolysis, and a postictal leukocytosis with primarily mature granulocytes and relative lymphocytopenia. A recent myocardial infarction can also cause an elevated CPK. An elevated prolactin level may occur following a complex partial or generalized tonic–clonic seizure, but can also be elevated after a syncopal event, therefore, limiting its usefulness unless a consistent clinical history is available.

Drug screens confirm the clinical suspicion of drug overdose or detect the presence of drugs, such as cocaine, that might precipitate a cardiac arrhythmia or epileptic seizure. However, these tests are usually more helpful in the evaluation of patients with altered mental status who are brought to the emergency room still unconscious or

delirious. It is uncommon that a diagnosis not thought of after a detailed history and examination is uncovered by the results of these laboratory tests.

A 12-lead ECG is standard in nearly all evaluations of syncope unless the diagnosis is obvious after the initial history and examination. The presence of heart block, short PR interval, or prolonged QT interval is evidence for an underlying conduction abnormality and a potential arrhythmia. Findings of atrial fibrillation, sinus bradycardia or tachycardia, ventricular arrhythmia, or changes of an acute myocardial infarction often only validate what is already suspected from the interview and examination. Patients without a history of heart disease, no symptoms suggesting a cardiac cause, and who have a normal ECG portend, more likely, a benign cause. Except for a tilt table test (which will be discussed later), these patients usually do not require further cardiac evaluation.

Prolonged cardiac monitoring either with outpatient ambulatory recorders such as a 24-hour Holter monitor or continuous inpatient monitoring is useful only with a history of heart disease, an abnormal ECG, symptoms suggesting an arrhythmia, or if the patient remains undiagnosed with recurrent syncope. If prolonged monitoring fails, referral to a cardiologist for electrophysiologic studies (EPS) is sometimes diagnostic, especially if the syncopal spell was preceded by palpitations, or there is a history of a recent myocardial infarction with the risk of a ventricular tachyarrhythmia or a family history of sudden death at a young age. Unfortunately, during EPS, arrhythmias unassociated with the patient's syncopal spells may be induced. Therefore, the results of these studies should be cautiously interpreted when a compatible history or positive response to medications is lacking.

Prolonged loop monitors that can be worn by the patient for weeks, months, or even longer have resulted in fewer undiagnosed events. The externally placed monitors are complicated by patient error when they forget to activate the monitor at the time of the event, inappropriately erase recorded information, disconnect or misplace leads, or develop an allergic reaction to the electrode pads. Implantable loop monitors avoid many of the patient errors, but are expensive and should be used when other tests are unrewarding and there is a high suspicion for an arrhythmia.

Echocardiograms are helpful in revealing structural disease when symptoms, examination, or ECG suggest a cardiac source. A valvular abnormality may be unrelated to the patient's symptoms, but the echocardiogram can assess the severity of the valvular disorder and help determine its role in the patient's syncope. Echocardiograms and stress ECG are particularly useful when evaluating exertional syncope.

Carotid massage may identify carotid hypersensitivity but has the risk of inducing ventricular fibrillation, asystole, stroke, or sudden death. It should only be carried out where the appropriate monitoring and resuscitation equipment are accessible. The technique is not standardized, and as many as 5–25% of asymptomatic elderly men may have a positive response. Carotid massage should be reserved for patients whose history suggests syncope occurring in a setting in which the carotid sinus might be stimulated (for example, while shaving, wearing a tight-fitting collar, or turning the head).

The tilt table test can be valuable in identifying patients with neurally mediated syncope. Its sensitivity in detecting disease in the adult patient may approach 80%, but is dependent on several variables including the angle and duration of the tilt, and if chemical stimulation with isoproterenol or nitroglycerin is used. The specificity of the test may be nearly 90%, but patients may have a positive response to tilt table testing while their spontaneous events could be due to an unrelated diagnosis. Tilt table testing is indicated for recurrent undiagnosed syncope in the patient with no evidence of heart disease (or for whom cardiovascular causes have been ruled out). If a patient has a history of heart disease, an abnormal ECG, or symptoms suggesting a cardiovascular source for syncope, other cardiac disorders should be excluded before proceeding to tilt table testing. The reproducibility of a positive test for neurally mediated syncope is low, therefore, it is not useful in appraising response to therapy.

Neuroimaging procedures such as computed tomography, magnetic resonance imaging, and cerebral angiography are only indicated when the initial examination suggests a disorder involving the central nervous system (CNS) that could produce a transient loss of consciousness. Rarely is an electroencephalogram (EEG) diagnostic of a seizure disorder unless the episode is occurring during the recording of the EEG. Usually, the diagnosis of a seizure disorder is dependent on the descriptions of the patient and any witness of the behavioral changes during the event, and the EEG is obtained to aid in the classification of the seizure type. Intensive neurodiagnostic monitoring with continuous inpatient EEG and video recording can differentiate seizures from nonepileptic events such as psychogenic unresponsiveness, anxiety attacks, or malingering. Unfortunately, the value of this highly diagnostic test is limited by the availability of special monitoring equipment, advanced technical and interpretive skills of the EEG technologist and electroencephalographer, expense of prolonged inpatient monitoring, and the variable frequency of the patient's spells. Prolonged EEG monitoring is more likely to be diagnostic if at least several spells occur weekly.

Diagnostic tests for evaluating syncope can be performed as an outpatient, but hospitalization for observation should be undertaken when the potential exists for serious risk to the patient. If this is an isolated or rare syncopal episode, the history and examination give no evidence for heart disease either suspected or known, and the ECG is normal, then there seems to be minimal and acceptable risk in discharging the patient from the emergency room or office and arranging for an outpatient evaluation. Inpatient admission for observation and initiation of diagnostic studies is often indicated in the following situations: (a) evidence of a cardiovascular cause for syncope from the history, examination, or abnormal ECG (e.g., acute ischemic changes, arrhythmia, increased QT interval, bundle branch block, or conduction defect), (b) normal ECG and no history of heart disease but the patient presents with chest pain or exertional syncope, (c) syncope due to severe side effects from medications, (d) severe orthostatic hypotension, (e) neurologic disorders, (f) syncope with a resultant injury that requires hospitalization for treatment of the injury, or (g) an associated diagnosed disorder that requires hospitalization (for example, a gastrointestinal hemorrhage, or a fractured hip incurred when the patient fell).

With a history of recurrent, undiagnosed syncope after extensive investigations, submitting the patient to a psychiatric interview might be rewarding. This is especially true in the setting of generalized anxiety, major depression, somatization, drug, or alcohol history. Video EEG with ECG monitoring, if the patient is experiencing frequent events, can be diagnostic for true seizures, nonepileptic psychogenic seizures, or pseudo-syncope.

Specific Causes

Neurally mediated syncope

Neurally mediated syncope, sometimes referred to as *vasovagal* or *reflex syncope*, may be the most common cause of syncope in patients without a history of heart disease. A reflex activated by stimulation of arterial or visceral mechanoreceptors causes this form of syncope. Mechanoreceptors located in the walls of the bladder, gastrointestinal tract, or carotid sinus are stimulated by pressure or distention and send afferent messages to the brainstem, which, in turn, transmits an efferent signal via the vagus nerve to the sinus node of the heart, producing bradycardia. Vasodilation, which is also part of the reflex and which contributes to the decrease in blood pressure, may be due to a reduction in efferent sympathetic activity.

The reflex can be precipitated by a sudden painful or emotionally charged experience. At other times, it occurs without any identifiable initiating event, usually while the patient is standing or walking. In this situation, venous pooling in the lower extremities causes a decrease in filling of the left ventricle and a compensatory increase in sympathetic stimulation to increase heart rate and maintain cardiac output. However, vigorous and rapid contractions of an incompletely filled left ventricle can stimulate mechanoreceptors, which produce paradoxical reflex bradycardia and peripheral vasodilation. Loss of consciousness in some cases is due to the cardioinhibitory response with bradycardia or even sinus arrest. In other events, it is due to the vasodilatory response with minimal or no reduction in heart rate, and in others hypotension is affected by mixed cardioinhibitory and vasodilatory responses.

Neurally mediated syncope may occur while a person is sitting or even lying down, but is most often experienced while a person is standing for a prolonged period of time, usually in a hot, crowded room while in a slightly dehydrated state. Symptoms of nausea, blurred vision, diaphoresis, generalized weakness, and the feeling of an impending loss of consciousness (presyncope) may precede the syncopal event. The patient then loses consciousness, becomes limp, and falls to the ground. A few arrhythmic myoclonic jerks or even incontinence may be observed and mistaken for a seizure (however, the myoclonus of neurally mediated syncope is quite brief, whereas a generalized tonic–clonic seizure may be prolonged for several minutes). The myoclonus is due to a momentary decrease in cerebral blood flow and cerebral hypoxia. Almost immediately after falling, a return of consciousness occurs, followed by a short period of confusion, and soon after an ability to return to regular activities without limitations (Table 5.2).

The diagnosis of neurally mediated syncope is based on a typical history, a normal physical examination, and the exclusion of other possible causes. For patients with an atypical history or recurrent episodes of syncope, a tilt table test may help identify neurally mediated syncope and distinguish it from other disorders. With neurally me-

diated syncope, immediately tilting the patient upright results in tachycardia and normal blood pressure, followed several minutes later by sudden bradycardia, peripheral vasodilation, or both, with a profound drop in blood pressure. In contrast, orthostatic hypotension causes an immediate and continuous drop in blood pressure when the patient is tilted upright from a reclined position.

Various management strategies for neurally mediated syncope have been employed. Unfortunately, most have only the strength of anecdotal reports or small series of patients to support their use. The most important first-line treatment for neurally mediated syncope is to educate the patient as to the cause of the disorder, help him to be aware of, and avoid when possible, precipitating events (e.g., hot crowded rooms, intramuscular injections, phlebotomy), recognize premonitory symptoms that may herald a loss of consciousness, and what they can do to abort the episode (sitting or lying down until the symptoms resolve). If symptoms are recurrent, volume expansion by increasing salt and fluid intake, moderate exercise to strengthen leg muscles and improve venous return, and waist high support stocking may help. Some patients may benefit from being taught isometric counterpressure maneuvers such as tightening the hand grip and arm muscles or crossing their legs while avoiding straining and causing a coinciding Valsalva maneuver (which can impair venous return to the heart and increase the risk for syncope). Tilt training, by having the patient stand against a wall for 15–20 minutes or as tolerated two or three times each day has been shown in some instances to reduce the frequency of syncope, but requires persistence and a highly motivated patient to continue the exercises.

For persistent neurally mediated syncopal events, drug therapy with β-blockers, scopolamine, disopyramide, angiotensin-converting enzyme inhibitors, selective serotonin reuptake inhibitors, theophylline, and ephedrine have been used with inconsistent or unsustained benefit. Addition of mineralocorticoids (for example, fludrocortisone) may be used to increase intravascular volume, but elderly patients should be carefully monitored for precipitation of congestive heart failure. Midodrine, an α-agonist, may help maintain vascular tone and prevent or dampen the vasodilatory effect of neurally mediated syncope. Its short effect requires that it be dosed two or three times each day, but should not be used before bedtime so as to avoid the sometimes serious problem of supine hypertension at night. Drug treatment for neurally mediated syncope should only be used for recurrent events that may result in injury when avoidance activities, maximum hydration, and physiologic maneuvers have failed.

Some reports show mixed benefits from insertion of a pacemaker for intractable neurally mediated syncope. However, it is not clear just what clinical features predict a successful outcome. For now, a pacemaker might be

---

Table 5.2 Neurally mediated syncope

Discriminating features

1 Evidence of an overactive autonomic nervous system
2 Positive tilt table test with reflex bradycardia and/or peripheral vasodilatation with reproduction of the syncopal episode
3 Sometimes triggered by specific circumstances (i.e., situational syncope)

Consistent features

1 Usually occurs in younger patients
2 Usually occurs while standing in a hot, crowded room
3 Physical examination, screening laboratory tests, and ECG are normal
4 Consciousness regained almost immediately after falling

Variable features

1 Presyncopal symptoms of blurred vision, nausea, diaphoresis, generalized weakness, and sense of impending loss of consciousness
2 Brief myoclonic jerks accompanying loss of consciousness

considered for patients with frequent and intractable neurally mediated syncope with risk for significant injury, who demonstrate a strong cardioinhibitory response rather than a vasodilatory response on tilt table testing, who fail to respond to nonpharmacologic and pharmacologic therapy, and for whom other diagnoses for syncope have been thoroughly investigated (for example, psychiatric and cardiovascular causes).

Situational syncope

When it is associated with specific circumstances, neurally mediated syncope is sometimes referred to as *situational syncope*. Syncope occurring during venipuncture may be the most commonly observed type of situational syncope. The sudden sharp pain of the phlebotomist's needle or the emotional shock of witnessing blood provokes reflex bradycardia, vasodilation, and brief loss of consciousness. Syncope can usually be avoided by placing the patient in a reclined position with their eyes diverted from the venipuncture site. Avoiding or modifying the offending situation that triggers reflex bradycardia and vasodilatation usually treats the other forms of situational syncope.

Micturition syncope occurs during or shortly following urination. Typically, the patient arises from bed in the middle of the night to go to the bathroom. Then, while urinating, mechanoreceptors in the wall of the contracting bladder are stimulated to produce reflex bradycardia and vasodilation. Standing adds an orthostatic component to the hypotension and contributes to the loss of consciousness. Treatment consists of recognizing the event as micturition syncope and having the patient urinate while sitting down.

Cough or *tussive syncope* occurs during a fierce bout of coughing, usually in the setting of chronic obstructive pulmonary disease. An increase in intrathoracic pressure brought on by coughing intensifies the hypotensive response by impairing venous return and decreasing cardiac output. Vigorous coughing may induce a gag response, leading to reflex bradycardia and vasodilation. Management consists of identifying and treating the underlying disorder that causes these uncontrollable coughing fits.

Swallow or *deglutination syncope* is a rare disorder caused by stimulation of esophageal mechanoreceptors during swallowing, notably of a large solid bolus of food. There is usually a history of an esophageal stricture or spasm, and management is directed toward treatment of the underlying esophageal disorder.

Defecation syncope, another rare form of situational syncope, occurs in the setting of a colonic disorder with episodes of painful defecation. Foreign bodies, such as ingested toothpicks, have been reported that may become embedded in the anus, causing painful defecation and reflex syncope. The obvious treatment is to recognize and to remove the offending agent. Defecation syncope

has also been reported to occur with functional obstruction of the inferior vena cava. Straining during a bowel movement increases intra-abdominal pressure and leads to obstruction of the inferior vena cava at the level of the diaphragm. A crural myotomy and surgical mobilization of the inferior vena cava may be curative, but should be reserved only for intractable cases in which syncope may result in serious injury.

Glossopharyngeal neuralgia rarely induces a reflex syncopal response. Sudden, severe, sharp pain extending along the course of the glossopharyngeal nerve in the posterior pharynx, neck, or external ear may produce reflex bradycardia, vasodilation, hypotension, and syncope. Sometimes a head or neck malignancy causing irritation of the nerve is discovered, whereas frequently no identifiable cause is found. Management consists of recognizing the disorder and its association with head and neck cancer, performing a detailed physical examination (supplemented with radiographic examinations when appropriate), and treating the underlying malignancy if discovered. If no cause is found, controlling the episodes of painful neuralgia by symptomatic treatment with phenytoin, carbamazepine, or gabapentin may prevent syncope. For extreme cases, either sectioning the glossopharyngeal nerve or implanting a cardiac pacemaker has been attempted with some success. However, implantation of a pacemaker to prevent reflex bradycardia does not abolish recurrent episodes of syncope if the mechanism for hypotension is primarily a vasodilatory and not a cardioinhibitory response. There have been reports of treating recalcitrant glossopharyngeal neuralgia and syncope with surgical exploration of the root entry zone of the vagal and glossopharyngeal nerves, and decompressing the nerves if there is evidence for compression due to an aberrant blood vessel.

Carotid sinus hypersensitivity is an exaggerated response to carotid sinus stimulation that causes syncope, usually occurring in elderly patients with a history of atherosclerotic vascular disease. Stimulation of the carotid sinus by external pressure or massage produces a vagally induced reflex bradycardia and vasodilation. The diagnosis is based on a positive response to carotid sinus massage and a history of syncope occurring only in situations in which the carotid sinus is stimulated, such as while wearing a tight collar, when shaving, or while turning the head. Treatment consists of avoiding situations in which the carotid sinus might be accidentally stimulated. For recurrent events, a pacemaker may be indicated.

Orthostatic hypotension

Orthostatic hypotension is a common cause of syncope in the elderly. A decrease in blood pressure, cerebral hypoperfusion, and loss of consciousness results if the cardiovascular system is unable to compensate quickly for sudden postural changes from lying (or sitting) to stand-

Table 5.3 Orthostatic hypotension

Discriminating features

1 Significant drop in orthostatic blood pressure
2 Often associated with a decrease in muscle tone

Consistent features

1 Most common cause of syncope in elderly patients
2 Occurs while standing or when making postural changes to a
   more upright position
3 Consciousness regained almost immediately after falling
4 Usually aborted if the patient can immediately assume a sitting
   or prone position

Variable features

1 Presyncopal symptoms of blurred vision, nausea, and disequilibrium

ing. Sometimes vague near-syncopal symptoms, characterized by blurred vision, dizziness, lightheadedness, disequilibrium, or nausea, may precede the syncopal event (Table 5.3).

Many conditions have been associated with orthostatic syncope. In the elderly, the most common cause may be medication effect from the overuse of diuretics, antihypertensives, sedatives, or various combinations of these drugs. Other causes include prolonged bed rest, dehydration, severe anemia, spinal cord disorders, autonomic neuropathies, neurodegenerative disorders associated with autonomic failure (for example, Parkinson's disease, or multiple system atrophy), postprandial hypotension, adrenal insufficiency, paraneoplastic syndromes, or hereditary disorders (such as dopamine β-hydroxylase deficiency or hyperbradykinism).

With a compatible clinical history, the diagnosis is established when the patient demonstrates a significant drop in orthostatic blood pressure associated with a recurrence of the syncopal event. The diagnosis is suspected if symptoms of near-syncope occur while standing, associated with an orthostatic decrease in systolic blood pressure of more than 20 mm Hg, or in an elderly patient, an absolute decrease in systolic blood pressure less than 90 mm Hg. A history of recurrent syncope, with events occurring either with the patient lying down or even sitting, generally indicates a disorder other than orthostatic syncope.

Therapy is directed toward identifying and correcting the condition or conditions predisposing the individual to orthostatic hypotension (for example, prolonged bed rest, dehydration, anemia), and educating the patient as to the adverse risks of hot weather, hot baths, rising quickly from a sitting to standing position, and the effects of meals and alcohol on orthostatic changes. When possible, diuretics,

antihypertensives, and sedatives should be discontinued or their doses modified. Other first-line measures include increasing sodium and fluid intake to expand plasma volume, providing waist-high support stockings to prevent venous pooling, elevating the head of the bed 6–8 inches at night to check nocturnal fluid loss and to increase vascular tone, moderate exercise to strengthen leg muscles, and ingestion of strong caffeinated coffee or tea.

Mineralocorticoids (for example, fludrocortisone) may be added to increase sodium and fluid retention and thereby help maintain an expanded plasma volume, but must be used cautiously so as not to produce supine hypertension or congestive heart failure. Desmopressin, which can prevent fluid loss at night, is another drug used to treat orthostatic hypotension. Midodrine, an α-agonist, increases vascular tone, is dosed two to three times each day, but should be avoided at night to prevent supine hypertension. The effects of other drugs such as prostaglandin synthesis inhibitors (for example, indomethacin or ibuprofen), metoclopramide, β-blockers, ergotamine nasal spray, clonidine, or yohimbine are too inconsistent or unreliable to readily recommend them as initial drug therapy for orthostatic hypotension.

Postural tachycardia syndrome (POTS), in which the patient experiences an exaggerated increase in his heart rate when changing to an upright position, may present with symptoms of palpitations, blurred vision, near, or complete syncope. Diagnosis is evident from the clinical features and measurement of the patient's heart rate and blood pressure lying and standing. Management includes avoiding volume depletion and treating similarly as for orthostatic hypotension.

Cardiac syncope

Cardiac causes for syncope often produce a sudden decrease in cardiac output, resulting in decreased cerebral perfusion and loss of consciousness. Symptoms that should lead to a suspicion of a cardiac cause include palpitations, chest pain, nonorthostatic position at the time of the syncopal event, or exertional syncope. Syncope from valvular heart disease such as aortic stenosis, idiopathic hypertrophic subaortic stenosis, and mitral stenosis, usually occurs in the setting of physical exertion and can be suspected by findings on physical examination. However, the presence of valvular heart disease may not necessarily indicate that this is the source for the patient's syncopal events unless severe outflow obstruction can be documented with ECG or cardiac catheterization.

Brief arrhythmias are a potentially serious cause for syncope, and sudden death may be a consequence if left untreated. Arrhythmias should be considered in any patient with a history of heart disease and no other apparent cause for syncope. Common examples include supraventricular tachyarrhythmias (for example, atrial fibrillation or flutter with a rapid ventricular response, and paroxysmal supraventricular tachycardia), sinus bradycardia, second- or third-degree heart block, ventricular tachycardia, or other ventricular arrhythmias sometimes associated with a congenital or acquired prolonged QT interval. The ECG may detect the rhythm disturbance at the time of the examination, but, in other instances, the rhythm disturbance may have resolved. In those cases, prolonged cardiac monitoring or EPS may be required to identify the arrhythmia, so that appropriate therapy can be started.

Other cardiac causes of syncope include severe cardiomyopathy, left atrial myxoma, cardiac tamponade, pulmonary hypertension, and pulmonary embolus. Diagnosis of these disorders relies on an appropriate history, physical examination, and confirmation by special studies.

Ictal asystole is a rare disorder due to induction of significant bradycardia or asystole as a result of a seizure, usually a partial seizure that involves limbic areas of the brain. The diagnosis may be made with video EEG monitoring, and treatment would be directed to controlling the seizures with anticonvulsants or a pacemaker.

Cerebrovascular disease

Cerebrovascular disease may provoke a syncopal attack by producing brainstem ischemia, with dysfunction of the ascending reticular activating system. This may occur, for example, with atherosclerotic cerebrovascular disease, migraine, or subclavian steal syndrome. Syncope secondary to a vertebrobasilar stroke or TIA usually occurs in the presence of other symptoms of brainstem ischemia, such as vertigo, diplopia, dysarthria, ataxia, incoordination, or focal motor or sensory symptoms (Table 5.4). In the absence of these accompanying symptoms, other causes of syncope should be considered. Vertebrobasilar or Bickerstaff's migraine is an uncommon cause of syncope, is most often seen in young women, and occurs with an associated headache and brainstem or cerebellar signs.

Subclavian steal syndrome typically presents with exercise-induced arm pain on the side on which the sub-

clavian artery is stenosed or occluded. Infrequently, syncope alone may accompany arm exercise, but the event usually occurs with other brainstem signs and symptoms. Physical findings of a diminished blood pressure or pulse amplitude in the involved arm and arteriographic findings of subclavian stenosis with reversal of flow through the vertebrobasilar artery help confirm the diagnosis.

Brainstem compression

Brainstem compression due to transient rises in intracranial pressure may produce loss of consciousness either by compressing and disrupting the reticular activating system, the brainstem vasopressor center, or by impairing vertebrobasilar blood flow. Congenital anomalies, such as Arnold-Chiari malformation, hydrocephalic attacks from a faulty ventricular shunt, or intermittent obstruction of the lateral ventricles by a colloid cyst, may create the necessary and temporary rise in intracranial pressure to cause syncope. The abnormal findings on neurologic examination, or history of a shunt placement for hydrocephalus, should raise suspicion for these disorders and lead to appropriate confirmatory neuroradiologic studies.

Seizures

Seizures are classified according to the behavioral change exhibited during the seizure and by the interictal EEG findings. The two major categories are primary generalized and *partial seizures*. The interictal EEG of primary seizures demonstrates generalized epileptiform discharges, whereas focal epileptiform discharges may occur interictally with partial seizures.

Primary generalized seizures include generalized tonic–clonic, absence, myoclonic, and atonic seizures. Primary generalized tonic–clonic seizures are characterized by rhythmic major motor activity occurring without warning, lasting 1–2 minutes, and sometimes associated with incontinence or tongue biting. The presence of tongue biting is more suggestive of a generalized tonic–clonic seizure than of other causes for syncope. *Absence seizures* are identified by a motionless stare lasting 5–10 seconds, sometimes accompanied by rhythmic eye blinking. Bedside hyperventilation for 3 minutes can sometimes evoke an absence seizure and validate the diagnosis. Myoclonic seizures are sudden, brief, irregular contractures of the extremities, often without loss of consciousness. An atonic seizure, or drop attack, is a brief, sudden loss of muscle tone, terminating in a fall if the patient is standing, and these usually occur without loss of consciousness. Patients with atonic seizures frequently have severe CNS abnormalities and exhibit other seizure types as well.

Partial seizures may begin with an aura (for example, focal sensory or motor symptoms, or experiential sen-

---

Table 5.4 Vertebrobasilar insufficiency

Discriminating features

1 Other brainstem signs and symptoms accompany syncope
2 Cerebral angiogram is abnormal

Consistent features

1 Usually takes place in elderly patients
2 Occurs in any position

Variable features

1 Recurrent episodes may lead to a fixed neurologic deficit

sations). As the seizure progresses, the patient may become confused or lose consciousness. Automatisms, such as chewing movements, swallowing, or picking at clothes, will sometimes occur during the seizures. A partial seizure without an alteration of consciousness is termed a *simple partial seizure*, whereas a partial seizure that is associated with an alteration or loss of consciousness is termed a *complex partial seizure*. Either type may evolve into a generalized tonic–clonic seizure, in which case it is termed a *partial seizure with secondary generalization*. For a more complete discussion of specific epileptic syndromes see Chapter 14.

Sometimes, it is difficult to distinguish an epileptic seizure from syncope. A syncopal event is usually described as a sudden loss of consciousness accompanied by generalized flaccid muscle tone. Brief myoclonic jerks may occur in the setting of cardiovascular and neurally mediated syncope and are believed to be due to cerebral hypoxia. However, major motor activity, like that which occurs with generalized tonic–clonic seizures, rarely happens during a syncopal event.

The diagnosis of an epileptic seizure is dependent on the detailed description of the event by the patient and a reliable witness. An EEG is helpful in classifying seizures as either primary generalized or partial seizures, but it is uncommon to record an epileptic seizure during a routine EEG. Exceptions to this are an absence seizure provoked by hyperventilation, or a nonepileptic psychogenic seizure brought on by suggestion techniques. It should be emphasized that a normal EEG does not rule out the possibility of a seizure disorder, nor does an abnormal EEG without a suitable clinical history confirm a diagnosis of a seizure disorder.

Transient Loss of Consciousness of Unknown Etiology

Although the cause of a patient's transient loss of consciousness can often be suspected after the initial interview and examination, if a source cannot be inferred and physical findings or a history of heart disease or abnormal ECG are present, a more comprehensive cardiac evaluation might be undertaken, as outlined previously. Patients without either underlying heart disease or symptoms suggesting a cardiovascular cause for syncope usually do not need further cardiac assessment because their prognosis for serious morbidity or mortality is low.

Patients who experience repeated events pose special management problems. How far should one proceed with an evaluation? Repeated attacks may not reflect a serious underlying disorder, but recurrent episodes of unconsciousness may, by themselves, threaten the patient's health if they occur at a time when the patient is engaged in an activity requiring intense concentration (for exam-

▼

Consider Consultation When...

▶ The cause of syncope is not clear after history, physical and neurologic examinations, and appropriate laboratory tests, particularly if a cardiac or neurologic basis is suspected (e.g., a history of cardiac or neurologic disease, and ECG abnormality, or focal neurologic deficit).

▶ Technical assistance is needed in interpreting or performing diagnostic procedures; or, further experience or expertise is needed to treat the diagnosed cause for syncope.

▶ The patient does not respond to treatment, or the patient's course is different from that expected.

ple, driving). In these situations, any alteration or loss of concentration might result in severe injury.

Patients with recurrent events should be reevaluated periodically. Over the course of time, repeated interviews and examinations may lead to the recognition of a specific disorder. Sometimes it is helpful to teach the patient's family or friends how to measure blood pressure and pulse rate, as well as what behavioral responses to observe when the patient is challenged with certain stimuli. A normal blood pressure and pulse immediately following an episode makes a cardiac arrhythmia less likely. Abrupt alerting immediately following the administration of a noxious stimulus (for example, inhalation of an ammonia capsule) raises suspicion for a psychogenic cause. Having the patient keep a diary to objectively quantify the frequency and pattern of the events allows the physician to decide if continuous, prolonged inpatient neurodiagnostic monitoring with EEG, ECG, and video would be worthwhile. The diary also provides a baseline against which the benefits of a therapeutic trial using, for instance, an anticonvulsant or psychotherapy, might be compared.

Finally, patients who remain undiagnosed after multiple events (especially if they have a history of a psychiatric disorder) may benefit from a psychiatric evaluation. Psychiatric disorders that may present with temporary loss of consciousness include anxiety disorder, panic attack, somatization disorder, malingering, or psychogenic unresponsiveness.

Annotated Bibliography

American College of Emergency Physicians. Clinical policy: Critical issues in the evaluation and management of patients presenting with syncope. *Ann Emerg Med* 2001;37:771–776. *Discusses the issues facing an emergency room physician when trying to decide what diagnostic tests are necessary and when the patient should be admitted to the hospital or discharged home.*

Brignole M, et. al. Guidelines on the management (diagnosis and treatment) of syncope—update 2004. *Europace* 2004;6: 467–537.
A summary of expert opinion in the approach to a patient with syncope. A review of the usefulness and indications for various diagnostic procedures and management options for specific causes of syncope.

Kapoor WN. Syncope. *N Engl J Med* 2001;343(25):1856–1862.
A comprehensive review of disorders associated with syncope; provides a critical analysis of the current diagnostic procedures and a thoughtful approach to the investigation of syncope.

Kaufmann H. Treatment of patients with orthostatic hypotension and syncope. *Clin Neuropharmacol* 2002;25(3):133–141.
Examines what is known about the pathophysiology of orthostatic and neurally mediated syncope, and provides an analytical review of currently available treatment options.

Sarasin FP, et al. Prospective evaluation of patients with syncope: A population-based study. *Am J Med* 2001;111(3): 177–184.
Reports the incidence of specific disorders presenting as syncope to an emergency department, with a description of a diagnostic algorithm in the investigation of syncope.

CHAPTER 6

Vertigo and Other Forms of Dizziness

Douglas J. Lanska

Outline

- ▶ Anatomy and physiology of the vestibular system
- ▶ History in the dizzy patient
- ▶ Examination of the dizzy patient
- ▶ Diagnostic tests
- ▶ Treatment
- ▶ Selected vertiginous syndromes and diseases

Dizziness is a very common problem in clinical practice, particularly among the elderly. Complaints of dizziness increase with age, due to age-related physiologic changes and age-associated diseases of the special sense organs and balance system. Although estimates vary depending on the study design and the characteristics of participants, 15–40% of persons over age 80 complain of frequent dizziness. Furthermore, compared to younger patients with dizziness, elderly persons with dizziness have greater disability, more chronic symptoms, and more frequent multifactorial etiologies.

From a neurologic standpoint, it is essential to distinguish vertigo from other causes of dizziness. To do this, it is necessary to understand the anatomy and physiology of the vestibular system, the symptomatology and clinical presentations of different categories of dizziness, and the general examination of the dizzy patient. This information will allow the practitioner to target further history, examination, diagnostic tests, and appropriate therapies.

Anatomy and Physiology of the Vestibular System

The vestibular receptors are housed in the bony labyrinth, a bilateral series of intercommunicating cavities and hol-

low channels in the petrous portion of the temporal bones. From a central cavity called the *vestibule* arise three semicircular canals and the cochlea. Within this bony labyrinth is the membranous labyrinth, a series of intercommunicating sacs and ducts filled with endolymphatic fluid and specialized structures for vestibular and auditory sensation. The vestibular portion of the membranous labyrinth includes the utricle and saccule within the vestibule, and the semicircular ducts within the semicircular canals. The space between the bony labyrinth and the membranous labyrinth contains perilymph, a connective tissue, and blood vessels. The membranous

Key Clinical Questions

Vertigo and other forms of dizziness

- ▶ Was the onset abrupt, subacute, or chronic?
- ▶ Is the course episodic or monophasic?
- ▶ If episodic, how long does the dizziness last?
- ▶ Can the dizziness be categorized as vertigo, disequilibrium, presyncope, or psychophysiologic (psychogenic) dizziness?
- ▶ Are there associated autonomic (e.g., nausea, vomiting), auditory (e.g., hearing loss, tinnitus), or central nervous system (CNS) signs or symptoms (e.g., diplopia, facial numbness, extremity weakness)?
- ▶ Can the symptoms be reproduced with provocative maneuvers (e.g., Dix-Hallpike positioning maneuver, hyperventilation, rotation)?
- ▶ Can any medications or drugs be implicated as a contributor to the dizziness?
- ▶ Is there evidence of vestibular imbalance on examination (e.g., nystagmus, past pointing)?

labyrinth and its neural structures receive their vascular supply from the internal auditory artery, which usually originates from a branch of the basilar artery.

Hair cells in the vestibular receptor organs transduce the mechanical forces associated with head acceleration into nerve action potentials. Hair cells are specialized sensory receptors from which protrude, on their apical sides, bundles of directionally sensitive protoplasmic filaments or "hairs." Deflection of the hairs in one direction decreases the resting membrane potential of the cell, resulting in an increase of the cell's spontaneous firing rate. Deflection of the hairs in the opposite direction produces hyperpolarization and a decrease in the spontaneous firing rate.

Receptor organs, called *macules*, in the utricle and saccule respond to linear acceleration and static tilt. Each macule consists of a mat of hair cells; an overlying gelatinous material embedding the hair cell projections, called the *otolithic membrane*; and a superficial covering of relatively dense calcium carbonate crystals called *otoconia*. Forces resulting from linear acceleration or gravity displace the dense otoconia and produce deflections of the directionally sensitive filaments protruding from the underlying hair cells.

Receptor organs called *cristae* in the semicircular ducts respond to angular acceleration. The cristae are located in enlargements of the semicircular ducts called *ampullae*. Each crista consists of a mat of hair cells and an overlying gelatinous mass called the *cupula*, which projects from the surface of the hair cells to the ceiling of the ampulla. Angular movements of the head produce flow of endolymph within the semicircular ducts, which displaces the cupulae and deflects the directionally sensitive filaments protruding from the underlying hair cells.

The three semicircular ducts are oriented orthogonally, with the lateral duct oriented roughly horizontally and the anterior and posterior ducts oriented vertically, so that the anterior duct on one side is in the same plane as the posterior duct on the opposite side. The lateral or "horizontal" duct is actually not quite horizontal, though, as it is tilted 30 degrees from the horizontal plane.

Sensory information from the vestibular receptor organs is conveyed centrally via the eighth cranial nerve, through the internal auditory canal in conjunction with the facial nerve, into the posterior fossa to synapse in the vestibular nuclei and cerebellum. The vestibular nuclei are situated in the brainstem on the floor of the fourth ventricle. The vestibular nuclei and brainstem reticular formation integrate inputs from the vestibular receptors, visual system, proprioceptive pathways, and cerebellum. The vestibular nuclei in turn project to the parietotemporal cerebral cortex, brainstem ocular motor and autonomic nuclei, and the spinal cord. Projections to the parietotemporal cerebral cortex are responsible for motion perception and spatial orientation. The connections

with the ocular motor nuclei mediate vestibulo-ocular reflexes (VOR). Vestibulo-ocular reflexes produce eye movements in the orbit that are equal in amplitude and opposite in direction to head movements, so that gaze remains steady. The projections to the spinal cord mediate vestibulospinal reflexes, which assist in maintaining posture and balance, particularly through tonic influence on the antigravity muscles.

Physiologic imbalances in neural discharges within the vestibular system are produced with head movements, rotation, and caloric stimulation. Pathologic imbalances in the vestibular system can be produced by impairments either in the vestibular inputs or in the central connections of the vestibular system. Vertigo results from a mismatch between the converging inputs and the expected sensory patterns. For example, acute unilateral labyrinthine dysfunction produces vertigo because the sensation of self-motion associated with the vestibular tone imbalance is inconsistent with expectations based upon visual and somatosensory information. The vertigo ultimately resolves, usually because of a rebalancing centrally, rather than a return of function peripherally: that is, central compensation corrects the mismatch between inputs and expectations.

The clinical manifestations of vestibular tone imbalance are produced through various vestibulo-ocular and vestibulospinal reflexes, as well as through the connections of the central vestibular system to cortical and brainstem centers. A disturbance of cortical spatial orientation produces the sensation of vertigo. Nystagmus is due to a direction-specific imbalance in the VOR. If eye movements do not match head movements, then images of the world move across the retina, producing blurred vision and an illusory visual sensation of environmental motion called *oscillopsia*. Postural imbalance is caused by abnormal activation of monosynaptic and polysynaptic vestibulospinal pathways. Finally, nausea and vomiting are due to activation of the medullary vomiting center.

History in the Dizzy Patient

Dizziness is a nonspecific term that describes an unpleasant sensation of imbalance or altered orientation in space. There are four major categories of pathologic dizziness: vertigo, disequilibrium, presyncope, and psychophysiologic dizziness. Careful history, provocative testing, and detailed examination will allow distinction of the major categories of dizziness in most cases and will often allow a specific etiologic diagnosis as well.

Vertigo is an illusion of movement due to an imbalance of tonic vestibular activity. It is usually rotatory, implying a disturbance of the semicircular canals or their central connections. Sensations of body tilt or impulsion indicate otolithic disturbances. Vertigo is commonly as-

Pearls and Perils

Dizziness

▶ There are four major categories of pathologic dizziness: vertigo, disequilibrium, presyncope, and psychophysiologic.

▶ Complaints of dizziness increase with age.

▶ Elderly persons with dizziness have greater disability, more chronic symptoms, and more frequent multifactorial etiologies.

▶ Drugs should be reviewed in all cases of dizziness.

▶ The elderly are particularly susceptible to drug ototoxicity.

▶ Careful examination of the eyes, ears, cardiovascular system, nervous system, and vestibular system is indicated.

▶ Provocative testing is often helpful in defining the subjective sensation and the often vague description of dizziness.

▶ Presyncope and disequilibrium may be exacerbated by antivertiginous medications.

▶ Patients with presyncope, disequilibrium, and psychophysiologic dizziness are unlikely to benefit from vestibular exercises or antivertigo medications.

sociated with nystagmus, oscillopsia, postural imbalance, nausea, and vomiting. Autonomic symptoms (e.g., sweating, pallor, nausea, vomiting) are generally more severe with vertigo of peripheral origin than with vertigo of central origin. Common causes of vertigo in the elderly include benign paroxysmal positioning vertigo, viral neurolabyrinthitis, trauma, toxins, and posterior circulation or labyrinthine ischemia. Common causes of vertigo in young adults include Ménière's syndrome, viral neurolabyrinthitis, trauma, and toxins.

Disequilibrium is a state of nonvertiginous altered static (e.g., standing) or dynamic (e.g., walking) postural balance. Patients with disequilibrium often complain of unsteadiness, imbalance, and falls. There are two types of disequilibrium: sensory and motor. Sensory disequilibrium is caused by altered spatial orientation, which may be due to proprioceptive impairment (e.g., from peripheral neuropathy or tabes dorsalis), balanced bilateral or compensated unilateral vestibular dysfunction (e.g., due to aminoglycoside toxicity or the residua of viral neurolabyrinthitis), visual–vestibular mismatch (e.g., due to impaired vision, ocular misalignment, or use of optic devices such as lens implants or new glasses), or multisensory impairment. Except in cases of visual–vestibular mismatch, patients with sensory disequilibrium generally do worse in the dark and frequently have a Romberg sign on examination. Motor disequilibrium is caused by impaired motor performance, which may be due either to mechanical factors (e.g., severe arthritis or prosthetic

limbs) or to dysfunction of central and peripheral nervous system motor pathways. The central motor pathways that may be affected in patients with motor disequilibrium include the pyramidal, extrapyramidal, and cerebellar systems, whereas the peripheral motor pathways include the peripheral nerves, neuromuscular junctions, and muscles. Motor disequilibrium, as from cerebellar dysfunction, is generally not exacerbated in the dark or with the eyes closed.

Presyncope is a syndrome characterized by a sensation of impending loss of consciousness, and is typically associated with weakness, diaphoresis, nausea, and epigastric distress. Other associated symptoms may include facial pallor or ashen-gray appearance, scotomata, visual dimming or "gray out," headache, tremulousness, and, depending on the cause, palpitations, acral and perioral paresthesias, and carpopedal spasms. Presyncope is due to diffuse and sudden impairment in cerebral metabolism, which may occur in isolation or as a precursor to loss of consciousness (i.e., syncope; see Chapter 5). The sudden cerebral metabolic dysfunction occurs due to generalized cerebral ischemia, or less commonly with hypoglycemia or hypoxia. Presyncope (and syncope) may occur with decreased cardiac output (e.g. arrhythmias, obstructive cardiomyopathies, pulmonary emboli), inadequate peripheral vasoconstrictor mechanisms (e.g., vasovagal response, sympatholytic drugs, primary autonomic insufficiency, central and peripheral nervous system diseases), cerebral vasoconstriction (e.g., hyperventilation), hypovolemia, mechanical reduction in venous return (e.g., cough, micturition), and with alterations in the oxygen or nutrient content of the blood (e.g., hypoxia, hypoglycemia). True syncope is rare with hyperventilation and hypoglycemia. Episodes of presyncope are generally relieved with recumbency.

Psychophysiologic (psychogenic) dizziness is a vague giddiness or dissociated sensation due to impaired central integration of sensory and motor signals in patients with acute and chronic anxiety. The dizzy sensation is typically protracted or continuous, with periodic exacerbations, often punctuated by episodes of hyperventilation-induced presyncope. Specific provocative factors may be identified, such as the presence of crowds, driving, or being in confined places (e.g., elevators). Episodes are not associated with facial pallor and are not relieved with recumbency.

Drugs should be reviewed in all patients with dizziness. Drugs associated with dizziness include alcohol and other central nervous system (CNS) depressant medications (e.g., benzodiazepines, barbiturates, phenothiazines), aminoglycoside antibiotics, anticonvulsants, antidepressant medications, antihypertensive medications, chemotherapeutic agents, loop diuretics (e.g., furosemide), and salicylates (see Table 6.1). The elderly are particularly susceptible to drug ototoxicity: (a) they

Table 6.1 Drugs associated with dizziness

Drug	Syndrome	Mechanism
Alcohol	1. Vertigo (positional) 2. Motor disequilibrium (ataxia)	1. Reversible changes in cupula specific gravity 2. Cerebellar dysfunction a. reversible after acute intoxication b. permanent after long-term abuse
Aminoglycosides	Sensory disequilibrium or vertigo, oscillopsia, and hearing loss	Irreversible damage to labyrinthine hair cells
Anticonvulsants	Motor disequilibrium (ataxia)	Cerebellar dysfunction 1. Reversible after acute intoxication 2. Potentially irreversible after chronic phenytoin intoxication
Antidepressants	Presyncope	Orthostatic hypotension
Antihypertensives	Presyncope	Orthostatic hypotension
Antimalarial agents	Sensory disequilibrium or vertigo, hearing loss, and tinnitus	Variably reversible damage to labyrinthine hair cells
Antipsychotics	Presyncope	Orthostatic hypotension
Cis-platinum	Sensory disequilibrium or vertigo, hearing loss, and tinnitus	Variably reversible damage to labyrinthine hair cells
Cytosine arabinoside	Motor disequilibrium (ataxia)	Variably reversible damage to cerebellar Purkinje cells
Ethacrynic acid	Sensory disequilibrium or vertigo, hearing loss, and tinnitus	Irreversible damage to cerebellar Purkinje cells
5-Fluorouracil	Motor disequilibrium (ataxia)	Reversible inhibition of cerebellar metabolism by metabolites
Furosemide	Sensory disequilibrium or vertigo, hearing loss, and tinnitus	Reversible inhibition of enzymes in cochlea
Minocycline	Sensory disequilibrium or vertigo, and tinnitus	Reversible vestibular toxicity
Salicylates	Sensory disequilibrium or vertigo, hearing loss, and tinnitus	Reversible inhibition of metabolic activity of labyrinthine hair cells and/or cochlear neurons
Sedative-hypnotics	Mixed disequilibrium	Reversible depression of CNS integration areas

are more likely to receive ototoxic drugs, (b) they have less reserve (due to age-associated vestibular end organ changes, preexisting sensorineural hearing loss, and previous treatment with ototoxic drugs), and (c) they are likely to have impaired renal function.

Helpful aspects of the history in the differential diagnosis of vertigo are outlined in Table 6.2. Particular attention should be given to the onset, duration, and course of the vertigo, as well as any associated autonomic, auditory, or CNS signs and symptoms. This information alone is often sufficient to suggest a specific etiologic diagnosis.

As outlined in Box 6.1, the neurologic symptoms associated with vertigo are particularly helpful in localizing the responsible lesions. Hearing loss and tinnitus generally imply peripheral dysfunction, usually involving the inner ear, but occasionally involving the internal auditory canal or the structures of the cerebellopontine angle. Since the motor fibers for facial expression pass in the seventh cranial nerve in close proximity to the vestibulocochlear sensory fibers in the eighth cranial nerve, peripheral-type facial paresis (involving both upper and lower facial muscles) may be associated with lesions of the internal auditory canal, cerebellopontine angle, or brainstem. Any of the following imply an intracranial basis for the dysfunction: diplopia, facial numbness, dysarthria, dysphagia, extremity weakness or numbness, or incoordination.

Patients with vertigo often give confusing and contradictory accounts of the directionality of their symptoms, probably because the vestibular and self-referred visual sensations of movement are oppositely directed. Therefore, it is helpful to determine the direction of the sensation of rotation of the body with the eyes closed, which is away from the side of a peripheral vestibular lesion.

Precipitating factors for vertigo may include head movements, coughing, sneezing, and loud noises. Head movements accentuate imbalance within vestibular pathways, and may produce vertigo even after compensation has occurred in response to a vestibular lesion. In addition, positional vertigo is frequently induced by ordinary head movements, such as looking up or to one side, lying down, sitting up, or bending over. Coughing and sneezing may precipitate vertigo, particularly by changing middle ear pressure in patients with a posttraumatic perilymph fistula. Loud noises may also precipitate vertigo in patients with inner ear disease, such as Ménière's disease. This is called the *Tullio phenomenon*.

Table 6.2 History in the differential diagnosis of vertigo

Condition	Onset	Duration	Course	Autonomic*	Auditory†	CNS
Benign paroxysmal positioning vertigo	Abrupt	Seconds	Episodic	+++	−	−
Seizures	Abrupt	Seconds/minutes	Episodic	−/+	−	++
Migraine	Abrupt	Minutes	Episodic	+++	−	++
Vertebrobasilar insufficiency/TIA	Abrupt	Minutes/hours	Episodic	+	+	+++
Ménière's syndrome	Abrupt	Hours	Episodic	+++	+++	−
Trauma	Abrupt	Days	Monophasic	++	++	++
Stroke	Abrupt	Days	Monophasic	+	+	++++
Vestibular neuronitis	Subacute	Days	Monophasic	++++	+++/++++	−
Toxic	Subacute/chronic	Days	Monophasic	+	+++	++
Posterior fossa mass	Subacute/chronic	Days	Varies	+	++	+++

−, never; +, uncommon; ++, common; +++, typical; ++++, universal; TIA, transient ischemic attack.
*Autonomic symptoms (sweating, pallor, nausea, vomiting) are much more common and much more severe with vertigo of peripheral origin (labyrinth or eighth nerve) than with vertigo of central nervous system (CNS) origin.
†Auditory symptoms generally only occur if the vascular event involves either the inner ear or the acoustic nerve.

Examination of the Dizzy Patient

Since patients' descriptions of dizzy sensations are often confusing, particularly when the events are episodic, provocative testing is often helpful in defining the subjective sensation and the often vague description of dizziness. Provocative testing can be used to produce physiologic sensations of vertigo or presyncope, which can then be compared and contrasted with the subjective sensations experienced by the patient.

Rotational or caloric testing can also induce physiologic vertigo in the office. To perform rotational testing in the office, the patient can be seated in a rotary office chair with the head tilted 30 degrees forward, and then rotated carefully 10 times over 20–30 seconds. Tilting the head forward 30 degrees places both horizontal semicircular canals parallel to the floor, and therefore perpendicular to the axis of rotation in the chair. As a result, both horizontal canals are affected with rotational testing, with output from one canal stimulated, while output from the other canal is inhibited. The mismatch between the resulting vestibular imbalance and visual and somatosensory information produces physiologic vertigo, which generally lasts less than 1–2 minutes. During this time, one can observe the typical peripheral vestibular nystagmus and past pointing (see later discussion). Because of the risk of falls and injury, patients should not stand until the vertigo has resolved. Vertigo can also be produced with caloric testing, for example, by injecting cold water into the patient's external auditory canal. However, this is generally much more uncomfortable for the patient than rotational testing, and is also more time-consuming and messier for the examiner. Caloric testing has specific indications, but is not recommended for provocative testing to determine the category of dizziness.

Hyperventilation produces presyncope with perioral and acral paresthesias and potentially carpopedal spasms. To produce these sensations in the office, the patient is asked to breathe deeply and quickly for 3 minutes through an open mouth with the lips not pursed. This is difficult to do even for cooperative patients, and considerable encouragement from the examiner is often required.

Other maneuvers are helpful in identifying certain specific pathologic conditions, rather than identifying the broad category of dizziness. Assessment of pulse and blood pressure with the patient both supine and standing is necessary to diagnose presyncope due to orthostatic hypotension. Orthostatic hypotension is defined as an orthostatic reduction of either systolic blood pressure of at least 20 mm Hg or diastolic blood pressure of at least 10 mm Hg, generally within 3 minutes of standing. Occasional patients with orthostatic hypotension may not manifest significant drops in blood pressure until they have been standing for at least 10 minutes. A fistula test is used to evaluate patients with vertigo from a suspected perilymph fistula, a disruption of the limiting membranes of the labyrinth. Patients with perilymph fistulas note the sudden onset of hearing loss with tinnitus and vertigo, usually following head trauma, coughing, sneezing, straining, or exercise. In the fistula test, an otoscope with an insufflator is used to transiently change the pressure in the external auditory canal. Alternatively, the tragus of the ear can be used to occlude the external canal, and ap-

Box 6.1 Neurologic symptoms associated with vertigo due to lesions at different anatomic sites

- ▶ Inner ear
  - Hearing loss
  - Tinnitus
- ▶ Internal auditory canal
  - Facial weakness
  - Hearing loss
  - Tinnitus
- ▶ Cerebellopontine angle
  - Facial numbness
  - Facial weakness
  - Hearing loss
  - Tinnitus
  - Extremity incoordination
- ▶ Brainstem
  - Diplopia
  - Facial numbness
  - Facial weakness
  - Dysarthria
  - Dysphagia
  - Extremity weakness
  - Extremity incoordination
  - Extremity numbness
- ▶ Cerebellum
  - Extremity incoordination

Pearls and Perils

Evaluation of vertigo

- ▶ Particularly in the elderly, great care should be taken in excluding a central cause for acute vertigo.
- ▶ Particular attention should be given to the onset, duration, and course of the vertigo, as well as any associated autonomic, auditory, or central nervous system signs and symptoms.
- ▶ Careful examination of the eyes, ears, cardiovascular system, nervous system, and vestibular system is indicated.
- ▶ Neurologic symptoms and signs are particularly helpful in localizing the responsible lesions.
- ▶ Vertigo due to peripheral vestibular dysfunction is often associated with severe nausea and vomiting.
- ▶ Hearing loss and tinnitus generally imply peripheral dysfunction, usually involving the inner ear.
- ▶ Peripheral vestibular nystagmus may be evident only when fixation is prevented.
- ▶ In central vestibular disorders, vertigo, autonomic, and audiologic manifestations are mild or absent, and there are frequently associated central neurologic signs or symptoms.
- ▶ Any of the following imply an intracranial basis for the dysfunction: diplopia, facial numbness, dysarthria, dysphagia, extremity weakness or numbness, or incoordination.
- ▶ A central cause is likely if the associated nystagmus has a pendular appearance, is purely rotatory or purely linear, changes direction with gaze in different directions, or is not suppressed with fixation.
- ▶ Small cerebellar strokes may mimic labyrinthine lesions clinically.

plying pressure to the tragus using the examiner's finger can alter pressure in the canal. In the appropriate clinical setting, a positive fistula test with transient vertigo and nystagmus is suggestive of a perilymph fistula and warrants referral to an otolaryngologist. The Dix-Hallpike positioning test is used to precipitate vertigo in patients with episodic symptoms, especially when the symptoms appear to be related to either head position or head movements. This technique, its application, and its interpretation will be discussed in detail later. Other provocative maneuvers that may be helpful in selected and controlled circumstances include carotid sinus massage and the Valsalva maneuver.

In all patients with dizziness or vestibular complaints, careful examination of the eyes, ears, cardiovascular system, nervous system, and vestibular system is indicated. The following discussion, though, will be limited to a review of the bedside examination of the vestibular system. Clinically, vestibular imbalance is indicated by nystagmus, past pointing, and postural and gait abnormalities.

Because different types of nystagmus have different clinical implications, it is important to carefully characterize nystagmus both by its appearance and by any pre-cipitating and inhibiting factors. For example, nystagmus may be characterized by the symmetry of the oscillations, whether the oscillations are linear or rotatory, and whether the oscillations are unidirectional or direction changing. Jerk nystagmus is identified by a clear slow-phase drift in one direction and a corrective quick phase in the opposite direction. Jerk nystagmus is traditionally described by the direction of the quick phases; for example, "down beat" nystagmus. In contrast, pendular nystagmus is characterized by smooth sinusoidal oscillations of the eyes.

Precipitating factors for nystagmus may include specific eye and head positions. Pathologic nystagmus may be present in primary position (spontaneous nystagmus), with a change in eye position (gaze-evoked nystagmus), or with a change in head position (positional and positioning nystagmus). Spontaneous nystagmus is assessed by direct observation of the patient's eyes while the patient is looking straight ahead, either fixating on a target or with fixation removed. Gaze-evoked nystagmus is assessed similarly with the patient fixating on targets 30 degrees to the right, left, up, and down. Extreme eye positions should be avoided because they can result in "end-point" nystagmus in normal individuals. Positioning nystagmus is assessed with the Dix-Hallpike positioning test.

An important inhibiting factor for peripheral vestibular nystagmus is fixation. While fixating, patients with peripheral vestibular nystagmus can use their visual pursuit system to counteract the nystagmus. In contrast, fixation does not suppress central vestibular nystagmus, since patients with central vestibular disorders cannot utilize their pursuit system to suppress the nystagmus. Central vestibular and visual pursuit pathways are highly integrated, so central vestibular lesions damage both systems, thereby precluding inhibition by fixation.

To visualize peripheral vestibular nystagmus, special techniques may be needed to suppress fixation. Ophthalmoscopy is a readily available way of preventing fixation when the nonviewed eye is covered. The direction of linear nystagmus when viewed with an ophthalmoscope is reversed from that observed by direct inspection of the eye, since (a) the axis of rotation of the eye is perpendicular to the line of sight, and (b) the retina lies behind the center of rotation to the eye, while the cornea lies in front. Torsional nystagmus can also be detected with an ophthalmoscope by observing the vessels around the macula. The direction of torsional nystagmus is not reversed when viewed with an ophthalmoscope, since the axis of rotation is parallel to the line of sight.

The clinical features of peripheral and central spontaneous vestibular nystagmus are contrasted in Table 6.3. Peripheral vestibular nystagmus is a mixed linear–rotatory jerk nystagmus that beats in one direction, away from a hypofunctioning labyrinth. With semicircular duct stimulation or dysfunction, eye movements occur in the plane of an affected semicircular duct. With all forms of peripheral vestibular nystagmus, nystagmus amplitude and frequency increase with gaze in the direction of the

quick phases due to summation of tonic driving forces and elastic restoring forces both moving the eyes in the direction of the nystagmus slow phases. The presence of any of the following suggests a central cause for the nystagmus: (a) the nystagmus has a pendular appearance, (b) the nystagmus is purely rotatory or purely linear, (c) the nystagmus changes direction with gaze in different directions, (d) the nystagmus is not suppressed with fixation, (e) vertigo is mild or absent, (f) nausea is absent, or (g) central neurologic signs or symptoms are present. Despite these helpful rules, small cerebellar strokes may mimic labyrinthine lesions clinically. Therefore, particularly in the elderly, great care should be taken in excluding a central cause for acute vertigo.

The Dix-Hallpike positioning maneuver tests for positionally induced nystagmus, particularly that associated with benign paroxysmal positioning vertigo. The patient is instructed to stare off into space and to try to avoid looking at any specific object during the procedure. The patient's head is turned to one side, and then the patient is rapidly moved backward from a sitting to a head hanging position. Turning the head to one side places the ipsilateral posterior semicircular duct in a parasagittal plane. When the patient is subsequently moved backward, the movement is in the plane of that duct. The examiner maintains the patient in the head hanging position for approximately 1 minute and observes the patient's eyes for nystagmus. Anticipation or the experience of vertigo may make patients very anxious. Calm but firm reassurance from the examiner is often necessary to complete the maneuver.

The clinical features of peripheral and central positional vestibular nystagmus are outlined in Table 6.4. Like peripheral spontaneous nystagmus, peripheral positional or positioning nystagmus is a mixed linear–rotatory jerk nystagmus. Peripheral positional or positioning vestibular nystagmus generally beats upward and toward the undermost ear, and has a latency of from 1 to 45 seconds (but typically only a few seconds) and a duration of less than 60 seconds. It lessens or disappears with repetition

Table 6.3 Clinical features of peripheral and central spontaneous vestibular nystagmus

	Peripheral	Central
Appearance	Jerk	Jerk or pendular
	Mixed linear and rotatory	May be pure linear or pure rotatory
	Unidirectional (beats away from hypofunctioning labyrinth)	May change direction with gaze in different directions
Fixation	Inhibits nystagmus	Little effect
Associated symptoms and signs	Severe vertigo	Mild or absent vertigo
	Severe nausea	Mild or absent nausea
	Hearing loss and tinnitus common	Hearing loss and tinnitus uncommon
	No central nervous system symptoms or signs	Central nervous system symptoms and signs common

Table 6.4 Clinical features of peripheral and central positional vestibular nystagmus

	Peripheral	Central
Latency	1–45 seconds	None
Appearance	Jerk	Jerk or pendular
	Mixed upbeat rotatory	May be pure linear or pure rotatory
	Unidirectional	May change direction with gaze in different directions
Fixation	Inhibits nystagmus	Little effect
Duration	<60 seconds	Persists
Fatigability	Lessens and may disappear on repetition	Persists
Associated symptoms and signs	Severe vertigo	Mild or absent vertigo
	Severe nausea	Mild or absent nausea
	Hearing loss and tinnitus common	Hearing loss and tinnitus uncommon
	No central nervous system symptoms or signs	Central nervous system symptoms and signs common

of the offending head positioning. The presence of any of the following suggests a central cause for the nystagmus: (a) the nystagmus begins immediately upon assumption of the offending head position, (b) the nystagmus has a pendular appearance, (c) the nystagmus is purely rotatory or purely linear, (d) the nystagmus changes direction with gaze in different directions, (e) the nystagmus is not suppressed with fixation, (f) the nystagmus continues indefinitely with maintenance of the offending head position, (g) the nystagmus persists with repetition of the offending head positioning, (h) vertigo is mild or absent, (i) nausea is absent, or (j) central neurologic signs or symptoms are present. As with spontaneous vestibular nystagmus, great care should be taken in excluding a central cause for acute vertigo, particularly in the elderly.

Corrective saccades are rapid conjugate eye movements that allow the patient's eyes to refixate on the target following a shift in gaze. Corrective saccades after single, rapid, small-amplitude head turns can be helpful in identifying the side of vestibular dysfunction, particularly when spontaneous nystagmus is absent. In this test, the patient's head is turned rapidly 5 to 10 degrees to one side by the examiner, while the patient attempts to maintain fixation on an object 6 feet or more away. The examiner observes the patient for corrective saccades. The gaze of a patient with unilateral labyrinthine dysfunction shifts only when the head moves quickly toward the dysfunctional side. An oppositely directed compensatory saccade corrects the gaze error. Thus, leftward saccades following rapid rightward head movements indicate right vestibular dysfunction, whereas rightward saccades following rapid leftward head movements indicate left vestibular dysfunction.

Caloric testing may also be helpful in determining the side of a peripheral vestibular lesion. Otoscopy must be performed prior to the test to ensure that the tympanic membrane is intact and that wax does not obstruct the external canal. The patient's head is elevated 30 degrees from a supine position to bring the lateral semicircular duct into a vertical orientation. Cold or warm water is instilled in the external canal, which induces convection currents in the endolymph of the lateral semicircular duct. Because of its ready availability, ice water is commonly used for bedside testing. Two to ten milliliters of ice water are usually adequate. A normal response to caloric stimulation with ice water consists of tonic deviation of the eyes toward the side of instillation plus nystagmus with corrective quick phases in the direction opposite to the tonic deviation. Warm water produces the opposite response. The onset is in 30–60 seconds, and the duration is usually 1–3 minutes. In comatose patients, only tonic deviation is observed. In labyrinthine or eighth-nerve lesions, neither cold nor warm water will elicit a normal response on the affected side. This is called *canal paresis*. Greater than 20% asymmetry in duration or frequency between the two sides suggests an abnormality on the side of the lesser response. If the dysfunction is mild, quantitative testing with electronystagmography may be necessary to establish the finding. If the ocular response to caloric stimulation is consistently greater in one direction than another, there is a directional preponderance of the vestibular system. This may occur with both central and peripheral vestibular disorders, particularly in the presence of spontaneous nystagmus. By itself, directional preponderance is not localizing.

Clinical disturbances of the vestibulospinal pathways are assessed with several tests including past pointing, stance, the Romberg test, and tandem gait with eyes closed.

When assessing a patient for past pointing, the patient is asked to sit facing the examiner with index finger extended and pointing at, but not touching, the examiner's extended finger. The patient is then asked to raise the arm to a vertical position with the index finger pointing at the ceiling, and subsequently return the arm to the initial position. This is repeated several times with the eyes closed. Consistent deviation of the arm to one side is called *past pointing*. If extralabyrinthine inputs are not minimized by keeping the eyes closed and the arm extended, visual or proprioceptive signals will permit accurate localization of the target even if vestibular function is impaired. For this reason, the standard finger–nose–finger test is not helpful in identifying past pointing. In acute vestibular lesions, patients past-point toward the affected side; however, the test can be misleading since CNS compensation rapidly corrects the past pointing and can produce a drift to the opposite side.

With acute unilateral vestibular lesions, patients have impaired postural control and may sway or fall toward the lesion. Although this is helpful diagnostically, the examiner must take great care when assessing stance and gait in patients with vestibular complaints, as patients may suddenly fall and could injure themselves. The examiner must provide adequate support for the patient to prevent falls and injuries. In patients who are unable to maintain their stance without support when their eyes are open, it is unnecessary and potentially dangerous to proceed with a Romberg test or an unsupported assessment of gait.

In patients with vestibular lesions, the tendency to fall toward the lesion is accentuated when they are prevented from using vision to compensate for the vestibular imbalance. This is the basis of the Romberg test. In the Romberg test, the patient is first asked to stand with eyes open and feet together. If the patient is unable to maintain balance in this position, the stance is widened until this is possible. The patient is then asked to close his or her eyes. Patients with proprioceptive or vestibular dysfunction may be unable to maintain this position. Patients with unilateral dysfunction usually sway or fall toward the side of the lesion, particularly if the dysfunction is acute. Because of CNS compensation, the test is less sensitive to chronic unilateral vestibular dysfunction. As with past pointing, overcompensation may result in falls toward the "good" side.

With eyes open, tandem walking may be impaired with acute vestibular lesions. It is, however, mainly a test of cerebellar function, because vision compensates for chronic vestibular and proprioceptive dysfunction. A better test of vestibular function is tandem walking with eyes closed. When cerebellar and proprioceptive function are normal, imbalance during this test indicates vestibular dysfunction. However, the direction of falling does not reliably indicate the side of the lesion. The test is also difficult for normal elderly people.

Diagnostic Tests

The history and physical examination are frequently sufficient to classify the dizziness into one of the four cate-

gories mentioned earlier, and perhaps even to suggest an etiologic diagnosis. In many cases, though, additional diagnostic tests will be required. These should be ordered selectively. The diagnostic evaluation of nonvertiginous dizziness is beyond the scope of this chapter. Discussion of the evaluation of disequilibrium can be found in Chapter 7 (Disorders of Gait), and discussion of the evaluation of presyncope and syncope can be found in Chapter 5.

Diagnostic studies that may be helpful in patients with vertigo include audiometry, electro- or video-nystagmography, bithermal caloric testing, brainstem auditory evoked potentials, and cranial imaging, optimally with magnetic resonance imaging (MRI). Consultation in problematic cases should be sought from neurology, especially in cases of CNS dysfunction, or otolaryngology, especially in cases of peripheral vestibular dysfunction.

Treatment

The treatment of dizziness varies by type and cause. In general, it is symptomatic and directed at the underlying cause. For example, vertigo may be alleviated with vestibular sedatives, whereas these agents may exacerbate presyncope and disequilibrium. Also, patients with acute persistent vertigo from peripheral vestibular lesions may benefit from vestibular exercises, whereas patients with presyncope, disequilibrium, and psychophysiologic dizziness are unlikely to benefit from these exercises.

Patients with any form of dizziness are at a significantly increased risk of falling (Box 6.2). Falls are the leading cause of both nonfatal injuries and unintentional injury deaths among older people in the United States, and dizziness is a major contributor to such falls. More than half of people age 65 or older fall each year, and 10% of these falls result in serious injury. Injuries from falls include hip fracture, other fractures, subdural hematoma, and other head injury. Many elderly people have multiple medical problems for which they are receiving medications, which in turn can often increase the risk of dizziness and falls (Box 6.3). The risk of falling and confusion increases with increasing number of medications, independent of the types of medications.

The risks of falls and fall-related injuries in patients with dizziness can be significantly decreased with appropriate management (Box 6.4). In particular, strategies utilizing multifactorial assessment and intervention can significantly reduce the rate of falling and the risk of fall-associated injury, including hip fractures, in dizzy patients, particularly those who are elderly, frail, and infirm. Although there is no consensus on which components are necessary in such multifactorial intervention programs, components can include educating and guiding staff, modifying the environment, implementing exercise programs, supplying and repairing aids, reviewing and mod-

▼

Box 6.2 Patient-related factors associated with an increased risk of falling

▶ History of previous falls (especially within the previous 6 months)
▶ Medication effects
  • Multiple medications
  • Specific medications
▶ Disease (Note: these are not mutually exclusive categories)
  • Sensory or motor disequilibrium
    – Impaired vision
    – Impaired hearing
    – Arthritis
    – Myopathy
    – Myasthenia gravis and other neuromuscular junction disorders
    – Motor neuron disease
    – Paraparesis (e.g., spinal cord injury)
    – Hemiparesis (e.g., stroke)
    – Other weakness
    – Neuropathy (especially sensory, motor, or sensori-motor polyneuropathy)
    – Tabes dorsalis
    – Spinocerebellar ataxia
    – Parkinson's disease
    – Other akinetic/rigid syndromes (e.g., progressive supranuclear palsy, multiple system atrophy, etc.)
    – Dyskinetic or hyperkinetic movement disorders (e.g., Huntington's disease)
    – Normal pressure hydrocephalus
    – Intoxications
    – Other impaired balance and gait
  • Vertigo
  • Orthostatic hypotension
  • Syncope
  • Neurocognitive impairment
    – Depression or treatment with antidepressants
    – Psychosis/Hallucinosis
    – Anxiety
    – Confusion or delirium
    – Alzheimer's disease
    – Other dementia
    – Frontal/subfrontal executive dysfunction
  • Infection (especially urinary tract infection)
  • Acute illness
▶ Other disability
  • Recent hospitalization
▶ Other
  • Error of judgment
  • Misinterpretation
  • Miscalculation
  • Misuse of equipment (e.g., ladder, roller walker, etc.)

▼

Box 6.3 Medications particularly likely to increase the risk of falling

▶ Antidepressants (especially tricyclics and serotonin-reuptake inhibitors)
▶ Anxiolytics (especially benzodiazepines)
▶ Antipsychotics (especially haloperidol and phenothiazines)
▶ Antihypertensives
▶ Antiarrhythmics
▶ Anticonvulsants
▶ Laxatives

ifying drug regimens, providing hip protectors, and post-fall problem-solving conferences. The choice of components should appropriately be targeted to the specific patient issues, including type of dizziness.

Other fall prevention methods may also be useful (Boxes 6.4 and 6.5), including exercise programs, evaluation and management of comorbid conditions predisposing to falls (e.g., orthostatic hypotension, parkinsonism, delirium, leg weakness, and arthritis), medication management (e.g., limiting or curtailing the use of certain medications, particularly those with sedative effects or those contributing to orthostatic hypotension, motor disequilibrium or ataxia), provision of appropriate footwear, use of assistive devices, elimination of home hazards, and the like. In addition, other approaches can decrease the risk of injury from falls (i.e., without necessarily impacting on the risk or frequency of falls), including evaluation and management of osteoporosis and the provision of protective orthotics (e.g., hip protectors).

At least on a yearly basis, medical care providers should ask elderly patients about any falls or difficulty with balance and gait. They should also observe their patients while rising from a chair, while standing, and while walking. Any elderly patients who have observed difficulty with getting around should be considered for professionally supervised balance, gait, and muscle-strengthening programs. Such programs, coordinated by physical, occupational, or kinesio-therapists, can decrease the risk of falls by 10%.

Commonly used antivertigo drugs and their dosages are shown in Table 6.5. In any given patient, it is often difficult to predict which drug or which combination of drugs will be most effective in alleviating the symptoms. The drug or drug combination is empirically chosen based on the known effects of each drug, and on the course and severity of the patient's symptoms. Severe forms of acute persistent vertigo are very distressing, particularly when accompanied by nausea and vomiting. Antivertigo medications with both sedative and antiemetic effects are very helpful in these situations. Chronic recurrent vertigo is

Box 6.4 Management of patients who fall

► Review all medications (including over-the-counter).
► Limit or eliminate problematic medications if possible, particularly those with sedative effects or those contributing to orthostatic hypotension or motor disequilibrium or ataxia.
► Decrease the total number of medications to four or fewer (if possible).
► Assess for orthostatic hypotension (i.e., pulse and blood pressure measured supine, standing, and standing after 3 minutes).
► Assess vision, hearing, heart, lungs, joints, muscles, and sensory function.
► Evaluate and manage comorbid conditions predisposing to falls (e.g., orthostatic hypotension, parkinsonism, delirium, leg weakness, and arthritis).
► Supply aids and assistive devices, including canes, ice gripper attachments for canes, walkers, lifts, etc.
► Observe patient rising from chair, standing, walking, and turning.
► Recommend an exercise program for patients who are suitable candidates, with professional supervision if necessary.
► Obtain appropriate blood tests (including complete blood count, serum electrolytes, calcium, phosphorus, alkaline phosphatase, 25-hydroxy vitamin D level, blood urea nitrogen, creatinine, glucose, vitamin B_{12} level, and thyroid stimulating hormone level).
► Obtain neuroimaging in presence of a head injury, new focal findings, or a suspected central nervous system process based on history or examination.
► Consider tests of bone mineral density (particularly of the hips and spine), especially in postmenopausal women or those at increased risk of osteoporosis or osteomalacia for other reasons (e.g., vitamin D deficiency, anticonvulsant use, steroids, cigarette smoking, etc.). Treat with appropriate agents and monitor if bone mineral density testing is significantly abnormal.
► Refer patients with observed difficulty ambulating to physical therapy for comprehensive evaluation and rehabilitation.
► Recommend appropriate footwear, e.g., comfortable, soft-soled shoes with adequate support, low or no heel, and appropriate tread (not smooth soled).
► Recommend hip protectors, which may decrease the risk of hip fracture by more than 50%.
► Refer to occupational therapy for an in-home safety evaluation.
► Eliminate home hazards to decrease fall risks.

Box 6.5 Environmental changes that can decrease falling include

► Removal of rugs
► Change to safer footwear (e.g., soft, flat-soled shoes)
► Use of nonslip bath mats
► Improvement of lighting (including use of a night light)
► Addition of stair, bathtub, and toilet rails
► Removal of low chairs
► Repair of pavement irregularities

less distressing and interferes less with daily activities. Agents with less sedating properties will help patients carry on with their normal routine. Agents that commonly cause confusion are best avoided in the elderly. Also, parenterally administered drugs that may produce hypotension or respiratory depression should generally be used only in a hospital setting.

In patients with acute persistent vertigo from peripheral vestibular lesions, recovery occurs more rapidly and more completely when vestibular exercises are begun as soon as possible after the onset of symptoms. The vestibular exercises shown in Box 6.6 are adapted from those proposed by Cooksey and Cawthorne in 1945. The exercises are intended to help the patient learn to use visual and proprioceptive information to compensate for the dysfunctional vestibular system. Eye and head movements are begun as soon as possible after the acute vertigo and autonomic symptoms subside. More complicated exercises involving head movements, bending, standing, and moving about are then gradually introduced as the patient improves. The exercises should be performed for at

Pearls and Perils

Vertigo management

► Antivertiginous medications with both sedative and antiemetic effects are very helpful in alleviating the symptoms of acute persistent vertigo.
► Antivertiginous medications with less sedating properties are least disruptive to the daily activities of patients with chronic recurrent vertigo.
► Antivertiginous medications that commonly cause confusion are best avoided in the elderly.
► In patients with acute persistent vertigo from peripheral vestibular lesions, recovery occurs more rapidly and more completely when vestibular exercises are begun as soon as possible after the onset of symptoms.

Table 6.5 Dosage and common effects of antivertigo medications

Drug	Dose	Sedation	Antiemetic	Anticholinergic	EPS*	Confusion†	Other
Diazepam (Valium)	5–10 mg po or IV q4–6h	+++	+	−	−	++	Respiratory depression
Dimenhydrinate (Dramamine)	50–100 mg po or IM q4–6h	++	++	++	−	+	
Droperidol (Inapsine)	2.5–10 mg IM or IV q12h	+++	+++	−	++	+	Hypotension, tachycardia
Meclizine (Antivert)	25–50 mg q4–6h	+	++	++	−	+	
Phenobarbital	30 mg po or IV q6–8h	+++	+	−	−	++	Respiratory depression
Prochlorperazine (Compazine)	5–10 mg po/IM q6–8h; 25 mg pr q12h; or 2.5–10 mg IV q6–8h	++	+++	+	++	+	Hypotension
Promethazine (Phenergan)	25–50 mg po/IM/pr q4–6h	+++	+++	+	+	+	
Trimethobenzamide	250 mg po q6–8h; 200 mg pr/IM q6–8h	+	+++	−	++	+	Hypotension

−, never; +, uncommon; ++, common; +++, typical
Anticholinergic effects include blurred vision, dry mouth, tachycardia, urinary retention, agitation, confusion. These manifestations may also occur with antihistamines (meclizine, dimenhydrinate), but to a lesser degree.
*Extrapyramidal (EPS) effects potentially include acute dystonia, parkinsonism, akathisia, and tardive dyskinesia.
†Confusion is particularly a problem in the elderly.

least 5 minutes several times per day. Specific head positions and movements that precipitate vertigo should be sought and repetitively performed to facilitate vestibular compensation. Antivertigo medications can be used during the exercises to help control both the vertigo and the autonomic symptoms. Although there are theoretical reasons to imagine that vestibular sedatives may limit the efficacy of vestibular exercises, no solid evidence suggests that such medications affect either the rate or degree of vestibular compensation.

Selected Vertiginous Syndromes and Diseases

Benign Paroxysmal Positioning Vertigo

Benign paroxysmal positioning vertigo (BPPV) is a mechanical disorder of the inner ear in which certain head movements or positions precipitate vertigo, with concomitant nystagmus and autonomic symptoms. In the vast majority of cases, the symptoms result from abnormal stimulation of the posterior semicircular duct. Benign paroxysmal positioning vertigo is particularly important to recognize because (a) it is very common, and indeed is probably the most common cause of vertigo in the elderly; (b) it can be disabling; (c) it can be accurately diagnosed by clinical examination; (d) extensive diagnostic studies are not indicated; (e) if untreated, it will usually

spontaneously remit, although manifestations may be protracted in some cases and recurrences are common; and (f) it is readily treatable and even curable. Specific conditions etiologically associated with BPPV include head trauma, middle ear and mastoid infections, middle or inner ear surgery, and labyrinthine ischemia. Most cases, however, are idiopathic.

The diagnosis of BPPV is clinical and depends on observing the characteristic manifestations, which are typically elicited with the Dix-Hallpike positioning test (see earlier description). Definite diagnosis of BPPV requires demonstration of linear–rotatory nystagmus with appropriate latency, duration, and fatigability. With adoption of the offending head position, vertigo and nystagmus begin with a brief latency of from 1 to 45 seconds, and typically 2 to 5 seconds. The nystagmus is mixed upbeat–rotatory and slightly disconjugate. For the rotational component of the *slow* phases, the dependent eye intorts and the upper eye extorts. The nystagmus varies somewhat in the two eyes and with the direction of gaze. It is more rotatory in the dependent eye and with gaze toward the dependent (affected) ear, and more upbeat in the upper eye and with gaze away from the dependent ear. The manifestations of BPPV subside in 10–60 seconds, even with maintenance of the precipitating position. If BPPV is elicited with the Dix-Hallpike positioning test, the vertigo and nystagmus may recur, usually less violently, when the patient returns to a sitting position. The

---

Box 6.6 Vestibular exercises

In bed
1 Move eyes up and down and then side-to-side, at first slowly, then quickly.
2 Move head forward and backward and then side-to-side, at first slowly, then quickly.

Sitting
1 Eye and head movements as above.
2 Rotate head and shoulders, at first slowly, then quickly.
3 Bend forward and pick up objects from ground.

Standing
1 Change from sitting to standing, at first with eyes open, then with eyes closed.
2 Eye and head movements as above.

Moving about
1 Turn around.
2 Walk across room, at first with eyes open, then with eyes closed.
3 Stand on one foot, at first with eyes open, then with eyes closed.
4 Climb up and down steps with eyes open.
5 Play games involving stooping, stretching, aiming (e.g., shuffleboard or bowling).

Pearls and Perils

Benign paroxysmal positioning vertigo (BPPV)

▶ BPPV is the most common cause of vertigo in the elderly.
▶ Extensive diagnostic studies are not indicated.
▶ Definite diagnosis of BPPV requires demonstration of positioning-induced linear–rotatory nystagmus with appropriate latency, duration, and fatigability.
▶ If typical nystagmus is observed with the Dix-Hallpike positioning test, the affected ear is the one undermost.
▶ The main differential diagnostic consideration is distinguishing BPPV from central causes of positional vertigo, which are more ominous.
▶ Cranial imaging, preferably with magnetic resonance imaging, is indicated if the clinical manifestations are not typical of BPPV, or if there is evidence of static neurologic dysfunction.
▶ Particle-repositioning or liberatory maneuvers and positioning exercises are highly effective therapies for BPPV.
▶ Drug therapy with vestibular sedatives is generally *not* helpful with the severe abrupt episodes of BPPV.
▶ Drug therapy may help suppress the nausea and nonspecific dizziness between episodes.
▶ Surgical procedures to correct BPPV are generally unnecessary and should be avoided.

---

duration of this nystagmus will also be less than 1 minute. With repeated assumption of the offending head position, the manifestations will rapidly and progressively decrease and may stop altogether. If typical nystagmus is observed, the affected ear is the one undermost. Generally, there should be no evidence of static neurologic dysfunction, particularly affecting the vestibular system, cerebellar pathways, and cranial nerves, although BPPV can also occur with Ménière's syndrome, labyrinthine ischemia, and head trauma, all of which may be associated with static neurologic or peripheral vestibular dysfunction (Table 6.6).

The main differential diagnostic consideration is distinguishing BPPV from central causes of positional vertigo, which are more ominous. Certain clinical findings can be very helpful in distinguishing central and peripheral forms of positional nystagmus (Table 6.4). However, despite the generally helpful clinical prediction rules, central lesions may rarely cause positional nystagmus that resembles BPPV clinically. Particularly in the elderly, great care should be taken in excluding a central cause for vertigo. Cranial imaging, preferably with MRI, is indicated if the clinical manifestations are not typical of BPPV, or if there is evidence of static neurologic dysfunction, particularly affecting the vestibular system, cerebellar pathways, or cranial nerves.

Several theories have been developed to explain the clinical phenomena of BPPV. In 1973, Schuknecht hypothesized that BPPV is produced by relatively heavy debris from degenerating otoconia of the utricular macule settling on the cupula of the posterior semicircular duct. As a result, the cupula of this duct would be transformed from a rotary motion sensor to a linear motion sensor. This "cupulolithiasis theory" was supported by some histologic evidence, but is not compatible with all of the clinical features of BPPV. In particular, this theory would predict sustained vertigo with maintenance of an offending head position. Generally, the debris floats freely within the endolymph of the duct in the form of loose particles or a congealed clot or plug. Since the particles or clot are heavier than endolymph, they gravitate toward the most dependent part of the duct. Movement of the particles or clot induces a flow of endolymph within the duct which pushes on the cupula, thereby producing a BPPV attack. This "canalolithiasis theory" can explain all of the clinical features of BPPV and provides the basis for effective approaches to treatment.

Currently, the preferred form of treatment is with various "particle repositioning" or "liberatory" maneuvers and exercises. If performed properly, these forms of therapy are highly effective in BPPV. The Semont and Epley maneuvers utilize a single sequence of head and

Table 6.6 Benign paroxysmal positioning vertigo

Discriminating features	Consistent features	Variable features
Episodic vertigo of abrupt onset, lasting seconds	Patients may estimate that vertigo lasts minutes	Onset following prolonged bed rest, head trauma, middle ear and mastoid infections, middle or inner ear surgery, or labyrinthine ischemia
Vertigo precipitated by Dix–Hallpike positioning test	Nausea and vomiting with episodes	Occurs more frequently in the elderly
Upbeat-rotatory jerk nystagmus	Nonvertiginous dizziness (disequilibrium) between episodes	Elderly cases are usually idiopathic
Nystagmus begins with latency of 1–45 seconds	No auditory manifestations	Vestibular paresis on bithermal caloric testing disease
Nystagmus duration is less than 1 minute	No symptoms or signs of central nervous system	
Nystagmus fatigues with repetition of Dix–Hallpike positioning test	No evident precipitating factors	
	Normal audiograms, brainstem auditory evoked responses, and cranial imaging	
	Electronystagmographic evidence of paroxysmal upbeat-rotatory nystagmus	

body positioning to remove debris from within the posterior semicircular canal and deposit it back into the utricular cavity. Complete resolution of symptoms with these maneuvers occurs after a single treatment in 80–90% of cases in most series. In contrast, the Brandt-Daroff exercises utilize a repetitive sequence of head and body positioning to facilitate central compensation.

The modified Epley liberatory particle-repositioning maneuver consists of four steps. The first two steps are basically a repeat of the Dix-Hallpike positioning test. In step 1, with the patient seated, the patient's head is turned horizontally 30 degrees toward the *affected* ear, so that the ipsilateral posterior semicircular duct is in a parasagittal plane. In step 2, the patient is tilted backward, so that both shoulders rest against the table, the head is slightly hanging off the opposite edge, and the nose is pointed to the side of the affected ear (i.e., the head is approximately 105 degrees back from the sitting position, with the head turn from step 1 maintained). Because of the head positioning, the movement in step 2 is in the plane of the affected semicircular duct. The resulting head-hanging position is maintained for 3 minutes. In step 3, the head is turned 90 degrees toward the unaffected ear. The head then continues turning another 90 degrees toward the unaffected ear, in conjunction with a 90-degree turn of the trunk. At this point, the patient is on his or her side, with the unaffected ear undermost and the nose pointed toward the table. Positioning nystagmus beating toward the uppermost (affected) ear predicts therapeutic success. In contrast, positioning nystagmus beating toward the undermost (unaffected) ear indicates that the plug of material within the duct has moved in the wrong direction, back toward the ampulla. This position is maintained for 3 minutes unless the nystagmus occurs in the wrong direction, in which case the entire procedure should be repeated. Finally, in step 4, the patient is moved

to the sitting position. A home-treatment version of these exercises is also available (see annotated bibliography), which is particularly helpful for patients with recurrences. If the Epley maneuver is unsuccessful, the procedure can be repeated, a Semont maneuver can be tried, or Brandt-Daroff exercises can be prescribed.

The Semont liberatory maneuver also consists of four steps. In step 1, with the patient seated, the patient's head is turned horizontally 45 degrees toward the *unaffected* ear, so that the contralateral posterior semicircular canal is in a coronal plane. In step 2, the patient is tilted laterally toward the affected ear, so that the ipsilateral shoulder rests against the table and the head hangs off the edge of the table with the nose up (i.e., the head is approximately 105 degrees from the sitting position, with the head turn from step 1 maintained). Because of the head positioning, the movement in step 2 is in the plane of the *affected* semicircular duct. The resulting head-hanging position is maintained for 3 minutes. In step 3, the patient is tilted laterally toward the opposite (unaffected) ear, so that the opposite shoulder rests against the table and so that the nose is down (i.e., the head is moved approximately 195 degrees from step 2, with the head turn from step 1 maintained). Positioning nystagmus beating toward the uppermost (affected) ear predicts therapeutic success. In contrast, positioning nystagmus beating toward the undermost (unaffected) ear indicates that the plug of material within the duct has moved in the wrong direction, back toward the ampulla. This position is maintained for 3 minutes unless the nystagmus occurs in the wrong direction, in which case the entire procedure should be repeated. Finally, in step 4, the patient is moved back to a sitting position. If the Semont maneuver is not successful, the procedure can be repeated, a modified Epley maneuver can be tried, or Brandt-Daroff exercises can be prescribed.

The Brandt-Daroff exercises were developed originally based on the cupulolithiasis model of BPPV. Although this model is no longer thought to explain the majority of cases of BPPV, Brandt-Daroff exercises are nevertheless effective in relieving the symptoms of BPPV. Indeed, the vast majority of patients experience complete relief of symptoms in 3–14 days. In addition, by showing patients that they may control their own symptoms, the Brandt-Daroff exercises provide considerable reassurance and greatly decrease the anxiety commonly associated with those symptoms. To perform the Brandt-Daroff exercises, the patient sits on the bedside, and then tilts laterally until the side of the head rests on the bed. This position is maintained until the vertigo subsides. The patient then sits up for 30 seconds or until the vertigo subsides. This maneuver is then repeated with the patient tilting to the opposite side. The entire sequence is repeated during a given session until vertigo is not elicited in the offending position. The exercises are done every 3 hours while awake, and are stopped after two consecutive vertigo-free days. If Brandt-Daroff exercises fail to eliminate the symptoms of BPPV after 2 weeks, the diagnosis should certainly be reviewed.

Drug therapy with vestibular sedatives is generally not helpful with the severe abrupt episodes of BPPV. Drug therapy may, however, help suppress the nausea and nonspecific dizziness between episodes. Whether use of vestibular sedatives delays recovery by slowing central compensation is controversial.

Surgical procedures to correct BPPV should be avoided. Surgical procedures, such as selective dissection of the ipsilateral posterior ampullary nerve, or transmastoid posterior semicircular canal occlusion, were advocated in the past. With the availability of the liberatory maneuvers and the Brandt-Daroff exercises, surgical procedures for BPPV are almost never needed now.

Vertebrobasilar Insufficiency

Vertebrobasilar insufficiency (VBI) is mainly a disease of the elderly. In VBI, ischemia of structures supplied by the vertebrobasilar circulation may produce a wide range of neurologic symptoms, including vertigo, diplopia, weakness, drop attacks, and visual field defects. The vertigo is abrupt in onset, usually lasts several minutes, and may be associated with nausea and possibly vomiting. A large proportion of patients with VBI have isolated episodes of vertigo at some time in their illness. However, recurring episodes of isolated vertigo over a period of months should suggest a diagnosis other than VBI.

The diagnosis of VBI is clinical, and depends on a history of recurrent episodes of transient neurologic dysfunction, generally lasting minutes, referable to the vertebrobasilar circulation. Neurologic examination, CT, and MRI scans are frequently normal unless there has been a prior stroke. Conventional and magnetic resonance angiography and transcranial Doppler ultrasonography may provide the most helpful diagnostic information in appropriate clinical circumstances. Limitations of angiography in VBI include the following: (a) angiographic findings may not correlate well with clinical symptoms and signs; (b) lesions are typically diffuse and inaccessible surgically, although newer interventional approaches may be helpful in selected cases; and (c) conventional angiography may cause further ischemia (Table 6.7).

The cause of VBI is usually atherosclerosis of the posterior cerebral circulation (subclavian, vertebral, or basilar arteries), which supplies the occipital lobes of the cerebral hemispheres, brainstem, cerebellum, eighth nerve, and labyrinth. Cerebral hypoperfusion (e.g.. from postural hypotension) can precipitate bouts of VBI, particularly in those with posterior circulation atherosclerosis. Unusual (and overdiagnosed) causes of VBI include subclavian steal syndrome and mechanical compression of the vertebral arteries from cervical spondylosis.

Treatment of VBI is usually directed at treating stroke risk factors and using antiplatelet agents, such as aspirin or clopidogrel. Anticoagulation is reserved for selected patients, including those with frequent incapacitating episodes and those with symptoms and signs suggesting impending basilar artery thrombosis, such as episodes of bilateral blindness or quadriparesis. Vestibu-

---

Table 6.7 Vertebrobasilar insufficiency/Transient ischemic attack (TIA)

Discriminating features	Consistent features	Variable features
Episodic vertigo of abrupt onset and duration of minutes to hours	Presence of stroke risk factors, including age over 55, hypertension, diabetes	Mild nausea and rarely vomiting
Central nervous system symptoms and signs during events, such as visual field deficits, diplopia, dysarthria, drop attacks, ataxia, or limb weakness	No auditory manifestations Normal neurological examination Normal audiograms, brainstem auditory evoked responses, electro- or video-nystagmography, and cranial imaging	Orthostatic hypotension Stenosis or occlusion of the subclavian, vertebral, or basilar arteries on angiography or ultrasonography Old infarcts on cerebral imaging

---

Pearls and Perils

Vertebrobasilar insufficiency

▶ VBI is mainly a disease of the elderly.

▶ Ischemia of structures supplied by the vertebrobasilar circulation may produce a wide range of neurologic symptoms, including vertigo, diplopia, weakness, drop attacks, and visual field defects.

▶ A large proportion of patients with VBI have isolated episodes of vertigo at some time in their illness.

▶ The vertigo is abrupt in onset and usually lasts several minutes.

▶ Recurring episodes of isolated vertigo over a period of months indicates a diagnosis other than VBI.

▶ The diagnosis of VBI depends on a history of recurrent episodes of transient neurologic dysfunction, generally lasting minutes, referable to the vertebrobasilar circulation.

▶ Neurologic examination, CT, and MRI scans are frequently normal unless there has been a prior stroke.

▶ Angiography should not be performed indiscriminately.

▶ Cerebral hypoperfusion from postural hypotension can precipitate bouts of VBI.

▶ Treatment of VBI usually involves treating stroke risk factors and administering antiplatelet agents.

▶ Anticoagulation is reserved for selected patients.

▶ Antivertiginous medications are not helpful and may exacerbate VBI by causing or exacerbating orthostatic hypotension.

Pearls and Perils

Ménière's syndrome

▶ The peak age of onset is in the fourth and fifth decades.

▶ Ménière's syndrome is characterized by episodic vertigo, fluctuating hearing loss and tinnitus, and a sensation of fullness or pressure in the ear.

▶ Each episode develops rapidly over minutes and then slowly subsides over several hours.

▶ The associated nystagmus quick phases are initially directed away from the affected ear.

▶ Early in the course of the illness, the hearing loss reverses completely, but later there is persistent and frequently progressive hearing loss.

▶ Bilateral involvement eventually occurs in about one-third of cases.

▶ Medical management includes symptomatic treatment of acute episodes, in conjunction with long-term prophylaxis with salt restriction and diuretics.

▶ In resistant cases, shunt surgery or ablative surgery can be considered.

▶ Ablative procedures are generally contraindicated in those with bilateral involvement.

---

lar sedatives are not helpful and may exacerbate the problem by causing or exacerbating orthostatic hypotension.

Ménière's Syndrome

Ménière's syndrome is characterized by episodic vertigo, fluctuating hearing loss and tinnitus, and a sensation of fullness or pressure in the ear. Each episode develops rapidly over minutes and then slowly subsides over several hours. The associated nystagmus quick phases are initially directed *away* from the affected ear, followed later by an oppositely directed secondary nystagmus. After the acute vertiginous episode is over, the patient frequently is dizzy and unsteady for several days. Early in the course of the illness, the hearing loss reverses completely, but later persistent and frequently progressive hearing loss occurs. Bilateral involvement eventually occurs in about one-third of cases. The peak age of onset of Ménière's syndrome is in the fourth and fifth decades.

Diagnosis is based on the characteristic clinical profile and documentation of fluctuating hearing loss. Audiologic evaluation shows sensorineural hearing loss usually worse at the lower frequencies, recruitment consistent with cochlear dysfunction, and relatively preserved speech discrimination. Electronystagmography may demonstrate a spontaneous peripheral vestibular nystagmus and either a vestibular paresis or directional preponderance on caloric testing. Brainstem auditory evoked responses are generally normal. Radiologic studies are not helpful (Table 6.8).

Ménière's syndrome can result from bacterial, viral, or syphilitic labyrinthitis, but the majority of cases are idiopathic. Genetic factors may be involved, as a positive family history is reported in up to 50% of cases. The principal pathologic finding in patients with Ménière's syndrome is an increase in the volume of endolymph, with dilation and distortion of the membranous labyrinth. The mechanism involved in the episodic symptoms of Ménière's syndrome is unknown, but is thought to involve rupture of utricular or semicircular canal membranes.

Medical management includes symptomatic treatment of acute episodes, in conjunction with long-term prophylaxis with salt restriction and diuretics. In resistant cases, shunt surgery or ablative surgery can be considered. Ablative procedures are generally contraindicated in those with bilateral involvement.

Viral Neurolabyrinthitis

Viral neurolabyrinthitis can occur at any age. It is typically manifested by the rapid onset over hours of either

Table 6.8 Ménière's syndrome

Discriminating features	Consistent features	Variable features
Episodic vertigo of abrupt onset, lasting hours	Nausea and vomiting with attacks	Loud noises may precipitate vertigo (Tullio phenomenon)
Ear fullness	Nonvertiginous dizziness between attacks	Family history of Ménière's syndrome
Fluctuating hearing loss and tinnitus, that increase during attacks	No central nervous system symptoms or signs	History of bacterial, viral, or syphilitic labyrinthitis
Spontaneous linear-rotatory jerk nystagmus during attacks	Audiogram demonstration of sensorineural hearing loss worse at lower frequencies, recruitment consistent with cochlear dysfunction, and relatively preserved speech discrimination	Electronystagmographic demonstration of spontaneous or positional peripheral vestibular nystagmus most prominent with eyes closed or open in darkness
Gait unsteadiness during attacks	Normal brainstem auditory evoked responses	Vestibular paresis or directional preponderance on bithermal caloric testing
	Normal cranial imaging	Superimposed BPPV

unilateral deafness, vertigo with associated nausea and vomiting, or some combination of the two. When vertigo occurs alone without audiologic manifestations, the condition may be called *vestibular neuronitis* or *vestibular neuritis*. When audiologic manifestations occur alone, the condition may be called *acoustic neuritis*. Only the syndrome with vertigo will be discussed further.

In viral neurolabyrinthitis, neurologic symptoms and signs are absent, other than those referable to the peripheral auditory and vestibular organs. Deafness, when present, is often profound but returns to normal in more than half of the cases. Vertiginous sensations typically peak within 24 hours and then gradually resolve over several weeks. Signs of acute unilateral labyrinthine dysfunction include both nystagmus with quick phases directed away from the affected ear and vestibulospinal dysfunction with postural imbalance and falling toward the affected ear. Since the labyrinthine dysfunction typically involves all of the ducts and otoliths of one labyrinth, the resulting nystagmus is horizontal-torsional, representing the balance of signals from the contralateral labyrinth.

The diagnosis is based on the following: (a) the presence of a characteristic clinical profile; (b) absence of neurologic signs and symptoms referable to the CNS; and (c) laboratory evidence of peripheral auditory and/or vestibular dysfunction using audiology, caloric testing, and electronystagmography. Audiograms may demonstrate unilateral sensorineural hearing loss. Bithermal caloric testing shows vestibular paresis and electronystagmography shows spontaneous nystagmus, most prominent with the eyes either closed or open in darkness. Brainstem auditory evoked responses and cranial imaging are normal (Table 6.9).

Viral neurolabyrinthitis must be distinguished from brainstem/labyrinthine ischemia, bacterial labyrinthitis, and perilymph fistula. In the elderly, vertebrobasilar ischemia should be carefully excluded. With vertebrobasilar distribution ischemia, there is usually a history of recurrent episodes of neurologic dysfunction. With brainstem ischemia or stroke, the onset is sudden or stuttering, there are typically, but not always, signs of brainstem or cerebellar dysfunction, and infarction may be evident on cerebral imaging studies. Infarction of the labyrinth results in *sudden* severe vertigo and deafness in contrast to the more gradual onset with viral neurolabyrinthitis. Bacterial labyrinthitis is usually associated with mastoiditis, which should be evident on examination with CT, using bone windows through the temporal bone. With a perilymph fistula, the onset of vertigo and deafness is abrupt;

Table 6.9 Viral neurolabyrinthitis

Discriminating features	Consistent features	Variable features
Monophasic vertigo with subacute onset lasting days	No central nervous system symptoms or signs	Unilateral hearing loss and tinnitus
Nausea and vomiting	Electronystagmographic demonstration of spontaneous nystagmus most prominent with eyes either closed or open in darkness	Audiogram demonstration of unilateral sensorineural hearing loss
Spontaneous horizontal-rotatory jerk nystagmus	Vestibular paresis on bithermal caloric testing	Vestibular neuronitis can occur at any age
Gait unsteadiness	Normal brainstem auditory evoked responses	
	Normal cranial imaging	

Pearls and Perils

Viral neurolabyrinthitis

▶ Patients experience the rapid onset over hours of unilateral deafness and vertigo, with associated nausea and vomiting.
▶ Central neurologic symptoms and signs are absent.
▶ Vertigo typically peaks within 24 hours and then gradually resolves over 1–2 weeks.
▶ Deafness is often profound, but returns to normal in more than half of the cases.
▶ Vestibular neuronitis must be distinguished from brainstem/labyrinthine ischemia, bacterial labyrinthitis, and perilymph fistula.
▶ Persisting vertigo beyond 2 weeks suggests CNS dysfunction with resulting inability to restore balance of vestibular tone.
▶ Patients with severe acute vertigo will be most comfortable lying in bed with the affected ear up.
▶ Antivertiginous medications can decrease both the sensation of vertigo and the accompanying nausea and vomiting.
▶ Initially, a parenterally administered antivertiginous medication with some sedative effects is preferable.
▶ Antivertiginous medications should be required only for a short period, usually less than 2 weeks.
▶ Vestibular exercises should be initiated as early as possible, usually several days after onset.
▶ Patients should gradually progress to more difficult vestibular exercises, even if they exacerbate the vertigo.
▶ Recovery in the elderly may be protracted.
▶ Recurrences occur in 20–30% of affected patients.

Consider Consultation When...

▶ The cause of dizziness is not clear after history, physical, and neurologic examinations, and appropriate laboratory tests.
▶ Further expertise or experience is needed to treat the underlying cause.
▶ The patient does not respond to treatment, or the patient's course is different from that expected.
▶ The patient has an intracranial mass lesion, the patient has an undiagnosed CNS disorder, or the patient has a positive fistula test.
▶ Technical assistance is needed in interpreting or performing diagnostic or therapeutic procedures.

there is usually a precipitating event such as head trauma, sudden strain (e.g., with lifting, coughing, or sneezing), or stapedectomy for otosclerosis; and a fistula test is frequently positive.

A large body of epidemiologic, pathologic, and experimental evidence supports a viral cause for most cases of neurolabyrinthitis. Vestibular neuronitis may be a component of a systemic viral illness or may occur as an isolated infection of the labyrinth and eighth nerve. In an individual patient with neurolabyrinthitis, a viral origin is difficult to document. Unless there is evidence to suggest another cause for acute persistent unilateral labyrinthine dysfunction, the patient should be managed as having viral neurolabyrinthitis.

The treatment is basically symptomatic and supportive. Vestibular sedatives can be helpful in decreasing the sensation of vertigo, and in decreasing the accompanying nausea and vomiting. Initially, a parenterally administered agent with some sedative effects

is preferable. Some commonly used agents are listed in Table 6.5. Vestibular sedatives should be required only for a short period, since acute vertigo due to peripheral vestibular disease typically resolves in 1–2 weeks. Persisting vertigo suggests CNS dysfunction, with resulting inability to restore balance of vestibular tone. In this circumstance, cranial imaging and neurologic consultation are indicated.

Initially, patients with severe acute vertigo will be most comfortable in bed, lying with the affected ear up. After several days, vestibular exercises can be initiated. These exercises are outlined in Box 6.6 (Chapter 6). The exercises should be performed for at least 5 minutes three times a day as long as vertigo persists. Patients should gradually progress to more difficult exercises even if they exacerbate the vertigo.

Recovery in the elderly may be protracted, with dizziness and unsteadiness persisting for years. Recurrences, which occur in 20–30% of affected patients, may represent reactivation of latent viruses.

Annotated Bibliography

Baloh RW. *Dizziness, hearing loss, and tinnitus.* Philadelphia: F.A. Davis, 1998.
  A readable review of neurotology, with concise discussions of the anatomy and physiology of the vestibular system, the evaluation of the dizzy patient, and the evaluation and management of common neurotologic problems.
Baloh RW, Halmagyi GM. *Disorders of the vestibular system.* New York: Oxford University Press, 1996.
  Monograph on disorders of the vestibular system, their evaluation, and management.
Baloh RW, Honrubia V. *Clinical neurophysiology of the vestibular system,* 3rd ed. Philadelphia: F.A. Davis, 2001.
  Monograph on the vestibular system and its disorders, with excellent discussions on the evaluation of the dizzy patient, and the evaluation and management of common neurotologic problems.

Brandt T. *Vertigo: Its multisensory syndromes*, 2nd ed. New York: Springer-Verlag, 1999.
Monograph on various vertigo syndromes, their evaluation, and management.

Brandt T, Steddin S, Daroff RB. Therapy for benign paroxysmal positioning vertigo, revisited. *Neurology* 1994;44:796–800.
A review of different treatment approaches for benign paroxysmal positioning vertigo. The article has excellent illustrations and clearly explains the mechanical basis for the liberatory and particle repositioning maneuvers.

The Consensus Committee of the American Autonomic Society and the American Academy of Neurology. Consensus statement on the definition of orthostatic hypotension, pure autonomic failure, and multiple system atrophy. *Neurology* 1994;46:1470.
Consensus definition of orthostatic hypotension.

Drachman DA. An approach to the dizzy patient. *Neurology* 1972;22:323–334.
Describes a broad medical approach to the evaluation of dizzy patients. Although the approach outlined is probably overly complex, the authors reached secure diagnoses in more than 90% of their patients.

Halmagyi GM, Curthoys IS. A clinical sign of canal paresis. *Arch Neurol* 1988;45:737–739.
Description of the head-thrust test for bedside evaluation of unilateral loss of semicircular canal function.

Lanska DJ, Goetz CG. Romberg's sign: Development, adoption, and adaptation in the 19th century. *Neurology* 2000;55:1201–1206.
Historical review of the origin, pathophysiologic basis, and utility of the Romberg sign.

Lanska DJ, Remler B. Benign paroxysmal positioning vertigo: Classic descriptions, origins of the provocative positioning technique, and conceptual developments. *Neurology* 1997;48:1167–1177.
Reviews the pathophysiology of benign paroxysmal positioning vertigo in a historical context, and provides a detailed explanation of the Dix-Hallpike positioning test.

Radtke A, Neuhauser H, von Brevern M, Lempert T. A modified Epley's procedure for self-treatment of benign paroxysmal positional vertigo. *Neurology* 1999;53:1358–1360.
A very useful approach for patients to employ self-treatment of recurrences of benign paroxysmal positioning vertigo. Illustrated instructions in English, German, French, and Spanish are available for patients at http://www.charite.de/ch/neuro/vertigo.html.

Disorders of Gait

Stephen J. Ryan

Walking on two feet requires simultaneous integration of several neurologic systems to overcome gravity, propel oneself forward, and compare motor performance with incoming data from several sensory systems. Many important neurologic diseases may manifest themselves partially or wholly as gait problems, since dysfunction at any level of the nervous system can upset these finely integrated systems and impair the act of walking. As a result, evaluation of disturbances of gait can reveal vital clues to diagnosis of neurologic disease.

Anatomy and Function

The initiation of motor activity is thought to arise in the frontal lobes and particularly the premotor cortex (Brodmann's area 6). The next step appears to involve activation and integration of a motor neural network, which includes the corticospinal system, the basal ganglia, and the cerebellum. The main component of the corticospinal tract arises from large pyramidal (Betz) cells in the precentral gyrus (Brodmann's area 4). These Betz cells give rise to fibers that descend ipsilaterally through the internal capsule to the cerebral peduncles of the midbrain, the basis pontis of the pons, and then the pyramids of the medulla. These fibers travel to the lower medulla to cross the midline at the decussation of the pyramids. The fibers then descend to terminate on the lower motor neurons in the anterior horn of the spinal cord. The lower motor neurons leave the spinal cord as the ventral root, which joins the (afferent) dorsal root to form the spinal nerve. The lower motor neurons then terminate at the muscles— the terminus forming the *neuromuscular junction* (NMJ).

The basal ganglia (the caudate, putamen, globus pallidus, and some other components) and the cerebellum are intimately involved in the process of movement as integrators and comparators of movement, motor function, and sensory input.

Proprioceptive sensory input is gathered from muscle and tendon stretch organs, and travels, along with joint position information, through the peripheral nerves

Key Clinical Questions

▶ Does the patient have medical conditions (e.g., diabetes) that might predispose to sensory or gait disturbance?
▶ Does the patient take any medications that might cause gait problems?
▶ Is the gait disorder associated with urinary incontinence?
▶ Is there evidence of associated unilateral or bilateral damage to the corticospinal tract?
▶ Is parkinsonism a feature of the gait disturbance?
▶ Is the gait disorder associated with foot deformities or foot drop?

to enter the posterior spinal cord via the dorsal root ganglia. Lower extremity proprioceptive information enters the spinal cord through the sacral and lumbar nerve roots and ascends to synapse in the nucleus dorsalis in the dorsal horn of segments C8 through L3. The nucleus dorsalis gives rise to axons ascending ipsilaterally in the ipsilateral dorsal spinocerebellar tract in the dorsolateral funiculus. The axons terminate at the nucleus Z portion of the nucleus gracilis in the medulla. Then fibers from nucleus Z enter the internal arcuate tract and cross the midline before rising to the ventral posterior nuclei of the thalamus in the medial lemniscus, and then to the primary sensory cortex through the internal capsule and the corona radiata. The axons traveling in the dorsal spinocerebellar tract send collateral branches through the inferior cerebellar peduncle to provide proprioceptive information to the cerebellum. Additional information is received from the visual and vestibular systems.

Mechanics of Walking

Normal walking is a complex task requiring maintenance of an upright posture while shifting the center of gravity from side to side to allow alternate raising and swinging of the lower extremities for forward motion (propulsion). The human body maintains resistance to gravity in part through antigravity reflexes that are mediated at the level of the spinal cord and brainstem. These reflexes preserve the legs and spine in extension and are controlled to some degree by the propriospinal and rubrospinal pathways. Additional reflexes at the level of the cervical cord and brainstem maintain and integrate neck and head position with limb movements while walking. The gluteal muscles, the quadriceps, and the paraspinous muscles are the most important muscles in producing extension. Weakness in these muscles (such as seen in muscular dystrophies) can severely impair stance, posture, and gait.

Walking consists of a repetitive *gait cycle*. The cycle is traditionally considered to begin at the strike of the right heel on the ground. The left toe is then lifted and the left leg swings forward at the hip with flexion of the knee. The right leg bears weight from its heel strike to the lifting of the right toe. Hence, this period is known as the right *support* or *stance phase*. The left leg movement is referred to as the *swing phase*. From the moment that the left heel returns to the ground until the right foot leaves the ground, the body is supported briefly by both feet. This is the *double support phase*. Running differs from walking in that both feet are off the ground briefly, so that propulsion is provided by a thrust of the hind leg. The entire sequence from one contact of the right heel to the ground to the next right heel strike is a *stride*. *Cadence* refers to the maintenance of a smooth rhythmic gait cycle. With normal walking, the arms swing freely and act as counterbalances for truncal and leg motion.

History and Examination

Evaluation of patients with gait problems begins with a complete neurologic history and examination. In particular, details of medical conditions that may predispose the patient to sensory or gait disturbance should be obtained. For example, diabetes commonly disturbs gait, with its frequent concomitant neuropathy and visual problems. Many medications (Box 7.1) can predispose patients to gait problems, especially if they produce orthostatic hypotension (e.g., propranolol), confusion (e.g., anticholinergics), ataxia (e.g., carbamazepine), or drowsiness (e.g., benzodiazepines).

Measurement of orthostatic blood pressure and pulse can detect orthostatic hypotension during standing. The neurologic examination closely evaluates strength, coordination, and sensation. The coordination examination should include testing of rapid alternating movements, stroking of the heel along the opposite shin from knee to ankle, and finger-to-nose testing. The five primary sensory modalities are tested in all limbs (light touch, pin-prick, temperature, position, and vibration) looking for focal sensory loss, graded distal (stocking–glove) sensory loss, or levels of decreased sensation, hyperesthesia, or dysesthesia.

Examination of strength should include particularly hip flexors (iliopsoas), hip extensors (gluteus maximus), hip abductors (gluteus medius), knee extensors (quadriceps), foot dorsiflexors (e.g., tibialis anterior), and foot plantar flexors (e.g., gastrocnemius). Strength can be measured and reliably recorded on a scale of 0–5 as recommended by the Medical Research Council (Box 7.2).

The focused gait examination (Table 7.1) detects both stance (or station) and walking abnormalities. Standing requires adequate strength to overcome gravity while maintaining appropriate control of balance and sway. The patient standing at rest can reveal an abnormality of posture or balance control. Walking requires forward propulsion while alternating weight support between each foot during alternate strides. Walking brings to light any problems disturbing the complex interaction of the various neurologic systems. The arms normally

---

▼

Box 7.1 Medications that commonly predispose to gait problems

► Antihypertensives
► Antidepressants
► Anxiolytics/sedatives
► Anticonvulsants
► Neuroleptics
► Anticholinergics

Box 7.2 Medical Research Council grading for strength

0   No muscle contraction
1   Flicker or trace of contraction
2   Active movement with gravity eliminated
3   Active movement against gravity but no resistance
4   Active movement against gravity and some resistance
5   Normal power

Box 8.1 Gait problems

▸ Normal elderly gait (senile gait)
▸ Frontal lobe gait
▸ Spastic gait
▸ Hemiparetic gait
▸ Scissors gait
▸ Spastic quadriparesis
▸ Extrapyramidal gait disorders
▸ Parkinsonian gait
▸ Choreic gait
▸ Cerebellar ataxic gait
▸ Sensory ataxic gait
▸ Steppage gait
▸ Myopathic gait
▸ Antalgic gait
▸ Functional gait disorders

---

swing freely during walking as a counterbalance, and lack of swing can be a very important diagnostic clue to gait abnormalities. Walking on the heel or toes may reveal weakness in foot dorsiflexion or extension. Tandem walking consists of walking in a straight line, alternately placing each foot in front of the other and pressing the heel of the leading foot against toes of the other. Tandem walking can be very sensitive for the detection of ataxias. However, minor difficulty in tandem walking is common even in the normal elderly person. Examining the pattern of wear on the sole of the shoes can suggest altered foot placement or foot dragging.

Later sections focus on the most common gait problems affecting adults, particularly the elderly. These gait problems (Box 7.3) include spastic, parkinsonian, cerebellar ataxic, sensory ataxic, steppage, myopathic, antalgic, and hysterical gaits. First, however, the gait changes in normal elderly persons bear discussion.

Senile Gait

Certain changes in gait can be expected with normal aging. These are sometimes referred to as *senile gait*. Stance changes occur to maximize stability: the feet tend to be spread wider, giving a broader base to support the center of gravity. With walking, there may be slowing in

Table 7.1 Gait examination

Station (stance)	Gait
Note posture, width of base	Free forward gait
Place feet together	Tandem (heel to toe) gait
Gentle forward and backward push (be ready to catch patient)	Heel walk
	Toe walk
	Walk around chair
Compare stance with eyes open and closed (be ready to catch patient)	Pattern of wear on shoe
Patient arises from chair	

speed, reduction in arm swing, and increased body sway. Normal cadence is preserved. These changes should be kept in mind when deciding if an elderly patient has a pathologic gait disorder (Table 7.2).

Frontal Lobe Gait

Dysfunction in the frontal lobes can lead to changes in gait broadly known as *frontal gait*. This gait disorder may stem from injury to the frontopontocerebellar tract (Arnold's bundle) that connects the frontal lobe and cerebellum. It is frequently associated with urinary incontinence. The stance is characterized by a wide base and poor balance control. The patient is slow to initiate the first step and then begins taking several small steps with very short strides. The patient may progressively lengthen the stride or stop abruptly. An interesting feature is "magnetic feet"—the patient seems to have difficulty lifting the feet, so that they appear stuck to the floor. As discussed in a following section, this gait disorder has some features in common with parkinsonian gait, but can be distinguished by relatively normal arm swing and the lack of other features associated with parkinsonism. Some neurologists feel that this gait disorder amounts to an apraxia—loss of voluntary control to begin a movement, although it can be elicited involuntarily, automatically (when the patient's attention is distracted from the task), or reflexively (Table 7.3).

Frontal gait is frequently seen in the context of diffuse or multifocal injury to the frontal lobes and the basal ganglia, as may occur with multiple infarcts or diffuse ischemic changes to the cerebral white matter (e.g., multi-infarct dementia or Binswanger's disease). Another entity

Table 7.2 Senile gait

Discriminating features	Consistent features	Variable features
Preservation of normal cadence	Widened base while standing	Arthritis of lower extremities
	Slowed speed	Depressed ankle jerks
	Mild reduction in arm swing	Loss of vibration sense in toes but not joint
	Increased body sway	position sense
	Age >65	

with this type of gait disorder is normal pressure hydro-cephalus (NPH), a form of communicating hydrocephalus without raised intracranial pressure. Normal pressure hydrocephalus typically manifests with the triad of dementia, frontal gait disorder, and urinary incontinence. It is important to recognize NPH, as it is treatable with thecoperitoneal or ventriculoperitoneal shunting, but the classic triad of symptoms is actually seen more commonly in multi-infarct dementia.

Spastic Gait

Damage to the upper motor neurons in the corticospinal tracts can lead to hemiparesis (weakness in two ipsilateral limbs), paraparesis (weakness in the lower extremities), or quadriparesis, depending on the location of injury. Upper motor neuron injury is associated with hyperreflexia, hypertonia, weakness, and also sensory deficits if nearby sensory pathways are injured. Long-standing injury to the upper motor neurons can lead to flexor contractures, posturing, and deformity (Table 7.4).

Hemiparetic Gait

Hemiparetic gait occurs when there is unilateral damage to the corticospinal tracts, usually cephalad to the decussation of the tracts at the base of the medulla and therefore contralateral to the side of weakness. This is a common gait problem and may be seen in such entities as stroke, cerebral palsy, and closed head injury. It may also occur with unilateral cervical spinal cord lesions producing ipsilateral hemiparesis. Injury to the spinal cord motor pathways on one side may be associated with ipsilateral deficits in discrimination, touch, and joint position sense, and contralateral deficits in pain and temperature sensation (the *Brown-Sequard syndrome*). When standing, the affected arm is usually held flexed at the elbow, and the leg can be held in extension. Walking frequently accentuates the abnormal posture of the arm, producing adduction at the shoulder, flexion at the elbow, and flexion of the thumb and fingers. Arm swing is often reduced. The leg swings first outward during forward motion and then returns in an arc. This important sign is known as *circumduction*. In contrast, the feet of normal young adults remain close to the midline during the swing phase, although the swing may be slightly widened in the normal elderly person. The upper body sometimes rocks away from the hemiparetic side during circumduction to aid balance. The sole of the shoe may scrape the floor and become excessively worn under the toe and along the outer edge of the sole on the affected side.

Scissors Gait

Spastic paraparesis generally results from injury to the corticospinal tracts in the spinal cord, below the level of the nerves to the upper extremities (i.e., below T1). This gait can be seen, for example, in patients recovering from spinal cord injury and in some patients with multiple sclerosis. The paraparetic patient will often stand with both legs held in stiff extension at the knees and hips. Move-

Table 7.3 Frontal gait disorders

Discriminating features	Consistent features	Variable features
Slow initiation of gait	Wide base stance	Dementia
"Magnetic feet" – feet appear stuck to floor	Very short stride	Urinary incontinence
	Normal arm swing	Increased tone in leg muscles
Poor balance control	Slow gait	Hyperreflexia
	En bloc turns	Babinski signs
		Tendency to fall backwards

Table 7.4 Spastic gait

Discriminating features	Consistent features	Variable features
Legs cross each other (scissoring)	Weakness	Sensory changes
Posturing of upper extremity (shoulder adduction, elbow flexion)	Hypertonia	Bladder problems
	Hyperreflexia	
	Babinski signs	
	Circumduction	

---

ments usually seem forced and stiff. The legs may cross in front of each other while walking (*scissors gait* or *scissoring*). The stride is short and the toes may scrape the ground. The trunk can sway sideways away from the leading leg in the stride.

Spastic Quadriparesis

Spastic quadriparesis requires injury to the motor control of the upper extremities (upper or lower motor neuron) in addition to the deficits noted above for spastic paraparesis. The arms can be held stiffly against the body with elbow flexion. This is seen most often in the setting of cerebral palsy (in this entity, it is often identified as spastic diplegia) or cervical spinal cord injury.

Extrapyramidal Gait Disorders

Parkinsonian Gait

A common gait problem presenting to the primary care physician is the parkinsonian gait. The problem relates to dysfunction within the basal ganglia and its connections, particularly the substantia nigra of the midbrain. The patient can stand with the head flexed forward (anterocollis or procollis), the spine bent forward, and the arms often held flexed at the elbows in front of the body. Because of impaired postural reflexes, the patient may begin to fall if pushed backward gently, or may take a series of quick small steps backward (*retropulsion*). The patient may be slow at initiating gait when asked, and may lean further forward once the patient starts walking. The arms are held stiffly at the side, often with greatly decreased arm swing. When asked to turn, the patient will turn rigidly like a block of wood, the *en bloc* turn. The stride is often very small and the shoes shuffle along the floor (*marche à petits pas*). A common feature is a gradual increase in forward leaning as the patient continues to walk, and the small steps begin to occur faster and faster. This is known as *festination* and can make the patient not only appear to be falling headlong but result in real falls. As noted by Oliver Sacks in 1983, in *Awakenings*, the inability to initiate movement can sometimes be overcome by visual or tactile stimuli, such as periodic tiling on the floor or another person touching the patient. Commonly associated features include a fixed, mask-like face; bradykinesia (difficulty in initiating and slow execution of movements); a 3- to 4-Hz tremor usually most evident in the upper extremities; and decreased blinking. Idiopathic Parkinson's disease is the most common cause of the syndrome of parkinsonism. The diagnosis is made when many of the listed features apply and no other cause is elicited by evaluation. Other common causes include parkinsonism induced by medications (most frequently neuroleptics) and strokes in the basal ganglia (atherosclerotic parkinsonism). Rarely, it can be seen after encephalitis, carbon monoxide poisoning, occupational exposure to manganese, or MPTP exposure. An uncommon disease, which can mimic some of the features of Parkinson's disease is *progressive supranuclear palsy*. This is an idiopathic neurodegenera-

---

Table 7.5 Parkinsonian gait

Discriminating features	Consistent features	Variable features
Masked faces with decreased blink	Bent forward at neck and waist	Bradyphrenia (slow thoughts)
3- to 4-Hz resting tremor	Slow to initiate gait	Micrographia (tiny writing)
Cogwheel rigidity	Arms held stiffly at side with decreased arm swing	Seborrhea
Feet shuffle on floor with small steps		Hypersalivation
Progressive forward leaning with faster steps (festination)	Bradykinesia (slow movements)	Whispering voice
Turns *en bloc*		
Falls easily if pushed or must make quick steps to avoid falling		

Table 7.6 Choreic gait

Discriminating features	Consistent features	Variable features
Rapid irregular limb movements	Frequent involuntary brief movements of face and extremities	Dementia
Twisting of neck and trunk		Neuroleptic or dopaminergic medication use
Sudden thrusts of trunk	Neck turns	

tive disease with axial rigidity, dysphagia, dysarthria, dementia, impairment of vertical and horizontal gaze, rigid extension of the neck (retrocollis), and resistance to levodopa therapy (Table 7.5).

Choreic Gait

Chorea is another manifestation of basal ganglia disease that may affect gait. Chorea is manifested by irregular, spasmodic movements of the face and limbs. The chorea affects gait by interrupting normal gait with rapid irregular limb movements, neck turns, and twisting of the trunk and neck. There can be sudden forward or sideward thrusts of the trunk and limbs. This entity is not common, but is seen most classically in adults with Huntington's disease, a neurodegenerative disease affecting particularly the caudate nuclei. A much more common cause of chorea in the elderly is chronic exposure to dopaminergic or antidopaminergic medications, although this is rarely severe enough to seriously affect gait (Table 7.6).

Cerebellar Ataxic Gait

Damage to the cerebellum can result in dramatic changes in gait, known as *ataxic gait*. The cerebellum is, in a general sense, an integrator and comparator of both sensory and motor information. The most significant diagnostic sign of cerebellar ataxia is difficulty standing with the feet together, regardless of whether the eyes are open or closed. On attempting this, the patient may fall or will promptly spread the feet to avoid falling. The gait ataxia is manifested by sudden uncontrolled lurching while walking and a need to grab onto objects for support. There is erratic foot placement, and stride varies considerably in length between steps. The patient is usually particularly poor at tandem walking. Cerebellar gait ataxia is manifested after injuries to the midline cerebellum. As an isolated finding in adults, this occurs most commonly in the setting of chronic alcoholism, whereas in children, midline cerebellar tumors are a frequent cause. If the lateral portions of the cerebellum (the cerebellar hemispheres) are also injured, other findings such as ipsilateral action tremor, limb ataxia, hyporeflexia, hypotonia, and breakdown of repetitive alternating movements (dysdiadochokinesia), may occur. If asked to walk around a large object, such as a chair, the patient may repeatedly veer toward the side of the lesion. This can be seen in such entities as cerebellar infarction, multiple sclerosis, cerebellar hemorrhage, and head injury (Table 7.7).

Sensory Ataxic Gait

It is important to differentiate cerebellar ataxia from sensory ataxia. Sensory ataxia arises when proprioceptive information is blocked from arriving at the sites of information integration in the brain (such as the cerebellum). This may arise from damage to the peripheral nerves, dorsal root ganglia, posterior spinal columns, or medial lemnisci. Such patients may stamp their feet to the ground, using both the sound and the greater neural impulses from the shock to overcome their impaired proprioception. In contrast to the foot slapping in the steppage gait (see following section), the feet are appropriately dorsiflexed when the knee is high. In addition,

Table 7.7 Cerebellar ataxic gait

Discriminating features	Consistent features	Variable features
Sudden uncontrolled lurching	Veering to side of lesion with unilateral disease	Loss of speech prosody or cadence
Erratic foot placement	Veering to both sides with midline or bilateral disease	Hyporeflexia
Wide variation in stride length	Falls if tries to stand with feet together (advanced disease)	Hypotonia
Grabs on to objects for support	Incoordination	Breakdown of repetitive alternating movements
Can stand with eyes closed	Ipsilateral intention tremor	
	Limb ataxia with hemispheric disease	

Table 7.8 Sensory ataxic gait

Discriminating features	Consistent features	Variable features
Feet lifted high but dorsiflexed appropriately at the ankle	Decreased vibration sense in lower extremity	Numbness in arms
No foot drop	Decreased temperature, pinprick, light touch in lower extremity	Worsens in dark room
	Can stand with feet together, eyes open, not closed	
	Foot slaps ground	

the patient may stand with feet together if the eyes are open, but falls or moves the feet quickly apart to avoid falling if the eyes are closed. Recall that the patient with cerebellar ataxia cannot stand with feet together even with eyes open. This occurs because the patient with sensory ataxia has a functioning cerebellum that is able to keep the patient upright as long as it continues to get some information—such as visual input. But closing the eyes removes this input source and the patient falls as the lack of proprioceptive information makes it impossible to tell where the feet or floor are. This difference was noted by the neurologist Moritz H. Romberg in the 19th century and is still known as *Romberg's sign*. Other signs that may aid in diagnosis include improvement with a cane (which broadens the effective stance and provides proprioceptive information about the floor through the often intact upper extremities) and worsening of the ataxia in a darkened room (which removes the visual clues to the patient). Nineteenth century physicians saw this entity frequently and called it "locomotor ataxia." In that era, the most common cause was tabes dorsalis, a neurosyphilitic degeneration of the dorsal root ganglia and the posterior columns of the spinal cord. The most common cause today is peripheral neuropathy. In the U.S., this is most frequently caused by diabetes mellitus but there are myriad other causes. Sensory ataxia is particularly prominent in patients with multiple sensory deficits, as for example, in a diabetic with peripheral neuropathy and cataracts. Such patients are particularly susceptible to nighttime injuries. Affected patients may benefit from the use of canes, and should be encouraged to use nightlights and to avoid moving about in the dark without turning on lights (Table 7.8).

Steppage Gait

Damage to the motor nerve fibers can also affect gait. Motor nerve injury leads to weakness limited to muscles in the distribution of the nerves affected, with associated muscular atrophy, hyporeflexia, and fasciculations. Peripheral motor neuropathy is generally associated with a predominately distal weakness. The most prominent changes related to gait occur when the ability to dorsiflex the foot is impaired. This leads to a "foot drop." The patient attempts to compensate by raising the knee quite high and taking a very high step, hence the name *steppage gait*. As the front of the foot hangs down, the toe is frequently caught on carpets, curbs, and other protuberances. To avoid tripping, the patient may kick the lower leg forward and then slap the foot to the ground. In any case, the front of the toe of the shoe may be scuffed or worn (Table 7.9).

This type of gait change may be seen in any condition with lower motor neuron involvement, including diabetes, Guillain–Barré syndrome (acute inflammatory demyelination of the motor nerves), early amyotrophic lateral sclerosis (degeneration of the upper and lower motor neurons), and lead intoxication. It is particularly common in younger adults with hereditary sensorimotor neuropathies. With the latter condition, motor complaints often predominate and are frequently accompanied by foot deformities, including a high arched foot and hammer toes (shortened extensor tendons displace the toes backward and up with a flexed appearance). Foot drop often benefits from various orthoses. Tendon transfer surgery can produce substantial improvement in some cases.

Table 7.9 Steppage gait

Discriminating features	Consistent features	Variable features
Knee lifted high	Distal weakness	Toe of shoe worn
Foot drop	Distal atrophy	Fasciculations
	Hyporeflexia	
	Foot slaps ground	
	Trips easily	

Table 7.10 Myopathic gait

Discriminating features	Consistent features	Variable features
Excessive lumbar lordosis	Proximal weakness	Gower's maneuver
Hyperextension of knees	Proximal muscle atrophy	Flattened clavicles
Exaggerated hip sway and	Preserved reflexes	Scapular winging
lateral pelvic movements	No sensory changes	Webbed appearance to neck
		Facial and palatal weakness

Myopathic Gait

Muscle diseases produce predominately proximal weakness in contrast to the distal weakness associated with neuropathic illnesses. Typically, there is proximal muscle atrophy, relative preservation of the reflexes, and no sensory changes. The pelvic girdle, the hip flexors, and the quadriceps muscles, as well as the paraspinal muscles of the back, which support the spine, are the muscle groups most affected. This leads to postural changes as the patient tries to preserve the stability of the center of gravity despite worsening axial weakness. In this position, bones and ligamentous structures, rather than muscle, largely support the body. With weakness of the hip and back extensors, there can be exaggeration of the lumbar lordosis with an associated protrusion of the abdomen. As the weakened quadriceps are no longer able to fully support the knees in their normal slightly flexed position, the knees become hyperextended while standing ("back kneeing"). Gluteal and other pelvic girdle muscle weakening prevents the pelvis from being held fixed and steady during gait (as the weight is shifted from one foot to the other). Thus, the pelvis tends to "waddle" as the patient walks. As a result, there is exaggerated hip swing, as well as lateral swing of the pelvis, as the patient shifts weight from side to side during the successive support phases. Associated shoulder girdle weakness is also readily apparent during walking, with hunching of the shoulders, rotation of the arms, so that the palms face backward rather than inward, and a floppiness of the arms due to impaired stabilization of the arm at the shoulder. Additional clues to the diagnosis include flattening of the clavicles (which normally curve down slightly from lateral to medial), a webbed appearance to the neck, and scapular winging (protrusion of the shoulder blade when the arm is flexed at the shoulder) (Table 7.10).

Many muscle problems tend to be rare, familial, and appear in children or young adults, including Duchenne's muscular dystrophy, facioscapulohumeral dystrophy, myotonic dystrophy, spinal muscular atrophy, and mitochondrial myopathies. Muscle diseases that first appear in adulthood include polymyositis, steroid myopathy, and myopathies related to hypothyroidism or hyperthyroidism.

Antalgic Gait

Walking may be affected by non-neurologic factors such as musculoskeletal pain or osteoarthritis. Stiffness of the lower back can reduce or eliminate lumbar lordosis and affect the stance and posture. If arthritis of the hip is severe, the patient may stand with the trunk leaning toward the affected side to reduce the weight load on the joint. The patient with knee problems may limp, favoring the affected leg by limiting the time of full weight bearing.

Functional Gait Disorders

Finally, gait can be affected in various ways in conversion disorders, other psychiatric disorders, and malingering. The result is often bizarre with very theatrical lurches, grabs for support, and even falls. The clinician must be very cautious in making a diagnosis of a functional gait disorder, however, in order not to miss an organic gait disorder, especially if some functional overlay is present. The patient may also demonstrate *giveaway weakness*, in which the patient is able to produce full muscular strength at first, but then quickly relaxes. With any of the so-called functional gait disorders, the patient's problems are maximized when they are witnessed and are greatly decreased or absent when the patient is unaware of observation by

Consider Consultation When...

▶ A patient presents with a frontal gait in the setting of urinary incontinence and a slowly progressive dementing disorder.

▶ A patient presents with acute or subacute spastic diplegia or quadriparesis.

▶ Huntington's disease is suspected in a patient with choreic gait.

▶ A patient presents with cerebellar gait ataxia.

▶ A diagnosis of functional gait disorder is considered.

▼

Pearls and Perils

Gait disorders

▶ Evaluation of patients with gait problems begins with a complete neurologic history and examination, with particular attention to medical conditions (e.g., diabetes) that may be associated with sensory or gait disturbances.

▶ Many medications can predispose to gait problems, especially if they produce orthostatic hypotension (e.g., propranolol), confusion (e.g., anticholinergics), ataxia (e.g., carbamazepine), or drowsiness (e.g., benzodiazepines).

▶ Tandem walking can be very sensitive for detection of ataxias; however, minor difficulty in tandem walking is common even in normal elderly.

▶ Patients with cerebellar ataxia cannot stand with feet together even with eyes open.

▶ Muscle diseases produce predominately proximal weakness, in contrast to the distal weakness associated with neuropathic illnesses.

▶ Walking may be affected by non-neurologic factors such as musculoskeletal pain or osteoarthritis.

the clinician. In patients with functional hemiparesis, there is no flexion or posturing of the upper extremity and no circumduction in the affected leg, the patient is able to use the leg for support, and there are no associated focal neurologic findings such as ipsilateral hyperreflexia or a Babinski sign. *Astasia-abasia* refers to the inability to stand (astasia) or walk (abasia) at all, despite the preservation of adequate strength and the demonstrated ability to voluntarily mimic all the movements necessary for walking. *Astasia-abasia* is highly suggestive of hysterical gait disorder. In cases of patients on long-term antipsychotic treatment, extrapyramidal gait problems due to medication effects should be considered in addition to hysterical gait problems.

Annotated Bibliography

Campbell WW. *DeJong's the neurologic examination*, 6th ed. Philadelphia: Lippincott Williams & Wilkins, 2005; pp. 526–533.
An excellent textbook detailing the neurologic examination in normal and disease states. The chapter on gait summarizes common gait changes relating to different neurologic problems.

Nutt JG, Marsden CD, Thompson PD. Human walking and higher-level gait disorders, particularly in the elderly, *Neurology* 1993;43:268–279.
Explores the neuroanatomic basis of gait and relates this to the various gait disorders. Particular emphasis is placed on normal and abnormal gait changes associated with aging.

Ropper AH, Brown RH. *Disorders of stance and gait, Adams and Victor's principles of neurology*, 8th ed. New York: McGraw-Hill, 2005; pp. 100–108.
A well-written chapter summarizing gait problems in several neurological illnesses.

Sudarsky L. Geriatrics: gait disorders in the elderly. *N Engl J Med* 1990;322(20):1441–1446.
Reviews common changes in gait among the elderly and frequent gait disorders seen in the aged population.

CHAPTER 8

Headaches

John T. Slevin and Melody Ryan

Outline

▶ General clinical approach
▶ Headache syndromes
▶ Symptomatic headaches

Headache is the most common painful state afflicting humans. Headaches were described by the ancient Greeks, and in the first century A.D., Galen described headache syndromes in detail. Throughout the Middle Ages, headaches were thought to be caused by an imbalance of one of four bodily fluids, or humors, and classified and treated accordingly. Treatment for the most part consisted of phlebotomy or the use of purgatives. However, it was not until the pioneering investigations of Harold G. Wolff in the early 1930s that migraine and other headaches were studied in a systematic and scientific manner.

Data from community surveys in the United States and Great Britain indicate that from 10–20% of the populations studied have at some time suffered from severe headache, whereas negligible numbers report having never suffered from headache. The epidemiology of headache has been described in more than 50 population-based studies, in which annual prevalence generally ranges from 60% to 90%. It has been estimated that more than 70% of the population of the United States will experience headache within a 1-year period. The economic burden on society in terms of medical costs and lost productivity from headaches is unknown. However, estimates of annual indirect costs in the United States have varied from $1.4 billion to as much as $17.2 billion for just migraine alone.

Although symptoms of head pain most often represent a primary headache disorder, many headaches may be due to underlying medical problems. Patients themselves may fear that headache indicates a sinister underlying problem, such as brain tumor, and seek reassurance as well as symptomatic relief. Accordingly, this chapter has been designed to aid the general practitioner in determining whether an individual patient's headache reflects a primary headache syndrome or is symptomatic of a more ominous medical or neurologic illness. The chapter begins with a general clinical approach to the evaluation of an individual complaining of head pain. The primary headache syndromes, criteria for their diagnoses, suggested laboratory evaluations, and treatment protocols are then described. Finally, symptomatic headaches as part of a variety of medical and neurologic illnesses will be discussed, including discriminating features that may aid in diagnosis.

General Clinical Approach

History

A large majority of individuals who come to physicians for relief of headache pain may have several types of headache, and it is incumbent on the care provider to delineate these if any success in treatment is to be achieved. For example, it is not uncommon for a patient to suffer from both migraine and tension-type headaches without really discriminating between the two.

Certain critical information elicited as part of the history will help determine the *types* of headache from which a patient is suffering. Where does the headache localize? Does it begin at a specific locus, or is it holoacranial? Migraine is typically hemicranial, whereas tension-type headaches are often occipital, retro-orbital, or frontotemporal. Does the patient gradually become aware of having a headache, as is common with tension-type headache, or does it begin more suddenly, in the fashion typical of migraine? Timing and frequency are also important. Tension-type headaches are more typical later in the day, whereas cluster headache is common within an hour of falling asleep. Migraine headaches rarely occur more than twice in a week, whereas cluster headaches can occur several times within a 24-hour period. What are the duration, severity, and character of the pain? A tension-type headache can last for days, and a typical migraine can last from 9 to 24 hours, but an individual cluster headache may last only 15–30 minutes. Severity is generally not a useful measure, since most patients in whom head pain is a primary symptom will complain that it is severe. However, pain severity is useful in a review of systems. More important is the character of the pain: tension-type headaches are often described as squeezing or a band-like pressure; migraine is typically described as throbbing; the pain of trigeminal neuralgia is shooting; and "lower-half" headaches are likened to being stabbed with an ice pick. What is the course of the pain? Does it have a well-defined beginning and end? How long does it take to reach a maximum level of discomfort? Are there precipitating factors? What attenuates the pain, and what exacerbates it? Are there any associated neurologic symptoms and signs? This is critical information and will be explored more fully when symptomatic headaches are discussed.

A query as to whether neurologic symptoms occur hours to days (prodromes) or minutes (auras) before the onset of a headache will help define types of migraine, perhaps broaden the differential to allow consideration of other conditions, and aid in neurologic localization of a lesion. Especially helpful in management is whether specific factors (food, environmental situations) may precipitate the headaches. Is there an association with sleep cycles, as in cluster headache or migraine, or are sleep patterns disrupted in association with the headache? To what

degree are emotional factors playing a role? Often, this information is crucial and takes an empathetic but critical listener to obtain it. Is there a history of prior head trauma, ophthalmologic or neurologic illness, or lumbar puncture? Is the patient taking medications or frequently exposed to substances that could contribute to the current headache syndrome; for example, nitroglycerin transdermal patches or job-site exposure to nitrates.

Examination

A good general physical examination, with emphasis on particular areas or systems dictated by the history, is an important aspect of the evaluation of a patient with headache. For example, an individual with a long history of chronic tobacco abuse with a new-onset headache needs a thorough examination of the chest for evidence of malignancy. As part of the physical examination of all headache patients, it is particularly important to obtain vital signs, including a blood pressure determination in both arms. A careful head and neck examination should include the following: a search for pain-eliciting trigger points, including percussion of the frontal and maxillary sinuses; palpation of the superficial temporal arteries for pulses and tenderness; palpation of cervical muscles for spasm or tenderness and evaluation of cervical range-of-motion; palpation of the mastoids; palpation of the temporomandibular joint with jaw opening and closing; auscultation of the head for bruits; examination of the oral cavity for masses or other lesions; examination of the teeth for signs of bruxism; percussion of the teeth with a tongue blade; and examination and palpation for cervical adenopathy. Since over half of headaches that originate with ear pain are caused by primary otalgias, an otoscopic examination of the external auditory canals should not be overlooked.

In both the emergency room and in the office of the general practitioner, there is seldom time to perform the detailed neurologic examination usually reserved for the specialist. If the following screening examination is normal, then the probability of finding an underlying neurologic or neurosurgical lesion as the cause of a symptomatic headache is low (Box 8.1). The examination should include a careful cranial nerve evaluation, including ophthalmoscopy. If not otherwise contraindicated, patients should be instructed to hop on either foot. The floor of our clinic is covered with 12-inch square tiles, within which we instruct the patient to hop. Successful performance requires essentially normal strength and sensation below the waist, as well as the ability to coordinate the activity. Patients are also asked to stand with arms abducted laterally to 90 degrees while standing with the heel of one foot in front of and touching the toes of the other foot, the so-called "tandem position." Most adults should be able to maintain balance in this position for 4 seconds. Lastly, the deep

Key Clinical Questions

Migraine

▶ Do you have nausea or feel sick to your stomach with your headaches?
▶ When you are with headache, does light bother you (a lot more than when you don't have headache)?
▶ Does your headache limit you from working, studying or doing what you need to do?

According to Lipton et al., in the primary care setting these three questions had a sensitivity of 0.81 and a specificity of 0.75, relative to an HIS-based migraine diagnosis assigned by a headache specialist.

▼

Box 8.1 Headache evaluation

History
▶ Types of headache
▶ Onset and location
▶ Timing and frequency
▶ Duration, severity, character
▶ Precipitating factors
▶ Associated signs and symptoms
▶ Course
▶ Prodromes and aura
▶ Sleep pattern
▶ Emotional factors
▶ Family history
▶ Medical/Surgical history
▶ Allergies/Medications

Physical exam
▶ Vitals
▶ Head/Neck/Ear exam

Neurological exam
▶ Cranial nerves
▶ "Hopping" and balance
▶ Reflexes

pend both on the setting and the individual's analytical style. In the emergency room, it is often more expedient to consider the headache course (Table 8.1). Is the patient complaining of an acute single headache? Is it an acute but recurrent headache? Alternatively, has the headache been present for days or weeks, and does it meet criteria for classification as a chronic daily headache. If the patient's headache can be easily classified under one of these categories, then certain etiologies can be considered based solely on headache course.

The flow diagram in Figure 8.1 represents an algorithmic approach to the evaluation of patients with headache. An algorithm will help the practitioner develop a differential diagnosis sufficiently accurate so that life-threatening illnesses will not be omitted from consideration. Perhaps the most important initial question is whether the headache is of new onset or different from prior headaches. A minimal evaluation and little change in management is usually necessary for an individual who has had migraine for years and is transferring care. However, this is in contradistinction to a middle-aged man with a long history of tension-type headaches who describes a new headache of recent onset that is highly different in character. Any recent history of trauma will require imaging studies appropriate for the type and degree of injury, but should, at a minimum, include a noncontrasted computed tomography (CT) scan to evaluate for the presence of blood (refer to the section on Symptomatic headaches: Trauma). If the patient is over 60 years of age, strong consideration must be given to the possibility of temporal arteritis. An erythrocyte sedimentation rate (ESR) should be measured emergently and appropriate steps taken if it is elevated (refer to the section Symptomatic Headaches: Inflammatory disease). If there has been progression in the character, severity, or frequency of a headache over weeks to months, or if there is a change in the neurologic examination, the possibility of an intracranial mass (e.g., tumor or expanding aneurysm) must be considered.

tendon reflexes are evaluated with particular regard to asymmetry and hyperactivity. This neurologic screening examination can be completed in fewer than 5 minutes. Of course, any abnormality must be pursued with a more detailed, but directed, examination.

Differential Diagnosis

The decision-making process that the practitioner uses in arriving at a differential diagnosis for headache will de-

Table 8.1 Differential diagnosis of headaches in Emergency Department patients

Acute single headache	Acute recurrent headache	Subacute headache (days or weeks)	Chronic headache
Subarachnoid hemorrhage	Migraine	Subdural hematoma	Chronic daily headaches
Systemic infection	Intermittent hydrocephalus	Temporal arteritis	Cervical spondylosis
Pressor reaction	Cerebrovascular insufficiency	Subdural hematoma	Brain abscess
Optic neuritis	Trigeminal neuralgia	Brain abscess	Psychiatric state
Glaucoma	Cerebral tumors	Pseudotumor cerebri	Analgesic rebound
Meningitis	Pheochromocytoma	Cerebral tumor	Paroxysmal hemicrania
Encephalitis	Subarachnoid hemorrhage		Cerebral tumor
(First) migraine	Cluster		Pseudotumor cerebri
Sinusitis	Pseudotumor cerebri		

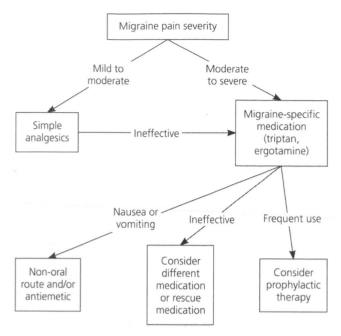

Figure 8.1 Migraine treatment algorithm/flowchart.

If there has been no recent change in the patient's headache profile, the clinician may determine that it fits a well-defined pattern of one of the primary headache syndromes. It is also helpful to inquire if either physical exertion or masticatory activity is consistently associated with headache. With exertional headaches, one should consider the possibility of aneurysm or other mass, especially in the posterior fossa. Developmental abnormalities of the posterior fossa, such as platybasia or Chiari syndromes, can also be associated with exertional headaches, without the presence of a mass-occupying lesion. Alternatively, pheochromocytoma should be considered in the patient with exertional headache. Chewing difficulty associated with headache raises the possibility of temporomandibular joint dysfunction or other oral abnormalities, including bruxism (refer to the section Symptomatic headaches: Pain of oral or dental etiology).

Although the algorithm presented here defaults to the primary headache syndromes, it is important to remember that tension-type, and even migraine, symptoms may be secondary to and reflect other underlying disease. For example, tension-type headache is commonly seen in patients with cervical degenerative joint disease or in patients suffering from depression. Patients with psychogenic headaches or with dependent personalities have underlying psychiatric illness which, when treated, may lead to resolution of headaches. Even with consistent use of this or other algorithms, there will always be a number of patients who remain difficult to classify and should be referred to a neurologist or headache specialist. Using this kind of approach, however, reduces the risk of missing a potentially life-threatening cause of headache.

No specific laboratory tests should be regularly ordered in all patients with headache. Laboratory tests, including chemistry panel, complete blood count, urinalysis, and drug screen, should be ordered as indicated. A lumbar puncture is critical in suspected cases of infection, including meningitis and encephalitis. Cerebrospinal fluid (CSF) examination may help ascertain the presence of pseudotumor cerebri or meningeal carcinomatosis. In cases of clinically suspected subarachnoid hemorrhage in which an imaging study is unrevealing, lumbar puncture is essential. Computed tomography should be performed for acute hemorrhage, clinical evidence of increased intracranial pressure, and if there is a deficit on neurologic examination. If available, magnetic resonance imaging (MRI) should be substituted for CT to image soft tissue and to better visualize the posterior fossa. An electroencephalogram (EEG) is necessary only in cases of headache believed secondary to an epileptic seizure, rare cases of epileptic equivalent headache, and suspected encephalitis. A chest radiograph should be obtained if the history or examination suggests malignancy. Sleep studies may be indicated in patients with headache who are overweight, snore, are heavy smokers, or otherwise raise a suspicion of sleep apnea (refer to the section Symptomatic headaches: Toxic and metabolic headaches).

Headache Syndromes

Migraine Headache

Migraine is the best defined of the idiopathic or primary headache syndromes. Typically, it is characterized by periodic, commonly unilateral, pulsatile headaches, which begin in late childhood or early adult life and recur with diminishing frequency during advancing years. With the gradual, widespread adoption of the classification and diagnostic criteria of the International Headache Society (IHS) first published in 1988 (Table 8.2), a coherent delineation of migraine prevalence is emerging. From several population-based studies using these criteria, it appears that migraine has its highest prevalence in individuals between 25 and 55, peaking at about age 40. The prevalence of migraine is about 6% among men and 16% among women, although this gender bias varies with age, increasing from menarche through the early fifth decade and declining thereafter. As might be predicted from these prevalence data, patients seeking health care for migraine tend to be women. The consultation is motivated by a need for pain relief among individuals with debilitating, persistent headache symptoms of recent onset. The migraineur's entry into the system is through the primary care physician in over half the cases; emergency rooms are a distant second, and only about 10% of migraineurs initially present to a neurologist.

Table 8.2 International Headache Society classification of migraine headaches (2nd Edition, 2004)

Classification No.	Name
1.1	Migraine without aura
1.2	Migraine with aura
1.3	Childhood periodic syndromes
1.4	Retinal migraine
1.5	Complications of migraine
1.6	Probable migraine

Table 8.3 Migraine without aura

Discriminating features	Consistent features	Variable features
At least five attacks	Moderate to severe intensity	Unilateral locus
Attacks lasting 4–72 hours	Aggravated by physical activity	Pulsatile
Either nausea and/or vomiting, or photophobia and phonophobia	Normal neurologic exam	Family history
No aura	Female > Male (3:1)	Environmental trigger

Classification

The classification of migraine using IHS criteria is presented in Table 8.2. The vast majority of cases will fall under *migraine without* (1.1) or *migraine with* (1.2) *aura*. The definition of migraine without aura, referred to in older literature as *idiopathic recurring headache* and *common migraine*, is comprehensive and requires five prior attacks. Much of the definition of migraine with aura concentrates on details of the aura, a symptom so clear and evident to most patients that only two prior episodes are required. The aura is not restricted to visual symptoms but may include a variety of neurologic symptoms. Not surprisingly, prior to the adoption of IHS criteria, such headaches were also described by their neurologic accompaniments (ophthalmic, hemiparetic, hemiplegic, and aphasic migraine). Ophthalmoplegic migraine consists of extraocular paralysis, which may include cranial nerves III, IV, and VI, occurring 6–10 hours after the onset of headache or as the headache subsides. Recovery is usually complete. Because this entity appears to overlap with Tolosa Hunt syndrome, in which the ophthalmoplegia is of longer duration (refer to the section Symptomatic headaches: Ophthalmologic headache), it was reclassified in 2004 under cranial neuralgias. Retinal migraine is defined as repeated attacks of monocular scotoma or blindness lasting less than 1 hour with or without an accompanying headache. It is necessary to exclude transient ischemic attack (TIA) in these individuals (Tables 8.3 and 8.4).

There are four major categories of "complications of migraine." In patients with status migranosis, the headache persists for more than 72 hours, despite conventional treatment. These individuals require more intensive treatment (see later). Persistent aura without infarction occurs when patients have episodes typical of prior attacks except that one or more aura symptoms persist for 1 week without radiographic evidence of infarction. Migrainous infarction is defined as one or more migrainous symptoms associated with an ischemic brain lesion in the appropriate territory, as demonstrated by neuroimaging. Remarkably, clinically evident infarction from migraine is quite rare: in the absence of other stroke risk factors, the incidence of "migrainous infarction" is estimated at 1.44 per 100 000 population per year. Several studies have compared head MR scans in headache patients and controls: small areas of increased signal on T2-weighted scans (*ischemic–gliotic changes*) appeared four to five times more commonly in patients with headache. The fact that clinically evident infarction does not occur more frequently in migraineurs may indicate that the clinically observed symptoms result from spreading decreased cerebral blood flow rather than cessation of blood flow at a fixed locus (see later) (Table 8.4). A last complication is the rare migraine-triggered epileptic seizure.

There are several different categories of migraine with aura. Migraine with typical aura includes those with scintillating scotomata, fortification spectra, and other homonymous visual disturbances previously termed *clas-*

Table 8.4 Migraine with aura

Discriminating features	Consistent features	Variable features
At least two attacks	Moderate to severe intensity	Prodrome
Reversible aura	Unilateral and pulsatile	Family history
Headache onset 5–60 minutes after aura begins	Nausea and/or vomiting, photophobia, phonophobia	Environmental trigger
	Normal neurologic exam	
	Female > Male (3:1)	

sic migraine. Additionally, headaches with auras consisting of either unilateral sensory disturbance or aphasia are also considered migraine with typical aura. Hemiplegic migraine, a rare type in which the aura includes motor weakness of up to 24 hours duration, can occur either sporadically or as an inherited disorder. Two specific genetic subtypes of *familial hemiplegic migraine* have been identified: mutations in the *CACNA1A* gene on chromosome 19 (FHM1) and in the *ATP1A2* gene on chromosome 1 (FHM2). Several other susceptibility loci for more common forms of migraine have been identified in genome-wide screens and candidate locus studies. The atypical aura of basilar artery migraine of Bickerstaff includes signs of brainstem or cerebellar dysfunction, such as diplopia, ataxia, dysarthria, other cranial nerve signs, and occasionally coma. Basilar artery migraine is more common in children and young adults, although the gender ratio of 4:1 favoring women is the same as for migraine with and without aura. Migraine aura without headache may include any of the neurologic deficits described previously and, in the past, has been termed *migraine equivalent*. It is critical that TIA and cerebral infarction are not overlooked in patients given a diagnosis of either "typical aura with nonmigraine headache" or "typical aura without headache."

Pathophysiology

According to Wolff's vascular theory of migraine, the aura is caused by intracerebral vasoconstriction, and the headache pain by reactive vasodilatation of the external carotid artery, enhanced by vasoactive polypeptides. This theory explained the throbbing quality of the pain, its varied localizations, and its relief with treatment by ergot preparations. However, it failed to explain either the prodrome or associated neurologic features of the migraine attack, and why some of the drugs used effectively to treat migraine have no effect on blood vessels.

In recent decades, the concept of the migraine syndrome has been expanded to include several distinct phases: prodrome, aura, headache, headache termination, and postdrome. Co-evolution of this concept and the IHS classification has led to the development of the neurogenic theory of migraine, for which the central tenet is a primary derangement of brain function. Investigations have studied serotonergic and noradrenergic pain-modulating systems originating in the brainstem, as well as the trigeminal and high cervical spinal neurons. A prodrome may begin hours to days before the aura or headache. Although the symptoms are vague, they tend to be specific for an individual migraineur. Although more introspective patients may report and recognize these, many are not aware of their prodromal features, hence, the importance of individuals maintaining a headache diary as part of their management. Similarly, during the postdrome, certain symptoms tend to recur as part of the migraine syndrome. These pre- and post-headache symptoms help the physician to separate types of headaches for an individual and may be useful in guiding pharmacologic management (Table 8.5).

Evidence from a variety of imaging (e.g., diffusion/perfusion MRI, functional MRI [fMRI], regional cerebral blood flow [rCBF] measured by Xe^{133}) and magnetoencephalography studies, suggests that the aura of migraine is a neuroelectric event similar to cortical spreading depression (CSD) induced experimentally in rodents. Cortical spreading depression is a spreading wave of neuronal depolarization, followed by a long-lasting suppression of neuronal activity and concomitant reduction in cerebral blood flow. Certain stimuli, including cortical trauma and high extracellular concentrations of glutamate, can induce CSD. However the initiating molecular events for migraine aura remain unknown. During migraine aura, cortical neuronal excitation followed by depression of normal neuronal activity spreads slowly from the site of initiation at 2–6 mm/min. Using fMRI to study migraines induced by visual stimulation, Cao and colleagues found that transient activation followed by spreading neuronal depression was accompanied by vasodilatation and hyperoxygenation. This brief increase in rCBF was followed by oligemia lasting approximately 1 hour after the wave of neuronal inhibition. Blood flow may decrease to 16–23 mL per 100 g of brain tissue per minute, well within the range associated with TIA. This spread of intracerebral oligemia may be bilateral, fail to respect territories of vascular supply, and evolve so that, as the leading edge advances, a return to normal occurs at the trailing edge. That stroke is such a rare complication of migraine may be explained by this phenomenon, which is distinctly different from stroke itself, in which the ischemic focus is fixed and obeys vascular territories. In a single report of cerebral blood flow during migraine with aura, oligemia began with the aura and persisted into the headache phase, consistent with a primary neurologic event producing secondary vascular changes, but not with reactive vasodilatation as a cause of headache.

Overwhelming evidence links serotonergic (5-HT) neurotransmission and trigeminal nerve activity with the

Table 8.5 Nonheadache symptoms of migraine	
Preheadache symptoms	**Postheadache symptoms**
Depression	Calmness
Drowsiness	Euphoria
Fatigue	Hyper-alertness
Hunger for sweets, thirst	Increased energy
IrritabilityLethargy	
Nervousness	
Yawning	

pain of migraine. Migraine-specific triggers induce a primary brain dysfunction (CSD, other?) that causes dilation of trigeminal nerve–innervated cranial blood vessels. These dilated blood vessels mechanically activate perivascular trigeminal sensory nerve fibers, causing both transmission of a pain response into the brainstem and peripheral trigeminal release of vasoactive peptides, particularly calcitonin gene-related peptide (CGRP) and substance P. These peptides exacerbate vasodilation and cause a *neurogenic inflammation*, characterized by plasma protein extravasation and mast cell degranulation within the dura mater. This further enhances activation of sensory trigeminal fibers, leading to increased CGRP release and causing increased inflammation and vasodilation; very quickly, a vicious cycle erupts leading to peripheral sensitization. Notably, CGRP has been detected in jugular venous blood during migraine attacks, and intravenous infusion of CGRP into susceptible individuals can elicit a migraine-like headache. Triptans (5-HT agonists) and ergotamines can significantly reduce this neurogenic inflammatory response. Moskowitz and colleagues have established a possible link between migraine aura and headache by demonstrating in a rodent model that CSD causes long-lasting extracerebral blood-flow enhancement selectively within the middle meningeal artery, dependent on trigeminal and parasympathetic activation, and plasma protein leakage within the dura mater.

A further tenet of the neurogenic theory of migraine pathogenesis is the concept of central sensitization that attempts to explain the later-stage temporal progression of a migraine attack and the development of migraine chronicity. In this model, central sensitivity is a reflection of neuronal hyperexcitability driven by peripherally sensitized trigeminal nociceptors (see earlier discussion). These sensitized trigeminal neurons abnormally bombard the downstream neurons with which they synapse in the trigeminal nucleus caudalis (TNC) in the brainstem. Although precise mechanisms are unknown, enhanced activity at glutamatergic synapses, as has been demonstrated in other hyperexcitability phenomena (e.g., long-term potentiation and kindling), is a leading candidate. Proposed loci of these pathologic changes are the TNC itself and perhaps brainstem periaqueductal gray matter. Once central sensitization has been established, subsequent attacks may occur in response to stress or excessive afferent stimulation, including light, noise, or odors, which are no longer appropriately modulated. It has been recognized for years that this susceptibility may have a hereditary basis: up to one-third of patients who have migraine with aura report migrainous family members, considerably higher than what is found in nonheadache controls.

Precipitating factors in migraine

Numerous foods and food additives can precipitate a migraine in susceptible individuals. Typically, nitrates and nitrites used in processed meats (e.g., hot dogs) can trigger migraines. Chocolate, aged cheeses, certain nuts, and wines can also induce a migraine, presumably due to their content of phenylethylamines. However, at least one blinded study has demonstrated that the phenylethylamine, tyramine, given intravenously to migraineurs, did not precipitate headache. Other food sources have included citrus fruits, dairy products, and shellfish. Caffeine and related substances are especially problematic in migraine patients who have headaches triggered by relative withdrawal states (such as in the early morning before resuming daily consumption). The physician needs to inquire about use of soft drinks, some of which contain considerable amounts of caffeine, as well as total daily intake of coffee, tea, and over-the-counter medications. Asian foods and many prepared foods contain monosodium glutamate, which can trigger headache (refer to the section on Toxic and metabolic headaches).

Bright or flickering light, noise, and odors have all been incriminated as precipitants of migraine. In addition to gastrointestinal symptoms (usually nausea and vomiting), the most common complaints among migraineurs during an attack are photophobia, sonophobia, and osmophobia. Although strenuous exercise can precipitate migraine in some individuals, the relationship to headache severity and frequency is variable, but may be reduced with a regular, moderate exercise schedule. Stress, as well as possible coexistent tension-type headache, may trigger migraine in some individuals, but this is not invariable among migraineurs. Attacks of migraine typically *follow* periods of stress (during the "let-down" phase), in contrast to tension-type headaches, which are more temporally correlated with times of greatest stress.

The association of sex hormones and migraine remains controversial. Not infrequently, attacks are linked to the menstrual cycle, and may be refractory to treatment. The documented peak in attack frequency occurring within several days of the onset of the menstrual period (and associated with drops in serum levels of both estrogen and progesterone) can be delayed with the administration of estrogen. Although migraine incidence generally decreases with advancing age, it may either regress or worsen at the time of menopause, and estrogen replacement therapy may exacerbate migraine. Thus, the relationship of estrogen level to headache is not straightforward. For replacement therapy, generally the lowest dose of estrogen required to control symptoms should be used. It sometimes helps to convert the dosing schedule from interrupted to continuous. In some women taking oral contraceptives, migraine attacks will be exacerbated, whereas in others they may improve or show no change. Consequently, women prescribed oral contraceptives must be followed for any change in their headache profile. Although the possible relationship between oral contraceptives, migraine, and stroke is controversial, the Collaborative Group for the Study of Stroke in Young Women found that a diagnosis of migraine did not increase the risk of stroke in women using oral contraceptives.

Comorbidity

Several disease states occur with higher frequency in at least some patients with migraine. Depression is more common in patients with migraine compared with those without migraine, occurring in approximately 40% of migraineurs. Migraines with aura have a relationship to cardiovascular and cerebrovascular disease in women. Data from the Women's Health Study demonstrated an approximate doubling of risk of myocardial infarction or ischemic stroke in women with migraines with aura. In contrast, those patients having migraine without aura do not appear to be at increased risk for ischemic disease. Some authors feel that having a patent foramen ovale with large right-to-left shunt not only predisposes patients to migraine, but may also explain the increase in stroke risk among patients with migraine with aura. Closure of the patent foramen ovale may decrease or stop migraines in up to 60% of patients with this condition. It has been suggested that migraines are more common in patients with epilepsy; however, the data are somewhat conflicting on this account. It appears that epilepsy is more likely in patients having migraine with aura (30.4%), but the relationship is not as clear for patients with migraine without aura. A large, case-control study has demonstrated that patients with migraine are 3.5 times more likely to have comorbid restless legs syndrome than are those without migraine. The pathologic link between these two disorders, if any, is unknown.

Treatment of Migraine

Management of the migraineur must include patient education, environmental modification, and medication considerations. Changes in the environment include alterations in diet, elimination of the precipitating factors just discussed, adoption of regular habits, and use of various nonpharmacologic interventions. Patient education and environmental modifications are intertwined. Migraineurs who better understand the nature of the illness will be more willing to adopt a lifestyle that will help to eliminate headaches. Pharmacotherapy has three facets: abortive treatment, adjunctive therapy, and migraine prophylaxis.

Patient education. The best form of treatment for migraines is preventative. Migraineurs should be encouraged to adopt a lifestyle that will help to eliminate or reduce headaches by reducing inciting agents or activities. Patients should be encouraged to initiate a wellness program that emphasizes regular exercise, balanced meals, and adequate sleep during headache-free intervals. The use of a headache calendar is an important component of this program. In addition to providing information useful in eliminating environmental triggers and assessing effectiveness of medications, it helps patients understand their disorder and its treatment. Many migraineurs feel their lives are controlled by their headaches. With understanding comes a greater sense of control over their headaches.

Environmental modification. Environmental modification is generally a slow process, taken on by the patient and physician during which efforts are made to identify precipitating factors. Alteration of some factors has been found to generally help migraineurs. For example, the frequency and severity of headaches may be reduced with regular exercise and sexual activity. Headaches can be brought on by both too much and too little sleep, and many migraineurs have learned that they feel better if they go to bed and get up at the same time every day. Complete elimination of caffeine from the diet is also advisable.

Migraineurs may experience an increase in severity and frequency of headaches during times of stress, loss (through death, separation or divorce), change of employment, and geographical relocation. For those individuals who appear to be under chronic stress and anxiety, or who are clinically depressed, individual or family counseling may be beneficial.

Sensory stimuli that may trigger migraines must be identified and eliminated or mitigated. These include strong or flickering lights, glue, paint, chemical or petroleum fumes, cigarette smoke, perfumes or other odors, and automobile exhaust fumes. As described earlier, numerous foods and food additives can trigger a migraine in those susceptible, although most authorities do not believe food allergies per se cause migraine. Foods to be eliminated from the diet should be determined on a systematic trial-and-error basis.

Pharmacotherapy

Abortive therapy. A Practice Parameter from the American Academy of Neurology (AAN) gives the following goals for acute treatment of migraine:

1. treat attacks rapidly and consistently to avoid recurrence;
2. restore the patient's ability to function;
3. minimize the use of backup and rescue medications;
4. optimize self-care and reduce subsequent use of resources;
5. be cost-effective for overall management; and
6. have minimal or no adverse effects.

Although no currently available medication meets all of these criteria, great strides have been made in the treatment of migraine in the past decade. Abortive therapies for migraine include simple analgesics, isomethep-tene, ergotamines, and triptans.

Simple analgesics include nonsteroidal anti-inflammatory drugs (NSAIDs), acetaminophen, and combination products (e.g., aspirin, acetaminophen, and caffeine). These simple analgesics are important first-line agents for treating mild to moderate migraine attacks. They are inexpensive and readily available without a prescription. A population-based survey in 1999 revealed that 57% of migraineurs treated their headaches exclusively with nonprescription medications. Therefore, the clinician should be certain to ask about prior use of these products and the efficacy and adverse effects experienced with their use. Acetaminophen products can be given according to the package directions for analgesia, not to exceed 4,000 mg/day from all sources of acetaminophen (including prescription combination analgesic products). However, acetaminophen alone has not demonstrated efficacy for migraine. The usefulness of NSAIDs may be due to inhibition of prostaglandin synthesis and platelet release of bradykinin and serotonin. Ibuprofen and naproxen are effective, and are rapidly and completely absorbed, reaching peak plasma concentrations in 1 hour. Because individual response to specific medications varies considerably, meclofenamate and indomethacin should also be considered. In an emergency room setting, an intramuscular injection of 60 mg of ketorolac may be an effective treatment. The dose of NSAIDs should be limited to the maximum listed in the prescribing information for each drug. Common adverse effects of NSAIDs include nausea, gastric upset, and diarrhea. Combination products include a combination of isometheptene, dichloralphenazone, and acetaminophen (e.g., Midrin, Isocom) or a combination of aspirin, acetaminophen, and caffeine (Excedrin). These products are effective for migraine and well tolerated. The isometheptene, dichloralphenazone, and acetaminophen product is contraindicated in patients with severe hypertension, glaucoma, and heart disease. One study has compared the efficacy of ibuprofen to the combination of aspirin, acetaminophen, and caffeine and to placebo. In this comparison, both medications were effective compared to placebo; however, the combination product had a 20-minute faster onset of action than ibuprofen. Similar numbers of patients became headache-free with either the combination product or ibuprofen at 1 or 2 hours postdose, but more subjects given the combination product were pain-free at 3 or 4 hours post-dose than subjects given ibuprofen. When given to patients with less severe migraines, the acetaminophen, aspirin, and caffeine combination was also more effective than 50 mg of sumatriptan given orally for pain relief at 4 hours post-dose, headache response, and use of rescue medications.

If a patient responds poorly to simple analgesics, or if the patient has moderate to severe migraine pain, the AAN Practice Parameter recommends proceeding directly to migraine-specific agents such as triptans or ergotamines. The triptans are effective treatments for migraine, acting on the specific serotonin receptors 5-HT_{1B} and 5-HT_{1D}. The effect of activation of these receptors is reversal of vasodilatation and decrease in neurogenic inflammation. A number of agents with various formulations are available (Table 8.6). Nonoral routes of administration have faster onsets of action and are important for patients who experience nausea, vomiting, and/or gastric stasis with migraine attacks. Subcutaneous sumatriptan is available in an auto-injecting device for self-administration. It has the fastest onset of action, the highest 2-hour response rate (76%), and the highest incidence of adverse effects of any triptan. Sumatriptan and zolmitriptan are also available in nasal spray formulations. The onset of action is faster for this administration form than for oral tablets. However, some patients dislike the taste of the nasal spray.

Orally disintegrating tablets are available for zolmitriptan and rizatriptan. These tablets are not absorbed sublingually. They disintegrate in the oral cavity, but are swallowed and absorbed in the intestinal tract. Therefore, they do not work faster than conventional oral tablets. The main use for these tablets is for patients who do not have access to water, or for patients who become nauseated if they consume water with a conventional tablet. However, in one study with zolmitriptan, 70% of patients preferred the orally disintegrating tablet to the conventional oral tablet.

Comparisons of efficacy generally consider two parameters: therapeutic gain 2 hours after administration and headache recurrence rate. The therapeutic gain is defined as the difference in headache response between placebo- and medication-treated subjects. The therapeutic gain is greatest for subcutaneous sumatriptan (51%) and lowest for frovatriptan (19%). The recurrence rates are highest for sumatriptan (38%), zolmitriptan (37%), and rizatriptan (47%). The lowest recurrence rates are for frovatriptan (7%) and naratriptan (17%). These differences may be somewhat explained by the different pharmacokinetics of the triptans (Table 8.6). Frovatriptan has the longest half-life of all the triptans at 26 hours; naratriptan follows with a half-life of 6 hours. This long half-life makes recurrence of migraine much less likely with these two agents. A combination product of sumatriptan 85 mg and naproxen sodium 500 mg is in development, and has demonstrated efficacy over placebo, naproxen, or sumatriptan alone in clinical trials. If a patient reports that a triptan is not efficacious, and further inquiry reveals that the medication has been used appropriately, it is reasonable to switch to another triptan. However, after the patient has failed three different triptans, it is unlikely that further trials will be effective.

Because of significant vasoconstriction, all triptans are contraindicated in patients with or at risk for coro-

Table 8.6 Abortive therapies for migraine

Agent (brand) Triptans	Dosage forms	T_{max}	$t^{1/2}$ (hours)	Dose	Maximum dose/ 24 hours (mg)
Almotriptan (Axert)	Tablets 6.25 mg, 12.5mg	1–3	2–4	1 tab, may repeat in 2 hours	25
Eletriptan (Relpax)	Tablets 20 mg, 40mg	1 hour	4–5	1 tab, may repeat in 2 hours	80
Frovatriptan (Frova)	Tablets 2.5mg	2–4 hours	26	1 tab, may repeat in 2 hours	7.5
Naratriptan (Amerge)	Tablets 1mg, 2mg	2–3 hours	6	1 tab, may repeat in 4 hours	5
Rizatriptan (Maxalt)	Tablets 5mg, 10mg	1–1.5 hours	1.8	1 tab, may repeat in 2 hours	30
	Orally disintegrating tablets 5mg, 10mg	1.6–2.5 hours	1.8	1 tab, may repeat in 2 hours	30
Sumatriptan (Imitrex)	Subcutaneous injection 6mg	12 minutes	1.9	1 injection, may repeat in 1 hour	12
	Intranasal 5mg, 20mg	30 minutes	2	1 spray in one nostril, may repeat in 2 hours	40
	Tablets 25 mg, 50mg, 100mg	2 hours	2.5	1 tab, may repeat in 2 hours	200
Zolmitriptan (Zomig)	Tablets 2.5 mg, 5mg	1.5 hours	3.75	1 tab, may repeat in 2 hours	10
	Orally disintegrating tablets	2.5 mg, 5mg 3 hours	3.75	1 tab, may repeat in 2 hours	10
	Intranasal 5mg	3 hours	3	1 spray in one nostril, may repeat in 2 hours	10
Ergots					
Ergotamine tartrate (Ergomar)	Sublingual tablets 2mg	unknown	2	1 tab under tongue, may repeat in 1 hour	6
Dihydroergotamine (DHE 45; Migranal)	Intranasal 4mg ampules	0.9 hours	10	1 spray (0.5 mg) in each nostril, repeat in 15 minutes	3
	Intravenous/intramuscular/ subcutaneous 1mg/mL	SQ 15–45 minutes	9	1 mL vials 1mL IV/IM/SQ, may repeat in 1 hour	2mg IV; 3mg IM/SQ

nary artery disease, stroke, uncontrolled hypertension, peripheral vascular disease, ischemic bowel disease, and pregnancy. They also should not be used in patients with hemiplegic or basilar migraines. Common adverse effects include a sensation of pressure, warmth, and/or tightness over the chest and neck areas, and tingling in the extremities.

All triptan administration is contraindicated within 2 weeks of treatment with monoamine oxidase inhibitors because of the potential for serotonin syndrome. They should not be given in patients using methysergide or methylergotamine, and they should be used with caution with other serotonin-active medications. Because of the risk of severe vasoconstriction, triptans should not be used within 24 hours of ergotamines. Likewise, different triptans should not be administered concomitantly, except for repeated doses at manufacturer-specified intervals (Table 8.6). Cimetidine increases the half-life of zolmitriptan, making dosage reductions of zolmitriptan necessary. Propranolol increases plasma concentrations of rizatriptan. Patients using both should be given 5-mg doses of rizatriptan. Because eletriptan is primarily metabolized by cytochrome P450 (CYP) 3A4, it is contraindicated in the presence of potent CYP3A4 inhibitors, including ketoconazole, itraconazole, erythromycin, clar-

ithromycin, ritonavir, nelfinavir, and indinavir. There have been case reports suggesting eletriptan should not be used with verapamil or fluconazole. Caution should be exercised when using eletriptan with any inhibitor of CYP3A4 metabolism.

Ergotamine has been used in the treatment of acute migraine attacks for over a century. Ergotamine and dihydroergotamine (DHE) are available in several dosage forms (Table 8.6). Dihydroergotamine (DHE) is an effective abortive treatment for acute migraine, offering excellent relief from severe headache, even when it is administered after the attack is well underway. DHE is available as a nasal spray and in a parenteral formulation. These nonoral routes of administration are particularly useful for patients who experience nausea and/or vomiting with their migraines. Although no longer considered a first-line therapy for migraine, ergotamine tartrate is available as a sublingual tablet, and combinations of ergotamine and caffeine are available as oral tablets and rectal suppositories.

Ergotamines are contraindicated in patients with or at risk for coronary artery disease, stroke, uncontrolled hypertension, peripheral vascular disease, ischemic bowel disease, and pregnancy. They should not be used in patients with hemiplegic or basilar migraines. With chronic, daily use, ergotamines have been associated with fibrotic complications. Unfortunately, a common adverse effect of ergotamine is nausea and/or vomiting. Because of this effect, many patients will require co-administration of an antiemetic. Other common adverse effects include diarrhea, cramps, paresthesias, tachycardia, and bradycardia.

Ergotamines should not be used within 24 hours of triptans because of the risk of severe vasoconstriction. There have been case reports of severe vasospasms leading to cerebral or extremity ischemia when ergotamines were administered with potent CYP3A4 inhibitors, including ketoconazole, itraconazole, erythromycin, clarithromycin, ritonavir, nelfinavir, and indinavir.

If these first-line therapies are ineffective, a rescue medication for the patient to self-administer may be added to therapy to alleviate pain and avoid frequent emergency department visits. Other conditions in which second-line therapies might be considered include intolerance or contraindications to first-line therapies. Opioid analgesics are occasionally chosen in these situations. However, the sedative adverse effects and the risk for abuse and/or dependence must be addressed before selection of an opioid analgesic. Butorphanol nasal spray and many oral combination products are available for these uses. Butorphanol nasal spray is prescribed as one spray in one nostril every 1 hour as needed for pain relief. The oral opiates should be administered according to manufacturer directions. Most of these combination products contain codeine. Therefore, it is necessary to inquire about allergies or intolerances (such as nausea) to codeine before the prescription is given. A possible alternative is the use of a tramadol-acetaminophen combination product, which has demonstrated efficacy in migraine compared to placebo. Another common component of the combination opioid analgesics is acetaminophen. It is prudent to also establish the amount of acetaminophen a patient receives from all sources, particularly nonprescription products, prior to prescribing additional acetaminophen.

Parenteral administration of other compounds may be necessary if the patient reports to the emergency department with unresolved migraine pain. In this instance, intravenous or intramuscular injections of an opioid analgesic or ketorolac may be required. An antiemetic is often helpful in these situations as well. Those patients with truly intractable headache, or *status migranosis*, should have a neurologic consultation. Many may require admission to the hospital for complicated treatment regimens, including repetitive DHE and corticosteroids.

Regardless of the therapy chosen for acute migraine relief, an assessment of efficacy is necessary. Rapoport and colleagues suggest the following questions to determine if a medication is optimal: (a) How quickly does the medicine begin to work? (b) When does the medicine reach its maximal effect? (c) When the medicine has reached its maximum effect, what percentage of the headache is gone? (d) Does the medication cause any adverse effects? (e) Does the headache recur or worsen within 24 hours after the patient is significantly improved? (f) How often can the patient become pain free and not have to take any further medicine? (g) How consistently does the medicine work?

Adjunctive therapy. Adjunctive therapy is directed at treating the migraine headache and associated symptoms. For some patients, the associated symptoms of migraine, especially nausea and vomiting, are more disturbing than the headache pain itself. Gastric stasis and delayed gastric emptying associated with migraine can decrease the effectiveness of oral medication. In addition, the medications used to treat migraine, especially ergotamines, can also produce nausea. Therefore, an antiemetic such as metoclopramide (10–20 mg), which will also enhance gastric emptying and the absorption of coadministered medications, should be given orally, intramuscularly, or intravenously at the onset of symptoms. Promethazine (25–50 mg), prochlorperazine (5–10 mg), and trimethobenzamide (100–250 mg) are all available in oral, rectal, and parenteral forms, and are also useful for control of nausea and vomiting, but do not enhance gastric emptying. These agents may cause sedation, an effect that should be discussed with the patient when prescrib-

▼

Pearls and Perils

Migraine headache

▶ The most common complaints among migraineurs during an attack are photophobia, sonophobia, and osmophobia.

▶ Attacks of migraine typically follow periods of stress during the "let-down" phase, in contrast to tension-type headaches, which are more temporally correlated with the time of greatest stress.

▶ Although the possible relationship among oral contraceptives, migraine, and stroke is controversial, a diagnosis of migraine does not increase the risk of stroke in women using oral contraceptives.

▶ Rebound headaches may occur with chronic overuse of ergot preparations.

▶ Prophylactic therapy is indicated if analgesics are needed more than two or three times per week, or if excessive amounts are required or are ineffective for treating a headache.

▶ Patients should be encouraged to initiate a wellness program that emphasizes regular exercise, balanced meals, and adequate sleep during headache-free intervals.

ing them. Serotonin receptor (5-HT$_3$) antagonists, such as granisetron, have not shown statistically significant clinical benefit for migraine relief.

Many patients are relieved of their migraine attack by sleep, and for them, even a mild analgesic coupled with a sedative-hypnotic or anxiolytic agent may be sufficient to allow sleep and the resolution of symptoms. The antiemetics discussed above may provide sufficient sedation, but for others a short-acting barbiturate (e.g., butalbital, 50 mg by mouth) or benzodiazepine (e.g., diazepam, 5–10 mg by mouth) may be necessary. Rest in a quiet, dark area must follow sedation. Patients must be warned of the danger of habituation.

A neuroleptic, especially in an emergency room setting, is an alternative for severe migraine attacks unresponsive to other therapies, but patients should be pretreated with 500 mL of normal saline to reduce the risk of hypotension. Effective agents include chlorpromazine (25 mg), haloperidol (5 mg), and thiothixene (5 mg).

Prophylactic therapy The need for prophylactic therapy depends on several factors including migraine frequency and severity, effectiveness and tolerability of abortive and interval therapy, and impact of the migraine syndrome on the patient's quality of life. The AAN Practice Parameter suggests the following criteria for initiating prophylactic therapy:

1. recurrent migraines that, in the patients' opinions, significantly interfere with their daily routines, despite acute treatment;
2. frequent migraines;
3. contraindication to, or failure or overuse of, acute therapies;
4. adverse effects with acute therapies;
5. cost of therapy is problematic;
6. patient preference; or
7. presence of uncommon migraine conditions (hemiplegic migraine, basilar migraine, prolonged aura, etc.).

The relationship between use of prophylactic therapy and health care expenditures has been examined in a large database from the U.S. Military Health System. This analysis found an increase in absolute expenditures for patients who were initiated on prophylactic therapy compared with those who were not given prophylaxis, largely due to increased ambulatory care visits and prescription medication costs. However, the overall cost of treatment for the prophylaxis group declined compared to their own pretreatment values, demonstrating that the expenditure for migraine prophylaxis for those with frequent and severe migraine headaches is cost-effective. General principles to guide the use of migraine prophylactic agents include using the lowest effective dose, giving an adequate

trial of therapy (2–3 months), and considering any coexisting conditions in the choice of agent (e.g., β-blockers are contraindicated in asthma patients, but beneficial in hypertension).

Many tricyclic antidepressants are used for the prevention of migraine. However, amitriptyline has the best clinical evidence for effectiveness. Over 60% of patients who benefit from amitriptyline show a response within 1 week, although it may take up to 6 weeks for full therapeutic effect. The usual starting dose is 10–25 mg at bedtime. If no adverse effects occur, the dose can be raised gradually, but as a rule, doses above 125 mg do not confer additional benefit. Common anticholinergic side effects include dry mucous membranes, constipation, blurry vision, confusion, and sedation. In older men, particularly, urinary retention is also a concern.

Among β-adrenergic blockers, propranolol, atenolol, metoprolol, nadolol, and timolol have all been shown to be effective. As a group, they are effective in up to 70% of migraineurs. β-Blockers with intrinsic sympathomimetic activity (acebutolol, pindolol) are not effective for migraine prophylaxis. A typical starting dose of propranolol is 20–40 mg twice per day. Usual therapeutic doses are 120–240 mg/day divided into three to four doses with a maximum dose of 320 mg/day. Guidelines for judging when a maximal tolerated dose has been reached include heart rate less than 50 beats per minute, systolic blood pressure less than 100 mm Hg, and a less than 10 beat per minute increase in heart rate following mild exercise. Full effectiveness of a given dose may take 4–6 weeks to occur. Adverse effects associated with β-blockers include fatigue, cold extremities, postural hypotension, and bradycardia. β-Blockers are contraindicated in those with asthma, congestive heart failure, or depression.

Among calcium channel blockers, verapamil, diltiazem, nicardipine, and nifedipine are all efficacious. The typical starting dose of verapamil is 80 mg three to four times per day. Because observable effects may not be apparent for 2–8 weeks, treatment should be continued for at least 2 months before evaluating efficacy. If either the response is not satisfactory or intolerable side effects arise, another calcium channel blocker can be tried. The most common adverse effects of these agents include constipation, drowsiness, and orthostatic hypotension.

Several different anticonvulsants have been used in the prophylactic treatment of migraine, including carbamazepine, phenytoin, gabapentin, topiramate, and divalproex sodium. Considered as a class, anticonvulsants decrease migraine events by about 1.3 attacks per 28 days compared to placebo. Divalproex sodium and topiramate have U.S. Food and Drug Administration (FDA)-approved indications for migraine prophylaxis. Divalproex sodium is absorbed through the gastrointestinal tract as the valproate ion. The usual starting dose is 250 mg twice daily or 500 mg once daily of the extended-release preparation. Liver function tests should be performed prior to therapy and at frequent intervals, especially during the first 6 months. Common side effects are nausea, alopecia, tremor, and weight gain. Topiramate 50 mg twice daily has also shown efficacy compared to placebo for migraine prophylaxis. This medication must be titrated slowly, no more than 25 mg increments weekly, to avoid excessive sedation and psychomotor retardation. Other common adverse effects of topiramate include dizziness and paresthesias. Uncommon, but serious, adverse effects include renal stones, oligohidrosis, hyperthermia, metabolic acidosis, secondary angle closure glaucoma, and acute myopia. Gabapentin demonstrated efficacy compared to placebo in one study, in which doses of 1,800–2,400 mg/day were used. Gabapentin was generally well tolerated, but some subjects reported dizziness, giddiness, and drowsiness.

Nonsteroidal anti-inflammatory drugs have been used as prophylactic, as well as acute, treatment for migraine. Naproxen and naproxen sodium have been most frequently examined as prophylactic agents. There are concerns, however, of rebound headaches when daily NSAID administration is stopped. Botulinum toxin has been injected into various muscles in the head to prevent migraine with some success. However, a patient would require referral to a practitioner with experience in these injections. Methysergide, an ergot alkaloid, has demonstrated efficacy, but is usually not used due to safety concerns. In addition to gastrointestinal symptoms and leg restlessness and pain, retroperitoneal and retropleural fibrosis have been associated with its use. Naratriptan, with its longer half-life has also been used for prophylaxis of menstrually related migraine. Using 1 mg twice daily for 6 days, starting 3 days before the onset of menstruation increased the percentage of patients without migraines during this period to 34-38% compared to 24-29% among patients who received placebo. However, it should be noted that most patients did not have complete prevention of their menstrually related migraines with this treatment.

A final comment on treatment and prevention of migraines when women may become pregnant or during pregnancy is in order. It is generally recognized that no medicine is completely without risk during the periconceptional and pregnancy stages. For abortive therapy of migraine, generally treatment with opioid analgesics or acetaminophen can be recommended. All of the prophylactic therapies have significant risk during pregnancy, and their use is not recommended.

Cluster Headache

Cluster headache is one of the most severe forms of head pain known to man. In contrast to migraine, cluster headache predominantly affects men, with a male-to-female ratio of at least 4.5:1. It accounts for only a small percentage of all headache sufferers and, unlike migraine, there is little evidence for a genetic factor. Peak incidence is in men aged 40–49 years and women aged 60–69 years. The age- and gender-adjusted incidence is 9.8 per 100,000 person-years. Patients with cluster headache are often heavy smokers and have a history of excessive use of ethanol. Periodicity is the main feature of cluster headache, with cluster periods lasting an average of 6–12 weeks. Cluster periods typically occur every year or two, are separated by periods of complete freedom from the headache, and tend to occur more frequently in spring and autumn. Recurrent clusters occur at the same site in over 75% of patients.

During a cluster, the headache tends to recur nightly, between 1 and 2 hours after onset of sleep, but may also occur several times during the night and day. Pain, described as excruciating, penetrating, and usually nonthrobbing, reaches a peak about 10–15 minutes after onset and lasts about an hour. It is usually felt unilaterally behind the eye, the temple, and in the maxillary area. In addition to pain, the cluster headache attack profile may include an ipsilateral blocked nostril followed by rhinorrhea, injected conjunctivum, and lacrimation, but there is no antecedent aura. Ptosis and miosis can also occur. Six percent of patients develop a permanent ipsilateral ptosis with repeated attacks. Patients may develop tenderness over the ipsilateral carotid artery, face, and scalp, as well as periorbital edema. The pain of a given headache may resolve as rapidly as it began, or it may fade away gradually. Ethanol commonly precipitates headaches during a cluster, but does not have this capacity during remissions. Patients who are aware of this frequently stop drinking during a cluster period. In a population-based study of Danish patients, 78% of cluster headache patients stated that the headaches restricted their activities, causing lifestyle changes for 96% of them. Thirty percent of these patients reported missing work within the last year because of a cluster headache attack.

Classification

The IHS classification groups cluster with other trigeminal autonomic cephalgias. The group includes cluster and paroxysmal hemicrania, both of which are subdivided into an episodic and chronic form, and *short-lasting unilateral neuralgiform headache attacks with conjunctival injection and tearing* (SUNCT) (Table 8.7). Chronic cluster is defined by absence of remission for more than a year. Over time, individual attacks tend to increase in frequency, and the syndrome becomes less responsive to therapy. The unilateral pain and autonomic features of paroxysmal hemicrania are similar to cluster, but attacks, which last only 5–10 minutes, may occur up to 30 times in a day. The chronic form is seen mostly in women, the episodic variant is without gender bias. Both forms of paroxysmal hemicrania show an absolute and specific responsiveness to indomethacin, typically 25 mg three to four times per day, making it both diagnostic and therapeutic. The unilateral pain and autonomic features of SUNCT, which occurs in men over 50, are similar to cluster. In contrast, attacks typically occur during the day, last 5 seconds to 40 minutes, and occur at a rate of 5–6 per hour. Lesions in the posterior fossa or involving the pituitary gland may mimic SUNCT. Patients may respond to corticosteroids, gabapentin, lamotrigine, or carbamazepine.

Pathophysiology

No unique and unifying pathophysiologic explanation exists for cluster headache. Indeed, migraine and cluster headaches share many clinical features, postulated mechanisms, and treatment. Two distinguishing clinical differences include the symptom localization and clock-like regularity of cluster. Based on the clinical features of cluster headache, it is reasonable to conclude involvement of ipsilateral trigeminal nociceptive pathways, activation of the cranial parasympathetic system, and dysfunction of the ipsilateral sympathetic nerves. Additionally, the clockwork consistency of attacks strongly suggests that a central pacemaker must be integrally involved in the genesis of this illness.

Cluster headache has traditionally been thought of as a "vascular" headache disorder. During an attack, extracranial, periorbital vasodilatation occurs. Vasodilators such as ethanol, nitroglycerin, and histamine are known to trigger cluster headache. However, other evidence suggests these vascular changes may be secondary to neuronal discharges in the area, as described earlier under the pathophysiology of migraine. Thus, the arterial and venous flow changes seen during cluster headache attacks are an epiphenomenon of trigeminal activation, are not specific, and do not play a large role in the genesis of cluster headache. To wit, pain drives changes in vessel caliber and not vice versa. Nevertheless, ample evidence supports involvement of both the trigeminovascular and parasympathetic systems in cluster headache. The excruciatingly severe unilateral pain is likely to be mediated by antidromic activation of the ophthalmic division of the trigeminal nerve, with release of calcitonin gene-related peptide (CGRP) into the cranial venous circulation. The autonomic symptoms are caused by activation of the cranial parasympathetic outflow from the seventh (facial) cranial nerve, associated with markedly elevated levels of vasoactive intestinal polypeptide (VIP). Of note, a functional reflex occurs between the trigeminovascular and cranial parasympathetic systems: stimulation of either the superior sagittal sinus or trigeminal ganglion results in the release of both CGRP and VIP into the cranial circulation.

The periodicity of clusters and the circadian regularity of headaches within a cluster suggest dysfunction of the biologic clock mechanism of the hypothalamus.

Table 8.7 Episodic cluster headache		
Discriminating features	**Consistent features**	**Variable features**
At least five attacks	Ipsilateral lacrimation	Ipsilateral ptosis
Attacks last 15–180 minutes	Conjunctival injection	Ipsilateral miosis
Frequency: eight per day to one every other day	Ipsilateral nasal fullness	Eyelid edema
Severe unilateral orbital and/or temporal pain	Ipsilateral rhinorrhea	Forehead/facial sweating
Circadian regularity	Recur 1–2 hours after sleep onset	Attack precipitated by alcohol during a cluster

Changes in a number of hormonal secretory circadian rhythms have been shown (e.g., in the levels of cortisol, β-endorphin, testosterone, and prolactin) between periods of cluster and remissions, leading to speculation that attacks may be linked to a disordered central pacemaker mechanism. In humans, this pacemaker is located in the hypothalamus, in an area known as the suprachiasmatic nucleus, which controls the rhythmic secretion of melatonin from the pineal gland. The 24-hour production of melatonin is reduced in patients with cluster headache, and the nocturnal melatonin peak is blunted during cluster periods. Low melatonin may be due to reduced availability of serotonin, which is needed for its synthesis. Furthermore, the biologic clock mechanisms in the hypothalamus are known to be modulated by serotonergic afferent neuronal pathways that may directly impact on certain treatment modalities.

Differential Diagnosis

The symptoms of cluster headache are so characteristic that its diagnosis is usually not a problem. However, the differential diagnosis should include other strictly unilateral headaches, such as episodic and chronic paroxysmal hemicrania, because of their unique response to indomethacin. Other considerations include SUNCT, trigeminal neuralgia, carotid dissection, temporal arteritis, pheochromocytoma, and the Tolosa-Hunt syndrome, which are all described elsewhere in this chapter.

Treatment

As with the migraineur, management of the patient with cluster headache must include patient education, environmental modification, and medication considerations. Patients should be apprised of the associations of cluster headache with heavy smoking and alcohol. Unlike migraine, other consistent precipitants are rare. Pharmacotherapy plays a much greater role, and, because of the relative brevity of individual headache attacks, has two facets: abortive treatment and prophylaxis.

Abortive therapy. Oxygen inhalation by a non-rebreathing mask at 6–10 L per minute for 15 minutes at the onset is effective in aborting cluster headache in about 70% of patients. Although oxygen relieves pain almost immediately, it may return after a brief respite, requiring repeated use. Because of the frequency of nocturnal attacks, maintenance of an oxygen tank at home during a cluster has proved to be effective, safe, and economical.

Subcutaneous administration of 6 mg of sumatriptan is an effective and well-tolerated treatment for acute attacks of cluster. Headache relief is achieved in about 75% of patients within 15 minutes. In at least one study, use of 12 mg led to increased side effects but no improvement in efficacy. Intranasal sumatriptan has also been shown to be effective; however, in a comparison trial with subcutaneous sumatriptan, only two of 26 subjects preferred the nasal form because of a slower onset of action. Zolmitriptan 10 mg nasal spray also showed efficacy compared to placebo as soon as 15 minutes following administration. Other triptans have shown greater efficacy only anecdotally. Intranasal dihydroergotamine has not been evaluated for cluster headaches.

Prophylactic therapy Treatment of cluster headaches should be directed toward prophylaxis, since the headaches are often too short for abortive medications to take effect and, if they occur multiple times per day, may lead to overmedication. Prophylactic medication should be started early in the course of a cluster episode and used daily until the headache has been absent for at least 2 weeks, after which it should be tapered. As a rule, medications can be completely discontinued during remissions but should be restarted with the first appearance of an exacerbation.

Calcium channel blockers are now widely used in the prophylactic treatment of cluster headache, and many authorities consider them the drugs of first choice. Verapamil has been used most commonly and appears to be the most effective, despite having little effect on cerebral hemodynamics. However, verapamil does influence hypothalamic adrenergic activity and affects a wide variety of biogenic amine receptors. The usual dose is 80–160 mg three times a day, or 240 mg of the sustained-release preparation once or twice a day. The common side effects are constipation, drowsiness, fluid retention, and hypotension.

Lithium is commonly used in the prevention of chronic and episodic cluster headaches. Doses of 600–900 mg/day, lower than those usually used for bipolar disorder, are effective. Headache suppression usually begins

---

▼

Pearls and Perils

Cluster headache

▶ Over 80% of patients with cluster headache are men.
▶ Alcohol commonly precipitates headaches during a cluster, but no longer has this capacity during remissions.
▶ Cluster headaches may only be delayed by abortive medications, are often too short for abortive medications to take effect and, if they occur multiple times in a day, may lead to overmedication; therefore, prophylactic medications are an important part of therapy
▶ A variant of cluster headache, chronic paroxysmal hemicrania, shows an absolute and specific responsiveness to indomethacin.

---

within a few days of treatment initiation. Common adverse effects include tremor, polyuria, and diarrhea. Serum lithium concentrations are sensitive to excessive intake of salt and to dehydration.

Corticosteroids have been used as prophylactic agents for cluster headache. Either prednisone up to 80 mg/day or dexamethasone up to 8 mg/day is usually effective within 1–2 days of initiation. Hyperglycemia, gastric upset, and mood swings are common adverse effects with short-term use. Because of the risk of serious, long-term adverse effects, such as osteoporosis and immunosuppression, the use of corticosteroids should be limited to 2–3 weeks duration. When stopping corticosteroids, a taper must be used, both because of the risk of headache recurrence and the risk of adrenopituitary axis suppression.

In contrast to migraine, there is a role for methylsergide in the prophylactic treatment of episodic cluster headache. The usual dose of 4–8 mg/day is most effective in the early course of the disease. With repeated exacerbations or evolution to chronic cluster, the medication loses efficacy. However, it does have an overall effectiveness of 70% in episodic cluster headache. The usual immediate adverse effects of methylsergide include leg swelling and muscle pain, acroparesthesia, chest pain, and nausea. Because of the usually short course of treatment during a cluster, commonly less than 3 months, fibrotic reactions are a minimal concern. It is, however, not advisable to treat clusters repeatedly.

Other agents have been utilized in small, open-label trials for cluster headache prophylaxis. These medications include valproic acid, topiramate, botulinum toxin, naratriptan, and baclofen. Although not proven in large, double-blind, placebo-controlled trials, they may prove effective in difficult-to-manage patients. Patients with repeated clusters, those who develop chronic cluster at the outset, and those in whom episodic headaches evolve into chronic cluster headache are best referred to a neurologist or other headache specialist.

Tension-type Headache

Tension-type headache (TTH) has been called by many other names, including muscle contraction headache, stress headache, ordinary headache, psychogenic headache, and tension headache. The TTH is the most common headache type, with a lifetime prevalence of 69% in men and 88% in women. In a Danish longitudinal study, the annual incidence rate for frequent TTH was calculated to be 14.2 per 1,000 population with a female-to-male ratio of 2.6:1. It is also the most common diagnosis among patients presenting to an emergency room with acute, nontraumatic headache. Tension headache has no prodrome or aura. The pain may be described as dull or achy, usually nonpulsatile, and is combined with a feeling of tightness, pressure, or constriction. It is typically mild to moderate in intensity, contrasting with the moderate to severe pain of migraine, although some patients with TTH report excruciating pain. Tension-type headache is usually bilateral, but can be unilateral in up to 20% of patients. In addition to involving any region of the head, it can involve the neck and jaw. Although TTH is no longer presumed to be caused by chronic muscle contraction, many patients will report pericranial and cervical muscle tenderness, as well as tenderness of the scalp (Table 8.8).

Classification

Under the IHS classification, TTH has been subdivided into infrequent episodic, frequent episodic, and chronic forms. At less than one headache day per month, infrequent episodic TTH seldom has impact on an individ-

ual. However, episodic TTH that occurs up to 180 days per year can cause considerable disability and often leads to *medication overuse headaches*. Because treatment of frequent episodic TTH and migraine without aura differ, the IHS made efforts to tighten criteria for their diagnoses (compare Tables 8.3 and 8.8). Frequent episodic TTH and migraine without aura often coexist and can be discriminated by a diagnostic headache diary. This will help to both direct appropriate therapy and selectively monitor treatment effectiveness for each headache type. More problematic for the clinician is discriminating between chronic migraine and chronic TTH, as well as determining whether medication overuse exists. It is possible to narrowly fit diagnostic criteria for both, suggesting that a small group of individuals may suffer from both. Again, a diary will help discriminate treatment and response to each headache type. Finally, chronic paroxysmal hemicrania (discussed under Cluster headache) is also a form of chronic daily headache, but relatively easily diagnosed by its specific responsiveness to indomethacin.

Chronic daily (migraine and tension-type) headache occurs in 2% of the population and is the most common problem seen at headache centers. Ninety per cent of patients with this disorder have a family history of headache. In addition to the causes mentioned above, chronic daily headache can have symptomatic origins including cervical spine disorders, oral or dental pain, and head trauma (refer to Symptomatic headaches, later). Despite IHS attempts to discriminate, there is apparent symptom overlap of the chronic forms of TTH and migraine supporting the view, first suggested by Raskin and Appenzeller, that both headache syndromes may belong to the same clinical continuum. Shared response to some of the same medications adds additional support to this contention. Such reasoning has led to the emergence of the *convergence hypothesis*, which postulates a single pathophysiologic mechanism to explain the clinical spectrum of primary headaches seen in migraineurs.

Treatment

Episodic tension-type headache. Episodic TTH is relatively easily treated. Almost all patients will demand some analgesics for pain. They should be strongly encouraged to use the milder analgesics: acetaminophen, aspirin, and NSAIDs. There is little evidence that more than standard nonprescription doses increase effectiveness. These medications should be taken as soon as the headache begins. Short-term use of muscle-relaxants such as carisoprodol, cyclobenzaprine, and methocarbamol at manufacturer-recommended doses are helpful in those patients with an element of cervical myalgia and spasm.

In many patients, episodic TTH may be associated with temporarily increased stress from direct environmental factors, including work, family, and marital prob-

Table 8.8 Frequent episodic tension-type headache		
Discriminating features	**Consistent features**	**Variable features**
12 and <180 headache days/year	Mild to moderate intensity	Bilateral or holoacranial
At least 10 prior attacks	Pressing/tightening quality	Family history
Attacks lasting 30 minutes to 7 days	Photophobia and phonophobia absent; or only one present	No aggravation by routine physical activity
No prodrome or aura	No nausea or vomiting	

lems. Discussion of any problems that surface is more therapeutic than is generally recognized. Many patients are anxious to discuss problems, and the physician serves as a counselor. Lastly, reassurance that their headache is a reflection of environmental pressures, that their physical examination is normal, and that they are not suffering from a brain tumor or other malignant illness, will help a number of patients.

Many individuals will respond to a course of home cervical traction, especially when the physiologic mechanism of stretching and relaxing tight cervical muscles is explained. Patients should be instructed to begin with 5 pounds and gradually increase to no more than 12 to 14 pounds of traction to the neck for 10 minutes three times per day. Use of more weight tends to encourage isometric contractions of cervical muscles that aggravates the pain. This form of physical therapy promotes relaxation and encourages the patient to take some direct responsibility for headache treatment.

Prophylactic treatment of TTH is a useful adjunct designed to reduce the frequency and severity of headache attacks. Its efficacy is often measured by reduced dependence on analgesics. An appropriate first choice is the tricyclic antidepressant, amitriptyline. The usual starting dose is 10–25 mg at bedtime. If no adverse effects occur, the dose can be raised gradually but, as a rule, doses above 125 mg do not confer additional benefit. Any of the other medications discussed earlier for migraine prophylaxis can also be tried, particularly in patients who have both TTH and migraine.

Chronic tension-type headache. Successful treatment of chronic tension-type headache (CTTH) is difficult, and the practitioner's goal should be directed toward control and not cure. Studies from most headache specialty centers report no better than 20% long-term cures of chronic daily headache regardless of therapy. Patients often exhibit physical and emotional dependency, low frustration tolerance, sleep disturbance, and depression.

Many headache patients tend to abuse a variety of medications. Frequent and excessive use of non-narcotic analgesics, such as aspirin and acetaminophen, leads to analgesic rebound headache (one of several categories under IHS code: Medication overuse headache). Several studies have reported marked improvement in patients with CTTH within several weeks after the withdrawal of analgesics and ergotamine. Whether analgesic abuse is a consequence, or a contributing cause of CTTH is not known. Curiously, however, nonheadache patients who take large amounts of analgesics for other conditions, such as arthritis, do not develop medication overuse headache.

Prophylactic medication is the mainstay of pharmacotherapy, but its efficacy is reduced by half in those patients who continue chronic analgesic use. Thus, an important first step in treatment involves the withdrawal of analgesic medication. A nonprescription medication may be withdrawn abruptly, but ergots, narcotics, and barbiturates must be tapered cautiously, sometimes in an inpatient setting. In the outpatient setting, controlled use of an NSAID may be used to withdraw a patient from aspirin and a tapering schedule of an isometheptene, dichloralphenazone, and acetaminophen formulation (e.g., Duradrin), beginning with one capsule four times per day and reducing the daily dose by one capsule per week, can be helpful in weaning patients from acetaminophen and, occasionally, from ergotamine. When narcotics or codeine-containing compounds are tapered, clonidine may be helpful in repressing some of the withdrawal symptoms. For many patients with chronic daily headache (whether CTTH or chronic migraine), detoxification requires hospitalization and the administration of repetitive intravenous DHE. This should be done with the help of a neurologic consultant or headache specialist. This is also the appropriate time to initiate psychotherapy, with a mental health specialist if feasible, and patient education. Botulinum toxin type-A has been used in a small study of 28 patients with CTTH. The medication was injected into pericranial muscles including frontalis, splenius capitis, trapezius, occipitalis, and temporalis. The number of headache days per month declined from a mean of 24.9 at baseline to 14.9 at one month, 9.1 at three months, and 5.1 at 1 year after the one-time injection.

As discussed earlier, for prophylactic medication to be effective, the patient must be withdrawn from any overused drug. Many authorities choose amitriptyline as the first choice for prophylaxis. Dosage is the same as that described for episodic TTH and migraine. Some patients with chronic daily headache respond to β-blockers, divalproex sodium, venlafaxine, or topiramate, at the same doses used to prevent migraine, reinforcing the concept that this entity can evolve from migraine as well as TTH.

▼

Pearls and Perils

Chronic daily headache

► Patients with chronic daily headache frequently abuse non-narcotic analgesics, such as aspirin and acetaminophen, which leads to analgesic rebound headache.

► Patients may show a marked improvement of headache frequency and severity within several weeks after the withdrawal of analgesics and ergotamine.

► Prophylactic medication is the mainstay of pharmacotherapy, but its efficacy is reduced by half in those patients who continue chronic analgesic use.

If the CTTH cycle can be broken, patients will often revert to their former episodic headache type. Education should continue into this phase. The phenomenon of analgesic rebound needs to be reiterated to patients: overuse of analgesics will itself cause daily headache, and daily analgesic medication will subvert the effectiveness of prophylactic medications. Behavioral modification, including reduction of stressors, is critical to ensure any degree of long-lasting control and prevention of recurrence of chronic daily headache. The use of a headache calendar by this group of patients is extremely important. As emphasized in the section on treatment of the migraineur, in addition to providing specific information helpful in management, using a calendar and learning about the nature of the illness gives the patient a greater sense of internal control over the headache and helps dispel some of the magical thinking concerning its treatment.

Symptomatic Headaches

A major concern to most physicians is that the patient coming to them with symptoms of headache will have some underlying medical or neurologic problem, for which headache is one of the symptoms. The following group of causes for headaches is certainly not complete, but it covers the majority of illnesses that may be seen in a general practice, among which headache is a major symptom.

Altered Cerebrospinal Fluid Dynamics

Increased intracranial pressure is often associated with headaches, either directly as in pseudotumor cerebri, or indirectly in association with space-occupying lesions, especially posterior fossa masses or deep cerebral tumors. Acute obstruction of CSF pathways always results in severe headache. This may be associated with Cushing's triad of hypertension, bradycardia, and respiratory slowing, which is almost always associated with deep coma. Cushing's triad appears more commonly in children than in adults. Although obstruction of CSF outflow anywhere along the ventricular system can produce headache, it is typified by colloid cysts of the third ventricle, an uncommon disorder accounting for less than 2% of all intracranial tumors. The headache pain is paroxysmal and precipitated or relieved by changes in posture, which has been postulated to be secondary to "ball valve" ventricular obstruction at the foramen of Munro. There may also be sudden falls or "drop attacks." A much more common cause of acute hydrocephalus and associated headache is ventriculo-peritoneal shunt malfunction, which is a neurosurgical emergency.

Ten to thirty percent of patients have been reported to develop headache 15 minutes to 4 days following a

---

Pearls and Perils

Symptomatic headache

▶ Refractory headache resulting from lumbar puncture will nearly always respond to an autologous blood patch injected into the epidural space adjacent to the puncture site.

▶ Persistent low-grade headache is a consistent feature of infectious mononucleosis.

▶ Headache and visual obscurations in a patient over 60 years of age should suggest temporal arteritis and demands an emergent Westergren sedimentation rate. If significantly elevated, treatment with steroids should be initiated immediately.

▶ Headache in a setting of slowly developing neurologic symptoms or signs should prompt consideration of an intracranial tumor as the cause.

▶ The most common cause of headache from dental disease is bruxism, or teeth clenching.

▶ Headache with nausea and vomiting occurring concurrently, rather than sequentially, among several family members should suggest carbon monoxide poisoning (e.g., from a faulty automobile exhaust or furnace) over a viral etiology.

---

lumbar puncture. Post–lumbar puncture headaches may last, on average, 4–8 days, but have been reported to last as long as several weeks or even months. They are twice as common in women than men. The pain is described as either a pounding or a dull ache, and is described equally as frontal, occipital, or diffuse. The headaches typically occur when the patient assumes an upright position and are abolished when lying flat. Over the years, a variety of risk factors have been evaluated; those that correlate with reducing headache risk are the use of a small-bore needle (21-gauge or smaller), use of atraumatic needles, replacement of the stylet, and the skill of the individual performing the procedure. Once headache is established, adequate hydration and remaining supine are sufficient for a resolution of symptoms over several days in most patients. Others respond to treatment with theophylline (300 mg t.i.d.). Refractory headaches respond to an epidural blood patch 90% of the time. Ten to 20 mL of autologous blood is injected into the epidural space adjacent to the dural sac, usually by an anesthesiologist. An attempt to prevent post–lumbar puncture headache with frovatriptan 2.5 mg/day for 5 days following the lumbar puncture was successful in a small, open-label, uncontrolled trial.

Pseudotumor cerebri, first described before the advent of readily available imaging studies, is generally an idiopathic illness, associated with increased intracranial pressure, in the range of 25–40 cm of CSF, as measured by lumbar puncture in the lateral decubitus position. The typical patient with pseudotumor cerebri is female, of childbearing age, obese, and amenorrheic. Over 80% of patients complain of headache, which is usually of insidious onset and generalized. The headache may be relatively mild, but 93% of patients in one study described it as the "worst ever." It is not uncommon for the headache to be present on awakening or at its worst in the morning or after exertion. The typical description fits the profile for TTH, although associated migrainous features often are present. Seventy per cent of patients with pseudotumor experience transient visual obscurations, 80% develop some degree of visual loss, and 10% become blind without treatment. The differential diagnosis for idiopathic pseudotumor cerebri includes venous sinus occlusion, hypoparathyroidism, hypervitaminosis A, systemic lupus erythematosus, renal disease, and treatment with tetracycline. Medical treatment, with help in management from the consulting neurologist, should begin with acetazolamide (Diamox), weight loss, and serial lumbar punctures. It is important to monitor vision closely with perimetry. Several authorities recommend optic nerve sheath fenestrations as a means of protecting vision. Although it is not certain by what mechanism this procedure is effective, it has been suggested that allowing the efflux of CSF through the surgical tear in the epineurium reduces pressure. An alternative treatment, which protects both vision and abolishes headache, is placement of a thecoperitoneal shunt. Unfortunately, these shunts are difficult to maintain and often require revision.

Cerebrovascular Disease

Subarachnoid Hemorrhage

Almost all patients suffering from subarachnoid hemorrhage will have an associated headache. It is typically described as the "worst headache of my life." Although this entity can occur at any age, the average age is 51 years. When the subarachnoid hemorrhage is due to a ruptured saccular aneurysm, patients may describe a sentinel headache that has occurred days to weeks before, and most likely represents a small hemorrhage, which spontaneously stopped. In most individuals, the primary rupture occurs during normal activity, but may be associated with exertion, including sexual intercourse. Neurologic abnormalities are common following subarachnoid hemorrhage, but may be absent. The patient may have nausea and vomiting and complain of photophobia or dizziness. More devastating hemorrhages are associated with amnesia, a decreased level of arousal, or coma. On examination, the patient may have ocular palsies, or pain with eye movements. Although nuchal rigidity is extremely common, absence of meningeal signs does not rule out subarachnoid

hemorrhage. After examination of patients with suspected subarachnoid hemorrhage, acute management begins with an unenhanced CT scan of the head. In the absence of contraindications, if the CT scan does not show evidence of intracranial hemorrhage, a lumbar puncture should be performed. If the CSF is xanthochromic, then the hemorrhage is at least 2–4 hours old. Patients with subarachnoid hemorrhage may also have nonspecific EKG abnormalities, and may have leukocytosis, albuminuria, glycosuria, and electrolyte disturbances. It is appropriate to obtain a consult from a neurologist or a neurosurgeon, who can help with further studies and management. Remember that patients with subarachnoid hemorrhage will occasionally provide a family history of cerebral aneurysm, subarachnoid hemorrhage, polycystic kidney disease, or coarctation of the aorta.

Intraparenchymal Hemorrhage

Three to ten percent of all strokes include hemorrhage into the brain parenchyma, and headache is a symptom in over 50% of these cases. Although many ischemic and hemorrhagic strokes include headache in the symptomatology, severe headache is a fair "predictor" of hemorrhagic stroke. Hypertension is present in at least 50% of patients with hemorrhagic strokes.

It is important for the generalist in the emergency room setting to be aware of hemorrhagic cerebellar stroke, which represents 10% of all intracranial hemorrhages. In over 75% of cases, patients complain of headache subsequent to the sudden onset of profound ataxia or syncope. Typically, patients are brought to a hospital emergency room and remain in the prone position without adequate testing of cerebellar function. Patients initially may have nothing more than an end-gaze nystagmus but, as the hemorrhage enlarges, they may experience an acute onset of brainstem compression and herniation, resulting in death. Patients with headache and cerebellar symptoms and signs should have an emergent

---

Pearls and Perils

Subarachnoid hemorrhage

▶ Most patients describe the headache of subarachnoid hemorrhage as the worst of their life.

▶ Up to one-third of patients may experience premonitory headaches due to leaking of an aneurysm for as long as a few weeks before a major rupture.

▶ Neither absent meningeal signs nor a normal head CT scan rules out subarachnoid hemorrhage.

▶ A lumbar puncture should be performed if the CT scan does not show blood and if there is no contraindication.

CT scan of the head. If a cerebellar hemorrhage is present, it should be treated as a neurosurgical emergency. Some neurosurgeons will follow small hemorrhages (less than 3 cm in diameter and not compromising the brainstem) with serial CT scans of the head. If the hemorrhage does not enlarge, patients can be managed conservatively without the need for surgery.

Ischemic Cerebrovascular Disease

Headache occurs acutely in 17–54% of persons with ischemic infarction. The headache is generally of mild to moderate intensity, and often occurs subsequent to the ischemic event, in contrast to the concurrent onset of headache with subarachnoid hemorrhage. These may have some localizing value: for example, if the headache is lateralized, it tends to occur frontally and ipsilateral to the symptomatic anterior circulation. Approximately a third of patients experiencing a TIA attack will experience headache, which tends to be more common with TIA in the vertebrobasilar than carotid system.

Carotid Artery Dissection

Carotid artery dissection is a rare cause of headaches, usually occurring in young adults. Eighty percent of cases have headache as a major symptom, which is usually in the frontoparietal region ipsilateral to the lesion. Patients also complain of pain in the anterior cervical region ipsilateral to the dissected carotid artery. A major diagnostic clue is an ipsilateral Horner's syndrome, including miosis, anhydrosis, ptosis, and pseudoexophthalmos, due to damage to the sympathetic plexus contiguous to the artery. One-third of patients with carotid artery dissection suffer ipsilateral cerebral infarctions several hours to days after the actual event. For this reason, it is advisable to obtain a neurological consultation and anticoagulate patients while the dissection is healing. Surgical intervention is generally not necessary. Some patients develop persistent headaches for years after the event. In a minority of these patients, treatment with antiepileptics, or possibly steroids, helps.

Cervical Disease

Beginning in middle or late life, disease of the cervical spine becomes a common cause of headache. A wide variety of disease processes have been implicated, including cervical radiculopathies. Radiculopathies generally produce neck pain and characteristic shooting (radicular) pain along the dermatome of the involved root, usually C6 or C7. In addition to radiculopathies (which may, in some cases, occur secondary to herniated discs), one should consider the possibility of hypertrophied ligamentum flavum, meningiomas of the foramen magnum, and other cervical tumors, including neurofibromas, ependymomas, and metastases. Changes in the bone caused by

rheumatoid arthritis, ankylosing spondylitis, and perhaps osteoarthritis, can be a source of headache, as can infectious processes such as tuberculous spondylitis.

The pain is usually described as occipital and is often asymmetric. It generally has a nonthrobbing, aching quality, and is associated with shoulder and low back pain. The course tends to be chronic and relapsing. Several treatment options are possible, including trigger point injections with local anesthetics, muscle relaxation techniques, NSAIDs, muscle relaxants, combinations of postural training, and cervical traction.

Hypertension

The association of hypertension with headache is controversial. Although as many as half of patients with hypertension complain of headache, the exact relationship is not clear. However, certainly there is a subpopulation in whom correction of the hypertension leads to resolution of headaches. If hypertension is severe, with diastolic blood pressures in the range of 120–130 mm Hg, or higher, headache is frequent and responds to reduction in blood pressure. In many of the patients with hypertension who also complain of headache, the pain is usually worse in the morning and located occipitally. Patients with chronic severe hypertension may develop hypertensive encephalopathy, characterized by impaired consciousness and severe headaches. These patients typically have papilledema and retinal hemorrhages on examination, abnormal electroencephalograms, and laboratory findings of uremia.

Infectious Disease

Headache is common in bacterial meningitis, where it is usually generalized. However, headache symptoms in bacterial meningitis are typically overshadowed by the often dramatic presentation of altered consciousness, fever, nuchal rigidity, and nonspecific neurologic signs. In contrast, headache is the most frequent symptom in viral meningitis, where it is often accompanied by photophobia, phonophobia, and fever, but a normal or only minimally altered level of consciousness. Infection by human immunodeficiency virus (HIV) can cause meningitis or impair immunity, so that individuals are subject to meningitis caused by unusual, as well as typical, pathogens. Among other viral infections, persistent, low-grade headache is a key feature of infectious mononucleosis. Headache with fever also occurs with uncommon infections involving the nervous system, including subdural empyema, epidural abscess, and brain abscess. In all cases of headache, altered level of consciousness, and fever, it is appropriate to obtain neurologic consultation.

Acute, but not chronic, sinusitis often causes a dull, nonpulsatile aching, the location of which depends upon the sinus involved. Most studies suggest that the pain in acute sinusitis arises from inflammation of tissues adjacent to the nasal structures, rather than from alterations in the sinus itself. There is some localizing value to the headache: in ethmoid sinusitis, patients complain of a pain that passes from the retro-orbital to the temporal region; sphenoid sinusitis produces headache symptoms referred to the vertex and orbits; maxillary sinusitis produces cheek, ear, and dental pain; and frontal sinusitis produces pain in the midfrontal region.

Inflammatory Disease

The most common inflammatory disease associated with headache is temporal arteritis. More than 85% of individuals who develop temporal arteritis are over 60 years of age. Women are affected much more commonly than men. Early symptoms include malaise, fever, weight loss, and jaw claudication. Many patients feel generally unwell and suffer weight loss. Some will complain of shoulder and hip girdle pain and stiffness secondary to polymyalgia rheumatica. Typically, the patient develops an increasingly intense headache, which may be throbbing or nonthrobbing, bilateral or unilateral, and usually localized to the site of the affected arteries. The headache is typically more severe at night and may be worse following exposure to cold. The affected superficial temporal artery and other scalp arteries are frequently swollen, red, tender, and without pulsation. It is important to diagnose temporal arteritis early because of the threat of blindness due to ischemic optic neuritis.

The Westergren erythrocyte sedimentation rate (ESR) is nearly always elevated, often to levels of 100 mm/hour or more. Treatment should be initiated immediately with steroids, typically 60–80 mg/day of prednisone, in divided doses. After 3–6 months, this can then be gradually reduced, typically to 20 mg/day, which will usually be required for at least 2 years. Unfortunately, alternate-day steroids have proved inadequate. The ESR is both a reliable index of therapeutic response and a bellwether of relapse. The decision to biopsy a symptomatic temporal artery remains controversial, but should always be done in cases in which the diagnosis is questionable. Typically, microscopic examination discloses an intense granulomatous or "giant-cell" arteritis, but its absence should not preclude treatment in patients suspected clinically of having temporal arteritis.

Other inflammatory diseases associated with headache include Henoch-Schönlein purpura, Takayasu's arteritis, systemic lupus erythematosus, and isolated central nervous system granulomatous angiitis. Pseudotumor cerebri and its associated headache is a common neurologic manifestation of Behçet's disease and probably reflects venous sinus thrombosis. Help with the diagnosis and management of these less common causes of headache should come from a consulting neurologist or rheumatologist.

Neoplastic Disease

About half of patients with intracranial neoplasms complain of headache at the time of diagnosis. Most studies suggest that headache is more likely to occur with faster growing masses. The pain of a brain tumor is usually deep, aching, dull, and nonthrobbing. It is often generalized, but tends to be frontal, intermittent, and not necessarily intense or severe. If unilateral, the brain tumor is invariably on the ipsilateral side. The headache tends to be intermittent until the tumor becomes sufficiently large to increase intracranial pressure or to cause pressure against pain-sensitive structures. Headaches in patients with brain tumors tend to be constant, severe, refractory to common analgesics, and associated with nausea or vomiting. The concept that brain tumor headache results from traction on intracranial pain-sensitive structures is supported by several recent CT and MRI studies, which relate headache to the size of the tumor and amount of midline shift.

When considering the diagnosis of intracranial tumor, probably more important than the quality and localization of the headache is the history of significant change from a prior headache pattern or occurrence of seizures, mental symptoms, and neurologic symptoms and signs. Patients fitting these criteria should be imaged and referred to a neurologist or neurosurgeon for consultation.

Neuralgia

Herpetic Neuralgia

Herpes zoster ("shingles") is a common viral infection of the nervous system that produces inflammatory lesions in the posterior root ganglia and is characterized clinically by a vesicular cutaneous eruption and radicular pain. The incidence rate is three to five cases per 1,000 persons per year, but rates tend to be higher in middle-aged and elderly patients. Involvement of the trigeminal ganglion occurs in about 20% of cases, in which the ophthalmic division is, by far, the most commonly affected. The Ramsey-Hunt syndrome, involving the geniculate ganglion, consists of a facial palsy in combination with herpetic eruption of the external auditory meatus. Other associated symptoms can include periauricular pain, tinnitus, vertigo, and deafness. Lastly, head pain, affecting palate, pharynx, neck, and the retroauricular region, can occur with herpetic infection of upper cervical roots or ganglia of the vagus and glossopharyngeal nerves. In all of these, a postherpetic neuralgia can develop with persistent, intense burning pain following the initial acute illness. It is more common in older individuals and can occur in as many as one-half of patients over age 60 years. The pain is localized over the distribution of the affected nerve, is associated with exquisite tenderness to even the lightest touch, and is usually described as sharp and shooting. The pain may persist for months or even years, although in younger patients, the discomfort usually subsides after several weeks. The incidence of postherpetic neuralgia is reduced if the acute infection is treated with an antiviral agent, such as acyclovir 800 mg five times per day for 7 days, beginning before the third day of symptoms. Although there remains some controversy about benefit, many practitioners also treat concurrently with steroids, such as prednisone 60 mg/day, with a rapid decrease over the following 2–3 weeks.

Trigeminal Neuralgia

A disorder of middle age and later life, trigeminal neuralgia is an intense, stabbing pain that occurs in paroxysms within the distribution of the mandibular and maxillary divisions (rarely, the ophthalmic division) of the trigeminal nerve. The most frequent of all neuralgias, it is usually unilateral, and the pain seldom lasts more than a few seconds to at most a minute, but may be so intense that the patient winces, leading to the alternate sobriquet "tic douloureux." An important characteristic feature is that the pain is induced even by the lightest touch to a particular area of the face, lips, or gums, as occurs with chewing, talking, yawning, or touching. Indeed, these trigger zones are reported to the physician by pointing, rather than touching, by the patient who carefully guards them. Affected individuals may go for days without eating or talking, to prevent the paroxysms of pain.

The etiology of trigeminal neuralgia is not well understood. Most cases are idiopathic, but a minority have been associated with multiple sclerosis, cerebellopontine angle tumors, aneurysms, and arteriovenous malformations. Usually, other objective signs of neurologic deficit help distinguish these symptomatic causes from idiopathic trigeminal neuralgia. Furthermore, the pain from these is often atypical and spreads beyond the distribution of the trigeminal nerve. The most widely used drug for treatment of trigeminal neuralgia is carbamazepine, at maintenance doses of from 600–1,200 mg/day. Uncontrolled observations and clinical practice indicate that clonazepam, gabapentin, lidocaine, oxcarbazepine, phenytoin, pregabalin, sodium valproate, and topiramate may also be effective. The maintenance dose of sodium valproate is 600–1,200 mg/day; the maintenance dose of pregabalin is 200–300 mg/day. There is evidence that baclofen (50–80 mg/day) alone provides pain relief and that lamotrigine (300–600 mg/day) has an additive effect in patients with insufficient relief using carbamazepine. Phenytoin or lidocaine can be used intravenously as emergency treatment if exacerbations are so severe that the patient cannot take anything by mouth. Often, the response to medica-

tion is dramatic, with either complete suppression of pain or a shortening of the duration of the attacks. Spontaneous remissions and recurrences are common, with a tendency for symptoms to occur more frequently as the disease continues. Consultation with a neurologist can help with the long-term management. Ultimately, some patients may require neurosurgery, usually stereotactically controlled thermocoagulation of trigeminal roots using a radiofrequency generator. Janetta has championed the hypothesis that idiopathic trigeminal neuralgia is, in most cases, due to compression of the trigeminal roots by a torturous blood vessel, and has performed microvascular surgery to relieve pain through decompression of the root. Gamma knife radiosurgery has become a treatment option for those unable to undergo more invasive surgical procedures. However, the long-term outcome is less effective. If trigeminal neuralgia recurs after surgical intervention, patients often respond to another trial of medical therapy.

Other Neuralgias

Other craniofacial neuralgias are much less common than trigeminal neuralgia, and include glossopharyngeal and occipital neuralgia, as well as neck–tongue syndrome, among others. The pain of glossopharyngeal neuralgia is intense and paroxysmal and may be provoked by swallowing, talking, chewing, yawning, or laughing. The pain may radiate in either direction between throat and ear and is characterized by cluster attacks, each lasting weeks to months. This is the only craniofacial neuralgia that may be accompanied by bradycardia, even to the point of causing syncope. In most cases, the pain is idiopathic. However, peritonsillar abscesses or neoplasms of the oropharynx have rarely been implicated. Medical treatment is the same as for trigeminal neuralgia.

Pain in the distribution of the greater or lesser occipital nerves gives rise to occipital neuralgia. Occasionally, patients experience extreme tenderness where the affected nerve crosses the superior nuchal line, and occasionally, scalp hypesthesia or paresthesias are present in the distribution of the affected nerve. Relief may be obtained with injection of local anesthetics with or without steroids, and with the use of oral NSAIDs or carbamazepine.

The neck–tongue syndrome has been attributed to compression of the second cervical root. In this syndrome, pain occurs unilaterally over the neck or occiput, in association with ipsilateral numbness of the tongue upon sudden rotation of the neck. Cervicofacial pain that can be elicited by pressure on the common carotid arteries of patients has been referred to as *carotodynia*. The pain produced is usually a dull ache, referred to the ipsilateral face, ear, jaws, and teeth. Most cases of carotodynia are thought to represent a migraine variant and are treated as such.

Otalgia

Pain from the ear, which may be primary or referred, can frequently generalize into a headache. Over half of headaches that originate with ear pain are caused by primary otalgias. Major causes include external canal foreign bodies (including excess cerumen), external otitis (e.g., swimmer's ear), acute infectious otitis media, trauma to the external or middle ear, and neoplasms (e.g., acoustic neuroma). Typically, acoustic neuroma causes ipsilateral hearing loss, tinnitus, and vertigo, but may also produce ear pain. Causes of referred otalgia include dental problems, sinus disease (particularly involving the maxillary sinus), glossopharyngeal neuralgia, tumors (e.g., tumors of the pharynx, larynx, and thyroid), and peritonsillar abscess.

Ophthalmologic Headache

A variety of ocular disorders have been associated with headache. A favorite but overdiagnosed etiology for headaches is eyestrain, due either to refractive errors or to an extraocular muscle imbalance. When actually present, the associated pain does indeed increase with increased use of the eyes. Optic neuritis, an acute inflammation of the optic nerve, frequently provokes slight pain in or behind the eye, especially with ocular movement or by pressure over the globe. Various types of visual defects can be found, including central scotoma and color vision impairment. Pupillary reactions are usually preserved, although abnormal. If the inflammation extends to the optic disc (papillitis), the funduscopic exam reveals blurred disc margins and, rarely, hemorrhages in the nerve head or adjacent retina. If the lesion is near the chiasm, the fundus may appear normal or only slightly congested.

Acute elevations of intraocular pressure, such as occur in narrow-angle glaucoma, frequently provoke episodic pain in or around the eye. Patients may also complain of nausea, tearing, and impaired vision. The lid and conjunctivae may be congested, and the globe is sometimes firm to palpation, although this is often difficult to assess reliably without tonometry. Other causes of pain include uveitis, episcleritis, and conjunctivitis. It is important to remember that pain in or around the eye that is produced by local causes seldom extends beyond the involved region.

Last, a number of eponymous syndromes exist, which include headache and restricted eye movements as prominent features. Probably the most common is the Tolosa-Hunt syndrome, which is characterized by single or recurrent attacks of unilateral, retro-orbital, continuous, boring pain, associated with ophthalmoplegia. Attacks, which can last from days to weeks, can show symptomatic improvement with prednisone within 48 hours.

Pain of Oral or Dental Etiology

The most common cause of headache from dental disease is bruxism, or teeth clenching. This is usually, but not always, related to anxiety. If asked, patients will often note that their spouse has heard them grind their teeth while asleep. If particularly bad, obvious wearing down of the teeth is apparent. Bruxism can often be helped by the fashioning of an oral prosthesis to serve as an occlusal bite-guard.

Temporomandibular joint (TMJ) dysfunction is an overdiagnosed cause of headache. Early in the development of the syndrome, there is pain in and around the TMJ. Commonly, the pain is described as in front of and behind the ear of the affected side, but it may also radiate over the cheek and face, and the ear may feel full. Pain in the TMJ may be confused with the pain of otitis media, tic douloureux, sinusitis, and arthritis, as well as the pain associated with tumors of the brain, head, or neck. Many patients with headache may have a lax TMJ, which is unrelated to the etiology of the headache. Initial treatment of TMJ dysfunction should include rest of the mandible, a softer diet, and use of NSAIDs and local heat. Plain x-rays of the TMJ are often normal. However, CT scans can show early bony changes. Long periods of remission from symptoms can occur. Patients should be managed by an oral or maxillofacial surgeon with special interest in TMJ disease.

Toxic and Metabolic Headaches

A variety of metabolic states or toxic exposures can result in headaches, in association with other signs and symptoms. A common pattern in this headache syndrome is a gradual intensification of the pain, followed by impaired consciousness, unless the cause of the disturbance is corrected.

A large number of toxins have been reported to cause headache, including carbon monoxide. Not uncommonly, when the weather turns cold, patients will appear in the emergency room with headache and nausea due to carbon monoxide poisoning from a furnace leak or faulty heating system. Invariably, some patients are sent back into that environment with the diagnosis of viral upper respiratory tract infection. A critical clue to correct diagnosis is that whole families will present to the emergency room with the same set of symptoms occurring at the same time. In contrast, a viral infection will be passed from one family member to another over a period of days to weeks.

Acute mountain sickness is a transient syndrome that includes headache, nausea, anorexia, and dyspnea. It can occur within several hours after reaching high altitudes, usually in excess of 10,000 feet. Rarely, coma or even death, associated with acute pulmonary edema, may occur. For mild cases, diuresis, induced by furosemide or acetazolamide, with return to lower altitudes, is sufficient.

Several vasoactive agents are commonly associated with headache syndromes. Headache can infrequently occur with facial and extremity flushing in the setting of mastocytosis, carcinoid, and serotonin-secreting tumors. Headache frequently occurs in patients on chronic hemodialysis and appears to be related to the dialysis procedure itself, as well as to low levels of renin and 18-hydroxy-11-deoxycorticosterone. Hypercapnia secondary to chronic respiratory insufficiency is frequently associated with headaches and drowsiness. Although monosodium glutamate (MSG) has been implicated as the cause of the "Chinese Restaurant" syndrome (headache, nausea, lightheadedness, and numbness, and burning of the neck, chest, and arms) and a trigger of migraine, clinical trials have failed to identify a consistent relationship between ingestion of MSG and the constellation of symptoms that comprise the syndrome.

Headaches also occur occasionally in association with endocrine disorders. Patients with hypoglycemia often complain of headache, in addition to lightheadedness, nausea, and sweating. Headache can be a prominent manifestation of hyper- and hypoparathyroidism, hypo- and hyperthyroidism (especially Hashimoto's thyroiditis), and Addison's disease. In the majority of these illnesses, headache is not a prominent feature.

A variety of medications may produce headache. Disulfiram, when combined with alcohol, produces a throbbing headache, which serves as part of the inducement to refrain from alcohol. Monoamine oxidase inhibitors can produce severe hypertension and headache if combined with tyramine-containing foods. Nitrates, used in the treatment of ischemic cardiovascular disease, can precipitate headache even in individuals not subject to migraine or similar headache syndromes. Headaches may also occur as a result of substance withdrawal. Typical examples include alcohol, caffeine, corticosteroids, ergot preparations, and narcotics. Withdrawal headaches can even occur following abuse of aspirin and acetaminophen. More commonly, abuse of these and other over-the-counter analgesics results in early morning rebound headaches, as discussed earlier.

Among drugs of abuse, migraine-like headaches have been associated with cocaine intoxication. Although the acute onset of new headaches in cocaine addicts can signal intracranial hemorrhage, ischemic stroke, or brain abscess, more commonly it can be attributed to acute intoxication or withdrawal. The presumed mechanism relates to cocaine's effect on noradrenergic and serotonergic systems. The most common headache syndrome among abused drugs is *hangover* after brief but excessive consumption of ethanol. Symptoms include headache, nausea, vomiting, malaise, nervousness, tremulousness, and sweating.

Trauma

The general internist will encounter headache associated with trauma, usually in two general situations. In the emergency room, patients with acute head trauma may have suffered intracranial hematomas. If conscious, patients with either epidural or acute subdural hematomas invariably complain of headache. Headache is one of the most frequent presenting symptoms, as high as 60% in some studies, in patients with subacute or chronic subdural hematomas. Subacute or chronic subdural hematomas should be suspected in patients who complain of headache and are on anticoagulant therapy or suffer from alcoholism, uncontrolled epileptic seizures, or renal disease requiring dialysis. It should also be considered in patients over 60 years of age, who have suffered recent intermittent confusion, even when the headache is described as minimal and no history of trauma can be obtained. In all of these cases, it is best to obtain a neurologic or neurosurgical consultation as soon as possible.

Patients with subacute or chronic subdural hematomas may first present in the outpatient office setting, as may patients with posttraumatic headaches. This latter is an immediate transient headache that follows almost all head injuries. Reported prevalence of chronic posttraumatic headaches is as high as 83% following head injury. However, many patients with posttraumatic headache take daily or near-daily medications to relieve the pain, raising the possibility that they are suffering from medication-overuse or rebound headaches. Posttraumatic headaches are often associated with irritability, concentration impairment, insomnia, memory disturbance, and lightheadedness. Although posttraumatic headaches typically resolve 4–8 weeks after trauma, it is

---

Consider Consultation When...

▶ A patient is in status migrainosis..

▶ A patient has an intraventricular shunt malfunction.

▶ Pseudotumor cerebri is suspected.

▶ An intracranial hemorrhage is suspected.

▶ Carotid artery dissection is suspected.

▶ A patient has headache associated with an altered level of consciousness and fever.

▶ A patient has had a significant change from a prior headache pattern or a headache in association with convulsive seizures, mental symptoms, nausea or vomiting; or there has been a slow development of neurologic symptoms and signs.

▶ Initiating long-term treatment plans for trigeminal neuralgia.

▶ A patient suffers acute head trauma with suspected intracranial hematoma.

▶ A patient with posttraumatic headaches has no resolution of symptoms after 2 to 3 months.

not uncommon for these headaches to persist as long as a year or more. Although the duration and severity of the headache and associated symptoms are usually related to the severity of the trauma, this is not invariable. Finally, the patient's long-term, functional recovery may be related both to premorbid status and level of functioning at the job site. Those individuals who are maximally challenged intellectually on the job may find that, upon returning to work, they are unable to perform at their prior level of activity. Indeed, some patients may ultimately require vocational rehabilitation. Because of the prospect of possible rehabilitation and litigation in many cases involving posttraumatic headaches, patients without resolution of symptoms after 2–3 months, if not sooner, should receive neurologic consultation.

Annotated Bibliography

Headache classification committee of the international headache society: the international classification of headache disorders, 2nd ed. *Cephalgia* 2004;24 (Suppl 1):1–160.
For nearly 20 years, the diagnostic criteria of the International Headache Society (HIS) have been the accepted standard. Awareness of the revised criteria in this second edition of The International Classification of Headache Disorders is a must for physicians who treat headache.

Pascual J, Mateos V, Roig C, et al. Marketed oral triptans in the acute treatment of migraine: A systematic review on efficacy and tolerability. *Headache* 2007;47:1152–1168.
A solid article comparing efficacy and adverse effect differences among triptans.

Silberstein SB. Practice parameter: Evidence-based guidelines for migraine headache (an evidence-based review). Report of the Quality Standards Subcommittee of the American Academy of Neurology. *Neurology* 2000;55:754–762.
A review of migraine diagnosis and neuroimaging criteria and brief review of acute and prophylactic medications for treatment.

Victor M, Ropper AH. Headache and other craniofacial pains. In *Adams and Victor's principles of neurology*, 7th ed. New York: McGraw Hill, 2001; 175–203.
A well-written chapter in one of the recognized standard textbooks of neurology that summarizes both primary headaches and those caused by other neurologic and systemic illnesses.

Welch, KMA. Contemporary concepts of migraine pathogenesis. *Neurology* 2003;61 (Suppl 4): S2–S8.
An excellent summary of how basic and clinical research have enhanced contemporary understanding of the etiology and pathophysiology of headache, particularly migraine.

Pain

Thomas C. Chelimsky

As our understanding of pain physiology and of the human pain experience evolves, so does our clinical approach to the patient with pain. Whereas some years ago, opiates were used only exceptionally in the person with chronic benign pain, narcotics are employed more frequently today. However, relieving the symptom of pain is a very short first step in the patient who has longstanding disabling pain with concomitant depression, sleeplessness, loss of function, and dysfunctional human relationships. Not only are we discovering new ways in which pain dramatically affects the function of distant parts of the nervous system, we are also finding new transmitters and factors that directly impact pain pathways. For example, several growth factors have been implicated in the generation of complex regional pain, and adenosine triphosphate (ATP), traditionally considered an energy-generating metabolite, has taken the lead as a major neurotransmitter in small afferent fibers and is a likely candidate for carrying pain signals from the peripheral nervous system.

At the same time, our society increasingly demands that physicians and scientists directly address pain issues. As an example of this new focus, pain was the cover story of the May 19th 2003 issue of *Newsweek*. Congress has considered a bill (H.R. 1863) to place pain care research, education, and treatment among our national public health priorities; the costs are staggering, with uncon-

ventional treatments alone accounting for several billion dollars expended by patients out of pocket each year, and U.S. business and industry losing about $90 billion annually to sick time, reduced productivity, and direct medical and other benefit costs. A recent meta-analysis estimated severe chronic pain at 11% of the general population. Approximately 23.5 million are disabled (National Institute on Disability and Rehabilitation Research), with pain directly causative in 75%. The high toll of pain in the United States has prompted the Joint Commission on Accreditation of Health Care Organization (JCAHO) to require all accredited organizations, whether inpatient or outpatient facilities, to develop and implement programs that screen for and effectively manage pain.

Physiology of Pain

The response to a single noxious sensation differs greatly from the experience of disabling pain. Only very recently has attention been drawn to models of chronic pain, and has technology sufficiently advanced to allow meaningful noninvasive investigation in humans. Most of what is known about pain physiology, however, derives from the

▼

Key Clinical Questions

Assessing the patient with pain

▸ What is the etiologic diagnosis (i.e., what is the illness)?
▸ What is the mechanistic diagnosis (i.e., what part of the illness is causing pain)?
▸ What is the impact of the pain on the patient's life?

intrinsically limited applicability of animal studies on pain *sensation* to *pain problems* in human beings. Based on these types of studies, one may conceptualize the pain system as comprising seven components (Figure 9.1):

1. the peripheral nervous system signaling unit;
2. the dorsal horn of the spinal cord, a processing "gate" featuring great synaptic plasticity;
3. the classical spinothalamic tract projecting to cortex, a sensory-discriminative afferent system that defines the physical properties of the pain;
4. the spinoreticular-limbic pathway, an affective or motivational system producing the negative quality of pain;

5. the reticulospinal descending modulating system, terminating in the dorsal horn;
6. the local modulating system, based on propriospinal connections; and
7. the neocortex providing cognitive and evaluative functions and controlling lower levels.

Peripheral Nervous System Signal

The *nociceptor* is a sensory neuron whose cell body resides in the dorsal root ganglion. Its process extends from the skin, where it is endowed with a specialized receptor, to the dorsal horn of the spinal cord, where it synapses. Although nociceptors specific for one type of injury (thermal, mechanical, or chemical) exist, the majority respond to many types of injury, hence the term "mechano-heat nociceptor." Most respond to the chemical mediators of inflammation such as prostaglandins, kinins, and substance P, with direct activation or *sensitization*.

This response reflects the important principle that tissue injury activates previously inactive fibers. For example, distention of the normal detrusor muscle of the bladder activates pressure-sensitive, non–pain-transmitting A fibers. With a urinary tract infection, or with an upper motor neuron lesion, an unmyelinated C fiber becomes the transducer, producing discomfort and a "full" signal at a much lower bladder volume. This change results in the clinical manifestations of dysuria and frequency.

Different nociceptor types activate at different *times* during an injury, rather than for different *types* of injuries. *Pain onset* is signaled by slowly conducting (unmyelinated) C-fiber mechano-heat nociceptors in glabrous skin, and in hairy skin, by a specific (type II) class of rapidly conducting (myelinated) A-fiber mechano-heat nociceptors (the "pricking pain" of a burn). *Continued pain* is signaled by another class of medium-speed A fibers (type I) in both types of skin.

Nociceptors exist in virtually all tissues, but are prominent in covering membranes (such as skin, periosteum, meninges, and peritoneum), vessels, ligaments, and tendons. Within the walls of hollow viscera, they signal distention almost exclusively. They are sparse or absent within the nonvascular and noncollagenous portions of parenchymal tissues such as brain, liver, and muscle. This distribution corresponds with the usual sites of chronic pain.

Dorsal Horn Processing "Gate"

Remarkably, the dorsal horn can process the same signal differently under different circumstances. Thus, the long popular *labeled-line theory* (holding that, for instance, a touch receptor always only transmits touch) has been put to rest. Although activation of a previously inactive neuron characterizes the peripheral component, changes in modality from one type of sensation to another are fre-

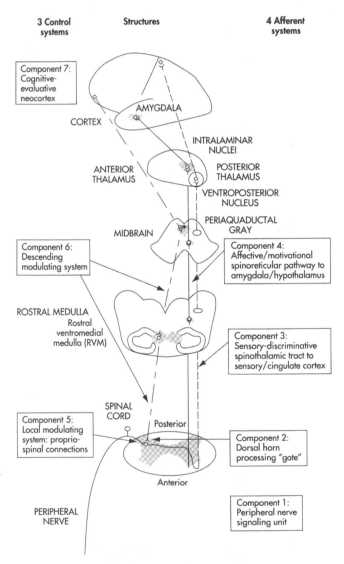

Figure 9.1 Overview of pain neurophysiology. The pain system is complex, but can be conceptualized in seven components, including four afferent systems and three control systems. This division is somewhat arbitrary, as all components clearly play a role in both functions, and it is ultimately impossible to truly separate them.

quent at the dorsal horn level. As a striking example, injection of capsaicin (the active ingredient of hot peppers; it produces a burning sensation by releasing substance P, one of the inflammatory neurotransmitters) next to a touch-sensitive, non–pain signaling receptor causes it to signal pain.

Such processing changes are well explained by the dorsal horn's four distinct operating modes (Table 9.1), each defined by the response to normally noxious and innocuous stimuli. The first is the "normal" or baseline state. The next two are temporarily altered states of pain suppression or *sensitization*, controlled by the on–off balance of the descending modulating system (see later discussion). The last—most relevant in chronic pain—is a pathologic state of reorganization due to irreversible injury. Dorsal horn neurons may undergo dramatic changes in their receptive field sizes in response to glutamate, substance P, and nerve growth factor.

Spinothalamic pathway

The second-order sensory neuron for pain originates in the dorsal horn ipsilateral to the body part represented. It crosses the midline two spinal segments above, ascending anterolaterally in the spinal cord, and dorsolaterally in the brainstem. These projections terminate in the ventroposterior nucleus of the thalamus, dispersed as clusters or islands throughout the nucleus.

Recently, a long-elusive specific nucleus for pain was identified in the ventrocaudal thalamus of the monkey. Positron emission tomography (PET) studies tell us that in patients with chronic pain, this same ventrocaudal nucleus is particularly active.

Spinoreticular pathway

Some dorsal horn neurons project to reticular formation nuclei throughout the dorsal brainstem. Reticular neurons, in turn, project to midline thalamic nuclei, the amygdala, and the hypothalamus. Because of its diffuse nature, the exact role and pharmacology of this pathway are not yet clear, and it is less well understood than the spinothalamic tract. Nonetheless, it may be the more important afferent pathway to the clinical management of

chronic pain. It may ultimately account for the aversive response to a painful state, including autonomic changes, and maladaptive and other behavioral responses, as well as mood and personality changes.

Reticulospinal modulating system

This crucial system is the target of nearly every oral analgesic. The lowest control level resides in a brainstem region, the rostral ventromedial medulla (RVM), which projects to the dorsal horn. Descending fibers travel through the dorsolateral funiculus of the spinal cord. The RVM, in turn, is modulated by the periaqueductal gray in the midbrain, the amygdala and ventromedial hypothalamus, and insular and frontal cortices.

The RVM includes two types of cells. The "off-cell" inhibits pain transmission, while the "on-cell" enhances pain transmission. The two cell types are in a physiologic balance. Through *collateral inhibition*, activation of one cell type directly inactivates the other. The state of this balance is controlled by higher centers through opioid peptides. Opiate inhibition of the on-cells increases the activity of the off-cells and reduces pain transmission. The major effect of this balance occurs at the dorsal horn. On-cells push the horn toward a *sensitized* state, while off-cells push it toward a suppressed state (Table 9.1).

Off-cells provide the main descending pathway, and on-cell activity is reflected by inhibition of the off-cell projection. Axons travel through the dorsolateral funiculus to reach the dorsal horn. Here, they inhibit second-order projection neurons of the spinothalamic system, using serotonin and norepinephrine, which interact respectively with the 5-HT2 and 2-adrenergic receptors. The inhibition of the spinothalamic tract projection neurons occurs through several mechanisms, including direct inhibition of this neuron and indirect inhibition through interneurons containing -aminobutyric acid (GABA) and opiates.

Propriospinal local modulating system

Evidence of the existence of a propriospinal local modulating system stems from the observation that a noxious stimulus reproducibly lessens the intensity of another one, if the two stimuli are in close proximity. This phenome-

---

Table 9.1 The operating modes of the dorsal horn

| Mode | Response to stimulus that is usually: | | Clinical syndrome | Example |
	innocuous	noxious		
Baseline	No pain	Pain	Normal	No injury
Suppressed	No pain	No pain	Hyposensitivity	Athlete continues sport, unaware of severe injury
Sensitized	Pain (allodynia)	Pain (hyperalgesia)	Inflammation	Hypersensitivity near gouty toe
Reorganized	Pain (allodynia)	Pain (hyperalgesia)	Neuropathic pain	Post-herpetic neuralgia

Adapted from Woolf CJ. *Textbook of Pain.* New York: Churchill Livingstone, 1994; pp. 101–112.

non may account for the expression "bite the bullet," and the practice of rubbing the area around a burn to lessen pain. Transsection of the dorsolateral funiculus of the spinal cord (containing the projection from the descending modulating system) does not abolish this phenomenon, and it is hence thought to be mediated by propriospinal pathways. Transcutaneous electrical nerve stimulation (TENS) units and aggressive mobilization may operate through this system.

Cognitive-evaluative neocortex

This system, although not well understood, involves the sensory and cingulate cortices. Perhaps the sensory cortex is involved with discriminative issues, while the cingulate cortex handles motivationally directed pain response, as the cingulate gyrus comprises a portion of the motivational/emotional limbic system.

General Principles of Pain Management

Acute versus Chronic Pain

Acute pain signals a threat, and its cause must be medically addressed. Once the problem is identified, the pain signal loses its usefulness and should be medically relieved until the process resolves. Chronic pain, however, serves no useful purpose. The problem is either diagnosed and irremediable, or unidentifiable. Thus, striking differences exist between acute and chronic pain that span physiology, behavior, and clinical approach (Tables 9.2 and 9.3). Although chronic pain can be defined as pain lasting longer than 3 months, the chronic pain *syndrome* is the more important clinical concept, and it can develop whenever chronic pain is not properly addressed. The chronic pain syndrome implies concomitant maladaptive behaviors that interfere with the patient's life. The degree of interference may be minimal, such as inability to perform a leisure activity, or dramatic, with loss of work, loss of social and family ties, and severe depression. Such a syndrome has an underlying neural basis, spanning

changes in the sensory, modulatory, and cognitive circuits previously described.

The management of acute and chronic pain differs entirely, as outlined in Table 9.3. The well-managed patient with *acute* pain has nearly total pain relief, whereas in *chronic* pain syndromes, such a goal is not even explicitly mentioned. Rather, chronic pain management focuses on maximum return of function and on coping strategies to reduce the effect the pain has on the patient's life, with regard to work, family life, and medical system dependency. The patient with a chronic pain syndrome must address many behavioral, functional, and medical issues, and is best handled by an integrated interdisciplinary pain team.

Pain Measurement

Although few human experiences are as overwhelming and distressing as pain, few aspects of clinical practice are as difficult to verify. Since health care providers tend to underestimate the level of pain experienced by patients, the patient's own report carries the greatest validity and should go undisputed. Generalized autonomic changes such as tachycardia and pupillary dilatation occur only in the acute setting, and these are not helpful in evaluating chronic pain. No benefit is gained by disputing the patient's report, and the greatest chance of successful treatment is based on face-value acceptance. Disbelief by the practitioner may compound a negative therapeutic impact onto a patient who is already struggling psychologically.

Two measures of pain have attained widespread use, with well-documented validity. The visual analog scale (VAS) is extremely simple, but measures only pain intensity. The McGill Pain Questionnaire takes longer to complete, but provides a deeper assessment of sensory, affective, and evaluative aspects of pain.

Patient Evaluation

In assessing the patient with pain, three questions need to be answered. First, what is the etiologic diagnosis (i.e., what is the illness)? Examples would include traumatic

Table 9.2 Differences in the characteristics of acute and chronic pain

	Acute pain	Chronic pain syndrome
Duration	≤2 weeks	>3 months
Dorsal horn physiology (see Table 9.1)	Baseline or sensitized	Reorganized
Autonomic changes	Generalized: rapid respiratory and heart rates, dilated pupils	No generalized effects
		Focal effects such as swelling or skin color change may occur
Long-term interference with life	None	Mild to severe
Maladaptive behavior	None	Present

Table 9.3 Differences in the approaches to acute and chronic pain

Management strategy	Acute pain: relieve pain	Chronic pain syndrome: return function
		Pain relief is not a goal
Management team	1–2 cooperating disciplines entirely adequate (multidisciplinary)	Requires interdisciplinary team, including at least patient, primary physician, psychologist, and occupational and physical therapists
Treatment	Primarily pharmacologic; blocks and opiates (if used) titrated to full pain relief, if possible	Primarily nonpharmacologic with blocks and drugs as adjuncts Opiates rarely used

injury, rheumatoid arthritis, and small-cell lymphoma. Second, what is the mechanistic diagnosis (i.e., what part of the illness is causing pain)? Various disease etiologies may be associated with many mechanisms, such as root compression, inflammatory pain, and spinal cord injury. Third, what is the impact of the pain on the patient's life? Answers may vary from none to total debilitation with major depression and anxiety. This last question is much less relevant in the patient with acute pain, where the goal of management is simply pain relief.

It is important to keep these three lines of thought separate, as each impacts on ultimate management decisions. For example, an etiologic diagnosis may indicate a short life expectancy, or may be entirely lacking at the initial visit due to an incomplete diagnostic evaluation. Either of these would contraindicate an intensive pain management program at that point in time. A mechanistic diagnosis frequently directs the pharmacologic and anesthesiologic approach to pain management. The impact of pain on life dictates the intensity and direction of psychological and behavioral intervention, psychiatric drug treatment, and, ultimately, lifestyle modification goals.

Acute Pain Management

The biggest single failure in acute pain management is inadequate dosing of pain relievers. Based on ethical, humanitarian, and quality-of-care issues, proper pain relief should be provided for patients with acute postoperative, posttraumatic, or post organ-failure pain. Yet this is not the case in 50–70% of such patients, mainly because caregivers either underestimate the intensity of pain or have an unfounded fear of addiction. Of 11,882 patients who were given opiate preparations in the hospital, one study could only find four cases of possible addiction. In contrast, unrelieved severe pain may produce major adverse consequences, including myocardial ischemia and irreversible nervous system damage, probably mediated by glutamate.

The available tools for acute pain management include systemic medications, administered orally or parenterally, and local anesthetic blocks of various types.

When oral agents cannot be given, or if they fail to provide complete relief, intravenous short-acting opioids such as morphine are administered through a patient-controlled analgesia (PCA) pump titrated to complete or (if side effects prevent this) near-complete pain relief. Local blocks are used when systemic administration cannot achieve adequate comfort levels. Once pain relief is achieved, oral medications are introduced at a dosage-equivalent level (Table 9.4). The duration of action for all drugs mentioned is around 3 hours, except for methadone and levorphanol, which are effective for as long as 8 hours.

Medications should be administered on a scheduled basis, and not as needed. Health care personnel frequently underestimate patient analgesic need, and the patient's knowledge of the time of the next dose may significantly relieve pain simply through anxiety reduction. Further, a regular dosage schedule keeps the analgesic levels constant and avoids the "roller-coaster" effect. Adjunctive agents such as nonsteroidal drugs and tricyclic medications are added when pain duration exceeds 1 week.

Chronic Pain Management

In contrast to acute pain, pain relief is rarely achieved in chronic pain syndromes. Long-term use of narcotics carries a higher risk of addiction and complications, al-

Table 9.4 Dosage of frequently used opioid agonist medications equivalent to 10 IM morphine sulfate

	Intramuscular dose (mg)	Oral dose (mg)
Codeine	130	200
Meperidine	75	300
Propoxyphene	50	100
Oxycodone	15	30
Morphine	10	30
Methadone	10	20
Levorphanol	2	4
Oxymorphone	1	10

though this tenet is coming under some scrutiny. Thus, the mainstay of treatment is the interdisciplinary program, in which an integrated team of health professionals focuses on improving the function of the patient to meet a preset specific goal. At most institutions, pain management teams include professionals from various disciplines, including neurology, psychology, anesthesiology, and physical medicine.

To be successful, pain management must break two traditional notions. First, the patient must relinquish the concept that increasing function must await pain relief and buy into the goal of controlling his life with high function in spite of pain. Although pain levels do drop with a pain program (presumably because greater fitness reduces the exertion required for a particular task), this is never explicitly stated as a goal. Second, caregivers must include the patient on their team, as an integral member with equal power. This approach differs from traditional Western medicine, in which the physician takes into account the patient's views and needs, then sets the management course. In pain management, the patient must truly set his own goals, and meet or alter them within the structured context of the team. If the patient cannot be motivated both to set the goals and to strive toward them in spite of pain, management will fail.

The complexity of the issues surrounding chronic pain has resulted in the use of the intensive interdisciplinary pain program lasting 8 hours a day for 3–6 weeks. Such a setting has many advantages. The patient is removed from his native environment, where maladaptive behaviors may have become ingrained to the point of going unnoticed. The management team, including the patient, can focus single-mindedly on one goal. Fruitful, problem-solving interactions occur between patients who are having similar problems. Finally, the uninterrupted contact time allows each discipline to address difficult issues concisely and effectively. Such a program is more cost-effective than trying to piece services together over a longer period of time, and it significantly reduces the use of medical resources in the long term.

The primary goal of the program is a more meaningful and satisfying life for the patient. The management tools that can help the patient toward this goal fall into three categories. First, the patient must learn the purpose, limitations, and proper use of medications, and be empowered to participate in educated self-management decisions. In parallel, when anesthetic blocks are suggested, the patient must understand their realistic limitations, purpose, and the patient's own active role in deriving maximal benefit. Second, the patient's lifestyle must be altered to incorporate pain and stress management strategies. Examples include self-pacing of activity levels, avoidance of pain-reinforcing behavior, reduction in covert pain signals (sometimes called "pain behaviors") along with improved open communication about pain, and fi-

nally, when appropriate, relaxation and biofeedback. Third, overall functional level and physical fitness must be gently and gradually increased, if the patient is to return to a productive life. Not only can a deconditioned patient not perform more strenuous daily activities, but his muscles also are more susceptible to spasm and even injury, both of which further increase pain.

The choice of medications is large. The particular agents selected depend in large part on the specific quality of pain (Table 9.5) and desired side effects. For example, a patient with sleep disturbance would benefit from a tricyclic agent, which will improve sleep patterns and reduce pain. In most cases, the mainstay of treatment involves some combination of a nonsteroidal anti-inflammatory drug (NSAID) and a tricyclic agent, with additional medications added to address remaining symptoms. For example, mexiletine could be added for severe tingling in a patient with arachnoiditis who is already on ibuprofen and amitriptyline. The tricyclics should always be pushed to tolerance, with gradual increases every second or third day, until either an unacceptable side effect (causing discontinuance) or the desired benefit ensue.

It is crucial that all pain-relieving medications be prescribed in a time-contingent, not pain-contingent fashion (that is, "scheduled," not "as needed"). Scheduled dosing provides constant levels of analgesic throughout the day; provides analgesia as the pain is beginning, not after hopelessly high levels have been reached; and takes much of the decision-making out of the patient's hands, thus reducing focus on pain levels and reducing the risk of improper use and addiction. Compared to as-needed dosing, scheduled dosing has been shown to reduce total drug used and enhance pain relief. If patients have difficulty with this concept, the analogy with treatment of high blood pressure, which also fluctuates from day to day, can be quite helpful.

Opiate use in chronic nonmalignant pain is controversial, but is finding some support. Careful adherence to some guidelines should avert abuse in most cases. Opi-

---

Table 9.5 Choice of analgesic medication based on symptoms and clinical context

Symptom	Medication
Deep aching	Nonsteroidal agent (NSAID)
Deep burning	Tricyclic antidepressants, clonidine
Surface burning	Capsaicin ointment
Spasms	Clonazepam, baclofen
Shooting pain	Carbamazepine, Dilantin, valproate
Paresthesias	Mexiletine, gabapentin, agents for "shooting pain"
Sympathetic pain	Phenoxybenzamine, prazosin

ates are never a first-line choice, and should be reserved for patients well known to the treating professionals after other measures, including a pain management program if appropriate, have been thoroughly tried. Opiates should generally not be used in a patient with a history of addiction, or out of frustration with noncompliance for other recommendations. Thus, opiates are appropriate in the patient who demonstrated complete and enthusiastic compliance with all control measures instituted, often including a pain management program, yet still cannot function at a reasonable level because of pain. If the entire team (including the patient) feels that function may be enhanced by an opiate, a carefully considered decision may be made to begin. At the outset, the team signs a formal contract containing the specific and individualized set of rules that govern that patient's opiate use, and this is placed in the patient's chart. With patient permission, a copy is made available to a single dispensing pharmacist. Any violation should result in discontinuation of the drug. Ultimate success is judged by whether the set functional goals are met and not by the patient's report of pain relief.

Only long-acting agents such as methadone or continuous-release morphine should be used. As with all other pain medications, and even more so with opiates, dosage should be scheduled regularly, never as needed. Changes are made once or at most twice per week, and the patient must not alter dosing up or down without explicit instruction from the physician. In addition, the patient must agree that no other physician will prescribe pain-relieving drugs for chronic pain. Most importantly, as in all pain management, specific *functional* goals must be set, such as returning to work or increasing the hours of a specific activity by 50%. An external observer, such as an employer, a fitness center attendant or, as the patient is often engaged in an active pain program, the rehabilitation staff, should validate the achievement of these goals. This last aspect of the contract provides a relatively solid safeguard, as true dependence invariably results in a decline in both work performance and family relationships. Most patients can tolerate long-term continuation without increasing dosage. An increase in dosage requirement suggests either drug dependence, requiring cessation of opiates, or physical tolerance requiring a 1-week drug holiday or switching to another equipotency opiate.

Certain frequently encountered issues must be resolved prior to the initiation of an intensive pain management program. Dependence on opiates, benzodiazepines, alcohol, or illicit drugs must be fully addressed, and the patient must be free from the offending agent for at least 6 weeks prior to beginning an intensive chronic pain management program. Simple measures, such as initiation of a tricyclic agent and physical therapy, may be used during this period, but a structured, aggressive program should be avoided since the patient would not maximally utilize it, and the patient's problem could be detrimental to other participating patients. Major depression and disabling anxiety are also best managed prior to beginning a program. Finally, if important legal issues are pending, these may alter the patient's ability to participate or provide a counter-incentive. Some programs require a minimum of 6 months' distance to any significant past illegal activity. Not resolving these issues prior to starting the intensive program significantly weakens its effectiveness, as the patient, staff, and other patients in the program become distracted from the main issue of pain, which in itself requires a full commitment of energy and motivation.

A nonspecialist may be able to treat the majority of milder cases of chronic back or limb pain by following some simple guidelines. The key is to be aggressive early and to refer within 3 months to an interdisciplinary program if the simpler uni- or multidisciplinary aggressive approach fails. A patient is appropriate for this approach if he has a process causing moderate pain that proves to be clearly nonremediable after a thorough evaluation. A referral to an interdisciplinary team should be made at the outset if the patient is not working because of pain only; if family or social relationships are threatened; if there is significant psychopathology, such as major depression; if the patient is thought to be drug-dependent; or if there are serious legal issues.

Treatment should begin with a simple generic compound such as ibuprofen, used at the highest recommended dosage and given on a scheduled, not as-needed basis. The patient should be monitored for gastrointestinal, liver, and kidney toxicities, and a gastric protective agent may be added if needed. Some type of activation of the body part experiencing pain should always accompany drug treatment. This is best done by referral to physical therapy for the low back and lower extremity, and occupational therapy for the neck and upper extremity. In more severe cases, both may be required. Depending on the severity of the problem, and the progress made by the patient, treatment time may be as little as two sessions to provide proper instructions and review for an independent program, or three sessions a week for several weeks. The eventual goal should always be an independent program. Passive modalities such as massage, ultrasound, and electrical stimulation hinder this goal, as they increase, rather than reduce, the patient's ultimate dependence on the medical system. Thus, these have no place in physiotherapy for chronic pain, except when they provide a window of opportunity for the patient to achieve a very specific goal in his active program.

The patient should be seen again in approximately 1 month. Absence of any progress at all should lead to referral to an interdisciplinary team. When improvement is satisfactory, the patient should continue his current regimen, with rechecks in physiotherapy at monthly intervals until no further progress occurs. This should then be followed by continuation independently three times a week in a fitness center for at least 1 year and, ideally, for life. When progress is neither absent nor satisfactory, a tricyclic agent should be added, as detailed later. Another follow-up should be scheduled in 1 month, and the same decision tree followed as with the first follow-up visit.

Amitriptyline is the best tricyclic agent for back, neck, and fibromyalgia syndromes, and when pain impairs sleep; 10 or 25 mg should be given 3 hours prior to bedtime, escalating the dose by one tablet every third day until improvement or an unacceptable side effect ensues. With limb pain, imipramine appears to be more effective, perhaps because it produces less sedation and can be given throughout the day. The usual starting dose is 5 or 10 mg three times a day, with the same gradual upward titration. In the elderly, nortriptyline and desipramine are better tolerated because of fewer side effects, and should be substituted for amitriptyline and imipramine respectively. Prolongation of Q-T interval should be checked by EKG in the elderly. Usual dosage is 20–150 mg/day for all agents mentioned, but clearly depends on response. Some elderly patients have responded dramatically to as little as 2.5 mg of desipramine once per day (achieved by having the pharmacist cut 10 tablets in four), and some young patients require several hundred milligrams per day. Doses in excess of 225 mg/day require blood level checks. Doxepin is available in a pediatric liquid formulation that allows administration of extremely low dosages down to 0.5 mg, which is very useful in excessively sensitive patients, including the elderly.

Specific Syndromes

Conditions Related to the Spine

Background and principles of management

Between 10% and 25% of all work injuries leading to temporary or total disability are due to back injuries, with an estimated cost of between $10 and $50 billion per year. Despite this enormous cost, there are few facts (and hence much opinion) regarding the true mechanism of pain, and most management decisions have no solid physiologic basis. One can begin to infer potential mechanisms with knowledge of pain-sensitive structures in the spine. These are listed in Table 9.6, based on intraoperative studies using progressive regional anesthesia.

In assessing a patient with neck or back pain, one considers two overarching questions. What symptoms or signs are worrisome and suggest further immediate investigation? And, would a surgical procedure be of any benefit? Table 9.7 outlines features that differentiate a benign lesion, such as arthritic or disk disease, from a malignant one such as an inflammatory or neoplastic process. If no features suggesting the latter are present,

Table 9.6 Pain-sensitive structures in the spine

Structure	Sensitivity to manipulation at surgery
Lumbar fascia	Insensitive
Supraspinous ligament	Mild tenderness
Muscles	Painful at neurovascular bundle entry and attachment site to bone
Nerve root	If normal, stimulation is completely painless; if swollen or compressed, stimulation reproduces "sciatica" symptoms
Annulus	1/3 of disks exquisite, 1/3 moderate, 1/3 no tenderness
Vertebral end plate	Severe deep pain
Facet joints	Sharp localized pain
Synovium/cartilage	Insensitive
Bones	Insensitive

Based on Kuslich SD, Ulstrom CL, Michael CJ. *Ortho Clin North Am* 1991;22:181–187.

one can follow the patient for 2–4 weeks, reserving sometimes unpleasant and costly examinations, such as imaging or electromyography (EMG), if no symptomatic improvement occurs. The exact roots involved can be determined using reflex, sensory, and motor abnormalities, as listed in Table 9.8.

The principles of surgical management are similar in the low back and in the neck. In clinical practice, at this time, two clear ends of the spectrum exist, along with a large, poorly defined gray zone. Most would operate for a clear-cut, acute neurologic deficit, and surgery is clearly indicated with disabling myelopathy or significant sphincteric dysfunction. In contrast, surgery is not indicated for chronic pain restricted to the spine in the absence of neurologic signs or a structural lesion. The ultimate decision is related to a balance of multiple factors (Table 9.9).

The acute episode of back and limb pain

Based on this information, how should one manage the common acute episode of uncomplicated back and (radicular) limb pain? A Finnish study of 187 patients suggested that telling patients to "go home and do what is comfortable" was much better than bed rest, and somewhat better than physical therapy. What follows is one of several viable approaches. Assuming a classical history and findings with a single root involved to a moderate extent, and without any of the "worrisome" characteristics listed in Table 9.7, no tests are ordered at the first visit. Assuming no contraindications, a 5-day course of prednisone (60 mg/day) is prescribed with rapid 2-day taper, then continuing with a nonsteroidal at maximum toler-

Table 9.7 Investigation of spine pain

Item	Comment
Pain severity	Severity itself has no etiologic implications
Pain location	Pain restricted to the spine suggests a mechanical process, while limb radiation implies root involvement. Referred pain must be distinguished from radicular pain. Radicular pain is suggested when the limb pain extends below the level of the elbow or knee, worsens with factors distinct from those affecting the spine pain or is accompanied by paresthesias, numbness or weakness
Temporal course	Rapid onset and a subsequent stable course suggests a mechanical cause. Progressive symptoms are worrisome for a neoplasm. A traumatic event can be the trigger to a serious process such as a pathologic vertebral fracture.
Exacerbating factors	1 Cough, sneeze or strain aggravating limb pain is a classic sign of an intraspinal lesion such as a disc or tumor made worse by rising venous pressure; helpful for localization, but not worrisome by itself.
	2 Supine, night-time back pain suggests a posterior cord lesion such as an ependymoma or meningioma.
	3 Hip extension or flexion reproducing limb pain on examination, termed positive reverse straight leg raise and straight leg raise, respectively, suggests midlumbar or lumbo-sacral root involvement.
	4 Isolated vertebral tenderness should always be investigated for infection or malignancy.
Number of roots involved	The likelihood of a malignant process increases as the number of roots involved increases unilaterally or across the midline. Noncontiguous root involvement (e.g., left L2 and right S1) is always worrisome for malignancy.
Sphincters	Urgency with severe pain and other mild stable sphincteric symptoms are not uncommon, but clear loss of function, such as reduced stream or incontinence, requires investigation.
Myelopathic signs	These range from minimal, an isolated equivocal Babinski response, for example, to severe, including bilateral clonus with severe weakness and spastic gait. The clinical impact ranges from minimal in a chronic indolent setting, to dramatic, if an acute progressive process warrants urgent action.
Associated signs	Fever and chills suggest an epidural or disk space infection, while weight loss occurs with malignancy.

ated dosage. If severe spasm is found on examination, muscle relaxants such as cyclobenzaprine, tizanidine, or benzodiazepines, among many, may be used for the first 5–10 days, although no strong evidence supports this practice. Two days into steroid treatment, the patient begins very gradual water jogging (5–10 minutes in the pool at the outset), progressing over 4 weeks to water aerobics. A tricyclic may also be added for sleep and pain control, as outlined earlier. Most cases of acute discs and

other new-onset uncomplicated mechanical or radicular pain benefit from this regimen.

The patient returns in 3 weeks. If no dramatic improvement is observed, investigations are then ordered, including EMG and magnetic resonance imaging (MRI) of the spine area involved. The EMG (see Chapter 3) provides *functional information* that (a) localizes the exact root(s) involved through distribution of muscles affected; (b) assesses severity of motor loss; (c) confirms the diagnosis of

Table 9.8 Physical findings for cervical and lumbar radiculopathy

Root	Reflex	Sensory loss	Motor loss (partial list)
C5	Brachioradialis	Lateral arm	Arm abduction, internal rotation
C6	Biceps	Thumb, lateral forearm	Forearm flexion, supination
C7	Triceps	Middle finger	Wrist extension, flexion, pronation
C8	Finger flexor	Fifth finger, medial forearm	Finger extension, flexion
T1	—	Medial arm	Hand intrinsics
L1	Cremasteric	Inguinal region	—
L3	Adductor	Medial thigh	Thigh flexion, adduction
L4	Knee (quadriceps)	Anterior thigh, medial calf and foot	Leg extension
L5	Internal hamstring	Great toe, dorsum of foot, lateral thigh, anterior calf	Thigh abduction, foot dorsiflexion and rotation
S1	Ankle and external hamstring	Small toe, plantar region, posterior thigh and calf	Thigh extension, leg flexion, foot plantar flexion
S2	Bulbocavernosus	Buttock	Anal sphincter

Table 9.9 Management of spine disease

Item	Appropriate operation may help	Surgery unlikely to benefit
Pain location	Radiates into the limb, especially into hand or foot.	Isolated to the spine
Duration	Days to weeks	Months to years
Neurologic findings	1 Reflex loss	None, or mild radicular
	2 Radicular weakness	
	3 Sphincteric involvement	
	4 Myelopathy	
Prior back surgery	None, or successful operation for different symptoms	Previous unsuccessful back operation for same symptoms
EMG	Denervation in appropriate myotome	Negative or mildly positive
Imaging	Clear and symptom-appropriate structural abnormality, such as herniated disc or spinal stenosis	Normal or mild changes

---

radiculopathy, if sensory nerve action potential amplitudes are unaffected; (d) reveals the degree of denervation through the presence of fibrillation potentials; and (e) defines any preexisting chronic lesions by enlargement of the electrical size of motor unit potentials, a process which begins at 6 weeks and takes 30 weeks to complete (and hence would be absent in the acute lesion). The MRI provides structural information that delineates any anatomic regions impinging on a root, such as spinal stenosis, a disc herniation or bulge, and facet hypertrophy. The severity of remaining symptoms, and the strength of the investigations in providing an appropriate specific diagnosis may prompt a surgical referral. The first section outlines nonsurgical management principles. A recent treatment guidelines by the American Academy of Neurology found no clear benefit for epidural injections in any clinical circumstance.

Spinal stenosis

Narrowing of the spinal canal may occur at either cervical or lumbar levels on a congenital basis, an arthritic basis or, most often, a combination of the latter superimposed on the former. Cervical stenosis causes a very slowly progressive myelopathy. One considers that the cervical canal is narrow when its anteroposterior dimension measured on a lateral plain film is less than 10 (Table 9.10).

Lumbar stenosis causes a specific syndrome known as *pseudoclaudication*. Pseudoclaudication consists of leg pain triggered by a specific amount of time spent in the erect posture, whereas the leg pain of true claudication depends on muscular effort. For example, standing in one place may precipitate pseudoclaudication but not true claudication, whereas bicycling may precipitate true claudication, but not pseudoclaudication. Lumbar stenosis usually involves the upper lumbar roots (L2–L4), and hence produces anterior and medial thigh pain. The pathophysiology is thought to be ischemia of these nerve roots in the upright posture due to the combination of further narrowing of the canal and venous engorgement.

Fibromyalgia and myofascial syndromes

Although the pathophysiology is not understood, the terms *fibromyalgia* and *myofascial syndromes*, when properly used, do not refer to "wastebasket" categories for otherwise nondiagnosable pain, but rather to fairly specific syndromes with specific diagnostic criteria. Fibromyalgia refers to a diffuse, total body pain syndrome with severe fatigue, whereas myofascial syndrome is localized to one or two extremities or body quadrants. The main physical finding in fibromyalgia is the "tender point," where palpation of specific tendinous structures produces a nonradiating pain. In contrast, in myofascial syndromes, a "trigger point" causes pain or numbness to radiate in muscle-specific patterns in response to palpation of the muscle belly. Despite differing clinical presentations, the two syndromes have several specific physiologic abnormalities in common. A particular disturbance of sleep appears to accompany both syndromes (Table 9.11).

Table 9.10 Lumbar spinal stenosis

Discriminating features
▶ Radicular pain in the legs associated with time upright. Prompt relief with sitting.
▶ Narrowed lumbar canal with impingement on nerve roots demonstrated by imaging studies

Consistent features
▶ Leg pain is not effort-dependent, for example, not due to bicycling
▶ Upper lumbar roots (L2–L4) involved, with anterior thigh pain, iliacus weakness, and a positive EMG.

Variable features
▶ Long symptom duration, with progressive decrease in pain-free upright time
▶ Back pain which is usually not time-dependent
▶ Sphincteric symptoms

Table 9.11 Fibromyalgia

Discriminating features
▶ Pain on digital palpation in 11 or more designated tender point sites, assessed separately on the right and left: occiput, low cervical, trapezius, supraspinatus, second rib, lateral epicondyle, gluteal, greater trochanter, knee

Consistent features
▶ Chief complaint of diffuse muscle aches, made worse by any activity
▶ Widespread, bilateral pain above and below waist for more than 3 months
▶ Stiffness
▶ Fatigue
▶ Nonrestorative sleep
▶ Functional disability

Variable features
▶ Associated psychological disorders, such as anxiety and stress reaction
▶ Headache
▶ Paresthesias
▶ Sense of swelling
▶ Irritable bowel syndrome
▶ Raynaud phenomenon

Whiplash injury refers to a flexion–extension injury of the cervical spine. The severity of the injury depends mostly on the total excursion and speed of the head, which relates poorly to the speed of a collision. Thus, when the injury results from a motor vehicle accident, as it does in more than 90% of cases, the apparent accident severity based on vehicular damage bears little relation to the severity of the whiplash injury. Symptoms may begin immediately or within several days. Between one-quarter and one-half of patients continue to have symptoms 5 years later, and these fall into two common symptom complexes. The first is a cervical myofascial syndrome with trigger points and nondermatomal radiating pain or numbness into the arms. The second may be termed *posttraumatic migraine syndrome*, characterized by severe headache, dizziness, nausea, scintillating scotoma, photophobia, phonophobia, and sometimes tinnitus or even recurrent syncope.

Treatment of these entities is similar, and similarly unsatisfactory. Standard pain management with an interdisciplinary team constitutes the best approach. Amitriptyline works better than imipramine. Other effective drugs include cyclobenzaprine and alprazolam. Trigger points, when present, should be injected with 1.5–2 mL of a solution containing half long-acting steroid and half long-acting anesthetic. Vascular headaches and concomitant symptoms may respond to high doses of verapamil (0.5–1 g/day), β-blockade, or anticonvulsants such as gabapentin or topiramate. Severe fatigue may re-

spond to amantadine or other stimulants. Pharmacotherapy is not helpful in isolation. The fitness and endurance training aspects of management are crucial.

Neuralgias and Related Conditions

Facial pain

Facial pain has traditionally fallen into the province of several unrelated specialties, based mainly on the presenting symptoms. No widely used cross-disciplinary classification scheme has been established, and the categories used here are somewhat arbitrary. The anatomically well-defined dental, gingival, and mucosal causes of pain are not addressed.

Tic douloureux (trigeminal neuralgia). The diagnosis of a classical facial neuralgia is based on the pain characteristics, presence of pain-free intervals, and absence of sensory or other neurologic findings. The pain is restricted to the face and consists of short trains of extremely brief jabs, commonly triggered by a non-noxious stimulus in a nearby location. The pathophysiology of the disorder is unknown, although the effectiveness of anticonvulsants suggests neural hyperactivity at some level. Most cases are idiopathic, but multiple sclerosis, infiltrative lesions, and vascular anomalies cause a minority. Cranial imaging should be performed if any atypical feature or neurologic finding is present. Many neurologists would advocate imaging even in typical cases (Table 9.12).

Treatment is initially pharmacologic, with carbamazepine, phenytoin, or baclofen. Other useful drugs in-

Table 9.12 Trigeminal neuralgia (tic douloureux)

Discriminating features
▶ Trains (1–2 min) of brief jabs (<1 sec) with sudden onset and offset
▶ Located on one side of face
▶ Stereotyped trigger area on same side but away from area of pain
▶ Trigger stimulus is innocuous, such as shaving, chewing or cold air

Consistent features
▶ Severe, incapacitating pain
▶ No pain between attacks. Pain may occur many times per day
▶ Spontaneous remissions lasting months to years
▶ Onset in fifth to eighth decade of life; earlier onset suggests multiple sclerosis or a structural lesion.
▶ Improvement with anticonvulsants, radio frequency lesion of the ganglion, and removal of a vascular loop, if present.

Variable features
▶ Background burning pain may be present
▶ Trigeminal nerve may be compressed by a crossing vessel
▶ Trigeminal nerve division involved is, in order of frequency: mandibular, maxillary, ophthalmic

clude mexiletine, valproate, and clonazepam. Approximately 25% of patients with typical tic douloureux eventually fail maximum tolerable doses of these medications alone or in combination. Imaging should be performed at this point if not previously done. Treatment options after failure of pharmacologic management then include injections of local anesthetic into the trigger zone, injection of alcohol into the gasserian ganglion, radio frequency ablation of the gasserian ganglion, and vascular decompression of the trigeminal nerve. Alcohol injection into the gasserian ganglion may produce relief of up to 1 year's duration. Repeated injections for pain recurrence are often unsuccessful. Radio frequency ablation may therefore be the procedure of choice, with reported benefit lasting 5 years in 50% of patients, good benefit from repeated procedures, and low surgical morbidity. Vascular decompression procedures are also advocated on the presumption that idiopathic neuralgia is related to vascular compression of the nerve. This procedure may be more effective than radio frequency ablation, but no study has prospectively compared the two procedures. The required suboccipital craniotomy for vascular decompression procedures carries greater surgical risk.

Temporomandibular joint dysfunction. Temporomandibular joint (TMJ) dysfunction refers to several different entities (which have in common pain in or around the TMJ or the muscles that act upon it) that are made worse by mastication. At least three conditions are recognized in association with these symptoms:

1. bruxism, or intermittent tight clenching of the jaw during sleep;
2. derangement of the joint itself, due to arthritis or displacement of the disc;
3. a myofascial syndrome with tenderness and trigger points found in the muscles.

In the elderly, these syndromes must be distinguished from true claudication of the jaw, which may be the presenting complaint of temporal arteritis. Diagnosis may be difficult, because many patients have symptoms that do not clearly fit one of the three conditions. Management depends on the diagnosis, and is most often handled by an oral surgeon. If needed, bruxism can be defined during a sleep study. Internal derangement of the joint may often respond to an intra-articular injection of steroid or may be demonstrated arthroscopically. Relief with trigger point injection suggests a myofascial syndrome. The pain management approach, with an oral surgeon and a speech therapist on the treatment team, may also be used in refractory cases.

Burning mouth syndrome. Burning mouth syndrome is classified as "atypical facial pain," but has enough char-

acteristic features to be treated separately. It is predominantly a disease of women over age 40. The major symptom is a continuous burning pain of either the tongue or the entire mouth, which may interfere with eating, swallowing, and sleeping. Examination is unrevealing.

Deficiencies of iron, zinc, and vitamins B_1, B_6, B_{12}, and E have been associated. It is helpful to check levels of all these substances, because patients often benefit from replacement of the deficient substance. In addition, the main alternative diagnosis is an associated covert or major depression. When depression is suspected, referral to a psychiatrist is frequently helpful, as proper treatment of the depression may produce resolution of the pain.

Atypical facial pain. Atypical facial pain is used to encompass nearly all other forms of facial pain. Unilateral pain, especially when progressive, may suggest an occult lesion and should prompt a more careful search than bilateral pain, for which a specific anatomic etiology is rarely found. The major caution in this group is avoidance of any irreversible treatments, such as ablations and operations of any type, without an incontrovertible indication. These patients respond poorly to the agents mentioned earlier. Biofeedback, relaxation, physiotherapy for facial exercises, and sometimes injections should be tried through the team approach, but success rates are low.

Postherpetic neuralgia

Shingles represents a reactivation of the herpes varicella zoster virus, which produces chickenpox. This virus remains dormant in the dorsal root ganglion cells, unless it becomes reactivated with aging or immune compromise related to cancer, acquired immune deficiency syndrome (AIDS), or pharmacologic immunosuppression. When pain persists or returns beyond 3 months after the initial attack, it is referred to as postherpetic neuralgia (PHN). No treatment has clearly been shown to be of benefit in the prevention of PHN, although steroids, acyclovir, and dimethylsulfoxide (DMSO) have received some attention (Table 9.13).

Postherpetic neuralgia remains restricted to the initially affected dermatome, commonly a thoracic one. The pain of PHN may be quite severe and debilitating. If the diagnosis is in doubt, a thermoregulatory sweat test demonstrates absence of sweating in the involved dermatome. Treatment follows the principles of pain management outlined in the first section of this chapter, with activation and exercise forming the basis of any successful treatment. Desensitization is often crucial and may be achieved with occupational therapy, water jogging, or the application of 0.075% capsaicin ointment. Anesthetic creams are also helpful, both directly for pain relief and in improving tolerance to capsaicin. Tricyclic agents constitute the core of pharmacologic intervention, with amitriptyline most commonly used. Carbamazepine and

Table 9.13 Postherpetic neuralgia

Discriminating features
- ▶ Pain more than 3 months after attack of shingles.
- ▶ Scar from healed vesicular lesions present
- ▶ Hypesthesia within affected dermatome and hyperesthesia in overlap zone

Consistent features
- ▶ Burning quality of pain, both deep and surface with tic-like jabs of pain

Variable features
- ▶ Occurs in 5–10% of patients with shingles
- ▶ Usually one root involved, but may be more.
- ▶ Thoracic dermatome or ophthalmic division of V most common, but may occur anywhere

Box 9.1 Differential diagnosis of painful neuropathy

I. Acquired disorders
- ▶ Diabetes
- ▶ Amyloidosis
- ▶ Paraneoplastic (breast, lung, lymphoma)
- ▶ Sjögren-associated ganglionopathy
- ▶ Human immunodeficiency virus (the third type of HIV-associated neuropathy occurring late in the disease)
- ▶ Vasculitis
- ▶ Hypothyroidism (LF)
- ▶ Idiopathic
- ▶ Drugs and toxins
- ▶ Gold
- ▶ Thallium
- ▶ Arsenic (often painless) (LF)
- ▶ Metronidazole
- ▶ Taxol
- ▶ Isoniazid (LF)
- ▶ Deficiencies
- ▶ Niacin (LF)
- ▶ B_1 (thiamine) (LF)
- ▶ Other B complex (B_{12}, folate) (LF)

II. Inherited disorders
- ▶ Fabry disease (α-galactosidase deficiency)
- ▶ Acute intermittent porphyria
- ▶ Riley-Day syndrome (HSAN III)
- ▶ Mitochondrial disorders
- ▶ Tangier disease

Most involve small fibers predominantly or in isolation, but some, labeled with "LF," involve large fibers.

mexiletine can reduce shooting pain. Finally, an epidural or sympathetic block is valuable in selected cases.

Pain associated with generalized neuropathies

Pain accompanying a sensorimotor neuropathy reflects involvement of the small sensory fibers at some level. Neuropathies involving only motor or large sensory axons often produce no pain. However, most "large-fiber" neuropathies have some degree of small-fiber involvement, and pain is more common than assumed. In addition, if the reduction in large fibers increases the utilization of small-fiber pathways, pain may ensue. Patients describe a burning or deep boring sensation in the feet and hands. The location of pain may also be spotty, with a dermatomal distribution, if the underlying neuropathy involves roots or dorsal root ganglion cells, as in shingles, diabetes, and Sjögren syndrome–associated neuropathy.

Diagnosis is straightforward in the patient with classical symptoms and findings, including reduction of sensation and deep tendon reflexes distally. Nerve conduction velocity (NCV) studies and EMG confirm the diagnosis. Some patients display small-fiber dysfunction only, such as reduction in pin-prick or temperature sensation, or reduction in sweating (often reflected by the complaint of excessive sweating in the normally functioning areas). The remainder of the examination may be normal, with preserved deep tendon reflexes. Since EMG and NCV do not test small fibers, and the diagnosis of isolated small-fiber neuropathy can only be made by autonomic testing, which defines the extent and severity of the condition.

Box 9.1 lists the causes of painful neuropathy. Involvement truly restricted to small fibers is rare enough that one must seriously consider a paraneoplastic syndrome in older patients. Diabetic neuropathies can be grouped by their temporal course. The slowly progressive, chronic neuropathy that continues for the duration of the disease, although sometimes uncomfortable, is usually not associated with severe pain. The subacute neuropathies, however, can be extremely painful. These come on over days to a few weeks, sometimes in association with disease onset, or paradoxically with improved treatment, such as a switch from an oral agent to insulin. Thoracic or abdominal radiculopathies often lead to cardiac and gastrointestinal evaluations, respectively. Weight loss may be severe, and often prompts a search for an occult neoplasm. The loss of weight may be profound enough to reduce insulin resistance to the point at which sugar levels normalize. It is crucial to appreciate that the severity of the syndrome may not correlate at all with the severity or duration of diabetes, which may even be marginal (Table 9.14).

Compressive mononeuropathies

Compressive mononeuropathies occur spontaneously or as a manifestation of an underlying diffuse neuropathy,

---

Table 9.14 Subacute diabetic neuropathies

Discriminating features
▶ Rapid onset of symptoms (1–12 weeks)
▶ Small fiber function involved out of proportion to large fiber function
▶ Autonomic testing abnormal in distribution of involved nerve

Consistent features
▶ Associated with change in glycemic control: disease onset or new treatment
▶ Prominent positive symptoms and pain
▶ Weakness and hypesthesia in same nerve distribution
▶ Significant weight loss
▶ Autonomic symptoms: hyper- or hypohidrosis, sexual or sphincteric dysfunction; orthostatic lightheadedness

Variable features
▶ Variable sites, with several well described syndromes:
  – Cranial nerve (especially III)
  – High lumbar root-segment disease (termed "diabetic amyotrophy")
  – Thoracic or abdominal involvement
  – Brachial plexopathy
  – Distal "stocking" neuropathy

Pearls and Perils

Complex regional pain syndrome (CRPS)

▶ In early CRPS (<6 months), very aggressive treatment may cure the syndrome.
▶ A 3-week course of steroids may dramatically relieve pain and reduce swelling.
▶ Sympathetic blocks (when effective) should be combined with aggressive physical and occupational therapy as the cornerstone of treatment.
▶ The affected limb heals poorly, and only an extremely strong indication should prompt surgery. When unavoidable, it is prudent to precede the operation with a program that optimizes limb function, administer a perioperative sympathetic block, and follow-up with an aggressive course of physiotherapy, accompanied by a sympathetic block series if needed.
▶ Immobilization fosters the development of CRPS and should be avoided at all costs.

---

such as that due to diabetes. The most common sites are the median nerve at the wrist (carpal tunnel syndrome), the ulnar nerve at the elbow, the tibial nerve at the ankle (tarsal tunnel syndrome), the peroneal nerve at the knee, and the plantar digital nerve between the metatarsal heads (Morton neuroma). Burning pain in the distribution of the nerve is associated with tingling when compression of the nerve increases. This phenomenon underlies two signs on physical examination, which elicit tingling or radiating pain in the distribution of the nerve: the Tinel sign is elicited when tapping the nerve at the presumed site of compression, whereas the Phalen sign is elicited when bending the joint at the presumed site of compression, for example, flexing the wrist for carpal tunnel syndrome or intorting the foot for tarsal tunnel syndrome. Patients also complain of a dull aching pain referred to limb areas proximal to the entrapment.

An EMG confirms the diagnosis of the compressive mononeuropathy, and defines any underlying generalized peripheral neuropathy. The presence of such a generalized process should prompt further evaluation to identify the cause. In addition, management of a compressive mononeuropathy in the presence of a generalized neuropathy should be more aggressive, with early surgical intervention, because the nerve's lowered metabolic reserve reduces its resistance to chronic pressure. Conservative management options include injection of steroid into the compressed area, a nighttime splint to immobilize the joint associated with the compression, and gentle physical therapy. The nonsteroidal and tricyclic agents are helpful. When conservative measures fail, or when a generalized peripheral neuropathy is present, surgical decompression of the nerve is usually effective. In fact, decompression should be entertained sooner when a compressive mononeuropathy occurs in the context of a generalized peripheral neuropathy, since the nerve may have far less regenerative reserve.

Limb Pain

Chronic limb pain may have many ligamentous, capsular, or muscular etiologies. When accompanied by obvious, visible changes of the limb, such as swelling or color changes, the term *reflex sympathetic dystrophy* (RSD) has been used. This term carries unwarranted pathophysiologic implications (the disease is not "reflex," minimally "sympathetic," and rarely "dystrophic"), which have prompted its replacement by the descriptive term *complex regional pain syndrome* (CRPS).

Complex regional pain syndrome can be defined based on four criteria: (1) pain out of proportion to, and out of the usual distribution of, any known pathology; (2) allodynia (pain induced by a normally innocuous stimulus); (3) alterations in limb function, which may be homeostatic, such as edema, and color, temperature, sweating changes, or may be motor, such as dystonia or spasm; and (4) alterations in limb structure, including hair, nail, skin, or bone changes (particularly periarticular bony demineralization). The diagnosis depends on the number of criteria present to a moderate or greater degree of severity: 4, definite; 3, probable; 2, possible; and 1, unlikely.

The term *sympathetically maintained pain* (SMP) is sometimes mistakenly used in reference to the same syndrome. Chronic regional pain syndrome is a clinical syndrome, requires no tests for diagnosis, and implies no underlying pain mechanism. Patients with CRPS may or may not respond to a particular treatment, such as a sympathetic block, in the same way that patients with chest pain radiating to the left arm may or may not respond to nitroglycerin. In contrast, SMP defines a pain mechanism, not a clinical syndrome. Sympathetically maintained pain refers to pain that stops when sympathetic outflow to the involved body part is stopped, by injection of anesthetic into the sympathetic ganglia or oral α-adrenergic pharmacologic blockade, for example. The diagnosis of SMP therefore requires one of these procedures, and its usefulness is restricted to defining the treatment course. Sympathetically maintained pain occurs with a variety of conditions, including CRPS; shingles, for example, may be supportive of a diagnosis of CRPS, but SMP is not a criterion for CRPS.

Although the diagnosis of CRPS requires no tests, some laboratory findings provide support when the diagnosis is unclear. Periarticular demineralization by X-ray studies establishes the fourth criterion for the diagnosis. A bone scan may show diffuse uptake in the involved limb, in support of the third criterion. Autonomic testing also correlates well with the clinical syndrome of CRPS, and limb temperature measurements predict the response to sympathetic blocks (that is, the presence of SMP) in CRPS. The term *pain/dysfunction syndrome* has been applied when no observable changes accompany disabling, diffuse limb pain.

In all types of limb pain, return of limb function is the goal and cornerstone of successful management. Compared with patients with other chronic pain syndromes, patients with limb pain, especially CRPS, require a more aggressive anesthesiologic approach, administered in the context of an interdisciplinary program. In the early stages (pain duration of less than 6 months), such aggressive treatment may sometimes cure CRPS. Specific measures include sympathetic blocks; systemic -adrenergic blockade, such as with phenoxybenzamine; and Bier blocks, which consist of filling the tourniquet-occluded venous system of the limb with an anesthetic, steroid, or sympathetic blocker for 20 minutes. The benefit of injections must be measured by *function* in physiotherapy, not only by the patient's own report of pain relief. When effective, injections are provided in a series, for example four to six times during an intensive 4-week program, and three times during the subsequent 4 months. Finally, in the early stage of CRPS, steroids can be nearly miraculous, especially in the lower extremity. A high dose, such as 60–80 mg of prednisone, is given daily for 1 week, and extended to a maximum of 3 weeks if effective the first week, with concomitant aggressive physiotherapy, or

while in a pain program. A paravertebral sympathectomy may be useful in carefully selected cases of CRPS who have SMP (a sympathetic block markedly reduces their limb pain), but who fail to respond to other measures. This procedure is falling out of favor because pain frequently returns 1–2 years after the operation, more severely than at the outset. Radio frequency ablation of the sympathetic ganglion has recently surfaced as perhaps the best alternative to surgical sympathectomy. This method provides about 3–6 months of functional disruption without destruction of the ganglion, and with consequent relief of pain. The procedure may be repeated.

Postamputation limb pain presents a different set of problems. More frequent than assumed, it occurs in almost three-quarters of all amputees in the first year after amputation. At 2 years, however, only a minority have significant pain. According to Jensen it may be divided, at least conceptually, into "(i) preoperative pain persisting after amputation; (ii) phantom pain; (iii) stump pain." Perhaps because it follows a surgical procedure, the pain is often managed surgically. No strong evidence suggests that this type of pain should be handled differently from other chronic pain states. Management aims to improve patient function in spite of pain. Anticonvulsants may be especially effective when stump pain arises from a neuroma. Opioids should be used early if improved function can be demonstrated and maintained. Calcitonin injections may also have a role here.

Visceral Pain

Chronic abdominal pain

The general physician may occasionally be called upon to manage the patient whose recurrent or chronic abdominal pain has no clearly identifiable etiology or no decisive treatment. In some cases, the pain may be attributed to chronic spasm of one of the duct sphincters (such as the sphincter of Oddi), to a chronic form of an acute disease (cholecystitis, appendicitis, pancreatitis), or simply to "irritable bowel syndrome." A thoracic or abdominal radiculopathy may also present with the chief complaint of abdominal pain, especially in diabetics. Although the evidence for some of these entities in an individual patient may be solid, the connection between the finding and the patient's complaint is frequently tenuous.

The best strategy with such patients is to use periods when pain is quiescent to train them in relaxation, endurance, and exercises that tone and strengthen the muscles near the site of pain. Periods of severe pain are then used to assess the response to these measures and to pharmacologic agents. All of the medications mentioned in the section on chronic pain management may play a role, depending on the quality and type of pain. Patients with abdominal pain, especially when it is due to spasm of a sphincter or viscus, may also respond to anticholinergic or adrenergic agents, such as glycopyrrolate, clonidine, or propranolol. In addition, clonazepam may relieve chest and abdominal wall spasms. Celiac plexus or ganglion blocks may also be helpful in selected cases.

The treating team should include a gastroenterologist as well as a dietitian, who can evaluate the impact of dietary habits on symptoms.

Pelvic pain

Undiagnosable pains of the pelvis, including anal pain, testicular and vulvar pain, and coital pain are difficult to treat. Although the usual maneuvers are clearly worth trying, the chances of success in this group of patients are low, possibly because of deep psychological disturbances inherent to pain in this area. A high frequency of sexual abuse precedes this disorder.

Oxalate-induced vulvodynia. Although uncommon, oxalate-induced vulvodynia deserves a mention because it is not well known, yet it is very easily treatable. It occurs in women in the second to sixth decades. The chief complaint is that of waxing and waning bilateral burning vulvar pain. Some patients have made the connection with high oxalate–containing foods, although most do not. High oxalate–containing foods include lamb, bitter chocolate, peanuts, pecans, wheat germ, and some of the edible weeds—dock, pokeweed, and purslane. Small amounts are also present in carrots, collards, kale, leeks, okra, parsnips, potatoes, and sweet potatoes. The finding of elevated 24-hour urinary oxalate excretion confirms the diagnosis. The pain can be relieved with calcium citrate supplementation. Recent literature has brought the existence of this disorder into question.

Cancer Pain

Conceptually, cancer pain should be handled in the same way as any other type of chronic pain. In addition, the presumed pain mechanism should dictate the choice of agent. What sets cancer pain apart is not the pain itself, but the poorer long-term prognosis and performance status of patients with metastatic cancer. Thus, many management strategies, such as endurance training, become impractical. Also, with so little time left to live, patients prefer not to spend weeks in a health facility. Given these considerations, opiates become the mainstay of treatment. Because of limiting toxicity in higher doses, it is crucial to implement other aspects of pain management to the extent feasible. These include physiotherapy and the adjunctive medications mentioned earlier, especially NSAIDs, tricyclic agents, and acetaminophen. Steroids may also be effective if tumor edema is compressing a pain-sensitive structure, and they possess intrinsic pain-relieving properties. Finally, when life expectancy is short, dramatic benefit can be gained by neurolytic procedures performed by an anesthesiologist, which destroy the responsible plexus or nerve.

Glossary of Pain Terms

The following terms are frequently used in the pain literature, but are seldom defined as a group. They are placed here for comparison and ease of reference.

Sensory Terms (in order of progressive complexity)

Sensory modality: Specific type of elemental sensation, which is thought to be directly transmitted by its own specialized receptors. Examples include temperature, joint movement, vibration, pain. A sensation requiring multiple elemental modalities, such as graphesthesia (discerning a letter traced on the skin) would not be called a modality.

Hypesthesia (from hypo, reduced, + esthesia, sensation): Reduced sensation to a particular modality, often included in the term (e.g., hypesthesia to temperature sensation), defined experimentally as *increased* threshold to that modality.

Hyperesthesia (from hyper, increased, esthesia, sensation): Heightened sensation to a modality, defined as a *reduced* threshold.

Hypoalgesia (from hypo, reduced, algesia, pain): Hypesthesia to the modality of pain.

Hyperalgesia (from hyper, increased, + algesia, pain): Hyperesthesia to the modality of pain. This may in turn be subdivided by pain submodalities, such as thermally, chemically, or mechanically induced pain.

Allodynia (from allo, other, + dynia, tenderness): Pain produced by a normally innocuous stimulus. This symptom represents, by definition, a *change in the modality* conveyed by a sensory pathway.

Hyperpathia (hyper, increased, + pathia, suffering): Hyperalgesia or allodynia, in the presence of hypesthesia. That is, an area shows reduced sensation to one or more modalities, while simultaneously having a heightened sensation to one of the pain modalities, or producing pain with a normally innocuous stimulus.

Paresthesia (para, beside, esthesia, sensation): Abnormal sensation, such as tingling, pricking, shooting, or tightness in the absence of any appropriate sensory stimulus. Such sensations are considered to be generated by an abnormality of the nervous system itself and suggest the diagnosis of neuropathic pain.

Neuropathic pain (neuro, nerve, + pathia, suffering): Pain generated by dysfunction of the nervous system itself, where such dysfunction is either proven or suspected. The dysfunction may be central or peripheral. The pain is burning, shooting, or associated with paresthesiae.

Neurophysiologic Terms (in alphabetical order)

Collateral inhibition: Inhibition of a neuron by a branch ("collateral") off the axon of its neighbor. The axon itself projects a long distance, whereas the collateral branch synapses close to the cell body. The nervous system uses this principle extensively, in two settings. Most commonly, collateral inhibition enhances contrast and sharpens a stimulus, such as an image or sensation, by inhibiting neighboring neurons with similar function to those firing. Less frequently, collateral inhibition reduces the function of neurons with a role opposite to those firing, producing a positive feedback loop.

Ephaptic transmission: Activation of an axon by "cross-talk" from a neighboring axon. Axons are normally shielded by their Schwann cells and by a purposely short length of contiguity between any two fibers. The nerve sprouts that follow a nerve injury have neither of these properties.

Labeled-line theory: The concept that a particular neuron, when activated, always results in the perception of the same modality (for example, vibration) through the same central synapses. Thus, the line, like a telephone line, which always conducts from the same house, can transmit nothing else, and is "labeled." This concept is not correct.

Sensitization: The response of a portion of the nervous system has increased over what is normally expected for a given stimulus. Sensitization refers to a quantitated nervous system response (such as the number of times a neuron fires), not a subjective patient report.

Wind-up: A type of sensitization that occurs in dorsal horn neurons: they increase their discharge rate in response to repeated identical C-fiber stimuli spaced at intervals of 3 seconds or less. This physiologic process matches subject reports that repeated identical noxious stimulations at less than 3-second intervals cause an

Annotated Bibliography

Jänig W, Stanton-Hicks M, eds. *Reflex sympathetic dystrophy: A reappraisal.* Seattle: IASP Press, 1996.
A small and inexpensive multiauthored text that nicely outlines many of the problems and controversies in reflex sympathetic dystrophy, including terminology, clinical aspects, and basic science issues.

Malmivaara A, Hakkinen U, Aro T, et al. The treatment of acute low back pain—bedrest, exercise or ordinary activity. *N Engl J Med* 1995;332:351–355.
A study of 186 Finnish patients randomly assigned to bedrest, exercise, or ordinary activity found that patients assigned to ordinary activity (the control group) did better than those assigned to the other two groups.

Melzack R, Wall PO. Pain mechanisms: A new theory. *Science* 1965;150:971–979.
The cornerstone hypothesis from which was derived much of the modern understanding of pain mechanisms.

Porter J, Jick H. Addiction rate in patients treated with narcotics (letter). *N Engl J Med* 1980;302:123.
Only four cases of possible addiction were found in 11,882 patients treated with opiates in the hospital for acute pain.

Wall PD, Melzack R. *Textbook of pain.* London: Churchill-Livingstone, 1994.
A superb multiauthored text covering nearly every aspect of pain physiology and management. Its 1,500 pages are divided into three sections: physiology, disease description, and therapy.

Consider Consultation When...

▶ The cause of the pain problem is not clear after history, physical and neurologic examinations, and appropriate laboratory tests.

▶ Pain is associated with new or unexplained neurologic symptoms and signs.

▶ Further expertise or experience is needed to treat the underlying cause.

▶ The patient does not respond to treatment, or the patient's course is different from expected.

▶ The only medication that is reported to relieve pain is an opiate.

▶ Complex regional pain syndrome (reflex sympathetic dystrophy) is not resolved within 6 weeks of the initial evaluation.

▶ A patient with chronic pain has new escalating pain levels.

▶ Interdisciplinary management is needed for disabling chronic pain.

▶ Technical assistance is needed in interpreting or performing diagnostic or therapeutic procedures.

CHAPTER 10

Sleep Disorders

Ruzica Kovacevic-Ristanovic and Tomasz J. Kuzniar

Outline

▶ Sleep architecture
▶ Sleep disorders

Disturbed sleep has plagued humankind for ages, and the elusive function of sleep has fascinated physicians and the public alike. Unfortunately, a search for a single "sleep center" in the brain has not been successful. Instead, lesion and stimulation studies have demonstrated the complexity of the sleep process, the multiplicity of structures involved in sleep, and the reciprocal interactions necessary for the initiation and maintenance of sleeping behavior.

Structures that have been found to facilitate sleep include the basal forebrain (i.e., preoptic area of the hypothalamus, specifically the ventrolateral preoptic nucleus [VLPO], promoting sleep via γ-amino-butyric acid [GABA/galanin] activity), the area surrounding the solitary tract in the medulla, the dorsal raphe nuclei, and the midline thalamus. The sleep-promoting role of the anterior hypothalamus results from its inhibitory effect on the posterior hypothalamic awakening neurons (mainly tuberomammillary-histaminergic neurons [TMN]) projecting widely to the cortex. Structures that have been found to facilitate waking are the newly discovered hypocretin (orexin) neurons in the dorsolateral hypothalamus, the ascending reticular activating system of the pons and midbrain, and the posterior hypothalamus. Although no direct interaction between the VLPO and hypocretin system has been reported, both innervate the main components of the ascending arousal systems (the adrenergic locus ceruleus [LC], serotonergic dorsal raphe [DR], dopaminergic ventrotegmental area [VTA], and histaminergic TMN). The VLPO [GABA/galanin] system inhibits, while the dorsolateral hypothalamic (hypocretin/ orexin) activates, these "arousal" systems. Destruction of the VLPO system results in insomnia, whereas destruction of the hypocretin system results in narcolepsy (hypersomnolence/sleep attacks and cataplexy). Integrity of the preoptic area of the anterior hypothalamus is not required for sleep onset, as sleep can be restored by inhibition of the posterior hypothalamus in cats made insomniac by preoptic lesions.

The control of alternating main sleep stages (non-rapid eye movement [NREM]/REM cycling) is attributed to a reciprocal interaction between two antagonistic systems: aminergic and cholinergic. Noradrenergic, histaminergic, and serotonergic neurons, which are active during the waking state, are virtually silent during REM sleep, whereas most other neurons are highly active. It has been accepted that the activation of forebrain structures during REM sleep is generated and transferred rostrally by brainstem cholinergic nuclei. The shut-off of dorsal raphe serotonergic neurons is one of the major factors underlying the activity of these cholinergic nuclei (disinhibition). Both systems, aminergic and cholinergic, are also involved in the process of cortical activation with arousal. The dopaminergic system (especially the ventral tegmental area) is specifically involved in the control of alertness. Dopaminergic neurons of the VTA, but not of substantia nigra (SN), are excited by hypocretins, and there is a greater hypocretin innervation of the VTA than the SN. Dopaminergic neurons in the ventral periaqueductal gray (PAG) are also activated during wakefulness. A descending dopaminergic projection may have an important role in sleep disorders accompanied by anomalies of sleep-related motor control (cataplexy, periodic limb movement disorder [PLMD], etc.).

Circadian sleep/wake rhythm is modulated by the hypothalamic suprachiasmatic nucleus (SCN). The SCN sets the body clock period to approximately 25 hours, with light and schedule cues ("time givers") entraining it to 24 hours. The retinohypothalamic tract conveys light stimuli to the SCN. This represents direct influence of light on the activity of the SCN. Melatonin has been implicated as a modulator of light entrainment, since it is secreted maximally during the night by the pineal gland ("hormone of darkness"). Thus, the anterior hypothalamus (VLPO) seems to serve as a center for "sleep switch" under the influence of the circadian clock (SCN).

Increasing understanding of the neurochemistry of sleep has raised the hope for more specific treatments of sleep disorders (e.g., hypocretin agonists and/or GABA/galanin antagonists for treatment of excessive daytime sleepiness or hypocretin antagonists/GABA/galanin agonists for treatment of insomnia). Rational design of new classes of stimulants/hypnotics will inevitably parallel better understanding of the intimate mechanisms of sleep physiology.

The important clinical, diagnostic, and therapeutic features of some sleep disorders are described in this chapter. Useful guidelines for diagnosis and therapy are also presented, although few universally accepted treatments are available for common sleep complaints.

Sleep Architecture

Since the evaluation of many patients with sleep disorders will involve the use of a sleep laboratory, it is important to understand the tests available and the parameters measured. Three basic parameters are needed to define the stage of sleep: an electroencephalogram (EEG), an electro-oculogram (EOG), and an electromyogram (EMG). The normal EEG of an alert, resting subject with closed eyes shows an 8–12-Hz posterior activity known as α (α). Two major sleep stages are distinguished: NREM and REM sleep.

Electroencephalographically, NREM sleep is composed of three stages. Stage N1 sleep is a stage of NREM sleep that directly follows the awake state. It is a very light sleep, and arousal threshold is low. The EEG shows a low-voltage tracing of mixed frequencies predominantly in the theta (θ) band, less than 50% α activity, vertex sharp activity, and slow eye movements. Stage N2 sleep is a stage of NREM sleep that is characterized by the presence of sleep spindles (12–14) and K-complexes against a relatively low-voltage, mixed-frequency background. It is considered "true" physiological sleep, because it is experienced by an individual as sleep onset. High-voltage delta (δ) waves may constitute up to 20% of stage 2 sleep. Stage N3 sleep combines what was previously described as stage 3 and 4 NREM and is defined by at least 20% of the period consisting of δ frequency EEG waves. The arousal threshold is highest during δ sleep.

Rapid eye movement sleep alternates with the NREM sleep at about 90-minute intervals in adults and

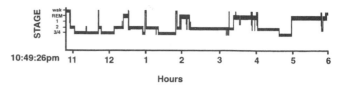

Figure 10.1 Hypnogram of a normal young adult. The progression of electroencephalogram stages of sleep demonstrates a concentration of stage N3 within the first half of the sleep period. Episodes of rapid eye movement (REM) occur at approximately 90-minute intervals, and the majority of REM appears within the latter half of the sleep period. Waking arousals are few.

60-minute intervals in infants. δ sleep is accumulated in the first third of sleep, whereas the proportion of REM sleep is highest in the last third of sleep (Figure 10.1). The EEG pattern during REM sleep resembles stage N1 sleep but is accompanied by rapid eye movements. In addition, EMG activity is low. There is a general activation of the autonomic system, with a higher average respiratory rate, heart rate, and blood pressure and, more importantly, much more pronounced variability throughout the REM period. In men with normal erectile function, penile tumescence (erection) occurs with each REM episode. In women, blood flow to the vagina is increased during REM sleep. People recall vivid dreams in about 80% of awakenings from REM sleep, compared to only 5% of awakenings from NREM sleep. However, in about 60–80% of awakenings from NREM sleep, people may recall stationary picture-like fragments.

Population studies have shown that the percentage of time spent in each stage varies with age and sex (Figure 10.2).

Sleep Disorders

The recently updated international classification of sleep disorders (International Classification of Sleep Disorders-2, ICSD-2, Table 10.1) divides sleep disorders into insomnias, sleep-disordered breathing, hypersomnias of central origin, circadian rhythm disorders, sleep-related movement disorders, and parasomnias. From the clinical standpoint, sleep disorders can be divided into those that produce a complaint of either insomnia or excessive daytime sleepiness, and those that intrude or occur during sleep but do not produce a primary complaint of insomnia or excessive daytime sleepiness.

Insomnia

Insomnia is a complaint (symptom) related to all conditions that lead to a perception of inadequate, disturbed, insufficient or nonrestorative sleep (despite an adequate opportunity to sleep), accompanied by daytime conse-

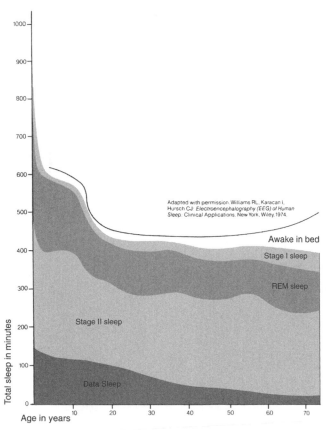

Figure 10.2 Development of sleep over lifetime. From Hauri P. *The sleep disorders.* Kalamazoo, MI: The Upjohn Company, 1982.

quences of inadequate sleep. A recent Gallup phone survey found that 35% of respondents reported experiencing at least one of the symptoms of insomnia every night or almost every night in the year preceding the survey.

Many intrinsic sleep disorders, such as persistent psychophysiologic insomnia, sleep-state misperception, restless legs syndrome (RLS), idiopathic insomnia, or even obstructive sleep apnea may present with a complaint of insomnia. Similarly, many extrinsic sleep disorders, such as inadequate sleep hygiene, environmental sleep disorder, altitude insomnia, adjustment sleep disorder, limit-setting sleep disorder, food allergy insomnia, hypnotic-dependent sleep disorder, and alcohol-dependent sleep disorder, may be accompanied by insomnia. Among circadian sleep disorders, delayed sleep-phase syndrome is associated with a complaint of sleep-onset delay, whereas advanced sleep-phase syndrome is accompanied by a complaint of an early morning awakening.

In general, the pattern of insomnia may consist primarily of (a) sleep onset delay (difficulty falling asleep), (b) early morning awakening (premature awakening with inability to fall asleep again), or (c) sleep fragmentation-sleep "maintenance" insomnia (repeated awakenings). These complaints are not mutually exclusive, and more than one component may coexist in the same patient. The

type of insomnia complaint seems to be age-dependent and related to age-dependent circadian rhythm tendency: sleep-onset delay is more prevalent among younger adults, whereas sleep-maintenance problems, such as frequent awakenings and early morning awakening, are more prevalent in later life.

Insomnias can be transient (less than 4 weeks), short term (1–6 months in duration), or chronic (more than 6 months in duration). Multiple factors can trigger transient insomnia, including life stress, brief illness, rapid change of time zones, drug withdrawal, use of central nervous system (CNS) stimulants, and pain. Transient insomnia is occasionally experienced by everyone, and recovery is usually rapid. These patients usually do not present to physicians. Chronic insomnia may be lifelong and is a widespread disorder.

The intrinsic insomnias include persistent psychophysiologic insomnia, sleep state misperception (paradoxical insomnia), and childhood-onset insomnia (true primary insomnia). Psychological factors are most important in the etiology of intrinsic insomnias. However, nonpsychological intrinsic sleep disorders (e.g., sleep apnea syndrome, alveolar hypoventilation syndrome, restless legs/periodic limb movements [PLMs]) may be responsible for insomnia in some cases. Among so-called extrinsic (i.e., secondary) insomnias, psychiatric disorders play a leading etiological role. Use of drugs (prescribed and recreational) and alcohol, and medical conditions, as well as other external/environmental conditions, are also frequent extrinsic etiologies of insomnia.

Sleep-onset delay

Sleep-onset delay is a common problem and probably accounts for most patients who present with a complaint of insomnia. It is usually due to psychological causes. In persistent psychophysiologic insomnia, sleeplessness may develop from a continued association of sleep time with stimulating practices and objects at bedtime ("learned sleep-preventing associations") and somatized tension. According to Spielman and colleagues, several groups of factors contribute to the emergence of a persistent psychophysiologic insomnia: (a) predisposing factors (personality, habits, heredity, etc.), (b) precipitating factors (any stressor), and (c) perpetuating factors (maladaptive conditioning, poor sleep hygiene, hypnotic and alcohol ingestion, worry about consequences of sleeplessness, etc.). Conditioning takes place between sleeplessness and stimuli normally conducive to sleep (bed/bedroom and bedtime rituals).

As a result, such patients sleep better away from their bedrooms and usual routines. In addition, somatized tension results from excessive focusing on insomnia. This in turn results in denial of the role of other personal problems in the etiology of the patient's problem. A conditioned internal factor may also develop in the form of

Table 10.1 American Academy of Sleep Medicine international classification of sleep disorders (2006)

1. Insomnia
Adjustment insomnia
Psychophysiological insomnia
Paradoxical insomnia
Idiopathic insomnia
Insomnia due to mental disorder
Inadequate sleep hygiene
Insomnia due to drug or substance
Insomnia due to medical condition
Insomnia not due to substance or known physiologic condition, unspecified
Physiologic (organic) insomnia, unspecified

2. Sleep Related Breathing Disorders
Primary central sleep apnea
Cheyne-Stokes breathing pattern
High-altitude periodic breathing
Central sleep apnea due to medical condition not Cheyne-Stokes
Central sleep apnea due to drug or substance
Central sleep apnea due to drug or substance obstructive sleep apnea, adult
Sleep-related nonobstructive alveolar hypoventilation, idiopathic
Sleep-related hypoventilation/hypoxemia due to pulmonary parenchymal or vascular pathology
Sleep-related hypoventilation/hypoxemia due to lower airways obstruction
Sleep-related hypoventilation/hypoxemia due to neuromuscular and chest
Wall disorders
Other sleep-related breathing disorders

3. Hypersomnias of Central Origin Not Due to a Circadian Rhythm Sleep Disorder, Sleep Related Breathing Disorder, or Other Cause of Disturbed Nocturnal Sleep
Narcolepsy with cataplexy
Narcolepsy without cataplexy
Narcolepsy due to medical condition, without cataplexy
With cataplexy
Narcolepsy, unspecified
Recurrent hypersomnia (including Kleine-Levin syndrome & menstrual-related hypersomnia)
Idiopathic hypersomnia with long sleep time
Idiopathic hypersomnia without long sleep time
Behaviorally induced insufficient sleep syndrome
Hypersomnia due to medical condition
Hypersomnia due to drug or substance (abuse)
For alcohol use
Hypersomnia due to drug or substance (medications)
Hypersomnia not due to substance or known physiological condition
Physiological (organic) hypersomnia, unspecified

4. Circadian Rhythm Sleep Disorders
Circadian rhythm sleep disorder, delayed sleep
Phase-type
Circadian rhythm sleep disorder, advanced sleep
Phase-type
Circadian rhythm sleep disorder, irregular sleep
Wake-type
Circadian rhythm sleep disorder, free-running type
Circadian rhythm sleep disorder, jet lag-type
Circadian rhythm sleep disorder, shift work-type
Circadian rhythm sleep disorder due to medical condition
Other circadian rhythm sleep disorder
Other circadian rhythm sleep disorder due to drug or substance

5. Parasomnias
Confusional arousals
Sleepwalking
Sleep terrors
Rapid eye movement
Sleep behavior disorder
Recurrent isolated sleep paralysis
Nightmare disorder
Sleep-related dissociative disorders
Sleep-related groaning (cataphrenia)
Exploding head syndrome
Sleep-related hallucinations
Sleep-related eating disorder

6. Sleep Related Movement Disorders
Restless legs syndrome
Periodic limb movement disorder
Sleep-related leg cramps
Sleep-related bruxism

7. Other Sleep Disorders
Other Physiological (Organic) Sleep Disorder
Other Sleep Disorder Not Due to Substance or Known
Physiological Condition
Environmental Sleep Disorder

REM, rapid eye movement; NOS, not otherwise specified.
From the American Academy of Sleep Medicine. *The International Classification of Sleep Disorders: Diagnostic and Coding Manual. Author, 2006, with permission.*

apprehension about unsuccessful and excessive efforts to sleep. Conscious efforts to fall asleep result in arousal (performance anxiety).

Patients suffering from persistent psychophysiologic insomnia consider themselves "light sleepers." They often have multiple somatic complaints, such as back pains, headaches, and palpitations that lead to occasional abuse of alcohol, barbiturates, and minor tranquilizers. The sleep of such patients in the sleep laboratory is usually good, because the conditioning factors that are active at home are reduced in the laboratory.

Many specific psychiatric illnesses associated with anxiety (e.g., anxiety and panic disorders, hypochondriasis, obsessive-compulsive disorders) and schizophrenia can be associated with sleep-onset difficulty, and sleep fragmentation as well.

Drugs can also compromise the initiation of sleep. When obtaining a history, the physician should inquire specifically about possible precipitants of drug-induced insomnia. Steroids, dopaminergic agents, xanthine derivatives (e.g., caffeine and theophylline), and β-adrenergic agonists (e.g., terbutaline and phenylethylamine derivatives used as stimulants, appetite suppressants, and decongestants) may cause sleep disruption. If such medications are taken late in the day, and in increasing amounts because of the development of tolerance, they can easily cause sleep-onset delay, as well as sleep fragmentation and "lightening" of sleep.

In addition to the psychological, psychiatric, and drug causes of sleep-onset delay, patients who have a disturbed circadian rhythm may have the same sleep complaint. In delayed sleep-phase syndrome, patients naturally fall asleep at 2 AM to 3 AM or later. They cannot fall asleep if they go to bed at conventional times. If they must then get up for a job or school at 6 AM, they will be sleepy in the morning because they did not get enough sleep. They have no trouble going to sleep and getting full rest if they can go to bed late and sleep until mid-day. A change in lifestyle, exposure to bright light upon awakening, melatonin taken 7–8 hours prior to presumed core temperature minimum (which usually takes place 2 hours before the awakening in the morning), and chronotherapy can correct this problem. With chronotherapy, the patient receives an individually designed sleep schedule to correct his sleep-onset delay, and the patient gradually attains a desired sleep-onset time and normal quality of sleep. Likewise, chronotherapy may help patients who have irregular sleep–wake patterns and who sleep for short and variable periods of time throughout a 24-hour period. These people often cannot fall asleep at conventional times because they have napped recently. Other groups of people presenting with a complaint of inability to fall asleep are shift workers and frequent travelers across different time zones who may experience "jet lag." Combined afternoon melatonin and morning bright light

therapy can be used to modify circadian rhythm in anticipation of a travel through time zones.

Although insomnia is typically related to psychiatric, medical, circadian or other sleep disorders, it can also be a primary sleep disorder. Primary insomnia may be present in 25% of all insomniac patients. It is hypothesized to be a disorder of hyperarousal, resulting from hypothalamic-pituitary-adrenal axis dysregulation. The insomnia is associated with a 24-hour increase in adrenocorticotropic hormone (ACTH) and cortisol secretion, consistent with a disorder of CNS hyperarousal. Also, chronic insomnia is associated with a shift of interleukin (IL)-6 and tumor necrosis factor (TNF) secretion from nighttime to daytime, which may explain daytime fatigue. Another contributory factor is low nocturnal melatonin production in chronic insomnia.

Treatment of chronic insomnia provides a significant challenge to the clinician. The physician should first identify the underlying condition(s) contributing to chronic insomnia. These may include psychiatric disorders such as depression, alcohol/substance abuse and chronic medical disorders, sleep apnea, aging, and alterations in the circadian rhythm. The clinician should individualize treatment based on concurrent medical problems, age, and hepatic and renal function. Pharmacologic treatment should be used judiciously and, if used, should be combined with nonpharmacologic interventions.

Counseling, particularly the promotion of good sleep hygiene practices, should be one of the first steps in the treatment of insomnia. Sleep hygiene includes setting a fixed hour for retiring each night, eliminating daytime naps, avoiding caffeine-containing beverages or anxiety-producing activities at night, and assuring that the bedroom is quiet, dark, and comfortable. Because patients may neglect to think of over-the-counter or herbal preparations as drugs, discussing the need to avoid sympathomimetic substances may prove fruitful.

Some patients who complain of insomnia may actually be attempting to discuss problems that they find difficult to raise, such as impotence, marital discord, or alcoholism in a family member. The complaint may be resolved if attention is given to these problems, regardless of whether sleep behavior is actually altered.

Only a few practical points concerning behavioral therapies need to be reviewed here. Techniques that attempt to increase relaxation, either through biofeedback or more conventional learning paradigms, may be valuable if they are aimed at a specific physiologic disturbance. For example, a patient whose polysomnogram indicates a large amount of muscle activity prior to falling asleep might benefit from EMG biofeedback. Other techniques aimed at reducing tension include progressive muscular relaxation and autogenic training. These techniques generally require the facilities of a sleep laboratory and the skills of a sleep specialist.

Sleep restriction relies on limiting time in bed to the estimated sleep time, and then gradually increasing it until an optimal sleep time is achieved. This approach is based on the observation that insomniacs spend too much time in bed in an attempt to obtain sleep. The latter technique introduces a state of mild sleep deprivation, which is likely to result in faster sleep onset, improved sleep continuity, and deeper sleep. Keeping a sleep log provides the clinician with a tool to assess sleep efficiency during treatment. Sleep logs can be validated and complemented by an *actigraph*—a device that is worn on the wrist of the nondominant hand and detects muscle activity that serves as a surrogate for wakefulness. If subjective sleep efficiency (perceived amount of sleep/time in bed × 100) over 5 days of sleep restriction exceeds 90%, the patient is instructed to increase bedtime by 15 minutes (i.e., by retiring 15 minutes earlier). If sleep efficiency remains less than 85% over 5 nights, time in bed is further restricted.

Cognitive therapy focuses on maladaptive thoughts that produce an emotional arousal, such as unrealistic expectations about sleep requirements, negative consequences of insomnia, and misattributions of daytime difficulties to poor sleep. The arousal elicited by maladaptive thoughts then acts as a perpetuating factor of insomnia. When compared head-to-head, psychological modalities are more successful in the treatment of insomnia than medications and give longer-lasting results.

Sleep-promoting medications can be used in the management of insomnia, but their use must be considered carefully. Most patients affected by sleep-onset delay do not require drug treatment. Hypnotics are most often appropriate for treatment of transient and short-term insomnias, to break the cycle of tension/anxiety in chronic insomnias, or as part of a comprehensive program of behavioral modification starting with improved sleep hygiene.

The choice of a sedative/hypnotic drug is dictated primarily by the duration of clinical effect. Ideally, hypnosedative effect should cease by the time the patient arises. An effective hypnotic drug should decrease sleep latency and increase the total sleep time, without producing daytime sedation. The efficacy of a hypnotic is defined by its ability to induce and maintain sleep, and directly depends on the drug's dose, absorption, and duration of action. Thus, an ideal hypnotic is rapidly absorbed and has a duration of action consistent with the sleep period (usually around 8 hours). Hypnotics with a duration of action that exceeds the sleep period usually lead to residual sedation during daytime, whereas the use of short-acting hypnotics in doses higher than required is often associated with undesirable adverse effects including rebound insomnia and anterograde amnesia. Development of dependence is also an undesirable possibility with the use of hypnotics. Its development can be minimized by intermittent use of low doses, together with limiting the duration of drug intake, and gradual withdrawal if the drug has been used continuously for more than a month.

Pharmacokinetic properties of a hypnotic (absorption rate, elimination half-life, etc.) determine the speed of sleep induction and the duration of the soporific effect, as well as possible daytime sedation. The onset of sleep induction after an oral dose depends on the rapidity of absorption from the gastrointestinal tract. The duration of action (sleep maintenance) of a single dose depends on the volume of distribution, elimination time, and clearance. With repeated administration at a fixed dosing rate, a drug will accumulate in plasma and brain until a steady state is reached. More than 90% of the time necessary to reach a steady-state condition depends only on the drug's elimination half-life. For a drug such as triazolam (Halcion) with a very short elimination half-life, accumulation will be complete within 1 day. That is, the mean plasma concentration will be no higher after multiple days of therapy than after the first day. At the other extreme is a drug such as flurazepam (Dalmane), which has a very long elimination half-life. Two weeks or more of long-term treatment will be necessary for a steady state to be attained. Hypnotics with longer half-lives (lasting more than 24 hours) show increased efficacy with 2 or 3 nights of administration, but they also show increased residual daytime effects. Some benzodiazepines produce persistent long-acting metabolites and cause impairment in alertness, motor performance, and cognitive function in the morning (a "hangover effect"). The rate of drug disappearance following discontinuation after long-term treatment will mirror the rate of accumulation. That is, the longer the elimination half-life, the more time will be needed for the drug to disappear.

Persistence of long-acting agents at the receptor sites throughout each 24-hour dosing interval increases the likelihood of a daytime anxiolytic effect, a potential benefit for patients with both anxiety and insomnia. In contrast, for short half-life hypnotics (e.g., triazolam [Halcion]), increased daytime anxiety has been reported in some studies, possibly attributable to wide fluctuations in plasma and receptor-site concentrations between doses.

Metabolism of hypnotic agents varies and is largely age-dependent. For example, the elimination half-life of diazepam in healthy men may increase three- to fourfold from 20 years of age to 80 years of age. The elimination of hypnotics is decreased in elderly people, who might have a low renal glomerular filtration rate, reduced hepatic blood flow, and decreased activity of hepatic drug-metabolizing enzymes. As a result, benzodiazepine dosage should be halved in the elderly, and even then daytime functioning may be impaired significantly.

The choice of hypnotics for elderly patients with sleep-onset delay, especially when they are acutely hospitalized, is further complicated by the risk of paradoxical excitation at night-time ("sun-downing"), which may be precipitated or exacerbated by medication. Although diphenhydramine has been useful in many of these patients, there is a risk of increasing their confusion because of its anticholinergic effect. These problems can be minimized by adjunctive measures such as leaving a light on in the patient's room and frequently reorienting the patient to their unfamiliar surroundings. A family member may occasionally be required to stay with the patient.

Pregnant women, alcoholics, and those with sleep apnea should not be given hypnotics, except in low doses and only in special circumstances. The prescribing of hypnotics to children is not recommended, except for rare use in the treatment of night terrors or severe somnambulism.

The choice of hypnotic may also be guided by its effects on particular sleep stages. The available hypnotic drugs have a surprisingly heterogeneous set of effects on sleep architecture. Although almost all agents employed as hypnotics will suppress REM sleep when given in sufficiently large quantities, two patterns of effects are seen at lower doses. Barbiturates, chloral hydrate, anticholinergics, tricyclics, and ethanol demonstrate REM suppression, whereas most benzodiazepines decrease stage N3. All of these agents appear to decrease sleep latency, reduce the number of spontaneous awakenings, and reduce wakefulness after sleep onset. Although the drugs that have the least effect on sleep architecture may offer a theoretical advantage in the therapy of insomnia, there is no clear demonstration that they induce "better, more natural" sleep.

There is seldom a reason to use more than a single agent in the treatment of insomnia. A failure to obtain an adequate response on the first night does not imply a need to increase the dosage immediately. A trial of at least 2 or 3 nights is indicated.

Discontinuation of treatment with hypnotics may result in a rebound insomnia (worsening of the original complaint) or even a frank withdrawal syndrome. Due to the intrinsic "tapering" effect of compounds with long half-lives, rebound and/or withdrawal phenomena appear to be unlikely. When they do occur, such effects are delayed in onset and are relatively mild. There is a much higher likelihood of rebound or withdrawal effect after abrupt discontinuation of short half-life hypnotics. Dose tapering is appropriate when short half-life hypnotics are discontinued.

Withdrawal from sedative drugs, especially barbiturates, is potentially dangerous and should be carried out under close supervision. These agents should never be discontinued abruptly (except in the rare case of hypersensitivity reactions).

In the last decade of the 20th century, benzodiazepines have almost completely replaced barbiturates in the treatment of insomnia. The preference for benzodiazepines is based on their lower toxicity (less respiratory and cardiac depression) and less marked tolerance, rather than on a superior hypnotic effect. All benzodiazepines reduce sleep latency, decrease the number and duration of awakenings, and increase total sleep time and sleep efficiency. Drug choices for sleep-onset insomnia and sleep-maintenance insomnia will be different: short half-life agents (e.g., triazolam [Halcion]) are preferred for sleep-onset insomnia, whereas long half-life agents (e.g., temazepam [Restoril]) are preferred for sleep-maintenance insomnia. It is important to note, however, that although many benzodiazepines have been marketed with emphasis on their short duration of action, many have long-acting active metabolites. This is often a problem in elderly patients and in those who experience a decrement in liver function.

Only five benzodiazepines are marketed as hypnotics in the United States: triazolam (Halcion), temazepam (Restoril), quazepam (Doral), flurazepam (Dalmane), and estazolam (ProSom). The newest of these agents, estazolam (ProSom), was introduced in 1990. Estazolam (ProSom) in a dose of 1–2 mg remains an effective hypnotic for at least 6 weeks of continuous administration with no evidence of clinically significant tolerance. It improves sleep latency and total sleep time, reduces the number of nocturnal awakenings, and improves both depth of sleep and sleep quality in adults with chronic insomnia. Various benzodiazepine anxiolytics (e.g., diazepam [Valium], alprazolam [Xanax], lorazepam [Ativan], or oxazepam [Serax]) are also prescribed for insomnia associated with anxiety disorders. Unfortunately, limited evidence supports their efficacy in treatment of insomnia.

Several nonbenzodiazepine hypnotics that were introduced over the turn of the century have now become the most commonly prescribed medications for insomnia. Zolpidem (Ambien) is an imidazopyridine hypnotic that is structurally unrelated to benzodiazepines, but which acts as a specific benzodiazepine receptor agonist. It has a mean elimination half-life of 3.5–5.1 hours (mean 4 hours). In young adults, zolpidem (Ambien) leads to a marked increase in slow-wave sleep with a reduction of stage N2 sleep. No change in REM sleep occurs. In middle-aged individuals, it reduces awake time and increases stage N2 sleep, without changing REM sleep. Zolpidem is also available in a slow-release form (Ambien CR).

Zaleplon (Sonata) is another nonbenzodiazepine hypnotic from the pyrazolopyrimidine class. In controlled trials, it has been shown to shorten sleep latency. It is metabolized by aldehyde oxidase and to a lesser degree by CYP450 3A4. Inhibitors of these enzymes may decrease its clearance and enhance sedative/hypnotic effect. Zaleplon has half-life of only 1 hour, so it may be used for initial or mid-period insomnia.

Zopiclone, a cyclopyrrolone compound, is another hypnotic, chemically unrelated to benzodiazepines, not available in the United States. Its isomer, eszopiclone

(Lunesta), a nonbenzodiazepine hypnotic, has been approved by the U.S. Food and Drug Administration (FDA) for treatment of insomnia. It has an onset of action of 1 hour and a half-life of about 6 hours. Eszopiclone has been shown to decrease sleep latency and improve measures of sleep continuity. It has not been associated with the development of tolerance over 6 months of use.

A structurally new compound with a distinct mechanism of action was recently introduced in treatment of insomnia. Ramelteon (Rozerem) is a nonsedating melatonin receptor agonist that is rapidly absorbed from the gastrointestinal tract, giving a peak concentration at 0.5–1.5 hours and a half-life of 1–2.5 hours. It then undergoes extensive liver metabolism, yielding weak, active metabolites that have an elimination half-life of 2–5 hours. Ramelteon produces modest shortening of sleep latency.

Several alternative therapies are widely used for treatment of insomnia, including valerian root, St. John's wort, and melatonin. The usefulness of valerian root (*Valeriana officinalis*) as a mild hypnotic is supported by a limited number of human studies. It seems to affect GABA metabolism and reuptake, mainly GABA A receptors, in addition to 5-HT_{1a} and adenosine receptors. St. John's wort (*Hypericum perforatum*) is popular as an herbal treatment for depression. Its use as a hypnotic has not been studied systematically, but it may promote "deep sleep." Melatonin is used to reset the circadian clock and help proper positioning of the sleep cycle within a 24-hour period, but it also has a direct, albeit mild, sedative/hypnotic effect. The most popular doses are 2–20 mg, approximately 30–120 minutes before bedtime. Caution should be exercised in patients with known cardiovascular disease, since melatonin is reported to cause vasoconstriction of the coronary and cerebral arteries in rats. Other possible side effects are inhibition of fertility, increased or induced depression, suppression of male libido, and retinal damage.

Early morning awakening

Early morning awakening can be seen in numerous clinical settings including depression, use of certain drugs, and advanced sleep-phase syndrome. Endogenous depression is characterized by premature awakening and an inability to fall asleep again, with variable sleep-onset disturbance, depending on the individual's component of agitation. A key polysomnographic finding is shortened REM sleep latency (considered by some experts to be a biologic marker of depression), in addition to increased intensity of REM sleep. δ sleep is also reduced, but this is a relatively nonspecific feature. In contrast, bipolar depression is frequently associated with hypersomnia. However, this state is again accompanied by a shortened REM latency and reduced stage N3 sleep. During the manic phase, the onset of sleep is delayed, and sleep is short. Insomnia may precede all other symptoms of depression, and restoration of sleep may be the first sign of recovery.

In patients with early morning awakening, sedative therapy is usually accompanied by an unacceptable degree of morning sedation ("hangover"). If the patient's workup suggests that depression is the cause of or contributes to the disorder, antidepressants appear to offer the best results and should be the initial form of therapy. Tricyclic antidepressants with a sedative effect are recommended if insomnia is associated with an affective disorder. Amitriptyline (Elavil) and trimipramine (Surmontil) reduce sleep latency and improve sleep continuity. Trazodone (Desyrel), a nontricyclic, is also widely used for treatment of insomnia in depressed patients. Although an improvement in sleep often precedes an improvement in mood, changes of affect should determine the end point in therapy.

Drug-induced early morning awakening may occur with the use of some short-acting benzodiazepines, such as oxazepam (Serax), or a short-acting nonbenzodiazepine, such as zaleplon (Sonata). Both have few residual morning after effects. Patients who drink alcoholic beverages prior to sleep may develop early morning awakening, apparently related to an increase in REM sleep ("REM rebound") after the alcohol is metabolized. An underlying psychiatric problem should be considered, as in any patient with an alcohol-related problem. Therapy involves a slow withdrawal of the causative agent.

Advanced sleep-phase syndrome is occasionally responsible for a complaint of early morning awakening and, as such, may mimic the typical pattern of sleep disturbance seen in depression. It is seen more frequently in elderly patients. There are few, relatively experimental treatments for this condition, including either reverse chronotherapy or exposure to light in the evening and light deprivation in the morning. Either treatment requires the skills of experts in sleep disorder centers. Usefulness of morning melatonin in treatment of advanced sleep-phase syndrome is limited due to its soporific effects.

Sleep Fragmentation

A complaint of frequent awakenings at night often signals the presence of an intrinsic dyssomnia, specifically sleep apnea or PLMD. Although multiple medical conditions can also interfere with sleep maintenance, psychiatric etiology is a less likely explanation for this complaint (Table 10.2).

In sleep apnea, sleep disruption is due to cessation of air exchange during sleep and subsequent frequent awakenings associated with occasional gasping for air or a choking sensation. Treatments of sleep-induced respiratory impairments are discussed in the section on disorders of excessive somnolence.

Periodic limb movement disorder is a condition in which insomnia is associated with the occurrence during

Table 10.2 Periodic limb movement disorder

Discriminating features
▶ Accurate description of the movements by a bed partner

Consistent features
▶ Repetitive and highly stereotyped limb muscle jerks during sleep
▶ Muscle jerks followed by a partial arousal
▶ Unawareness of movements by patient who instead may report frequent nocturnal awakenings, unrefreshing sleep and aching of the legs upon awakening

Variable features
▶ Association with restless legs syndrome (dysesthesias relieved by movement, triggered by rest and worse in the evening or at night)
▶ Association with identifiable medical problems, dietary substances or medications
▶ Response to dopaminergic drugs, opioids, benzodiazepines or gabapentin

sleep of repetitive and highly stereotyped limb muscle jerks. They are frequently followed by a partial arousal. Patients are often unaware of the movements at night. Rather, they report frequent nocturnal awakenings and unrefreshing sleep. A history from a bed partner is important, because they usually provide an accurate description of the movements. Insomnia characterized by marked sleep onset delay may result from a related disorder, RLS, in which disagreeable sensations of creeping occur deep inside the calves whenever sitting or lying down, causing an almost irresistible urge to move the legs and thus interfering with sleep onset. Almost all patients with RLS also have PLMs. Coincident PLMs are not required for the diagnosis of RLS. Diagnosis of RLS relies entirely on the patient's symptoms. Revised criteria emphasize the onset of symptoms with rest and a clear circadian pattern to the symptoms. The four essential criteria for the diagnosis have been published and widely accepted: (a) a sensation of an urge to move the limbs (usually legs), (b) motor restlessness to reduce sensations, (c) onset or worsening of the symptoms at rest, and (d) marked circadian variation in occurrence or severity of the symptoms, with evening predominance.

Many RLS patients experience periodic leg movements while awake (PLMW), especially in sedentary situations. These waking movements are typically seen in patients with RLS. The prevalence of RLS is 5–10%. The prevalence increases with age, and may be higher in women.

The large majority of patients afflicted by RLS represent idiopathic cases, unrelated to any other medical condition as a possible cause.

Several secondary associations with RLS have been well documented, including pregnancy, iron deficiency,

and end-stage renal disease. Differential diagnosis of RLS includes positive symptoms of neuropathies and radiculopathies, specifically neuropathy associated with rheumatoid arthritis and diabetes mellitus. Other conditions that may cause symptoms similar to RLS include peripheral vascular disease causing claudication, fibromyalgia, nocturnal leg cramps, and arthritis.

The exact pathophysiology of RLS/PLMD is unknown. However, several studies suggest dysfunction of the subcortical dopamine system, which results in reduction of the spinal and possibly cortical inhibition that may be state-dependent. Positron emission tomography (PET) and single-photon emission computed tomography (SPECT) studies show small decreases in dopaminergic function in the striatum of RLS patients compared with controls.

The accepted and usually successful treatments for restless legs and PLMD include dopaminergic drugs and opioids, among others. The dopaminergic agent carbidopa/levodopa (Sinemet) improves all of the cardinal features of both RLS and PLMD, including discomfort in the legs, involuntary periodic movements during the waking state, periodic limb movements during sleep, and sleep discontinuity. Side effects include gastrointestinal discomfort, nausea, and vomiting. Typical doses of carbidopa/levodopa (Sinemet) are 25/100 mg to 100/400 mg taken at bedtime, and occasionally during the night as well. If higher doses are used, the phenomenon of augmentation may be seen, which consists of increased intensity of symptoms, and earlier onset in the day, reduced time at rest before the symptoms start and, in some cases, widespread dysesthesias and restlessness. Rebound is a phenomenon of reappearance of RLS symptoms in the morning, after the effects of a dose of levodopa wears off.

Direct dopamine agonists, pramipexole (Mirapex) and ropinirole (Requip), are very effective in RLS and are currently the treatment of choice. Typically, either medication is started at a low dose and then titrated up, over a period of days to weeks, to achieve control of symptoms. Side effects are rare and include nausea, dizziness, and sleepiness. Numerous opioids have been used, such as codeine, propoxyphene (Darvon), oxycodone (Percodan), pentazocine (Talwin), Levo-Dromoran, and methadone. Their effectiveness has been tested formally by only a few studies. Trials using gabapentin (Neurontin) demonstrated also significant subjective and objective improvement in patients with RLS/PLM syndrome. Clonazepam, although widely prescribed for PLM, appears to have only a modest effect. Additionally, it has not been shown to reduce the symptoms of RLS to any significant degree. Adequate body iron stores (to reach ferritin levels higher than 50 g/L) appear to ameliorate some of the symptomatology but may require iron supplementation.

Sleep fragmentation/frequent awakenings often signal the presence of medical conditions such as alveolar hypoventilation, which, in adults, may be secondary to massive obesity (obesity-hypoventilation syndrome), chronic obstructive pulmonary disease, stroke, myopathy, cordotomy, or lesions involving structures that control sleep and breathing. Primary alveolar hypoventilation (previously termed "Ondine's curse") is usually reported in infants and is associated with a further worsening of hypercapnia and hypoxemia in sleep. Other conditions capable of causing severe sleep fragmentation include gastroesophageal reflux with regurgitation, heartburn and dyspepsia, nocturnal angina, sleep-related asthma, nightmares, and cluster headache. Numerous other medical and neurologic conditions can be associated with this form of insomnia, including CNS infections, head trauma, nocturnal epilepsy, fibromyalgia, cardiovascular disorders, pulmonary disease, any painful condition, toxic conditions, and endocrine abnormalities. Hypercortisolism (especially iatrogenic) should be considered if sleep fragmentation is prominent. Additional causes of sleep fragmentation include various nocturnal disruptions, such as bruxism (teeth grinding). Generally, if sleep fragmentation is due to a known etiology, treatment of the underlying disorder can be expected to alleviate the sleep disturbance and thus obviate the need for hypnotics.

Sleep Disorders Associated with Hypersomnolence

In a strict sense, the term *hypersomnolence* should be reserved for those patients who have a demonstrable tendency to fall asleep in the waking state when sedentary, or who have sleep "attacks." There may also be diminished alertness in waking, described as subwakefulness. In all cases presenting with these symptoms, it is important to separate excessive daytime somnolence from less specific symptoms of fatigue, malaise, or depression.

Included in this category are intrinsic and extrinsic dyssomnias as well as parasomnias and disorders associated with medical-psychiatric disorders. The chief symptoms of this group of disorders are an inappropriate and undesirable sleepiness during waking hours, decreased cognitive and motor performance, an excessive tendency to sleep, unavoidable napping, an increase in total sleep over 24 hours ("true" hypersomnia), and a difficulty in achieving full arousal on awakening. The major causes of excessive daytime sleepiness are sleep apnea syndrome (43%), narcolepsy (25%), and insufficient sleep.

Sleep apnea

A potentially lethal condition, sleep apnea is an abnormal breathing pattern during sleep characterized by cessation of airflow at the level of the nostrils and mouth lasting for at least 10 seconds. The estimated prevalence of clinically significant apnea (apnea/hypopnea index of >5/hour associated with a symptom of daytime sleepiness)

ranges from 1% to 4% of the adult population. It is the most frequent diagnosis in sleep disorder centers and the most frequent cause of daytime sleepiness.

Sleep apneas are subdivided by type. Obstructive or upper airway apnea occurs secondary to a sleep-induced obstruction of the airway. Central apnea occurs secondary to decreased respiratory muscle activity. Mixed apnea combines both phenomena. It usually starts as a central apnea (with no respiratory effort) and develops into an obstruction later. Either obstructive or, much less frequently, central apnea predominates in every patient.

Obstructive sleep apnea (OSA) seems to be caused by a concentric pharyngeal collapse and is not due to active musculature contraction. Contributing factors may include abnormal anatomic relationships among the muscular or bony structures of the nasopharynx, oropharynx, or hypopharynx (e.g., a short thick neck, macroglossia, micrognathia, retrognathia, a relatively small and low-positioned hyoid bone, or a narrow pharynx); inappropriate involuntary respiratory control of pharyngeal and diaphragmatic muscle tone; increased compliance of the pharyngeal walls, especially fatty or redundant pharyngeal and submucosal folds; and the amount of inspiratory, intraluminal negative pressure. Apneas are more prevalent with increasing age and worsen with alcohol or sedative drug intake.

Diagnosis of sleep apnea relies on history (best supplied by a bed partner), physical signs, presence of risk factors, and results of polysomnographic evaluation. Clinical symptoms usually include snoring, persistent daytime sleepiness, tiredness and fatigue, unrefreshing sleep attacks, restless sleep/frequent awakenings, abrupt awakenings with choking/gasping sensations, deterioration of memory and judgment, early morning confusion, automatic behavior at times (i.e., amnestic attacks), morning headaches, personality changes, sexual dysfunction, intermittent nocturnal enuresis, and a generally depressed outlook. Although many patients with OSA are moderately overweight, morbid obesity is present only in the minority. Large neck circumference is frequently observed (>16 inches in females and >17 inches in males). Abnormal development of the mandible in the form of micro- and retrognathia, a crowded upper airway because of a voluminous tongue, a large uvula, enlarged tonsils, evidence of hypothyroidism, hypertension, erythrocytosis, sleep-related arrhythmias, and congestive heart failure may be noted. Waking respiratory function is usually within normal limits. Hypertension has been reported in 48–96% in patients with OSA. Alveolar hypoventilation, associated with an elevated waking $Paco_2$, occasionally accompanies OSA. An increased $Paco_2$ of 45 mm Hg or higher has been reported in 23% of obese patients with OSA. Typically, marked cyclic sinus arrhythmia appears during sleep apnea. This rhythm pattern is characterized by progressive sinus bradycardia during apnea (heart rates of less than 30 beats/minute are not uncommon) with an abrupt reversal and sinus tachycardia at the onset of ventilation. The latter is due to an arousal and a surge of catecholamines. Second-degree atrioventricular (AV) block, prolonged sinus pauses, limited runs of ventricular tachycardia, and paroxysmal atrial tachycardia episodes also occur. Furthermore, systemic and pulmonary artery pressures rise in association with each obstructive apnea. When episodes of apnea occur in rapid succession, pressures do not return to baseline but show a stepwise increase. About 22–30% of patients with systemic hypertension were found to suffer from OSA. In large-scale studies, presence of OSA is a known, independent risk factor for systemic hypertension.

Risk factors for development of sleep apnea are age, male gender, anatomic abnormalities of the upper airway, family history of snoring and sleep apnea, history of smoking, and alcohol or sedative use. All apneas are more frequent with increasing age and following alcohol or sedative drug intake. A suspected diagnosis of sleep apnea is confirmed by polysomnography (Table 10.3).

Central sleep apnea is not a single disease entity, but may result from any one of a number of processes that produce instability of respiratory control. In contrast to patients with OSA, patients affected predominantly by central sleep apnea are older, primarily complain of sleep fragmentation (i.e., insomnia), are not overweight, and have less pronounced oxygen desaturation and a more moderate hemodynamic impact. There is no definite gender distribution. Central apnea in the Cheyne-Stokes pattern may complicate congestive heart failure (CHF), and, if present, worsens prognosis in CHF. Coexistence of obstructive and central apnea, with an "appearance" of central apneas upon control of obstructive events by therapy has recently been termed "complex sleep apnea."

Upper airway patency does not need to be fully compromised for symptoms of daytime sleepiness to occur. The upper airway resistance syndrome is accompanied by subjective and objective evidence of pathologic daytime sleepiness. In some people, even a minor reduction of airway patency with sleep onset may lead to a modest increase in upper airway resistance and a slight drop of tidal volume without hypoxemia. In response to increased resistance, inspiratory muscles increase their effort to maintain normal tidal volume. Compensatory increased respiratory effort usually triggers a brief EEG arousal (3–14 seconds in duration), interrupting further development of obstruction before oxygen desaturation occurs. If the α EEG arousals are frequent, clinically significant daytime sleepiness may result. Snoring is noted in most, but not all, of these individuals.

Both central apnea and OSA can be complications of other medical or neurologic disorders. These include brainstem infarction, bulbar poliomyelitis, medullary neoplasms, syringomyelia and syringobulbia, olivopontocerebellar atrophy, Alzheimer disease, encephalitides, Creutzfeldt-Jakob disease, postencephalitic parkinsonism, cervical cordotomy, neuromuscular disorders affecting the intercostal muscles and diaphragm (e.g., myasthenia gravis), higher cervical spinal poliomyelitis, Guillain–Barré syndrome, limb-girdle dystrophies, and especially myotonic dystrophy. Hypoventilation and daytime sleepiness are prominent in all of these disorders. Predominantly, OSA may result from enlarged tonsils (an especially important factor in the etiology of sleep apnea and snoring in children); myxedema; micrognathia and other facial or mandibular abnormalities; platybasia; neck infiltration secondary to Hodgkin disease, lymphoma, or radiation therapy; acromegaly; and familial or acquired dysautonomia (usually mixed central and OSA).

An evaluation of the patient suspected of having sleep apnea syndrome includes a history from the patient and (most importantly) their bed partner. Physical examination should concentrate on blood pressure, evidence of right heart failure, nasal and pharyngeal abnormalities, as well as abnormal facial, neck, and skeletal or muscle configuration and function. Pulmonary function studies may be necessary to identify primary hypoventilation during the waking state and to evaluate responsiveness to carbon dioxide (CO_2). Chest radiographs and electrocardiograms are useful in evaluating pulmonary hypertension, determining the status of the right and left ventricles, and establishing the coexistence of other cardiopulmonary disorders. A hemogram will document the presence of polycythemia. In selected patients, thyroid studies are necessary to rule out hypothyroidism.

Table 10.3 Obstructive sleep apnea

Discriminating features
▶ Cessation or 70% reduction in airflow due to pharyngeal collapse lasting for at least 10 seconds

Consistent features
▶ Snoring
▶ Sinus bradycardia during apnea with acceleration at the onset of ventilation
▶ Daytime sleepiness and fatigue
▶ Increased frequency of apneas with age and alcohol or sedative drugs
▶ Normal waking respiratory functions

Variable features
▶ Morbid obesity
▶ Associated atrial and ventricular arrhythmias
▶ Associated hypertension
▶ Morning headaches
▶ Deterioration of memory and judgment
▶ Nocturnal hyperhidrosis

The initial medical workup should be followed by an all-night polysomnographic study, which is essential for an accurate diagnosis and an estimation of the severity of oxygen desaturations. The severity of sleep apnea and the presence of significant arrhythmias will be derived from the sleep study and will guide future treatment. The severity of sleep apnea is defined by the number of episodes per hour of sleep (the apnea-hypopnea index [AHI] or respiratory disturbance index [RDI]), and the degree of oxygen desaturations (the oxygen desaturation index, lowest oxygen saturation, and percentage of time in bed [TIB] occupied by a particular range of oxygen saturation).

Treatment of sleep apnea. The treatment of sleep apnea syndromes depends on the associated abnormality, which must be defined before it can be treated. An important general treatment is weight loss. Weight loss is the only potentially curative measure, provided weight loss is not only achieved, but maintained. Abstinence from alcohol and avoidance of sedative-hypnotic drugs should be encouraged.

Pharmacologic approaches, including acetazolamide, theophylline, naloxone, medroxyprogesterone, and clomipramine have not been studied systematically on a large number of subjects. Protriptyline may exert a beneficial effect in an occasional patient with OSA. Its effect may be due to a reported direct action on the muscle tone of the upper airway. A recent crossover unblinded trial of protriptyline and fluoxetine suggested equal effectiveness of the two drugs, with about 30–50% of patients showing improved oxygenation during sleep. Similar results have been reported with mirtazapine.

A number of studies suggest that the administration of oxygen may be a useful method of treating central sleep apnea, although the mechanism by which it reduces central apneic events has not been established. It is hypothesized that the potential destabilizing influence of the hypoxic ventilatory response on respiratory control may in fact be counteracted by the administration of oxygen. However, in some cases, hypercapnia and the frequency of the OSA may increase.

The most widely used treatment of OSA is nasal continuous positive airway pressure (CPAP), which acts by establishing a "pneumatic splint" to the upper airway. Nasal CPAP causes elevation of the intraluminal pressure in the oropharynx, thus reversing the transmural pressure gradient across the oropharyngeal airway. Nasal CPAP is the only treatment as effective in controlling apnea as tracheostomy. The major reasons for occasional CPAP failure are poor compliance due to nasal obstruction or psychosocial or cosmetic reasons. Some patients whose apneas are eliminated with CPAP continue to have non-apneic desaturations, especially during REM sleep. Usually, these patients are obese, with chronic obstructive pulmonary disease (COPD) in addition to sleep apnea. In

such situations, supplemental oxygen may be beneficial. The benefits derived from oxygen treatment should be polysomnographically verified.

Bilevel positive airway pressure–spontaneous (BPAP-S) offers an effective alternative to patients who are uncomfortable while expiring against the high pressures delivered by CPAP. This device allows independent titration of expiratory and inspiratory airway pressure and has been very helpful in conditions associated with hypoventilation such as comorbid obesity, intrinsic lung disease, and chest deformity.

Several modes of PAP therapy are available for patients requiring ventilatory support for hypoventilation (neuromuscular diseases) or central sleep apnea (periodic breathing, central apnea syndrome, complex sleep apnea). Bilevel positive airway pressure–spontaneous-timed (BPAP-ST) or adapt-servo ventilation can be used with success for these conditions.

Sometimes correction of nasal obstruction can result in significant reduction of sleep apneas. Adenoidectomy, tonsillectomy, and surgical correction of maxillofacial anomalies may abolish or significantly reduce the number of apneas. Patients with serious mandibular deformities can undergo surgical procedures of maxillary, mandibular, and hyoid bone advancements, but a significant number of failures occur, primarily in patients with the most severe mandibular deficiencies.

Attempts to promote uvulopalatopharyngoplasty (UPPP) as an alternative surgical treatment of sleep apnea have not been successful. Multiple studies indicate at best a variable success rate, ranging from 33 to 70%. More encouraging are results of trials of UPPP as a treatment for snoring. A 75–100% success rate in elimination of snoring has been reported. Cessation of snoring is not surprising, since the structures generating the sounds of snoring are surgically removed. However, if apneas are also present, they may persist despite the disappearance of snoring.

Laser-assisted uvulopalatoplasty (LAUP) involves partial resection of the uvula and soft palate using a laser. LAUP is a simple surgical procedure that does not require anesthesia and can be done on an outpatient basis in two to seven sessions. It seems to be highly effective in eliminating habitual snoring, with success rates of 70–84%. However, it is not recommended for treatment of sleep apnea.

Surgical procedures comprise bypass surgery (tracheostomy); *upper airway reconstructions—soft tissue modifications* (uvulopalatopharyngoplasty, laser-assisted uvulopalatoplasty, somnoplasty, placement of plastic rods in the soft palate, radio frequency volumetric reduction of the tongue, laser-assisted lingual resection, tongue base suspension, tonsillectomy, and adenoidectomy) and *upper airway reconstructions-skeletal modifications* (mandibular osteotomy with genioglossal advancement and hyoid suspension, maxillomandibular osteotomy and advancement, hyoid myotomy and suspension to mandible, hyoid myotomy and suspension to thyroid cartilage, anterior hyoid advancement, transpalatal advancement pharyngoplasty, and nasal surgery).

The use of prosthetic devices focuses on the nasopharyngeal inlet and the position of the base of the tongue. Several oral appliances have been shown to improve sleep apnea, but are generally recommended only for mild to moderate apneics. Even in these subgroups, their efficacy in controlling sleep apnea is in the range of 50–60%.

For some positional apneics, training them to sleep on their sides may produce an effective cure. Wearing a T-shirt with a sewn-in pocket in the back filled with tennis balls or an inflatable backpack may prevent patients from sleeping in the supine position.

An association between OSA and cardiovascular disease was recognized early. Several studies reported a significant correlation between blood pressure and the frequency of apneas and hypopneas. In contrast to the fall in blood pressure during NREM sleep in nonapneic individuals, blood pressure rises in patients with OSA. Obstructive sleep apnea can aggravate or precipitate myocardial ischemia in patients with coexisting coronary artery disease. Obstructive sleep apnea has been associated with higher prevalence of arrhythmias, including atrial fibrillation; stroke; and coronary artery disease.

Positive effects of CPAP in patients with OSA on cardiovascular outcomes are widely accepted, although less well supported by clinical studies. Elimination of OSA by CPAP for 1 month led to dramatic improvements in the left ventricular ejection fraction and cardiac functional status of patients with idiopathic dilated cardiomyopathy and congestive heart failure. Compliance with CPAP treatment might be an essential factor determining the success rate. Nocturnal CPAP treatment of Cheyne-Stokes respiration in patients with congestive heart failure led to significant improvements in cardiac function and quality of life, but had no effect on their survival. The effect of newer treatment modalities on survival of central sleep apnea patients is unknown.

Polysomnography should be considered an integral part of the diagnostic evaluation of patients with cardiovascular disease, because treatment of concomitant sleep-disordered breathing with CPAP can lead to an improvement in cardiovascular function, particularly in patients with congestive heart failure.

Narcolepsy

Narcolepsy is a syndrome consisting of excessive daytime sleepiness and abnormal manifestations of REM sleep (Table 10.4). The latter includes frequent sleep-onset REM periods, which may be subjectively appreciated as hypnagogic hallucinations, and dissociated REM sleep inhibitory processes, such as cataplexy and sleep paralysis.

The cardinal symptoms of narcolepsy include excessive daytime sleepiness, sleep attacks, and cataplexy. Ex-

---

Table 10.4 Narcolepsy

Discriminating features

▸ History of excessive daytime sleepiness, sleep attacks, cataplexy, and other auxiliary symptoms

▸ Mean sleep latency of ≤5 minutes on Multiple Sleep Latency Test (MSLT)

▸ Two or more REM sleep onsets on MSLT

▸ Dreaming during the naps

Consistent features

▸ Daytime sleep attacks lasting about 15 minutes

▸ Patient awakens refreshed

▸ Autosomal dominant inheritance with variable penetration

▸ Low cerebrospinal fluid hypocretin-1 levels in narcolepsy with cataplexy

Variable features

▸ Associated cataplectic attacks with abrupt loss of muscle tone initiated by emotion

▸ Sleep paralysis usually accompanied by intense fear

▸ Hypnagogic hallucinations

▸ Fragmented nocturnal sleep

▸ Association with HLA types DR2 and DQ1

▸ Appearance of REM sleep within 20 minutes of nocturnal sleep onset

---

cessive sleepiness may manifest as a permanent impairment of vigilance that can be profound between attacks. Sleep attacks usually last about 15 minutes. The patient awakens refreshed and there is a definite refractory period of 1–5 hours before the next attack in some patients. Cataplexy is a sudden reduction or abrupt loss of muscle tone that is either generalized or limited to particular muscle groups. Cataplexy ranges from weakness in the muscles supporting the jaw, or a sense of weakness in the knees, to a complete muscular weakness causing the patient to slump to the floor, unable to move. Cataplectic attacks are characteristically initiated by laughter, surprise, outbursts of anger, or a feeling of exaltation. These attacks can last anywhere from several seconds to as long as 30 minutes.

Auxiliary symptoms of narcolepsy include sleep paralysis, which occurs while the patient is falling asleep or waking from sleep. Consciousness is preserved and the episode is usually accompanied by intense fear. Hypnagogic or hypnopompic hallucinations also occur at the onset of sleep or on awakening, respectively, and are usually frightening. Automatic behavior, sometimes reported as "blackouts," is a reflection of severe sleepiness. Nocturnal sleep is also disturbed with frequent awakenings, frequent sleep-onset REM periods, and vivid dreams. The combination of excessive daytime sleepiness and cataplexy is pathognomonic for narcolepsy.

Diagnosis of narcolepsy is based on (a) a history of excessive daytime sleepiness, sleep attacks, cataplexy, and other auxiliary symptoms; (b) objective documentation of pathological sleepiness by the Multiple Sleep Latency Test (MSLT) showing a mean sleep latency of 5 minutes or less; (c) two or more sleep-onset REM periods documented by the MSLT; and (d) nocturnal REM latency shorter than 20 minutes.

Narcolepsy is familial, and transmission seems to follow an autosomal dominant inheritance pattern with variable penetrance. Narcolepsy is also strongly associated with human leukocyte antigens (HLAs) DR2 and DQ1. The usefulness of HLA typing in clinical practice is limited by the fact that up to 30% (depending on ethnic group) of asymptomatic people are also DR2-positive (DR15-positive according to more recent HLA nosology). More recent studies have further demonstrated that HLA DR2 is not the best HLA marker for narcolepsy, especially in the African-American population, since some 30% of African-American narcoleptics are DR2 negative. It now appears that susceptibility to narcolepsy might be related more to the DQ region than to the DR region. A specific HLA DQ1 subtype (DQB1*0602) appears to be a better marker for both Caucasian and African-American patients. It is found in 95–98% of all narcoleptic patients with cataplexy in all ethnic groups. DQB1*0602 may represent a genetic marker for the disorder, indicating possible presence of a "narcolepsy-susceptibility" gene on chromosome 6. If a patient is DR2-negative, a request for DQB1*0602 typing may help support the diagnosis. A negative test for DQB1*0602 does not rule out a diagnosis of narcolepsy, however. Only 8–10% of narcoleptics are aware of another member of the family with narcolepsy/cataplexy. Prevalence studies have shown that the risk for a first-degree relative to develop narcolepsy/cataplexy is 1–2%. This risk, although low, is 10–40 times higher than the risk observed in the general population. Twin studies, however, have demonstrated only 25–31% concordance for narcolepsy in monozygotic twins. Thus, although genetic factors may define susceptibility, other (perhaps environmental) factors may trigger disease onset.

A crucial role for the hypocretin (orexin) system in the genesis of narcolepsy was suggested by the discovery of a mutation in the hypocretin-2 receptor gene in a canine model of narcolepsy. Almost simultaneously, a mouse model of narcolepsy was described in the homozygous preprohypocretin (the precursor to two neuropeptides: hypocretin-1 and hypocretin-2) knock-out mouse.

Both discoveries prompted intense research in humans. Hypocretin-containing neurons are localized in the dorsolateral hypothalamus around the perifornical nucleus. These cells project widely to the entire brain, including the cerebral cortex, basal forebrain structures such as the diagonal band of Broca, the amygdala, and brainstem areas such as reticular formation, raphe nuclei, and locus ceruleus.

Hypocretin deficiency seems to be involved in the pathogenesis of narcolepsy. The cerebrospinal fluid (CSF) content of hypocretin-1 (hcrt-1) is very low in narcolepsy patients with cataplexy. Neuropathologic studies have demonstrated absent hcrt-1 and hcrt-2 in the brains of narcoleptic patients compared to controls, in addition to increased numbers of astrocytes in the hypothalamus, suggestive of neuronal degeneration there.

Treatment of narcolepsy. Treatment of narcolepsy focuses on the two most disabling symptoms of narcolepsy: excessive daytime sleepiness/sleep attacks and cataplexy. In rare patients, successful treatment is achieved by improved sleep hygiene: obtaining adequate sleep at night, regulating sleep phase, maintaining a regular daily schedule of bedtime and rising time, and therapeutic naps. Most patients, however, will need stimulants in addition to good sleep hygiene and scheduled naps. Stimulants primarily include dextroamphetamine (Dexedrine) and methylphenidate (Ritalin). Stimulants are likely to reduce but not eliminate excessive daytime sleepiness and performance deficits. Methamphetamine (Desoxyn) in doses higher than those recommended for treatment of obesity was found to almost normalize sleepiness and performance in eight subjects studied, but its use is rare due to concerns about abuse and related adverse behaviors. Side effects and the potential for development of dependence often limit the use of stimulants. Dose-related, clinically significant side effects include irritability, agitation, headache, and peripheral sympathetic stimulation. A novel wake-promoting agent, modafinil (Provigil) is usually grouped with the stimulants, but seems to have a different mechanism of action, not fully understood at present. Unlike amphetamines and methylphenidate, modafinil does not appear to significantly alter the release of dopamine and noradrenaline. Although it does not stimulate the release of noradrenaline directly, it does require an intact -adrenergic system for its stimulant effect to occur. The advantage of modafinil over other stimulants is the lower frequency and severity of side effects (especially irritability and agitation), although headache may emerge if rapidly titrated. Mazindol (Sanorex or Mazanor), an anorectic imidazoline derivative with pharmacologic activity resembling the amphetamines, and selegiline (Eldepryl), a monoamine oxidase (MAO)-B inhibitor that is converted to L-amphetamine, improve daytime alertness and may have fewer side effects than amphetamines, but neither has been shown to be more effective than amphetamines in treating narcolepsy. This long list of stimulants has been recently supplemented by a medication with a completely different mechanism of action: sodium oxybate (Xyrem). This compound has been shown to markedly decrease the frequency of cataplexy and significantly reduce daytime sleepiness. Sodium oxybate has a short half-life and has to be given twice at night. In spite of this cumbersome dosing schedule, it is now considered a treatment of choice in cataplexy.

In addition to sodium oxybate, tricyclic antidepressants can also effectively treat cataplexy. Cataplectic attacks respond to imipramine (Tofranil), nortriptyline (Pamelor), and protriptyline (Vivactil). One of the most effective drugs for treatment of cataplexy is clomipramine (Anafranil), a potent serotonin reuptake inhibitor. Side effects of tricyclics, due primarily to their anticholinergic properties, may limit their use in some patients. The most frequent side effects are dry mouth, increased sweating, sexual dysfunction (impotence, delayed orgasm, erectile and ejaculatory dysfunction), weight gain, tachycardia, constipation, blurred vision, and urinary retention. Sudden discontinuation of tricyclics is likely to result in severe worsening of cataplexy, even occasionally status cataplecticus. Newer antidepressants with more exclusive inhibition of serotonin uptake (fluoxetine [Prozac], paroxetine [Paxil], and sertraline [Zoloft]) can also be useful in the management of cataplexy, with fewer anticholinergic side effects. The anticataplectic effects of these drugs most likely related to their desmethyl metabolites, which are potent noradrenaline reuptake inhibitors.

▼

Pearls and Perils

Sleep disorders

▶ Evaluation of a patient presenting with complaints of a sleep disorder relies not only on the patient's history, but also on that of their bed partner.

▶ Chronic insomnia is a symptom of a variety of psychiatric, psychological, medical, neurologic, and circadian rhythm sleep disorders.

▶ Multiple factors may contribute to sleep disorders.

▶ Insomnia resistant to a combination of behavioral and pharmacologic interventions may require all-night polysomnography to identify a possible primary sleep disorder.

▶ Obstruction of the upper airway varies in severity from primary snoring, to upper airway resistance syndrome, to obstructive sleep apnea characterized by repetitive partial or complete occlusions of the upper airway, with desaturations and arousals.

▶ Obesity, hypertension, a large neck circumference, and reduced dimensions of the oropharynx frequently accompany the sleep apnea syndrome.

▶ Sleep apnea and insufficient sleep are leading causes of daytime sleepiness.

▶ Insufficient sleep should not be neglected in the differential diagnosis of a sleep disorder associated with excessive daytime sleepiness.

Patients refractory to other treatments may benefit from monoamine oxidase (MAO) inhibitors.

Idiopathic CNS hypersomnia is a condition resembling narcolepsy, but without sleep-onset REM periods, cataplexy, or auxiliary symptoms. Treatment with stimulants is usually less effective.

Insufficient sleep

Insufficient sleep is a frequent cause of daytime somnolence. The individual is voluntarily, but often unwittingly, chronically sleep deprived. Although this relation may seem self-evident, most of the patients are unaware that their chronic sleep deprivation is responsible for their continuous excessive sleepiness. When these individuals obtain adequate sleep, their complaint of somnolence during the day disappears.

Various other medical and medicinal causes of excessive daytime somnolence deserve mention. Sedative-hypnotics, anticonvulsants, antihypertensives, antihistamines, and antidepressants are common causes. Withdrawal from stimulants may also give rise to severe sleepiness. Multiple medical and toxic conditions may be associated with drowsiness, such as hyperglycemia (prior to ketoacidosis or nonketotic coma), hypocorticalism, hypoglycemia, hypothyroidism, panhypopituitarism, hepatic encephalopathy, hypercalcemia, renal insufficiency, vitamin B^{12} deficiency, chronic subdural hematoma, encephalitis, intracranial neoplasm, meningitis, or head trauma. *Hypersomnolence* is a misnomer in many of these conditions, since more often a state of obtundation occurs.

There are also two rare periodic disorders of excessive sleepiness. *Kleine-Levin syndrome* is characterized by recurrent periods of extended sleep, megaphagia, sexual disinhibitions, and social withdrawal if awake. *Menstruation-associated hypersomnia* is a period of sleepiness during a patient's menstrual period. No other changes in behavior are observed with this syndrome.

Parasomnias

Parasomnias include a heterogeneous group of behavioral disturbances that occur only during sleep or are exacerbated by sleep. They do not have a common pathophysiologic mechanism. They represent disorders of arousal, partial arousal, and sleep stage transitions. Disorders of arousal include confusional arousals, sleepwalking, and sleep terrors, which arise from NREM sleep (usually δ sleep), and are prevalent in childhood. Disorders of arousal start with a confusional arousal from sleep. Such arousals are characterized by confusion, disorientation in time and space, and slow speech and mentation. They occur usually in children and may progress into sleepwalking (somnambulism) or sleep terror (*pavor nocturnus, incubus*). Typically, there is very little if any recall for the event the following morning, and minimal if any recall of dream-like mentation. Most somnambulistic episodes last a few seconds to a few minutes.

A sleep terror is an arousal from NREM sleep accompanied by a piercing scream or cry and behavioral manifestations of intense anxiety indicating autonomic arousal. Autonomic manifestations include mydriasis, perspiration, piloerection, rapid breathing, and tachycardia. Morning amnesia for the episode is the rule. There is often a concurrence of more than one of these disorders in the same child, and a hereditary predisposition to parasomnias has been noted. Several factors contribute to the occurrence of disorders of arousal including predisposing factors (genetic factors), increased amounts of sleep or difficulty awakening (age, recovery from prior sleep deprivation, fever, CNS depressant drugs), and sleep fragmentation–triggering factors (pain, environmental stimuli, stimulants, stress). Somnambulism and/or sleep terrors in children are not considered to be caused by psychological factors, although persistence into adulthood or new onset in adulthood may be associated with diverse forms of personality disturbance and psychopathology. Most children grow out of this condition between the ages of 7 and 14 years.

It is important to protect patients against injury by installing safety rails at the head of stairways, and by placing locks on windows. If predisposing (and especially triggering) factors are identified, every effort should be made to minimize or avoid them. Many patients respond to benzodiazepines before sleep. Tricyclic drugs, such as imipramine, desipramine, and clomipramine, may also be effective.

Sleep-related *enuresis* is involuntary micturition beginning usually during deep NREM sleep in an individual who has or should have gained voluntary waking control of the bladder. In contrast to this idiopathic nocturnal enuresis, symptomatic enuresis is due to urogenital or other diseases and is generally less benign. Idiopathic enuresis and somnambulism/sleep terrors tend to disappear by late childhood or adolescence, and probably represent a phenomenon of delayed maturation. At 5 years of age, 15% of boys and 10% of girls are still enuretic. With regard to treatment, tricyclic antidepressants, specifically imipramine (Tofranil) 10–25 mg at bedtime are valuable, as are daytime "bladder exercises" aimed at increasing bladder capacity. Oxybutynin chloride (Ditropan) has been used with variable success. Intranasal desamino-d-arginine vasopressin (DDAVP, Desmopressin) at low doses has been shown to have a definite effect, especially in adults and children over the age of 9 years. Conditioning with a buzzer and pad is the most successful modality of treatment for the enuresis, but success may not be maintained when the buzzer is discontinued.

Nightmares are due to an arousal from REM sleep with the recall of a disturbing dream, accompanied by anxiety and much less prominent autonomic arousal. The awakened patient is momentarily oriented and alert. Vocalization, fear, and motor activity are less intense than in sleep terrors. Nightmares are likely to occur in the second half of the night, when more prolonged REM episodes are likely to occur. Withdrawal from alcohol, amphetamines, or hypnotics at the time of the REM rebound is frequently a cause of nightmares.

REM sleep behavior disorder (RBD) is a parasomnia characterized by vigorous motor activity (instead of atonia) in response to dream content. Manifestations of acting out dreams include laughing, talking, chanting, singing, yelling, swearing, gesturing, reaching, grabbing, arm flailing, punching, kicking, sitting up, jumping out of bed, crawling, and running movements. Not surprisingly, RBD can result in injury. One-third of people with RBD have a demonstrable underlying neurologic disorder. These include degenerative (e.g., amyotrophic lateral sclerosis, Parkinson disease, progressive supranuclear palsy, multiple system atrophy, olivopontocerebellar degeneration), developmental/congenital/familial (narcolepsy, Tourette syndrome, fatal familial insomnia), vascular (subarachnoid hemorrhage, vasculitis, ischemia), neoplastic (acoustic neuromas, pontine neoplasms), and postinfectious (Guillain–Barré syndrome) disorders. Acute RBD can result from drug intoxications (tricyclic antidepressants, monoamine oxidase inhibitors) or from drug withdrawal (butalbital, meprobamate, pentazocine, nitrazepam). Drugs may be associated with a chronic form of RBD as well (tricyclic antidepressants, fluoxetine, venlafaxine, mirtazapine, selegiline, anticholinergics). Most of the cases are, however, idiopathic and tend to occur in the elderly. Clonazepam (Klonopin) is the drug of

Key Clinical Questions

▶ What is the patient's sleep/wake schedule like? Poor sleep hygiene or a pattern of significant rebound sleep on weekends is likely to contribute to a patient's symptoms of either insomnia or hypersomnolence.

▶ What is the patient's sleep pattern like on vacation? This will provide the examiner with an estimate of the individual patient's need for sleep and its timing.

▶ Does the patient have a bed partner? The history is markedly enhanced and validated by a collateral source of information.

▶ How does the patient function during the day? Both insomnia and hypersomnolence will adversely affect daytime mood, performance at work, and social interactions.

▶ Is there any family history of similar symptoms? Many sleep disorders or predispositions for them run in families: restless legs, snoring, narcolepsy, parasomnias, etc.

Consider Consultation When...

▶ Signs and symptoms of sleep apnea (e.g., loud snoring, observed respiratory pauses, and excessive daytime sleepiness) are reported by the patient or the patient's bed partner.

▶ The apneic patient continues to report excessive daytime sleepiness after being given appropriate treatment (e.g., CPAP, surgery, or dental appliance), or following a period of satisfactory control of sleepiness becomes very sleepy again or starts snoring.

▶ Surgical treatment for snoring or sleep apnea is considered. Surgery usually eliminates or markedly reduces snoring, but may allow (inapparent) sleep apnea to persist.

▶ A patient with chronic obstructive pulmonary disease complains of insomnia or excessive daytime somnolence.

▶ Signs and symptoms of narcolepsy are present, including excessive daytime somnolence, refreshing sleep attacks, cataplexy, sleep paralysis, hypnagogic hallucinations, and vivid dreams.

▶ A narcoleptic patient becomes refractory to prescribed stimulants, or reports worsening of sleepiness.

▶ Signs and symptoms of restless legs syndrome with periodic limb movement disorder interfere with the patient's ability to function adequately during the day and fall asleep at night.

▶ A patient reports symptoms of sleep–wake schedule disorder (e.g., disorganized timing and variable duration of sleep and waking episodes) or complains of inability to fall asleep and wake up spontaneously at the desired times.

▶ Chronic insomnia does not respond to either simple behavioral modifications (improved sleep hygiene) or short courses of pharmacotherapy.

▶ A patient presents with a complaint of violent or injurious behavior during sleep, suggesting a diagnosis of REM sleep behavior disorder.

▶ It is not clear whether nocturnal behaviors are epileptic or nonepileptic (parasomnias).

choice for treatment of RBD (initial dose 0.5–1.0 mg). Anecdotal reports also suggest effectiveness of compounds such as desipramine, levodopa, clonidine, L-tryptophan, gabapentin, MAO inhibitors, and melatonin.

The pathophysiology of RBD has not yet been fully elucidated. One hypothesis is that RBD results from injury to the pedunculopontine nucleus (PPN) or from abnormal afferent signals in the basal ganglia transmitted via the pallidotegmental tracts. Single-photon emission tomography imaging demonstrates significantly reduced striatal dopamine uptake in RBD patients. Positron emission tomography imaging shows reduced striatal dihydrotetrabenazine binding, indicating loss of dopaminergic midbrain neurons.

Parasomnias also include cluster headaches and the related (but more chronic) condition of paroxysmal hemicrania. Cluster headaches occur in REM sleep and may be related to increased cerebral blood flow. Cataphrenia (nocturnal groaning) and exploding head syndrome are less frequent parasomnias.

Sleep-related eating disorders may occur in patients with OSA, somnambulism, eating disorders, medication abuse, or in isolation. They are characterized by almost nightly eating episodes during which most patients are only partially conscious. Two-thirds of patients are women who are generally concerned about the weight gain. Daytime binge eating or obsessive-compulsive disorder is absent. Treatments include clonazepam (Klonopin), L-dopa/carbidopa (Sinemet), and fluoxetine (Prozac). Case series associated sleep-related eating are reported with use of certain medications, including zolpidem (Ambien).

About 45% of patients with seizure disorders have seizures primarily during sleep. Generalized seizures are markedly activated by NREM sleep, especially stages N1 and N2. Partial seizures may occur during NREM and REM sleep. Prolonged EEG monitoring may be necessary in some difficult cases, in which it is necessary to distinguish epileptic from nonepileptic episodic behavior.

Other parasomnias that may occur in childhood as well as in adulthood include head banging (jactatio capitis nocturna), abnormal swallowing, and painful penile erections. Whether these conditions require a polysomnographic evaluation and treatment depends entirely on the persistence of the symptoms and the degree of the patient's disability. Bruxism affects up to 15% of children. This condition may contribute to periodontal disease and temporomandibular joint dysfunction.

Annotated Bibliography

American Academy of Sleep Medicine. *International Classification of Sleep Disorders–2 (ICSD-2)*. Author, 2006.

Bradley TD, Logan AG, Kimoff RJ, et al. Continuous positive airway pressure for central sleep apnea and heart failure. *N Engl J Med* 2005;353(19):2025–2033.
Large scale trial of application of CPAP in patients with central sleep apnea.

Hauri P, Linde S. *No more sleepless nights*, 2nd ed. New York: John Wiley and Sons, 1996.
Excellent "consumer-level" resource for insomnia sufferers.

Kryger MH, Roth T, Dement WC. *Principles and practice of sleep medicine*, 2nd ed. Philadelphia: WB Saunders, 2000.
This book is an invaluable resource covering fundamental as well as clinical aspects of sleep medicine. It is organized in sections covering a broad range of issues from characteristics

of normal sleep to sleep breathing disorders. References are abundant and appropriate.

Littner MR, Kushida C, McDowell Anderson W, et al. Practice parameters for the dopaminergic treatment of restless legs syndrome and periodic limb movement disorder. An American Academy of Sleep Medicine Report. Standards of Practice Committee of the American Academy of Sleep Medicine. *Sleep* 2004;27(3):557–559.

Morgenthaler TI, Kapur VK, Brown TM, et al. Standards of Practice Committee of the AASM. Practice parameters for the treatment of narcolepsy and other hypersomnias of central origin. *Sleep* 2007;30(12):1705–1711.

Morgenthaler T, Kramer M, Alessi C, et al. Practice parameters for the psychological and behavioral treatment of insomnia: An update. An American Academy of Sleep Medicine report. *Sleep* 2006;29(11):1415–1419.

Morin CM. *Insomnia, psychological assessment and management.* New York: The Guilford Press, 1993.
This book represents a clear and well-organized review of the problem of insomnia and a scientifically validated treatment approach.

Morin CM, Bootzin RR, Buysse DJ, et al. Psychological and behavioral treatment of insomnia: Update of the recent evidence (1998–2004). *Sleep* 2006;29(11):1398–1414.
This is an updated summary of behavioral treatments of insomnia.

Parish JM, Somers VK. Obstructive sleep apnea and cardiovascular disease. *Mayo Clin Proc* 2004;79(8):1036–1046.
Thorough review on cardiovascular consequences of obstructive sleep apnea.

Silber MH. Chronic insomnia. *N Engl J Med* 2005;353:803–810.
Excellent and concise review for a practitioner caring for patients with insomnia, with discussion of medical and psychological aspects of treatment.

Taheri S, Zeitzer JM, Mignot E. The role of hypocretins (orexins) in sleep regulation and narcolepsy. *Ann Rev Neurosci* 2002;25:282–313.
This article reviews the role of the hypothalamus in the regulation of sleep; the discovery of hypocretins; clinical aspects of narcolepsy including epidemiology, symptoms, genetics, diagnosis, and treatment; animal models of narcolepsy; hypocretin deficiency in human narcolepsy; the role of hypocretins in normal sleep and arousal; and other biologic functions of hypocretins.

Acute Confusional States

Douglas J. Lanska

Definition and Importance

A confusional state is an acquired mental disorder characterized by cardinal deficits in attention and coherence of thought and action, and is often associated with an altered level of arousal, global cognitive dysfunction affecting multiple cognitive domains, perceptual disturbances, sleep–wake cycle disruption, affective disturbances, and emotional lability. Acute confusional states typically develop over a short period of time, generally hours to days. The disturbances fluctuate during the day and are typically worse at night. Acute confusional states are usually reversible if the underlying cause can be identified and adequately treated (Table 11.1).

Acute confusional states are very common: 10–25% of patients on acute medical and surgical wards have acute confusional states. These patients typically have markedly prolonged hospital stays, frequent associated complications, much higher in-hospital and post-hospital mortality rates, and higher medical care costs. Acute confusional states greatly increase the risk of seizures, decubitus ulcers, deep venous thromboses, aspiration pneumonia, fractures and subdural hematomas from falls, and complications related to the inappropriate removal of intravenous (IV) lines, nasogastric tubes, endotracheal tubes, and arterial lines by agitated patients. In addition, in some studies, one-quarter to as many as three-quarters of elderly patients who developed confusional states in the hospital died during the hospitalization. Those who survived the hospitalization had a very high mortality rate in the months immediately after discharge. Moreover, some of the survivors had residual focal or diffuse brain injury.

Groups at high risk of developing confusional states include those who are elderly, demented, postsurgical, drug or alcohol abusers, those taking certain medications (including particularly anticholinergic and central nervous system (CNS) depressant medications), and those with preexisting brain damage, significant medical illness, or acquired immunodeficiency syndrome (AIDS). Additional factors that are important in postsurgical patients include the complexity of the surgical procedure, time on bypass for cardiac surgery, presence of hip fracture, severity of the postoperative illness, postoperative respiratory failure, serum levels of anticholinergic drugs, presence of electrolyte disturbances, decreased cardiac output, tobacco exposure, and nutritional status as measured by serum albumin levels.

Clinical Features

Two major categories of acute confusional states are recognized: lethargic (hypokinetic) confusional states and delirium or agitated (hyperkinetic) confusional states (Table 11.2). Patients with lethargic confusional states are typically somnolent, apathetic, and quietly confused. The confusional state in such patients is often unrecognized, or these patients are thought to be depressed or uncooperative. Misdiagnosis leads to further morbidity and increases the risk of mortality, since the underlying causes of the confusional state remain untreated and, in addition, the frequent inappropriate administration of antidepressants with anticholinergic properties compounds

Table 11.1 Acute confusional states

Discriminating features

▶ Inattention with reduced ability to focus, sustain, or shift attention to external stimuli
▶ Loss of coherence of thought or action
▶ Dysfunction developed over a short period of time, generally hours to days
▶ Dysfunction fluctuates over the course of the day, and is often worse at night

Consistent features

▶ Altered level of consciousness, including lethargy or hyper-alertness
▶ Disorganized thinking, as indicated by rambling, irrelevant, or incoherent speech
▶ Disorientation to time and place
▶ Memory impairment, with difficulty learning new material or remembering past events
▶ Impaired language function, particularly naming difficulty (anomia) and writing impairment (agraphia)
▶ Perceptual disturbances, including illusions and hallucinations
▶ Disturbances of the sleep–wake cycle with daytime sleepiness or insomnia
▶ Affective disturbances and emotional lability
▶ Impaired judgment and impulse control

Variable features

▶ Onset may occur at any age
▶ Dysarthria
▶ Increased or decreased psychomotor activity
▶ Tremor, asterixis, or myoclonus
▶ Seizures
▶ Ataxia
▶ Autonomic disturbances
▶ Focal or lateralizing neurologic signs
▶ Abnormal cranial imaging
▶ Abnormal cerebrospinal fluid

Table 11.2 Differential features of hypokinetic and hyperkinetic acute confusional states)

	Hypokinetic	Hyperkinetic
Level of arousal	Alert or somnolent	Alert or hyperalert
Autonomic disturbances	No	Prominent*
Psychomotor activity	Decreased	Increased
Affect	Apathetic, dysphoric, or less commonly euphoric	Apprehensive or angry

* Note: Autonomic disturbances in hyperkinetic acute confusional states are typically those of adrenergic hyperactivity: tachycardia, hypertension, mydriasis, and tremor.

nificance (impaired vigilance) and yet are easily distracted by extraneous environmental stimuli (distractibility), and are often unable to inhibit irrelevant or inappropriate responses. As a result, confused patients are unaware of much that goes on around them and are unable to grasp their immediate situation. Their speech is often rambling, with abrupt shifts from topic to topic. Thinking is slow and incoherent. Skilled movement sequences also show signs of disintegration, impersistence, and perseveration, although fragments may be performed correctly.

Other common features of acute confusional states include alterations in level of arousal, disorientation, memory difficulty, language impairment, abnormal perceptions, disrupted sleep–wake cycles, affective disturbances and emotional lability, psychomotor abnormalities, abnormal adventitious movements and other motor disturbances, and reflex and tone changes.

It is a common misconception that confusional states are simply disorders of wakefulness and arousal, and certainly in their more severe forms confusional states may precede or follow stupor or coma. However, the mechanisms of wakefulness and attention do not overlap completely. Acutely confused patients may be fully alert and, especially in the early stages, attention is impaired out of proportion to any changes in level of arousal. Nevertheless, confused patients frequently do have alterations in level of arousal, which may vary from hyperalertness in delirious or hyperkinetic confusional states, to lethargy and somnolence in apathetic or hypokinetic confusional states.

To be oriented, patients must attend to environmental stimuli, update memory information on time and place, and reason appropriately. Such abilities are defective in confused patients. As a result, confused patients are typically, but not always, disorientated to time and are often disoriented to place. Confused patients, however, do not become disoriented to person. In addition, the ability to learn, that is to incorporate new information into short- or long-term memory, is impaired in confused patients, because the information to be learned cannot be attended to

the problem. In contrast, delirious or hyperkinetic confused patients are typically agitated and hypervigilant, have prominent psychomotor hyperactivity, and manifest signs of adrenergic hyperactivity (e.g., tachycardia, hypertension, dilated pupils, tremor). Agitation and hyperactivity may preclude a thorough evaluation of cognitive, neurologic, and general functions.

As already noted, the fundamental deficits in all types of acute confusional states are impaired attention and loss of coherence of thought and action. Confused patients are unable to grasp a normal amount of information in a short period of time (decreased attention span), have difficulty persisting at an activity (impaired perseverance, or impersistence) and yet may persist in thoughts or actions that are no longer appropriate (perseveration), are unable to monitor the environment for events of sig-

and registered in immediate or working memory in the first place. The memory defect involves inadequate perception or registration of information, rather than impairment of retentive memory. Thus, memory often improves if a confused patient is allowed sufficient drilling during the acquisition portion of a learning task. Confused patients are also susceptible to certain distortions of memory, or paramnesias. One common form of paramnesia in confused patients is reduplicative paramnesia or delusional misidentification. For example, confused patients commonly believe they are at home or some other familiar place, despite the obvious evidence to the contrary around them (reduplicative paramnesia for place). Less commonly, they may believe that an imposter has been substituted for someone they interact with, often a spouse (reduplicative paramnesia for person, or Capgras syndrome). If evidence to the contrary is presented to a confused and delusional patient, he may go to elaborate lengths to justify the conflicting information with fabricated explanations (confabulation). In this situation, the patient is not intentionally being deceptive, and has no insight or ability to comprehend that the confabulated material is not true.

In confused patients, fluency, grammar, and word choice of spoken language are generally essentially normal. Repetition and comprehension may be impaired, but are usually fairly normal when the material to be understood or repeated is within the span of attention. Both in spontaneous speech and confrontationally, confused patients may have naming difficulty (anomia) with word-finding pauses and paraphasic errors—that is, substituting one word for another, incorporating incorrect syllables into words, or creating entirely new word-like strings of meaningless syllables (neologisms). Confused patients may also involuntarily repeat words or syllables (palilalia). In addition, writing, even in mild cases, is often disturbed (agraphia): the writing may be scrawled in many different directions on the page with letters and words of various sizes and spacings, may incorporate many incorrect words and misspellings that make the writing incoherent, may contain sections consisting entirely of letters or portions of letters repeated incessantly, particularly those than contain multiple loops, or may contain omissions such as undotted "i"s and uncrossed "t"s.

Abnormal perceptions are common in acutely confused patients and may include illusions and hallucinations. Whereas illusions are the distortion or misinterpretation of an actual physical stimulus, hallucinations are unprovoked perceptual experiences, which occur in the mind in the absence of an external physical stimulus. Hallucinations in acute confusional states are typically visual or a combination of visual and auditory. Tactile (haptic) hallucinations occur less commonly, but are typical of delirium tremens and delirium secondary to anticholinergic (e.g., atropine) and some other drug toxicity (e.g., chloral or trichloroacetaldehyde). Tactile hallucinations are also seen commonly with either cocaine or amphetamine intoxication. Indeed, as many as 15% of regular cocaine users experience a variety of tactile hallucinations, often involving a sensation of small insects crawling on the skin (formication or colloquially "cocaine bugs"). Particularly with delirious states, hallucinations of any type may be terrifying and associated with paranoid delusions. Psychotic hallucinatory-delusional behavior may at times obscure the deficit in attention.

Confused patients frequently have disrupted sleep–wake cycles, typically with daytime somnolence and nighttime agitation. The confusional state varies throughout the day as well, being most pronounced in the evening or night (sundowning). Sleep disruption is both a manifestation of the confusional state and a contributor to it.

Affective disturbances are common in confused patients and include a wide spectrum of types and intensities. Categories of affective disturbances in confused patients may include anger, apprehension, apathy, dysphoria, or euphoria. Within each of these categories, patients may manifest a wide range of intensities, as for example, from irritability or hostility to anger to rage, from anxious or fearful to terrified or panicked, from dull to apathetic, from sad to despondent, and from happy to euphoric. These affective disturbances may fluctuate quickly in confusional states, for example, with irritability and excitability alternating with apathy, drowsiness, and diminished vigilance. Such patients are considered to be emotionally labile.

The patient's level of activity can vary tremendously from a marked motor restlessness (hyperactivity) to slowed and infrequent movements (bradykinesia and hypokinesia, respectively) to virtually no movement (akinesia). In addition to changes in psychomotor activity, confused patients may have a variety of motor disturbances including slurred speech (dysarthria), various adventitious movements (e.g., tremor, asterixis, and myoclonus), and incoordination (ataxia). The tremor associated with confusional states is generally a fine postural tremor, most prominent distally with sustained antigravity muscular activity, present throughout movements, not increased with proximity to a target, and not present at rest. Asterixis is an irregular asymmetric flapping movement of the limbs in which the flaps correspond to loss of muscular tone and sudden electrical silence in the muscles as assessed by electromyography. Asterixis was originally described in hepatic encephalopathy, but it may be seen in a wide variety of metabolic encephalopathies; occasionally, asterixis may be seen unilaterally with focal brain lesions. Myoclonus is a sudden, brief twitch of a muscle or group of muscles. Like asterixis, it is seen in a wide variety of metabolic encephalopathies. Multifocal myoclonus is particularly prominent with uremia, postanoxic states, and hypocalcemia. Ataxia is an inability to coordinate the muscles in the execution of voluntary movement. In confused patients, it is particularly common with intoxications and with various metabolic encephalopathies.

Accompanying the motor disturbances is a variety of reflex and tone changes. Lethargic confused patients typically have normal or decreased muscle tone and normal or decreased muscle stretch reflexes. In contrast, delirious patients may have variable hypertonicity and hyperreflexia, including clonus and bilateral Babinski signs. These "long tract signs" indicate dysfunction of corticospinal pathways, but do not necessarily indicate permanent structural damage. Indeed, they are fairly common in a variety of metabolic and toxic states, including hypocalcemia, hypomagnesemia, hepatic encephalopathy, and sedative withdrawal.

Causes

Confusional states are commonly associated with medical and surgical illness, intoxication and withdrawal states, and CNS disease. Some of the common causes of hypokinetic confusional states are shown in Box 11.1, and some of the common causes of hyperkinetic confusional states are shown in Box 11.2.

Medical and surgical illnesses associated with confusional states include metabolic disturbances, infections and fever, endocrine dysfunction, and cardiopulmonary,

hepatic, or renal failure. Many different metabolic disturbances are implicated as causes of confusional states, including hypoxia, hypercarbia, acidosis, hypo-/hyperglycemia, hyperammonemia, uremia, hypo-/hypernatremia, and hypercalcemia. Common infections associated with confusional states include septicemia, urinary tract infections, and pneumonia. Endocrine disturbances associated with confusional states include hypo- and hyperthyroidism, hyperparathyroidism, and Addisonian crisis. Most often, these metabolic disturbances produce confusion by interfering with either neuronal metabolism or synaptic transmission.

Intoxications and withdrawal states may be seen with prescription or over-the-counter medications, alcohol and illicit drugs, and, less commonly, with environmental or occupational toxins. A list of prescription medication categories and specific examples of medications associated with confusional states is given in Table 11.3. Many drugs and toxins cause confusional states by interfering with neurotransmitter function. In

---

Box 11.1 Common causes of hypokinetic acute confusional states

A Associated with medical and surgical illness
  1 Metabolic disorders
  2 Infections/fever/sepsis
  3 Congestive heart failure
  4 Postoperative
  5 Hip fracture
B Associated with drug intoxication
  1 Alcohol
  2 Opiates
  3 Benzodiazepines
  4 Barbiturates
  5 Other sedative drugs
C Associated with central nervous system disease*
  1 Structural parenchymal lesions (stroke, tumor, abscess, contusion)
  2 Subdural hematoma
  3 Meningitis
  4 Encephalitis

* Note: Acute confusional states associated with central nervous system disease will have focal or lateralizing neurologic signs, abnormal cranial imaging, or abnormal cerebrospinal fluid.

Box 11.2 Common causes of hyperkinetic acute confusional states

A Associated with medical and surgical illness
  1 Pneumonia
  2 Sepsis
  3 Postoperative
  4 Thyrotoxicosis
B Associated with drug intoxication
  1 Alcohol
  2 Scopolamine
  3 Atropine
  4 Other anticholinergic drugs
  5 Cocaine
  6 Amphetamine
  7 Other adrenergic drugs
C Associated with drug withdrawal
  1 Alcohol (delirium tremens)
  2 Barbiturates
  3 Benzodiazepines
  4 Other sedative drugs
D Associated with central nervous system disease*
  1 Structural parenchymal lesions (stroke, tumor, abscess, contusion)
  2 Subdural hematoma
  3 Meningitis
  4 Encephalitis, especially herpes simplex encephalitis

* Note: Hyperkinetic acute confusional states associated with central nervous system disease will generally have focal or lateralizing neurologic signs, abnormal cranial imaging, or abnormal cerebrospinal fluid.

Table 11.3 Medications associated with acute confusional states

Category	Examples	Category	Examples
Antibiotics		**Anti-parkinsonian agents**	
	Acyclovir (Zovirax)	Anticholinergic	Benztropine (Cogentin)
	Amphotericin B (Fungizone)		Biperiden (Akineton)
	Cephalexin (Keflex)		Trihexyphenidyl (Artane)
	Chloroquine (Aralen)	Dopaminergic	Amantadine (Symmetrel)
	Isoniazid		Bromocriptine (Parlodel)
	Metronidazole (Flagyl)		Levodopa/carbidopa (Sinemet)
	Rifampin		Pergolide mesylate (Permax)
Antispasmodics and anticholinergics			Selegiline (L-Deprenyl; Eldepryl)
	Atropine	**Cardiovascular agents**	
	Belladonna alkaloids	ACE inhibitors	Captopril (Capoten)
	Dicyclomine (Bentyl)		Fosinopril (Monopril)
	Hyoscyamine (Levsin)		Lisinopril (Prinivil; Zestril)
	Scopolamine	Antiarrhythmics	Disopyramide (Norpace)
Anticonvulsants			Lidocaine (Xylocaine)
	Carbamazepine (Tegretol)		Mexiletine (Mexitil)
	Phenobarbital		Procainamide (Pronestyl)
	Phenytoin (Dilantin)		Quinidine
	Primidone (Mysoline)	Beta-blockers	Atenolol (Tenormin)
	Valproate (Depakote)		Metoprolol (Lopressor)
Antihistamines			Nadolol (Corgard)
	Chlorpheniramine		Propranolol (Inderal)
	Diphenhydramine (Benadryl)	Central adrenergic	Clonidine (Catapres)
	Hydroxyzine (Atarax; Vistaril)	stimulants	Methyldopa (Aldomet)
	Promethazine (Phenergan)	Inotropic agents	Digoxin (Lanoxin)
Anti-inflammatory and analgesic agents		**Psychotropics**	
Narcotics	Butorphanol (Stadol)	Antianxiety agents	Alprazolam (Xanax)
	Codeine		Buspirone (BuSpar)
	Hydrocodone (Lortab; Vicodin)		Clonazepam (Klonopin)
	Hydromorphone (Dilaudid)		Clorazepate (Tranxene)
	Meperidine (Demerol)		Chlordiazepoxide (Librium)
	Morphine		Diazepam (Valium)
	Oxycodone (Percocet; Tylox)		Lorazepam (Ativan)
	Pentazocine (Talwin)		Oxazepam (Serax)
	Propoxyphene (Darvocet)		Prazepam (Centrex)
Nonsteroidal	Etodolac (Lodine)	Antidepressants	Amitriptyline (Elavil)
	Ibuprofen (Motrin; Advil)		Amoxapine (Asendin)
	Indomethacin (Indocin)		Imipramine (Tofranil)
	Ketorolac (Toradol)		Nortriptyline (Aventyl, Pamelor)
	Nabumetone (Relafen)		Trimipramine (Surmontil)
	Naproxen (Naprosyn; Anaprox)		Doxepin (Sinequan, Adapin)
Salicylates	Aspirin	Antipsychotics	Chlorpromazine (Thorazine)
	Diflunisal (Dolobid)		Molindone (Moban)
	Salsalate (Salflex)		Thioridazine (Mellaril)
Steroids	Adrenocorticotropic hormone	Psychostimulants	Dextroamphetamine
	Methylprednisolone (Solu-Medrol)		Methylphenidate (Ritalin)
	Prednisone		Pemoline (Cylert)
Antineoplastics		Other	Lithium
	Fluorouracil		*(continued on next page)*

Table 11.3 Medications associated with acute confusional states *(continued)*

Category	Examples	Category	Examples
Sedative-hypnotic agents		**Other**	
Benzodiazepines	Flurazepam (Dalmane)		Aminophylline
	Temazepam (Restoril)		Chlorpropamide (Diabinese)
	Triazolam (Halcion)		Cimetidine (Tagamet)
Other	Chloral hydrate		Disulfiram (Antabuse)
	Phenobarbital		Insulin
Sympathomimetics			Metoclopramide (Reglan)
	Dextroamphetamine		Theophylline
	Ephedrine		Thyroxine
	Methylphenidate (Ritalin)		Timolol ophthalmic (Timoptic)
	Phenylephrine		
	Phenylpropanolamine		
	Pseudoephedrine		

particular, anticholinergic, dopaminergic, adrenergic, and CNS depressant medications (e.g., opiates and benzodiazepines) all produce confusional states, at least in part, by their actions on selected CNS synapses. Central cholinergic pathways, in particular, are critical for vigilance and arousal, and many different categories of drugs contain agents with anticholinergic properties.

Primary CNS causes of confusional states include head injury, subarachnoid hemorrhage, stroke, raised intracranial pressure, intracranial infection (e.g., meningitis, encephalitis), and epilepsy (e.g., postictally). Most of these conditions affect the brain either diffusely or multifocally and are thus able to disrupt the widely distributed neuroanatomical network subserving attention. Focal CNS lesions can also occasionally produce confusional states when they disrupt certain critical heteromodal association areas of the cerebral cortex.

Confusional states, particularly in the elderly, may have multiple causes. In addition, relatively minor systemic illness may produce confusion in the elderly and in demented patients.

Pathogenesis and Pathophysiology

Spotlight Model of Attention

A flood of external and internal stimuli constantly bombards the brain. Since the brain can attend to only a limited number of stimuli at a given time, the brain must filter this onslaught of information if effective learning and action are to occur.

An often employed (albeit imperfect) model of attention is that of a spotlight at a play. According to this conceptualization, the brain focuses attention on critical external or internal stimuli, like the spotlight that illuminates the appropriate character in the play. Stimuli out-side the focus of attention are suppressed and generally ignored, unless they are of sufficient intensity, novelty, or importance to reach attention despite the filter. Thus, stagehands dressed in black are not perceived as they work quietly in the darkened area of the stage, while a brightly dressed character entering the stage singing would trigger a shift in the spotlight from the previous character to the new one. Similarly, someone watching a television show might not be aware of the noise from the dishwasher or the neighbor's lawnmower, but would shift attention immediately if the telephone rang.

The "spotlight model" can also be used to help understand impairments in attention. If the entire stage was illuminated, the selectivity of the spotlight would be lost, and all of the activity on the stage would be seen by the audience. The audience would be unable to focus on the appropriate character and might perceive a disorganized jumble of activity as their focus wanders from character to character or as attention is given to inappropriate stimuli, such as the stagehands. If, instead, the person operating the stage spotlight is drunk, the spotlight may shift haphazardly across the stage, the operator may try to follow each new person who enters the stage, or the operator may try to follow an attractive looking person even when that person does not have an important role. The unfortunate audience would be unable to follow the action on the stage or develop any coherent idea of the story. Similarly, an inattentive person cannot isolate the appropriate stimuli for attention, may shift attention when it is inappropriate (distractible), or maintain attention after it is inappropriate (perseveration). As a result, action and thought lose their normal coherence, and the patient responds inappropriately. Thus, to achieve coherent thought or action, only selective stimuli can be allowed to reach attention, and this selectivity must be maintained over a period of time.

Distributed Neural Network

The neuroanatomic network subserving attention is widespread and heavily interconnected. Structures participating in this network include the reticular activating system of the upper brainstem tegmentum and its projections, the thalamus, the basal ganglia (particularly the striatum), and specific areas of neocortex. The cortical areas include prefrontal, posterior parietal, and midtemporal heteromodal cortical association areas, as well as some limbic areas, such as the cingulate gyrus. The strong relationship between confusional states and toxic-metabolic-multifocal brain dysfunction probably occurs for two reasons. First, since attention is a widely distributed function in the brain, involving multiple brain areas, it is susceptible to diffuse or multifocal insults. Second, the neuroanatomic network subserving attention requires extensive polysynaptic chains of information processing, which again makes attention vulnerable to diffuse or multifocal insults. Some agents, which might be thought to act diffusely, actually relatively selectively affect specific areas of the network. Alcohol and anesthetic agents, for example, exert their greatest depressant effect on the reticular formation and on multimodal association cortex.

Confusional states are not restricted to diffuse or multifocal neuronal insults, however. Acute infarcts in certain cortical areas can also produce confusional states, particularly when the infarcts involve either heteromodal association cortex or connections of heteromodal and limbic cortex. Such damage to a single component of the network often produces an array of symptoms referable to several components of the network as a result of the heavy interconnections among the components. Hypokinetic confusional states are most likely with right-sided fronto-striatal lesions, particularly with inferior prefrontal lesions in the distribution of the superior division of the middle cerebral artery or with lesions of the striatum, involving either the head of the caudate nucleus or putamen. These areas modulate the motor-exploratory aspects of attention. In contrast, hyperkinetic or delirious confusional states are more common with lesions of either the right middle temporal gyrus in the distribution of the inferior division of the middle cerebral artery or the left temporal-occipital junction in the distribution of the posterior cerebral artery. These areas receive heavy input from limbic areas and serve in part to modulate the motivational and affective aspects of attention.

Evaluation and Diagnosis

History

A detailed medical history is often difficult or impossible to obtain from acutely confused patients, particularly those who are agitated, hallucinatory, or delusional. A calm but firm and persistent interrogation is often helpful, using a systematic series of questions that the patient can answer with brief responses. Often, though, it is necessary to rely on surrogate respondents and previous medical records for information.

When acute confusional states develop outside of the hospital, it is important to review the patient's previous medical diagnoses and medications, occupational and residential exposures to toxic chemicals, and use of alcohol and illicit drugs. Medical illnesses associated with confusional states include a very wide spectrum of disorders: neurologic, pulmonary, cardiac, renal, gastrointestinal, and endocrine.

When acute confusional states develop in the hospital, it is important to review the chart, noting other medical diagnoses, medications, present and past vital signs, abnormal behavior, and laboratory data. If the patient has recently had surgery, carefully review the operative report and the anesthesiology log of the operation. The nurses' notes, medication records, and order sheets should not be overlooked, as the nurses' notes are often more informative than physician progress notes regarding the onset and character of abnormal behavior, and, as do all of these sources, have important details about the initiation and discontinuation of medications. If possible, attempt to correlate the abnormal behavior with clinical events (e.g., prolonged hypotension or hypoxia) or the initiation of medications.

Examination

Since systemic illness is very often a cause of acute confusional states, physical examination should be thorough and should include assessment of temperature, pulse, blood pressure, respiratory rate and pattern (including episodes of apnea), signs of meningeal irritation, and signs of volume depletion, as well as careful examination of the lungs, heart and vascular system, abdomen, skin, and lymph nodes. Medical alert bracelets and signs of IV drug abuse should be sought. Standardized assessment tools may improve the accuracy of delirium diagnosis, especially in postsurgical and intensive care unit patients.

Since the assessment of certain cognitive functions depends on the integrity of other functions, mental status examination is necessarily hierarchical. Mental status examination should proceed systematically and sequentially from assessment of both appearance and spontaneous behavior to assessment of level of arousal, attention, language, orientation, recent and remote memory, and visuospatial function. Affect, reasoning, judgment, and insight are also important, but are often best assessed by simple observation rather than formal bedside testing.

The level of arousal reflects the integrity of the brainstem reticular activating system and its projections to the two cerebral hemispheres. Level of arousal is as-

Pearls and Perils

Evaluation of confused patients

▶ Groups at high risk of developing confusional states include the elderly, postsurgical patients, drug abusers, and those with preexisting brain damage or acquired immunodeficiency syndrome.

▶ The fundamental deficits in all types of acute confusional states are impaired attention and loss of coherence of thought and action. Confusional states are not simply disorders of wakefulness and arousal.

▶ Abnormal perceptions are common in acutely confused patients, and may include illusions and hallucinations.

▶ Confused patients frequently have disrupted sleep–wake cycles, typically with daytime somnolence and nighttime agitation.

▶ Confused patients may have a variety of motor disturbances including slurred speech, various adventitious movements, and incoordination.

▶ Confusional states are commonly associated with medical and surgical illness, intoxication and withdrawal states, and central nervous system disease.

▶ The patient's previous medical diagnoses and medications, exposures to toxic chemicals, and use of alcohol and illicit drugs should be reviewed.

▶ Since systemic illness is very often a cause of acute confusional states, physical examination should be thorough.

▶ Acute confusional states are frequently misdiagnosed as dementia, aphasia, amnesia, or psychosis. Misdiagnosis leads to further morbidity since the underlying causes remain untreated and, in addition, the frequent inappropriate administration of medications compounds the problem.

▶ The most helpful laboratory studies are those used to identify systemic illnesses commonly associated with acute confusional states.

▶ Particularly in elderly patients, confusional states may herald a serious medical illness, and at the same time may impair clinical recognition of the underlying medical problem.

sessed by noting both the patient's spontaneous activity and activity in response to stimulation. An alert patient is awake, aware of internal and external stimuli, and able to interact appropriately with the examiner. Note, though, that alertness does not imply a capacity to focus attention. Lethargy or somnolence is a state of less than full alertness in which the patient tends to drift off to sleep unless constantly stimulated, and even when alerted is inattentive and less than fully aware. Obtundation, stupor, and coma represent progressively lower levels of arousal that are considered in Chapter 13. At the other end of the spectrum, hyperalert individuals are awake, but appear overly watchful as they frequently scan the room, shifting attention to each novel stimulus. They are unable to relax, and are often anxious and easily startled.

In hypoalert cases, both the intensity of stimulation needed to arouse the patient and the patient's responses should be noted and recorded. To arouse a hypoalert patient, the intensity of stimulation can be increased progressively from saying the patient's name in a normal conversational tone, to speaking in a loud voice, gentle or vigorous tapping or shaking the patient's shoulder, and noxious stimulation. If noxious stimulation is needed, only appropriate techniques should be employed, such as supraorbital pressure, sternal rub, or nail bed pressure with a pen or similar object. Techniques such as nipple twisting are never appropriate, may damage tissues, and are certain to be misinterpreted if witnessed by family members or others. The patient's highest-level responses can be graded in terms of the quality of the motor response, vocalizations, and eye opening. Motor responses can vary from purposeful movements, to semipurposeful movements (e.g., localizing pain or withdrawal), posturing (abnormal flexion or, even worse, extension), and no response. Verbal responses can vary from normal conversation to progressively incoherent but still interactive conversation, inappropriate words (including profanities), meaningless or unintelligible sounds, and ultimately no vocalization. Eye opening responses can vary from spontaneous eye opening with normal eye contact with the examiner to eye opening only in response to sound or pain, or no eye opening. Simple scales, such as the Glasgow Coma Scale, are available for grading such responses and, when performed serially, these provide a ready way of monitoring the level of arousal over time, noting either regression or response to treatment.

Although attention is very much dependent on the level of arousal, attention is a separate function that depends on a distributed neural network, which, as noted earlier, includes the brainstem reticular activating system, the thalamus, the basal ganglia, and specific heteromodal cortical association areas. Impaired attention can in moderate or severe cases be assessed observationally by noting incoherence of thought and action, decreased attention span, impaired perseverance or impersistence, perseveration, impaired vigilance, distractibility, and inability to inhibit irrelevant or inappropriate responses.

Some aspects of attention can also be assessed more formally at the bedside, and such assessments may be particularly valuable both in supporting a diagnosis in mild cases and in following patients over time. Particularly important are assessments of span and perseverance. Span is remarkably uniform: most people can grasp seven (plus or minus two) discrete items of information in a short period of time. The simplest and most clinically useful index of this is the forward digit span; that is, the number of digits that a patient can repeat in forward order should be close to seven. If the span is reduced, learning, memory, and language comprehension will all be secondarily affected, since the patient will not even be able to register all of the information that has been presented. Perseverance, an aspect of sustained attention, can be assessed with sequential tasks of various levels of difficulty. "Serial sevens" is one of the most familiar tests of perseverance, although it is relatively difficult, very education-dependent, and not a pure test, requiring mathematical operations in addition to sustained attention. In this test, the patient is asked to count backward from 100 by sevens for at least five sequential subtractions. Mistakes are noted but not corrected by the examiner. Similar but simpler tests are "serial threes," usually assessed by asking the patient to count backward from 20 by threes, and counting backward (i.e., by ones) from either 20 or 100. Alternative tests, which are less educationally dependent and often more readily accepted by patients, are saying the days of the week in reverse order, or somewhat more difficult, saying the months of the year in reverse order. Patients should be encouraged to complete each of these tasks, going backward through all seven days or all 12 months, as it is often the later responses that become muddled, with the patient skipping days or months, or switching to forward order.

Vigilance and inhibition of irrelevant responses are other aspects of attention that can be assessed. Vigilance can be assessed with a "continuous performance, signal detection" paradigm. For example, the patient can be asked to raise his right hand each time the examiner says the letter "A." The examiner then presents a random sequence of various letters orally to the patient, so that the distracters (i.e., non-A's) are generally more numerous than the signals (i.e., A's) in a ratio of approximately 4 to 1. As an index of vigilance, the examiner notes particularly the proportion of signals in which the correct response was given (i.e., sensitivity). The proportion of distracters in which the response was not given (i.e., specificity) is also important, and can be considered as an index of ability to inhibit irrelevant responses. Ability to inhibit irrelevant responses can also be assessed with a related "go/no-go" paradigm. For example, with palms placed flat on a surface, the patient is instructed to raise the right index finger (i.e., "go") in response to a single tap by the examiner, but not raise the finger (i.e., "no-go") in response to two taps. The examiner then presents a random sequence of single and double taps, and notes particularly the proportion of double taps in which the patient did not raise the finger.

In right-handed individuals, language function is localized to the left cerebral hemisphere in the area around the sylvian fissure, which is supplied by the middle cerebral artery. This hemispheric lateralization of function is called *dominance*. In contrast, most left-handed individuals have considerable language representation in both cerebral hemispheres. Language function should be assessed systematically by evaluating verbal comprehension, verbal repetition, verbal fluency, naming ability, writing, and reading. Comprehension can be assessed by asking patients to perform simple motor tasks. One-step tasks and tasks involving midline body parts (e.g., "close your eyes," or "stick out your tongue") are easier and therefore less sensitive than tasks involving multiple steps or crossed-body parts (e.g., "point at the ceiling and then at the door," or "take your left little finger and touch your right ear"). The more complex tasks, though, may exceed the attention span of confused patients, resulting in apparent deficits in language comprehension. If attention span is reduced, this needs to be considered in assessments of language function. Another approach that may be helpful with confused patients is to ask simple short-answer questions (e.g., "Is a hammer good for cutting wood?" or "Do dogs fly?"). One may have to ask a series of such questions in order to determine if comprehension is preserved or impaired, especially if the patient has a tendency to perseverate. Repetition can be assessed by asking patients to repeat simple phrases, particularly those that involve mainly nonsubstantive words (e.g., "over, under, and upon," or "no ifs, ands, or buts"). Palilalia can be elicited by asking the patient to repeat the word "hippopotamus" (a possible response: "hip-hip-hippo-po-potamus") or the expression "tip top" (a possible response: "tip-tip-top-top"). Fluency is assessed by observing the patient's responses and spontaneous speech. Nonfluent speech is effortful, sparse, often poorly articulated and difficult to understand (dysarthric), nonmelodic and dysrhythmic (dysprosodic), and agrammatic. The sparseness of nonfluent speech is manifest by decreased phrase length (e.g., responses often limited to a single word) and decreased word output (less than 50 and often less than 10 words per minute), whereas the agrammatism is manifest by deletion of syntactic language structures (e.g., prepositions, articles, adverbs) and difficulty in handling relational words, plurals, pronouns, possessives, and verb tenses.

Each of the examined language functions may be affected in isolation or in combination with other functions. True comprehension difficulty (i.e., not due to impaired arousal or attention) implies posterior hemisphere dysfunction, often involving the Wernicke area in the posterior portion of the superior temporal gyrus, whereas impaired fluency implies anterior hemisphere dysfunction, often involving the Broca area in the posterior portion of the inferior frontal gyrus. Impaired repetition is seen with damage to the Wernicke area, Broca area, or the fiber tract connecting them, the arcuate fasciculus. Naming difficulty may be seen with any perisylvian lesion of the dominant hemisphere. Finally, agraphia accompanies both aphasic and nonaphasic disorders, such as confusional states, whereas alexia usually results either from disconnection of visual input from language areas with lesions of the occipital lobe and adjacent splenium of the corpus callosum (alexia without agraphia), or from lesions of the angular gyrus (alexia with agraphia).

Orientation should be assessed, particularly in regard to time and place. Many individuals are normally unable to give the exact time or date, but errors of more than 2 hours in time of day, 1 day in day of the week, or several days in day of the month, confusion of weekdays and weekends, and incorrect month or year (except at transitions) are abnormal. Despite the frequency with which orientation to person is apparently assessed in clinical medicine as indicated in clinical records, confused patients rarely, if ever, are disoriented to person. Severely inattentive and agitated patients or very somnolent patients may not respond to a question about their name, but in such cases, patients will generally attend briefly when their name is called.

Learning and memory reflect the integrity of another distributed neuroanatomic network, which includes both limbic and neocortical areas. The most important components are the medial temporal lobes, which include the hippocampus and amygdala, the basal forebrain, and the diencephalon, which includes the dorsomedial and paramedian thalamic nuclei, as well as the mamillary bodies. Memory may be assessed by asking patients to register and recall several unrelated objects, such as pizza, dog, and Chevrolet. More difficult tasks are asking the patient to remember several items with specific modifiers, such as white rose, speeding Buick, and Elm Street, or asking the patient to remember more than three objects. In any case, in order to compensate for the confounding effects of poor attention, the information presented should be within the immediate span of the patient. In addition, the material to be learned should be repeatedly drilled to ensure that it has been acquired and encoded. The objects should be repeated as necessary until the patient is able to recall them immediately after presentation. The number of trials required to register the items is a measure of attention, but not a particularly sensitive one, as usually only moderately to severely inattentive persons have difficulty registering three simple items. Once the patient has registered the items, the patient should be distracted for several minutes with either other questions or assessments of other cognitive functions. After distraction, the patient is asked to recall the items. Many confused patients flippantly indicate that they are unable to recall any of the items. Firm, persistent reassurance and encouragement should be given to ensure that patients make a maximal effort to recall the objects. Cues, such as category prompts (e.g., "One was a kind of food.") or phonemic prompts (e.g., "sh" for Chevrolet) can be given if the patient seems unable to recall the presented information. Alternatively, the patient can be asked to recognize the correct item from among a set of distractors

(forced-choice testing). A marked improvement with prompting or forced-choice testing indicates that the patient was able to learn the material but had difficulty retrieving it due to lack of effort, depression, or possible basal ganglia and frontal lobe disorders. Failure to recall the material even with prompting, if originally presented so as to be within the patient's span and adequately drilled so that the information was clearly registered, indicates a true impairment in ability to store or learn new material (amnesia), and likely dysfunction within the neuroanatomic network subserving memory.

Constructional apraxia is impairment in the ability to copy figures, despite preservation of muscle power, coordination, and sensibility. It can be assessed by asking patients to copy geometric figures, such as intersecting pentagons or a two-dimensional projection of a cube (Necker cube). Marked impairment in such copying tasks is usually attributed to dysfunction of the right cerebral hemisphere, but some impairment results with lesions of either hemisphere. Patients with right hemisphere dysfunction typically fluently produce copies that are detailed but have a fragmented or disrupted shape, with impaired orientation and disrupted spatial relations, whereas patients with left hemisphere dysfunction slowly and effortfully produce copies lacking detail, but preserving overall shape, orientation, and spatial relations. Very simple figures, such as a triangle, a rectangle, or a circle, should be avoided in assessments of constructional praxis, as these objects may be recognized, verbally encoded, and drawn from memory without copying.

Visuospatial abilities can also be assessed readily at the bedside by asking patients to imitate gestures and finger positions in space. One surprisingly simple and effective technique is to ask patients to imitate the examiner while he forms a rectangle by joining the right thumb to left index finger and the left thumb to right index finger. Impaired patients typically form a diamond shape by joining the same fingers—thumb-to-thumb and index-finger-to-index-finger. They may have trouble recognizing their effort as incorrect, even when pressed, or, if they recognize their error, they may be unable to correct it and may struggle with various fingers and orientations. Although this task undoubtedly involves a number of cognitive functions, it seems to correlate fairly well with difficulty copying geometric figures on paper.

Various brief mental status screening instruments, such as the Mini-Mental State Examination (MMSE), are useful adjuncts to bedside mental status testing and may improve recognition of deficits, enhance clinical judgment, and facilitate monitoring. However, such instruments cannot be used as substitutes for a careful bedside mental status examination. Test scores on such instruments do not, of themselves, establish a diagnosis of an acute confusional state, nor do they determine the etiology of an acute confusional state if one is present. Low scores are not specific for acute confusional states. Scores on such screening tests may be abnormal when any form of cognitive impairment exists, whether such impairment is congenital or acquired, focal or diffuse, or associated with a clear or clouded sensorium. Moreover, some impaired patients may score in the "normal" range. Indeed, all of the available screening instruments are relatively insensitive for ascertaining mild confusional states. These instruments can, however, be useful in following confused patients over time, to assess both progression of illness and clinical response to therapy.

The neurologic examination may also reveal important clues to the etiology of an acute confusional state, particularly if focal or lateralizing findings are present. Careful attention should be given to examination of visual fields, pupils, other cranial nerves, limb strength, gait, coordination, reflexes, and cortical sensory functions. Alterations in psychomotor activity and adventitious movements (e.g., tremor, asterixis, or myoclonus) should be noted. Tremor in confusional states is demonstrated by having the patient close his eyes and hold the arms and hands outstretched forward (flexion at the glenohumeral joint and neutral position at the wrist), whereas asterixis is most easily demonstrated in the hands by having the patient holds the arms outstretched forward with the wrists extended ("as though you're stopping traffic": flexion at the glenohumeral joint and extension at the wrist).

Differential Diagnosis

Generally, the diagnosis of an acute confusional state is straightforward, based simply on history and examination. However, a careful consideration of other diagnostic possibilities is important, as acute confusional states are frequently misdiagnosed as dementia, aphasia, amnesia, or psychosis.

Although acute confusional states and dementia are both syndromes characterized by loss of function in multiple cognitive domains, impaired attention is the most salient feature of acute confusional states, whereas attentional deficits in demented persons are either not evident or are overshadowed by other cognitive deficits, such as memory loss. In addition, although acute confusional states may be associated with alterations in the level of arousal, demented patients are generally fully alert in the absence of a superimposed confusional state (so-called *beclouded dementia*). Other helpful, but less fundamental, discriminators between these conditions include patterns of onset, diurnal variation, and duration. Confusional states generally have an acute or subacute onset, a course that fluctuates during the day and is typically worse at night, and a duration of days to at most months, whereas dementia often (but not invariably) begins insidiously, varies little over the course of a day, and has a duration of months or years.

Posterior aphasias, such as Wernicke aphasia, may occasionally be mistaken for acute confusional states, since the coherence of verbal output may be impaired in both conditions, and indeed in Wernicke aphasia may be reduced to a series of meaningless syllables. Here again, though, the most salient feature of acute confusional states is impaired attention, whereas the most salient feature of aphasias is a language disturbance. Relatively preserved attentional abilities, normal nonverbal behavior, difficulties in auditory comprehension but relatively preserved gestural comprehension, and prominent paraphasic errors and neologisms in spontaneous speech are characteristics of aphasic patients, but not confused patients. Outside the sphere of language, the behavior of aphasic patients is natural and appropriate to the situation.

In the acute stage of alcoholic amnestic syndromes (Wernicke encephalopathy) many patients are confused, but in the chronic state (Korsakoff psychosis), patients typically are attentive, alert, and able to use environmental information effectively. In contrast, confused patients are inattentive, frequently have an altered level of arousal, and are unable to use environmental information effectively. Whereas a confused patient lying in a hospital room may believe that he is at home, despite the obvious evidence to the contrary, an amnestic patient will immediately recognize that he is in a hospital. In addition, the nature of the memory deficits in confusional states differs from that in amnestic syndromes. In confused patients, the memory defect involves inadequate perception or registration of information, rather than impairment of retentive memory, whereas in amnestic patients, retentive memory is impaired and the perception and registration of information are preserved. Thus, memory often improves in confused patients, but not amnestic patients, if sufficient drilling is allowed during the acquisition portion of a learning task.

The prominence of secondary psychotic behavior in a confused patient may result in the incorrect diagnosis of a functional psychosis. Although confused patients present acutely with impaired attention and often with an altered level of arousal, memory impairment, and disorientation, patients with functional psychoses, such as schizophrenia and manic-depressive psychosis, have a history of preexisting abnormal behavior and are alert and generally attentive (unless attention is disrupted by active hallucinations), with preserved memory and orientation. In general, psychiatric illness does not cause severe confusion, disorientation, or an altered level of consciousness. In addition, the hallucinations in confusional states are generally visual or mixed and vary throughout the day, generally being worse at night, whereas the hallucinations of functional psychoses are generally auditory and less susceptible to diurnal variation. Furthermore, the delusions of confused patients are commonly paranoid, but generally relate to the immediate situation and change rapidly in content, whereas the delusions of paranoid schizophrenics are stable and systematized, typically concerning expansive, global ideas such as worldwide plots or the FBI.

Laboratory Studies

Once a clinical diagnosis of an acute confusional state is established, a number of laboratory studies are helpful in establishing the etiologic factors responsible. As outlined in Box 11.3, the most helpful studies are those used to identify systemic illnesses commonly associated with acute confusional states. Therefore, routine studies should include arterial blood gas or oxygen saturation, blood urea nitrogen and creatinine, complete blood count with differential, electrolytes (including sodium, calcium, magnesium, and phosphorus), glucose, liver function studies, urinalysis, an electrocardiogram, and a chest X-ray. Sec-

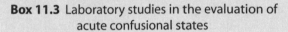

Box 11.3 Laboratory studies in the evaluation of acute confusional states

Routine studies
- Electrolytes, including sodium, calcium, magnesium, and phosphorus
- Blood urea nitrogen, creatinine, and estimated glomerular filtration rate
- Complete blood count with differential
- Glucose
- Liver function studies
- Arterial blood, gas or oxygen saturation
- Urinalysis
- Electrocardiogram
- Chest X-ray

Additional studies depending on clinical circumstances
- Albumin
- Arterial ammonia
- Antinuclear antibody
- Vitamin B_{12} and folate levels
- AM and PM cortisol levels
- Human immunodeficiency virus (HIV) serology
- Porphyria screen
- Syphilis serology
- Thyroid-stimulating hormone and free thyroid index
- Westergren sedimentation rate
- Toxicology screen, including alcohol level
- 24-hour urine for heavy metals
- Cultures of blood, urine, sputum, feces, cerebrospinal fluid
- Electroencephalogram
- Neuroimaging (computed tomography or magnetic resonance imaging)
- Lumbar puncture

ond-line studies that can be employed depending on the results of the routine studies and the clinical circumstances include a serum albumin level, ammonia level, antinuclear antibody, vitamin B_{12} and folate levels, a.m. and p.m. cortisol levels, human immunodeficiency virus (HIV) serology, thyroid-stimulating hormone and free thyroid index, syphilis serology, porphyria screen, Westergren sedimentation rate, toxicology screen, 24-hour urine for heavy metals, electroencephalogram (EEG), neuroimaging (computer tomography [CT] or magnetic resonance imaging [MRI]), and lumbar puncture.

Although EEG is often considered a routine or standard diagnostic test in the evaluation of acute confusional states, and while EEG has fairly characteristic abnormalities in such circumstances, it is unusual for the results of an EEG either to provide important diagnostic insights in someone diagnosed clinically as having a confusional state or to prompt significant changes in the management of a person with an acute confusional state. Therefore, EEG should generally be employed selectively in the evaluation of confused patients, and EEG should certainly never substitute for a careful clinical assessment. The EEG is often valuable in confused patients with a history of seizures or epilepsy, particularly in patients who have had recent seizures and may be having subclinical seizures, or in rare patients who present with absence or partial complex status epilepticus. Clues to the latter conditions include repetitive blinking, clonic movements of face or limb muscles, and repetitive stereotyped complex motor phenomena (automatisms). The EEG can also be helpful in evaluating cases of suspected encephalitis or when doubt exists about a diagnosis of a confusional state, particularly when superimposed on other preexisting medical or psychiatric problems, such as dementia, manic-depressive psychosis, or schizophrenia. If EEG is employed diagnostically, it is important to note that clinical changes often precede the changes on EEG and, in any case, the EEG in confused patients may not become recognizably abnormal. For example, an initial high-frequency pattern may be slowed during a confusional state, but still fall within the range of normal. Thus, a single EEG that is apparently normal does not exclude an acute confusional state. If there is diagnostic confusion, serial EEGs may be helpful in establishing the diagnosis.

Slowing and disorganization of cerebral rhythms are the most consistently reported changes on EEG in confused patients, particularly in hypokinetic confused patients. Slowing indicates a decrease in the frequency of the cerebral rhythms due to a corresponding decrease in the overall level of cortical excitation, whereas disorganization indicates a disturbance in the brain's synchronizing mechanisms due to a decrease in tonic activity of the reticular activating system and to disruption of corticothalamic interactions. Early on, the frequency of the normal background rhythm (8–13 Hz) slows and then is intermixed with less regular θ activity (4–7 Hz). Later, the slower activity becomes generalized and less reactive to external stimuli. Eventually, the activity slows into the δ range (less than 4 Hz) with waves of variable, but often higher, amplitude. The degree of slowing in hypokinetic confused patients generally correlates with the degree of depression in the level of consciousness, and recovery is accompanied by a corresponding acceleration of the cerebral rhythms. In contrast, low-voltage fast activity is often found in hyperactive, agitated patients with heightened arousal, particularly those withdrawing from sedative drugs, including alcohol. In these patients, recovery is associated with slowing of the background cerebral rhythms.

Other common EEG abnormalities in confused patients include triphasic waves, intermittent rhythmic δ activity, and multifocal or generalized epileptiform activity (i.e., spikes and sharp waves) superimposed on a background of widespread bisynchronous or asynchronous slow waves. Triphasic waves are high amplitude, bilaterally synchronous, anteriorly predominant waves named for their three-component deflection alternating about the baseline. They occur most commonly with toxic-metabolic encephalopathies, especially hepatic encephalopathy. High-voltage bursts of synchronous (θ or δ) activity may occur in mild or moderate diffuse encephalopathies, and generally attenuate with eye opening or other alerting stimuli. They occur particularly over anterior head regions and are often referred to as *frontal intermittent rhythmic delta activity* or FIRDA. A number of toxic, metabolic, and endocrine disorders are associated with multifocal and generalized epileptiform activity, including Addison disease, alcohol or barbiturate withdrawal, anoxia, dialysis encephalopathy, hypocalcemia, hypoglycemia, hyponatremia, tricyclic antidepressant overdose, and uremia. In contrast to these abnormalities, asymmetric δ activity, asymmetric or localized decrease in amplitude, or localized paroxysmal features (e.g., spikes, sharp waves, or spike-and-wave complexes) generally indicate primary intracerebral disease. However, although such intracranial disease may be the cause of a confusional state, it may also be incidental, as with a chronic abnormality caused by earlier damage.

Neuroimaging with CT or MRI should be employed if either the history or examination of a confused patient suggests the possibility of structural intracranial disease. A history of any of the following should prompt consideration of cranial neuroimaging: severe headaches, alcohol or other drug abuse, HIV infection, cancer, head injury or recent trauma, recent cardiothoracic surgery, previously diagnosed CNS disease, or focal CNS dysfunction. Neuroimaging should generally be employed if focal or lateralizing signs of CNS dysfunction are present in an acutely confused patient. Neuroimaging should also be considered if no cause for the confusional state has been identified with routine studies.

Assuming there are no contraindications, lumbar puncture should be employed in the evaluation of acutely confused persons if there is fever, headache, signs of meningeal irritation (e.g., nuchal rigidity and photophobia), elevated white blood cell count, HIV infection or other immunosuppression, cancer, or the cause of the confusional state is unclear. Contraindications for lumbar puncture include clinical or radiologic evidence of structural intracranial disease, increased intracranial pressure, and significant coagulopathy. In these circumstances, lumbar puncture should not be performed until it can be judged by a neurologically knowledgeable and experienced physician to pose no significant risk to the patient. In any case, cranial neuroimaging (usually with CT) should be performed prior to lumbar puncture if either focal neurologic signs or signs of increased intracranial pressure are present. If meningitis is suspected and a lumbar puncture cannot safely be performed, the patient should be started immediately on appropriate antibiotics.

In patients with medical and surgical illnesses, and in intoxication and withdrawal states, generally no focal abnormalities are apparent on neurologic examination, brain imaging, or electroencephalography, and the cerebrospinal fluid is clear. Such cases are often referred to by the term *toxic-metabolic encephalopathy*, particularly when the specific etiology has not been determined. Actually, this somewhat nonspecific term refers to a broad spectrum of neuropsychiatric disturbances resulting from toxic or metabolic derangements, including confusional states, but also organic hallucinosis, organic psychosis, stupor, and coma. This terminology presumes (probably correctly) that confusional states associated with medical and surgical illness, intoxication, and withdrawal states all have their basis fundamentally in diffusely disrupted neuronal metabolism. In contrast, focal abnormalities on neurologic examination, brain imaging, or electroencephalography, and abnormal cerebrospinal fluid are typical of confused patients with CNS disease. By analogy with the term toxic-metabolic encephalopathy, confused patients with focal or multifocal neurologic abnormalities could be said to have a *focal* or *multifocal encephalopathy*.

Management

If the evaluation has identified a cause or causes for the confusional state, these should obviously be directly addressed. When an etiology has not been identified, serial physical and laboratory examinations are essential. Particularly in elderly patients, confusional states may herald a serious medical illness and at the same time may impair clinical recognition of the underlying medical problem.

All patients with confusional states should have their vital signs and fluid status monitored closely. In addition, confused patients should be observed closely for deterioration and for dangerous behaviors. Restraints should be employed only as necessary and with appropriate monitoring to protect the patient from potentially dangerous behaviors, such as climbing over the bed rails or pulling out lines, tubes, and catheters. All nonessential medications should be discontinued. Medications that are deemed essential should be carefully reviewed to determine if the dose can be lowered or if less toxic alternatives can be substituted. In particular, agents with sedative or anticholinergic properties should be discontinued or substituted whenever possible. Fluid and electrolyte balance, and adequate oxygenation and nutrition need to be ensured.

With few exceptions, agitated psychotic behavior in confused patients that either creates hazards for the patient or interferes with ongoing medical treatment is best managed with high-potency traditional antipsychotic medications, such as haloperidol (Haldol), or atypical antipsychotics, such as risperidone (Risperdal) and olanzapine (Zyprexa).

Haloperidol is a potent antipsychotic medication that has no anticholinergic properties and is rarely associated with hypotension or respiratory depression. In addition, haloperidol may be administered orally, intramuscularly, or intravenously. Intravenous haloperidol has been widely used in seriously ill patients without harmful effects, and administration intravenously is associated with more rapid action and less severe extrapyramidal effects. Regardless of the route of administration, the usual initial dosages are the same, and are determined as a function of the patient's age and the severity of agitation (Table 11.4). The dosage may be repeated every hour until the patient is either calm or sedated. Subsequent doses are usually administered at 4- to 8-hour intervals, depending on the response of the patient. If parenteral administration is used initially, the oral form should be substituted as soon as is practical. The parenteral dose administered in the previous 24-hour period is used as an approximation of the total daily oral dose required, which is administered in three or four divided doses. In some cases, the total daily dose may be split nonuniformly, so that a larger portion is given in the evening to facilitate return to a regular sleep–wake cycle.

With administration of potent traditional antipsychotic medications, clinical signs and symptoms must be

---

> ▼
>
> **Pearls and Perils**
>
> **Management of confused patients**
>
> ▶ All patients with confusional states should have their vital signs and fluid status monitored closely.
> ▶ Confused patients should be observed closely for deterioration and for dangerous behaviors.
> ▶ Restraints should be employed as necessary to protect the patient from potentially dangerous behaviors.
> ▶ All nonessential medications should be discontinued.
> ▶ Medications that are deemed essential should be carefully reviewed to determine if the dose can be lowered or if less toxic alternatives can be substituted.
> ▶ Agents with sedative or anticholinergic properties should be discontinued or substituted whenever possible.
> ▶ Fluid and electrolyte balance, and adequate oxygenation and nutrition need to be ensured.
> ▶ With few exceptions, agitated psychotic behavior in confused patients that either creates hazards for the patient or interferes with ongoing medical treatment is best managed with high-potency traditional or atypical antipsychotic medications.
> ▶ Environmental interventions can be helpful, particularly in relatively mild cases.

monitored closely, with particular attention directed at efficacy, sedation, extrapyramidal effects, and blood pressure. With sedation, extrapyramidal manifestations, or hypotension, neuroleptic medication should be held until the side-effect resolves, and subsequent dosages should be decreased or an alternative pharmacologic agent should be sought. Use of anticholinergic medications to resolve extrapyramidal manifestations such as dystonia should generally be avoided in acute confusional states, because of the risk of exacerbating the confusional state. Although hypotension is rare with high-potency neuroleptics, such medications should nevertheless be administered cautiously to patients with severe cardiovascular disorders, because of the possibility of precipitating angina. If hypotension develops, it generally responds to IV saline. Epinephrine should not be used to treat neuroleptic-induced hypotension, since neuroleptics may block epinephrine's vasopressor activity and further paradoxical hypotension may occur.

Although the role of atypical antipsychotic medications in the treatment of delirium remains uncertain, limited data suggest they may have similar efficacy to haloperidol, with less side effects than high-dose haloperidol. Limited data suggest that, in certain circumstances, atypical antipsychotic medications may be used to prevent postoperative delirium: for example, a single 1 mg dose of risperidone administered shortly after cardiac sur-

---

Table 11.4 Usual initial dosages of haloperidol in agitated adults

Degree of agitation	Young	Elderly
Mild	2 mg	0.5 mg
Moderate	5 mg	1 mg
Severe	10 mg	2 mg

▼

Key Clinical Questions

▶ Does the patient have a reduced ability to focus, sustain, or shift attention to external stimuli?

▶ Is there a loss of coherence of thought or action?

▶ Did the cognitive dysfunction develop over a short period of time (hours or days)?

▶ Does the cognitive dysfunction fluctuate over the course of the day?

▶ Is the cognitive dysfunction worse at night?

▶ Is there an altered level of arousal (e.g., somnolent or hyperalert)?

▶ Are autonomic disturbances present (e.g., tachycardia, hypertension, mydriasis)?

▶ Is psychomotor activity increased or decreased?

▶ Is affect altered (e.g., apathetic, dysphoric, apprehensive)?

▶ Does the patient have altered perceptions or hallucinations?

▶ Does the patient have active medical or surgical issues (including recent surgery) that may be contributing?

▶ Can any medications or drugs (including alcohol) be implicated as a contributor to the confusional state, either due to intoxication or withdrawal?

▼

Consider Consultation When...

▶ It is not clear whether a patient has an acute confusional state or another condition, such as dementia, aphasia, amnesia, or psychosis.

▶ The cause of an acute confusional state is not clear after history, physical and neurologic examinations, and appropriate laboratory tests.

▶ Further expertise or experience is needed to treat the underlying cause.

▶ The patient's course is different from that expected.

▶ Technical assistance is needed in interpreting or performing diagnostic or therapeutic procedures.

gery with cardiac bypass may reduce the incidence of postoperative delirium. Atypical antipsychotic medications have lower frequencies of extrapyramidal effects, particularly compared with high-potency traditional antipsychotics such as haloperidol. Reasonable starting dosages for atypical antipsychotics in confused patients are risperidone (Risperdal) 0.5 mg twice daily, olanzapine (Zyprexa) 5 mg/day, and quetiapine (Seroquel) 25 mg twice daily. Quetiapine has a relatively low frequency of extrapyramidal side effects, and is therefore particularly useful in patients with parkinsonism, including those with Lewy body dementia. Clozapine (Clozaril) is not generally used in confused patients because of its anticholinergic activity, potential fatal toxic effects (e.g., agranulocytosis), and required blood monitoring.

Other types of pharmacologic agents are indicated in a few specific circumstances, such as drug withdrawal states, severe anticholinergic intoxication, hepatic encephalopathy, and AIDS encephalopathy. Benzodiazepines are the agents of choice in treating alcohol withdrawal delirium. Physostigmine salicylate (Eserine; Antilirium), a reversible anticholinesterase, is indicated in the treatment of severe anticholinergic intoxication. Oxazepam (Serax) or lorazepam (Ativan) can be used in hepatic encephalopathy, combined with aggressive treatment of precipitating factors, facilitation of ammonia clearance from the body with lactulose and nonabsorbable antibiotics, dietary protein restriction, and correction of fluid and electrolyte imbalance, acid–base disturbances, and coagula-

tion defects. Intravenous lorazepam (Ativan) in combination with haloperidol can be safely and effectively used to treat delirious AIDS patients.

Environmental interventions can be helpful, particularly in relatively mild cases. Nurses and family members can reassure agitated patients and reorient confused individuals to time and surroundings. Improving sensory input by having patients wear their eyeglasses and hearing aids helps patients understand their surroundings and decreases agitation and paranoia. A quiet, well-lit room with a visible clock and calendar may help to reduce anxiety, agitation, and disorientation. In addition, a room with a window will help to reorient patients to diurnal clues and may limit disruption of the sleep–wake cycle. A night-light may decrease nocturnal agitation and frightening illusions.

Several factors, including age and cause, determine the clinical course. For patients with toxic or metabolic confusional states, removal of the underlying cause when that is possible results in clinical improvement. Particularly in young patients without structural brain disease, recovery can be rapid and dramatic. In the elderly and in patients with CNS disease, clinically evident improvement may be delayed for days or even weeks, recovery may be protracted for weeks or months, and residual dysfunction is not uncommon. Among medical inpatients, quicker in-hospital recovery is associated with better outcomes.

Annotated Bibliography

American Psychiatric Association: Practice guideline for the treatment of patients with delirium. *Am J Psychiatry* 1999; 156(Suppl 5):1–20.
Guideline for treatment of delirium.
American Psychiatric Association. *Diagnostic and Statistical Manual of Mental Disorders* (DSM-IV-TR 2000). Washington, D.C.: American Psychiatric Association, 2000.
The American Psychiatric Association's classification of psychiatric and neuropsychiatric conditions, as well as clinical de-

scriptions of the entities and semioperationalized diagnostic criteria. As is typical of a psychiatric viewpoint, hypokinetic and hyperkinetic acute confusional states are subsumed under the term "delirium." Although attentional deficits are incorporated into the diagnostic criteria, delirium is incorrectly considered fundamentally as a disturbance of consciousness.

Casarett DJ, Inouye SK, for the American College of Physicians–American Society of Internal Medicine End-of-life Care Consensus Panel. Diagnosis and management of delirium near the end of life. *Ann Intern Med* 2001;135:32–40.

Cole MG, Primeau FJ, Elie LM. Delirium: Prevention, treatment, and outcome studies. *J Geriatr Psychiatry Neurol* 1998;11:126–137, 157–158.

Meta-analysis of available studies concerning the prevention, treatment, and outcome of delirium.

Elie M, Cole MG, Primeau FJ, Bellavance F. Delirium risk factors in elderly hospitalized patients. *J Gen Intern Med* 1998;13:204–212.

Meta-analysis of studies to 1995 concerning risk factors for delirium in hospitalized patients.

McCusker J, Cole M, Dendukuri N, Han L, Belzile E. The course of delirium in older medical inpatients: A prospective study. *J Gen Intern Med* 2003;18:696–704.

CHAPTER 12

Dementia

Douglas J. Lanska

Outline

- ▶ Definition and diagnosis
- ▶ Criterion-based diagnosis
- ▶ Staging of dementia severity
- ▶ Diagnostic workup and differential diagnosis
- ▶ Management

Definition and Diagnosis

Dementia is a clinical state characterized by a significant loss of function in multiple cognitive domains that is not due to an impaired level of arousal. The term *dementia* does *not* necessarily imply irreversibility, a progressive course, or a specific underlying cause. This chapter addresses general features of the dementia syndrome. For discussion of specific dementing and degenerative syndromes, including disease-specific management see Chapter 22.

Diagnosis of dementia requires either (a) assessing an individual's current level of mental function and documenting a higher level of intellectual function in the past, or (b) documenting a decline in intellectual function by serial examination over a period of time (usually 6–18 months). Cognitive deficits due exclusively to delirium, restricted brain lesions (e.g., aphasia), and psychiatric disorders (e.g., depression) must be distinguished and excluded. An initial diagnosis of dementia cannot be made when consciousness is impaired or when conditions exist that prevent adequate evaluation of mental status. If dementia is identified, further evaluation is necessary to determine the etiology of the dementia and to stage its severity.

Individuals who should be evaluated for evidence of dementia include those with memory or other cognitive complaints with or without functional impairment, elderly patients in whom the question of competency exists, depressed or anxious patients with cognitive complaints, and patients who arouse physician suspicion of cognitive impairment during their interview despite the absence of complaints. Because of their increased risk of developing dementia, patients with identified mild cognitive impairment should be monitored for cognitive and functional decline. Current evidence does not support screening asymptomatic individuals for dementia, regardless of age, a position supported by analyses from the U.S. Preventive Services Task Force, the American Academy of Neurology (AAN), and the Canadian Task Force on Preventive Health Care. However, as recommended by the American Medical Association and the American Academy of Family Physicians, physicians should be alert for evidence of cognitive and functional decline in elderly patients.

Depending on the severity of the dementia, a skillfully taken history may reveal deficits in several areas of intellectual function. For most patients, this information should be obtained from, or at least substantiated by, an informant. In taking a history, certain functional items, such as difficulty with recalling recent events, preparing a meal, playing games of skill, filling out business forms, handling financial records, and shopping alone, are helpful in confirming the presence of a significant intellectual impairment. It is also useful to inquire about a family history of Alzheimer disease or other dementia, presence of depression, evidence of vascular disease, and previous social and occupational functioning.

Cognitive or mental status testing should include assessment of orientation, recent and remote memory, language, praxis, visuospatial function, calculations, and judgment. The neurological examination may also reveal important clues to the etiology of the patient's dementia. Careful attention should be paid to the existence of focal abnormalities, extrapyramidal signs, and gait disorders.

Various brief mental status screening instruments, such as the Mini-Mental State Examination (MMSE), are useful adjuncts to bedside mental status testing, and may improve recognition of deficits and enhance clinical judgment. However, test scores on such instruments do not, of themselves, establish a diagnosis of dementia, nor do they determine the etiology of the dementing illness if one is present. Scores on such screening tests may be abnormal when any form of cognitive impairment exists, and mildly demented patients may score in the "normal" range. In addition, age, education, ethnicity, and language of the respondent have all been shown to influence responses to mental status test items. The clinician must make allowances for each of these in assessing patients with cognitive difficulties. Although cut-off points have been recommended for some of the standardized, well-known mental status tests, they are not definitive.

Criterion-based Diagnosis

Routine clinical diagnoses of dementia are inherently less reliable and are also less accurate than clinical diagnoses using standardized criteria, particularly when made by clinicians with little neurologic or psychiatric training. In available studies of community diagnoses, dementia was both unrecognized in a large portion (21–85%) of affected patients receiving care for other conditions, and commonly misdiagnosed in others.

Dementia is commonly unrecognized (a) in elderly patients, particularly if they are not regularly seen by the same physician; (b) in patients with dementia of mild severity; (c) in patients with coexistent psychiatric dysfunction; and (d) in patients with mental retardation.

Common causes of false positive clinical diagnoses of dementia include: (a) failure to recognize functional psychiatric disorders, particularly depression, as a cause of cognitive impairment in the elderly; (b) failure to distinguish delirium from dementia; (c) failure to distinguish focal from global intellectual impairment; (d) misapplication of dementia diagnosis to poorly educated individuals and individuals with lifelong intellectual impairment (e.g., mental retardation) without documented intellectual decline; and (e) misapplication of dementia diagnosis to those with cerebral atrophy on computed tomography (CT) without clinical dementia (Table 12.1).

Given that dementia is a syndrome, or group of signs or symptoms that occur together, the diagnosis of dementia is dependent on the specific criteria utilized in a given syndromic definition. Diagnosis of dementia requires documentation of (a) a decline in cognition involving multiple cognitive domains, including memory; (b) clinically significant cognitive dysfunction interfering with activities of daily living, work, usual social activities, or relationships with others; and (c) preserved

---

Table 12.1 Diagnosis of dementia

Discriminating features

▶ Decline in cognition, involving multiple cognitive domains, including memory

▶ Cognitive disturbances are clinically significant, as demonstrated by interference with activities of daily living, work, usual social activities, or relationships with others

▶ Consciousness is not impaired by delirium, drowsiness, stupor, or coma

▶ Cognitive impairments cannot be attributed to depression or focal brain disease

Consistent features

▶ Personality change, including apathy, irritability, and cantankerousness

▶ Impairment in abstract thinking

▶ Impaired judgement and impulse control

▶ Impaired language function (aphasia), such as naming difficulty (anomia)

▶ Impaired performance of motor activities, despite intact comprehension and motor function (apraxia)

▶ Impaired recognition of objects, despite intact sensory function (agnosia)

▶ Impaired ability to copy intersecting two-dimensional figures of projections of three-dimensional figures

▶ Psychiatric disturbances, including agitation, anxiety, depression, or paranoia

Variable features

▶ Onset may occur at any age

▶ Onset may be abrupt or insidious

▶ The course may be static, stuttering, or gradually progressive

▶ Cognitive impairments may be reversible, partially reversible, or irreversible, depending on the etiology, and the magnitude and duration of the deficits before institution of appropriate treatment

---

alertness and attention. In addition, cognitive impairments cannot be attributable to depression or focal brain disease. Involvement of multiple domains of cognitive function helps distinguish the demented patient from a patient with a discrete focal lesion. Memory impairment is required for diagnosis of dementia, since the neural circuits subserving memory are distributed widely in the brain and therefore are likely to be affected by diffuse and multifocal pathologic processes. A clinically significant decline ensures that the change is not an artifact of the testing circumstances and helps to distinguish dementia from the relatively minor cognitive changes that occur with normal aging. A clear sensorium is helpful in distinguishing dementia from an often-reversible acute confusional state. Finally, dementia must be distinguished from the cognitive effects of depression and focal brain disease, because these latter problems are managed differently.

The most widely used and most fully operationalized criteria for dementia are those developed by the American Psychiatric Association for the *Diagnostic and Statistical Manual of Mental Disorders* (DSM). These criteria are recommended by the AAN as a clinical guideline for routine use in the diagnosis of dementia. To fulfill DSM-III-R diagnostic criteria for dementia: (a) cognitive impairment must involve several domains, including short- and long-term memory and one or more of the following: abstract thinking, judgment, higher cortical function, and personality; (b) the cognitive disturbance must interfere with work, usual social activities, or relationships with others; (c) the cognitive disturbance cannot occur exclusively during the course of delirium; and (d) a specific etiologic factor must be identified, or in the absence of such a factor, nonorganic mental disorders (e.g., depression) must be excluded as possibilities. The newer fourth revision of the DSM does not include separate diagnostic criteria for the dementia syndrome, but does include criteria for individual types of dementia. These recent criteria essentially incorporate the criteria for dementia into criteria for each major clinical type of dementia.

Unfortunately, existing criteria are not fully operational: they allow considerable latitude in judgment as to which cases fulfill the criteria. There are still no uniform standards for determining how intellectual function is to be assessed, how intellectual decline is to be documented, or what degree of decline in intellectual function is sufficient for the diagnosis of dementia. Available criteria include considerations about functional performance that can result in inconsistencies, because some individuals may continue to function adequately despite a clear deterioration from their premorbid abilities, whereas others in more demanding environments may come to attention because of problems at work, even before performance on standard cognitive assessment instruments becomes abnormal.

Some patients may not meet diagnostic criteria for dementia, even though they or their families are concerned about changes in intellectual functioning. This group may include well-educated, high-functioning individuals and patients with psychiatric problems (e.g., depression or anxiety), and patients with early or very mild dementia. These patients should be encouraged to return for reevaluation, since observation over time, often 6–12 months, may help to document cognitive decline. For these patients, neuropsychological testing is often valuable to detect subtle cognitive difficulties.

Identification of mild cases of dementia is especially difficult. The commonly used screening tests for dementia are insensitive to mild cognitive dysfunction. Diagnosis of mild cases is further hampered by the lack of consistent, established values for what constitutes "normal" cognitive impairment associated with aging. As a result, dementia is frequently unrecognized or its severity underestimated, particularly in older subjects. Less intelligent or less educated individuals are more likely to be diagnosed as mildly demented, particularly because performance on the simple cognitive instruments is strongly influenced by education. In addition, both depression and delirium are likely to be confused with mild dementia.

Staging of Dementia Severity

Applying the label "dementia" or "dementia syndrome" is not the final product of the diagnostic process, since it says nothing about the functional or anatomic extent of involvement, or the underlying pathologic process. Once a person is recognized as demented, it is necessary to determine which domains of cognitive function are impaired, to give some measure of the severity, and to identify the specific disease(s) causing the dementia.

Diagnostic criteria for dementia have traditionally considered the syndrome categorically as present or absent. However, the care needs of affected individuals vary greatly as a function of severity. To deal with this, many clinicians apply one set of criteria to establish the presence of dementia and another set of criteria to establish the severity of the dementia.

Because dementia is a clinical syndrome, it cannot be graded by the severity of a pathologic change, although measures of pathologic change in a specific type of dementia may correlate with measures of impairment or disability. Severity of dementia can be categorized in terms of impairment of cognitive function, the functional disability resulting from the cognitive impairment, or some combination of the two.

The World Health Organization (WHO) has defined impairments as "any loss or abnormality of psychological, physiological, or anatomical structure or function." Earlier studies particularly tried to categorize dementia in terms of impairment by establishing various cut-off scores on lengthy psychometric tests; however, the groupings were generally arbitrary and unreliable, and the prolonged assessments were difficult to complete with demented patients. More recent studies have used overall scores or section scores from brief cognitive assessment scales. Some clinicians use the overall score from the MMSE to indicate the severity of cognitive impairment. For example, impairment may be judged minimal or mild for scores of 20 or better, moderate for scores of 15 to 19, and severe for scores of 14 or less.

Disabilities, in contrast, represent "any restriction or lack (resulting from an impairment) of ability to perform an activity in the manner or within the range considered normal...". Investigators have assessed functional abilities or care needs using simple rating scales or performance on functional measures. Some of the instruments employed were developed as overall functional assessments and, as such, they do not concentrate on cognitive function, but assess overall disability, including that arising from other medical, social, and emotional problems. Data sources used in determining a patient's functional ability are not interchangeable. Patients may overstate their abilities (especially early in the course), and family members may overstate or understate them, relative to assessments made by skilled nurses. A simple and clinically important way of categorizing the severity of disability is by rating the patient's capacity for independent functioning. In mild dementia, the patient can live independently; in moderate dementia, some degree of supervision is necessary; and in severe dementia, continual supervision is required.

Diagnostic Workup and Differential Diagnosis

Diagnostic tests are necessary in the differential diagnosis of dementia to identify readily treatable metabolic and structural causes. The detailed workup depends on the suspected diagnosis, but generally should include a complete blood count, serum electrolytes including calcium, glucose, blood urea nitrogen (BUN) and creatinine, liver function tests, thyroid-stimulating hormone level, serum vitamin B_{12} level, and structural cranial neuroimaging (Box 12.1).

Neuroimaging studies facilitate identification of many potentially treatable conditions, including tumors, subdural hematomas, hydrocephalus, and strokes. Although relatively uncommon when not anticipated clinically, these conditions are easily detected radiologically and often treatable. Therefore, a structural cranial neuroimaging procedure should generally be performed once during the initial evaluation of patients with dementia. Since most of the potentially reversible conditions requiring a neuroimaging procedure for diagnosis are large structural lesions, either noncontrast CT or magnetic resonance imaging (MRI) is indicated.

Other tests may be helpful in certain circumstances, but are not recommended as routine studies: apolipoprotein E genotyping, sedimentation rate, serum folate level, free thyroid index, human immunodeficiency virus (HIV) testing, syphilis serology, chest X-ray, urinalysis, 24-hour urine collection for heavy metals, toxicology screen, neuropsychological testing, electroencephalography, lumbar puncture, volumetric CT or MRI, single photon emission computed tomography (SPECT), and positron emission tomography (PET).

Although not generally necessary, neuropsychological testing may be helpful in (a) demonstrating cognitive impairment in individuals whose initial evaluation is borderline or suspicious; (b) distinguishing depression from dementia; (c) determining competency for legal purposes;

Box 12.1 Diagnostic tests in evaluation of dementia

Standard tests
- ▶ Complete blood count
- ▶ Serum electrolytes (including calcium)
- ▶ Glucose
- ▶ Blood urea nitrogen (BUN), creatinine, and estimated glomerular filtration rate
- ▶ Liver function tests
- ▶ Thyroid-stimulating hormone
- ▶ Serum vitamin B_{12} level
- ▶ Neuroimaging (noncontrast head computed tomography [CT] or magnetic resonance imaging [MRI])

Additional testing*
- ▶ Apolipoprotein E genotyping
- ▶ Erythrocyte sedimentation rate
- ▶ Serum folate level
- ▶ Free thyroid index
- ▶ Human immunodeficiency virus testing
- ▶ Syphilis serology
- ▶ Chest X-ray
- ▶ Urinalysis
- ▶ 24-hour urine for heavy metals
- ▶ Toxicology screen
- ▶ Neuropsychological testing
- ▶ Electroencephalography
- ▶ Lumbar puncture
- ▶ Cerebrospinal fluid 14-3-3 protein
- ▶ Head CT with and without contrast
- ▶ Volumetric head CT or MRI
- ▶ Single photon emission computed tomography (SPECT)
- ▶ Positron emission tomography (PET)

*Dependent on clinical circumstances

---

and (d) assisting in the evaluation of early dementia, particularly when major decisions need to be made with regard to a patient's job or other personal affairs. Neuropsychological testing is most valuable in making a longitudinal diagnosis of dementia when the presence of significant cognitive decline is difficult to establish, as it often is in extremely high-functioning individuals, in individuals with mental retardation, or in individuals with very limited educational backgrounds.

Lumbar puncture is not indicated routinely in the evaluation of dementia. Assuming there are no contraindications, a lumbar puncture should be performed when the following are present: cancer, suspicion of central nervous system (CNS) infection, reactive serum antitreponemal syphilis serology, communicating hydrocephalus, dementia in a person under age 55, a rapidly progressive or unusual dementia, suspicion of Creutzfeldt-Jakob disease (CJD), immunosuppression, and suspicion of CNS vasculitis (particularly in patients with connective tissue diseases). Specific cerebrospinal fluid (CSF) studies depend on the diagnostic considerations in a given case.

An electroencephalogram (EEG) is not recommended as a routine study, but may assist in distinguishing depression or delirium from dementia, and in evaluating cases of suspected encephalitis, CJD, metabolic encephalopathy, or seizures.

In a small percentage of cases (less than 10% on average), a specific treatable or potentially reversible etiology of the dementia syndrome will be identified, usually with the assistance of the diagnostic studies noted. The most important examples are medication-induced encephalopathy, depression, thyroid disease, CNS infections (e.g., neurosyphilis or cryptococcal meningitis), vitamin deficiencies (especially vitamin B_{12} deficiency), and structural brain lesions (e.g., tumors, subdural hematomas, and hydrocephalus). Nevertheless, truly reversible dementia is rare, and occurs in only about 1% of presenting cases. When such conditions have been excluded, the remaining causes of dementia consist mostly of Alzheimer disease, fronto-temporal dementias, vascular dementia, and other uncommon degenerative dementias (see Chapter 22).

Management

A balanced humane combination of environmental, behavioral, and (when necessary) pharmacologic treatments is likely to be the most effective management approach to improving the health, functional status, behavior, and quality of life of patients with dementia. Unfortunately, problematic behaviors in demented patients are often addressed by aggressive pharmacologic intervention and institutionalization in environments with little physical or social stimulation.

The first step in the management of a patient with dementia is to ensure that readily treatable causes of dementia are identified and appropriately treated. However, regardless of whether a readily treatable cause is identified, it is important to monitor demented patients for treatable causes of excess disability—that is, more impairment than can be explained by the primary disease process. In the last year of life, most demented patients require assistance with multiple basic activities of daily living, have severe impairments in cognitive functioning, and receive some care in general medical-surgical hospitals. Frequent causes of excess disability in demented patients include systemic illness, depression, medications, delirium, pain, and poor hearing or vision. In particular, frequent falls or an acute or subacute change in behavior or cognitive function should suggest medication toxicity, orthostatic hypotension, or an intercurrent illness. Intercurrent illnesses are frequently treatable, and medication

---

Pearls and Perils

Dementia management

▶ Patients with dementia may have treatable causes of excess disability, particularly systemic illness, depression, medication toxicity, delirium, pain, and poor hearing or vision.

▶ Frequent falls or an abrupt change in behavior or cognitive dysfunction should precipitate an evaluation for medication toxicity, orthostatic hypotension, or intercurrent illness.

▶ Behavioral changes present considerable challenges for caregivers, are often amenable to therapy and, unless treated, frequently precipitate institutionalization.

▶ If coexistent depression is suspected, an empiric trial of antidepressant medication should be considered.

▶ Delusions, paranoia, and hallucinations will often respond to antipsychotic medications.

▶ Changes in personality tend to be resistant to pharmacologic therapy, but may respond to behavioral modification.

---

toxicity is generally amenable to discontinuation or substitution of medicines. Appropriate management of such problems can result in significant cognitive and functional improvement and may allow demented patients to return to their previous functional level.

In general, the more home-like the environment, the better patients with dementia do on measures of depression, aggression, social withdrawal, and depression, even when adjustments are made for the degree of cognitive impairment, prescription drug use, caregiver training and experience, and the like. Even in institutional environments, certain design characteristics and behavioral management approaches greatly impact on the frequency of disruptive behaviors among demented patients. Privacy, personalized bedrooms, and common areas where residents can socialize are all associated with fewer psychotic symptoms, and less agitation and aggression. Common areas that vary in ambiance and camouflaged exit doors are associated with reduced levels of depression, social withdrawal, misidentification, and hallucinations. Such design characteristics produce less conflict over trying to leave the unit, a greater sense of control and empowerment, and greater independence of movement. In part, this is because caregivers tend to consider such environments safer and so allow greater autonomy among residents.

Graded assistance, practice, positive reinforcement, and an exercise program can help to maintain and increase functional independence, physical health, and mood among dementia patients. The goal of an exercise program should be to have patients participate in at least

30 minutes of moderate-intensity exercise per day, including aerobic/endurance activities (e.g., walking), strength training using light hand weights, balance exercises, and stretching and flexibility training. Caregivers should also be encouraged to identify pleasant patient activities to encourage positive patient–caregiver interactions and to increase patient physical and social activity.

Some common behaviors of demented patients present considerable challenges for caregivers, are often amenable to therapy, and frequently precipitate institutionalization if left untreated. These behaviors include insomnia and disrupted sleep cycles, delusions, paranoia, hallucinations, falling, depression, changes in personality, wandering, and incontinence.

When insomnia is not stressful to the patient, and when the patient's awakenings do not interfere with the caregiver's sleep, no treatment is necessary. Unfortunately, although demented patient's are seldom troubled by their sleep disruption, night-time wakening is often very disruptive for the caregiver, and may result in fatigue, anxiety, depression, or medical illness in the caregiver. The effects of most pharmacologic therapies for insomnia last only weeks or months, so that a sequential therapeutic approach is generally best, limiting the number of simultaneous interventions (Box 12.2). Initial interventions can include:

- ▶ Evaluate and treat underlying conditions such as hunger, pain, leg cramps, fear, and environmental disruption.
- ▶ Encourage moderate physical exercise during the day.
- ▶ Minimize naps during the day without depriving the patient of needed rest.
- ▶ Restrict fluids after 6 pm.
- ▶ Avoid diuretics in the afternoon and evening.
- ▶ Avoid caffeinated beverages and medications, including over-the-counter medications that contain caffeine.

Box 12.2 Management of insomnia

- ▶ Evaluate and treat underlying conditions.
- ▶ Encourage moderate daily physical exercise.
- ▶ Minimize naps.
- ▶ Restrict night-time fluids.
- ▶ Avoid nighttime diuretics.
- ▶ Avoid caffeinated beverages and medications.
- ▶ Try bedtime snacks with a warm beverage.
- ▶ Give bedtime back rubs.
- ▶ Read to the patient at bedtime.
- ▶ Avoid sedative medications, particularly those with prominent anticholinergic effects.

- ▶ Avoid alcohol, particularly before bedtime.
- ▶ Provide bedtime snacks with a warm beverage such as milk, decaffeinated tea, or herbal tea.
- ▶ Give bedtime back rubs.
- ▶ Read to the patient at bedtime.

Daytime wakefulness may be facilitated by getting patients dressed and out of bed in the morning. In hospital or nursing home settings, keeping the bed rails up during the day may deter napping and thereby facilitate an improved sleep–wake cycle.

When these techniques of managing sleep problems in demented patients prove ineffective, medications can provide some, although often limited, relief. These agents increase total sleep time and decrease nocturnal awakenings, but do not decrease sleep latency. Unfortunately, drug therapies (e.g., short-acting benzodiazepines or zolpidem) have frequent and significant side effects in demented patients (Box 12.3), and the medications eventually lose their effectiveness as patients become tolerant. Such agents may have significant carry-over effects and may result in increased confusion, agitation, and drowsiness in demented patients. These effects may increase over a period of several weeks. Even drugs with short half-lives may produce daytime sedation and increase confusion and agitation, especially with more than 2 weeks of repeated daily dosing. In addition, withdrawal of these agents may be associated with increased insomnia, confusion, and agitation. Sometimes the need for a sedative/hypnotic can be avoided by adjusting other medications. For example, if patients are also being treated for depression or delusions, antidepressant (e.g., trazodone or mirtazapine) or antipsychotic medications (e.g., quetiapine) with sedating properties can be chosen and administered in the evening. Since cholinergic neural systems are important for learning, and since these systems are preferentially involved in Alzheimer disease, anticholinergic agents may exacerbate memory problems and confusion. Therefore, agents with significant anticholinergic properties, such as diphenhydramine or tricyclic antidepressants, are best avoided in demented patients.

Antipsychotic agents can be considered to treat agitation or psychosis in demented patients when environmental modification is not effective. Aggression, delusions, paranoia, and hallucinations that are causing distress may respond to either traditional or atypical antipsychotic medications. However, the efficacy of antipsychotic medications for control of such behavioral manifestations of dementia is at best limited, and these agents can be associated with many side effects, some of which are severe. Pharmacologic treatments of dementia-related behavioral symptoms should therefore be used cautiously at minimum dosages, monitored closely for side effects and efficacy, and evaluated for tapering or dis-

▼

Box 12.3 Problems with sedative/hypnotic medications

- ▶ Confusion, agitation, drowsiness
- ▶ Hangover effects
- ▶ Tolerance
- ▶ Withdrawal
- ▶ Falls and fall-related fractures and other injuries
- ▶ Paradoxical excitation

▼

Box 12.4 Side effects of atypical antipsychotic medications

- ▶ Tardive dyskinesia (rare)
- ▶ Parkinsonism (less common than with typical antipsychotics)
- ▶ Dystonia (less common than with typical antipsychotics)
- ▶ Akathisia
- ▶ Asthenia
- ▶ Lethargy/sedation
- ▶ Worsened cognition
- ▶ Agitation
- ▶ Headache
- ▶ Dizziness
- ▶ Orthostatic hypotension
- ▶ Weight gain
- ▶ Hyperlipidemia (hypercholesterolemia and hypertriglyceridemia)
- ▶ Impaired glucose tolerance and type II diabetes mellitus
- ▶ Cerebrovascular events (strokes and transient ischemic attacks)
- ▶ Death (particularly from cardiovascular diseases and pneumonia)

continuation within 6 months of stabilization of symptoms and every 6 months thereafter.

Over the past decade or so, atypical antipsychotic drugs (e.g., risperidone, olanzapine, and quetiapine) rapidly became the preferred agents to manage behavioral and psychotic symptoms of dementia, including delusions, aggression, and agitation. In part, this shift was because of the perceived relative safety of atypical antipsychotic agents compared to traditional antipsychotic agents, particularly in terms of fewer extrapyramidal manifestations. However, evidence supporting the efficacy of atypical antipsychotic agents for control of the behavioral manifestations of dementia is at best weak, and such agents may be associated with significant side effects, including worsened cognition, lethargy, orthostatic hypotension, and extrapyramidal effects (Box 12.4). Furthermore, such agents are frequently used inappropriately, especially in nursing homes, where studies have documented that less than half of treated residents receive antipsychotic therapy in accordance with prescribing guidelines.

Increasing evidence suggests that potentially serious risks are associated with atypical antipsychotic medications. Since 2003, the U.S. Food and Drug Administration (FDA) has issued a series of advisories concerning the use of atypical antipsychotic medications in demented patients, initially because of an increased risk of cerebrovascular disease adverse events (strokes and transient ischemic attacks) noted with these agents. Atypical antipsychotics used to treat behavioral aspects of dementia have also been associated with a small increased risk of death, which precipitated the most recent advisory from the FDA concerning these agents in April 2005 (http://www.fda.gov/cder/drug/advisory/antipsychotics.htm). In randomized placebo-controlled trials of atypical antipsychotic medications, the FDA estimated the death rate from all causes to be 1.6 to 1.7 times higher among demented patients taking an atypical antipsychotic medication than among demented patients taking a placebo.

Clinicians should be cautious about employing atypical antipsychotic agents for management of behavioral aspects of dementia, particularly given their limited efficacy, recognized risks, the black-box warnings, and the lack of an FDA-supported indication. Clinicians would be prudent to obtain and document informed consent before initiating these agents for the control of behavioral manifestations of dementia. When such agents are used, the clinician must document the specific condition that warrants use of antipsychotic medications and must closely monitor and document side effects and efficacy. Periodic attempts at drug withdrawal should be considered for most nursing home residents (and others) taking atypical antipsychotic medications for the control of behavioral symptoms associated with dementia.

Reasonable starting dosages for atypical antipsychotics in demented patients are risperidone (Risperdal) 0.5 mg daily or twice daily, olanzapine (Zyprexa) 2.5–5 mg daily, and quetiapine (Seroquel) 25 mg twice daily. Quetiapine has a relatively low frequency of extrapyramidal side effects and is therefore particularly useful in patients with parkinsonism, including those with Lewy body dementia. The use of clozapine (Clozaril) in demented patients is limited by its anticholinergic activity, potential fatal toxic effects (e.g., agranulocytosis), and required blood monitoring.

The side-effect profiles of traditional antipsychotic medications vary by potency. High-potency agents, for example haloperidol (Haldol), have a high frequency of extrapyramidal effects, but are less sedating and have few anticholinergic effects. Low-potency agents, such as thioridazine (Mellaril), are sedating and have more anticholinergic effects, but few extrapyramidal effects. Occasionally, traditional antipsychotic drugs with intermediate potency (e.g., perphenazine [Trilafon]), may have the fewest undesirable effects in demented patients. Conventional antipsychotic agents are also at least as likely as atypical agents to increase the risk of death in elderly patients. Indeed, conventional antipsychotic medications are associated with a significantly higher adjusted risk of death (37–56% greater risk) than are atypical antipsychotic medications within 6 months of therapy initiation. The higher risk of death for those treated with conventional antipsychotic medications applies to patients with or without dementia and those in or out of nursing homes. The greatest increased risk of death occurs soon after initiation of therapy and with higher dosages of medications. Therefore, conventional antipsychotic drugs should not be used to replace atypical agents that are discontinued in response to the FDA advisory.

Before prescribing conventional antipsychotic agents, caregivers, guardians, and patients should be informed of the risks, including tardive dyskinesia, parkinsonism, sedation, orthostatic hypotension, and an increased risk of death (Box 12.5). Reasonable starting dosages for these agents are haloperidol (Haldol) 0.5 mg daily or twice daily, thioridazine (Mellaril) 10 mg at bedtime or twice daily, and perphenazine (Trilafon) 2 mg daily or twice daily. Some evidence suggests that higher doses (e.g., 2–3 mg/day) of haloperidol may be more effective than lower doses (<1 mg/day) in controlling symptoms.

Some patients will improve behaviorally with treatment using acetylcholinesterase inhibitors or memantine. It is reasonable to defer use of antipsychotic medications for control of behavioral symptoms until the effect of acetylcholinesterase inhibitors has been evaluated, unless safety considerations warrant urgent treatment with antipsychotic medications to attempt to control intolerable behavioral symptoms.

Depression alone may produce cognitive impairment in older individuals. Depression is also a common concomitant of dementia, particularly Alzheimer disease. If coexistent depression is suspected, an empiric trial of antidepressant medication should be considered, although limited data support the efficacy of antidepressants for patients with depression and dementia. Antidepressants with relatively few anticholinergic effects include venlafaxine (Effexor), trazodone (Desyrel), fluoxetine (Prozac), bupropion (Wellbutrin), desipramine (Norpramin), amoxapine (Asendin), and maprotiline (Ludiomil). Trazodone should be used cautiously in men following documented discussion of risks due to the rare association with priapism. Trazodone, amoxapine, and maprotiline are moderately sedating. If antidepressant medication proves ineffective, electroconvulsive therapy is safe and may be effective in treating depressed, elderly demented patients.

Changes in personality tend to be resistant to pharmacologic treatment, but may respond to behavioral modification. Manifestations of personality changes are often minimized by approaches that avoid confrontation and utilize regular routines. Calmness, firmness, and a sense of authority help minimize combative and aggressive behaviors.

Wandering may be problematic. Pharmacologic management of wandering is generally not helpful. Helpful approaches to the management of wandering in demented patients are outlined in Box 12.6. Childproof doorknob covers, sequential locks on doors, a fenced yard, and alarm systems set to alarm when a patient leaves a given area can be of assistance. The patient's name and address and the telephone number of the responsible person should be put in the patient's wallet or purse. Identification bracelets or necklaces may also be considered. Address labels and telephone numbers should be put on clothes. Strips of 100 or more address labels for clothes can be ordered inexpensively through mail order companies or sewing supply shops. Police and neighbors should be alerted to the patient's possible wandering and need for assistance. Caregivers should keep current photographs of the patient to use in a search if the patient wanders off. Restraints should be avoided.

Box 12.5 Side effects of traditional antipsychotic medications

▶ Tardive dyskinesia
▶ Parkinsonism
▶ Dystonia (acute or tardive)
▶ Akathisia
▶ Sedation
▶ Dizziness
▶ Hypotension
▶ Orthostatic hypotension
▶ Death

Box 12.6 Management of wandering

▶ Use childproof doorknob covers.
▶ Place sequential locks on doors.
▶ Fence the yard.
▶ Install alarm systems.
▶ Provide personal identification.
▶ Notify police and neighbors.
▶ Have current photographs available to use in a search.
▶ Avoid restraints.

> **Box 12.7** Management of urinary incontinence

- ▶ Dress patients in easily removable clothing.
- ▶ Exclude urinary tract infection, diabetes, and bladder outlet obstruction.
- ▶ Restrict nocturnal fluid intake.
- ▶ Avoid diuretics and caffeine.
- ▶ Install a night light in the bathroom.
- ▶ Provide a commode.
- ▶ Consider diapers.
- ▶ Utilize behavior modification, scheduled toileting, and prompted voiding.

> **Box 12.8** Safety management

- ▶ Monitor medications.
- ▶ Fix or remove unstable furniture and rugs.
- ▶ Supervise or restrict access to alcohol, other toxic substances, matches, cigarette lighters, stoves, and electrical appliances.
- ▶ Ensure that stairs are well lit with solid hand rails.
- ▶ Place combination locks on doors to the outside.
- ▶ Dismantle bathroom and closet locks.
- ▶ Provide bathtub rails and place nonskid mats or appliques in the bathtub.
- ▶ Adjust the water heater temperature to avoid scalding.
- ▶ Remove firearms.
- ▶ Restrict or prohibit driving.

The management of urinary incontinence in demented patients is outlined in Box 12.7. Patients with incontinence should be dressed in easily removable clothing and kept clean and dry. Treatable causes of incontinence should be sought and managed appropriately. In patients with urinary incontinence, a fasting blood sugar should be obtained to identify diabetes, and a urinalysis should be obtained to exclude infection. In men, a rectal examination should be done to evaluate the prostate. If nocturnal enuresis is a problem, a number of steps may minimize the problem: restrict nocturnal fluid intake; avoid diuretics, including caffeinated beverages and medications, particularly in the afternoon and evening; install a night light in the bathroom; provide a commode; and consider diapers. Behavioral modification, scheduled toileting, and prompted voiding may help reduce urinary incontinence. With fecal incontinence, a rectal examination should be done to assess for fecal impaction. It may be necessary to regulate elimination with either dietary aids, laxatives, suppositories, or enemas.

The physician should reassess safety issues regularly, and encourage the patient and family to correct potentially hazardous situations (Box 12.8). Medications should be adequately supervised. Unstable furniture and rugs should be fixed or removed. Access to alcohol, toxic substances, matches, cigarette lighters, stoves, and electrical appliances should be adequately supervised or restricted. Stairs should be well lit and have solid handrails. Combination locks on doors to the outside should be recommended in wandering patients. Bathroom and closet locks should be dismantled. The bathtub should be fitted with rails, and nonskid mats or appliqués should be placed on the floor of the tub. The water temperature in the water heater should be adjusted to avoid scalding. Objects that can be used as a weapon should be placed out of reach of demented patients. Firearms, in particular, should be removed from the house.

Patients with dementia have a substantially increased rate of motor vehicle accidents and driving performance errors. Driving should be restricted or prohibited if judgment, emotional control, geographic orientation, visuospatial abilities, or motor function are significantly impaired. Current guidelines from the AAN state that patients with Alzheimer disease of mild or worse severity (as judged by a Clinical Dementia Rating score of 1 or greater) and their families should be told that, because of their condition, they have a substantially increased risk of accidents and driving performance errors, higher than society tolerates for any group of drivers. Therefore, as a practice standard, "discontinuation of driving should be strongly considered." Even patients with "very mild" Alzheimer disease (as judged by a Clinical Dementia Rating scale score of 0.5) have an increased risk of accidents compared with other elderly drivers, although similar to that which society accepts for 16- to 19-year-old drivers and drivers intoxicated with alcohol at a blood alcohol concentration of less than 0.08%. Patients and their families should be told of this increased risk of traffic safety problems compared with other elderly drivers, and referral of the patient for a driving performance evaluation "should be considered." Because patients with early Alzheimer disease are likely to worsen, as a practice standard "clinicians should reassess dementia severity and appropriateness of continued driving every 6 months." No specific guidelines on driving for other types of dementia are available, but it is reasonable to apply the AAN guidelines to patients with other types of dementia.

The physician should guide the family in coping with the patient's illness, encourage family members to provide an appropriate and supportive care environment, and anticipate and, to the extent feasible, prevent stage-dependent problems. Clinicians should encourage caregivers to use graded assistance, practice, and positive reinforcement to increase functional independence. A sta-

▼

Key Clinical Questions

▶ Has there been a decline in cognition, involving multiple cognitive domains, including memory?
▶ Are the changes in cognition clinically significant, as manifested by interference with activities of daily living, usual social activities, or relationships with others?
▶ Is consciousness impaired?
▶ Can the cognitive dysfunction be attributed to depression, focal brain disease, or delirium?
▶ Was the onset insidious or abrupt?
▶ Is the course static, stuttering, or gradually progressive?
▶ What activities of daily living are impaired?
▶ Are there any problem behaviors (e.g., wandering, incontinence, agitation, aggression, insomnia, delusions, paranoia, or hallucinations)?
▶ Are there any safety concerns at home?
▶ Does the patient still drive?
▶ What are the living arrangements and social supports?
▶ Does the patient have a durable power of attorney document, guardianship, or living will?
▶ Does the patient have active medical or surgical issues that may be contributing?
▶ Can any medications or drugs (including alcohol) be implicated as a contributor to the cognitive dysfunction?

▼

Consider Consultation When...

▶ It is not clear whether the patient has dementia or another condition, such as mental retardation, age-associated memory impairment, amnesia, aphasia, acute confusional state, or depression.
▶ The cause of the dementia is not clear after history, physical and neurologic examinations, and appropriate laboratory tests (see Box 12.1).
▶ Further expertise or experience is needed to manage complex behavioral and social problems, or to treat the underlying cause.
▶ The patient's course is different from that expected.
▶ Technical assistance is needed in interpreting or performing diagnostic or therapeutic procedures.

well-being and quality of life, and delay institutionalization of patients with dementia. Such interventions include education, support groups, and respite care (e.g., adult day care or in-home services). The Alzheimer's Association, senior citizen centers, social workers, and various Alzheimer disease and dementia support groups can provide information on available services in each locality. Meals on Wheels, day care programs and other respite services, paid caretakers, and Adult Protective Services are supports should be considered depending on the clinical circumstances and community availability.

Annotated Bibliography

American Geriatrics Society and American Association for Geriatric Psychiatry. Consensus statement on improving the quality of mental health care in U.S. nursing homes: management of depression and behavioral symptoms associated with dementia. *J Am Geriatr Soc* 2003;51:1287–1298.
Consensus statement on management of dementia in nursing homes.
American Psychiatric Association: *Diagnostic and Statistical Manual of Mental Disorders* (3rd ed.–revised: DSM-III-R). Washington, D.C.: Author, 1987.
Diagnostic criteria for dementia.
Bains J, Birks JS, Dening TR. The efficacy of antidepressants in the treatment of depression in dementia. *Cochrane Database Syst Rev* 2002;(4):CD003944.
Systematic review of available evidence concerning antidepressants as a treatment for depression in patients with dementia.
Clarfield AM. The decreasing prevalence of reversible dementias: An updated meta-analysis. *Arch Intern Med* 2003;163: 2219–2229.
Systematic review of available evidence concerning the frequency of reversible dementias.
Doody RS, Stevens JC, Beck C, et al. Practice parameter: Management of dementia (an evidence-based review). Report of

ble, dependable setting can be facilitated by maintaining regular schedules; by minimizing changes in the daily routine, the care environment, and the caregivers; by keeping the patient's possessions in the same place; by keeping stimulation (e.g., activities, conversations, visitors, television) to tolerable levels; and by providing and enhancing multiple sensory cues with increased lighting levels, night lights, large clocks, large calendars, and seasonal decorations. Caregivers should schedule demanding tasks, such as bathing, for the patient's best time of the day. Expectations of the patient's role in various tasks need to be periodically readjusted to the patient's fluctuating or declining functional capacity. External stimulation needs to be reduced when the patient becomes tense, agitated, hostile, or belligerent. Communication with patients is particularly important. Caregivers should avoid confrontation; communicate with simple, concise, and concrete statements; avoid negative statements such as "don't do that!"; and use distractions as a response to perseveration and undesirable behavior. The physician should regularly review the patient's capacity for independent function. As early as possible, the physician should also encourage patients and families to obtain a durable power of attorney for healthcare decision-making.

Psychosocial interventions directed toward caregivers may decrease caregiver stress, improve caregiver

the Quality Standards Subcommittee of the American Academy of Neurology. *Neurology* 2001;56:1154–1166.
Current guidelines for management of dementia, although increasingly out-of-date concerning medication management.

Dubinsky RM, Stein AC, Lyons K. Practice parameter: Risk of driving and Alzheimer's disease (an evidence-based review). Report of the Quality Standards Subcommittee of the American Academy of Neurology. *Neurology* 2000;54:2205–2211.
Systematic review and practice guideline concerning driving and Alzheimer disease, which is likely applicable to dementia in general.

Knopman DS, DeKosky ST, Cummings JL, et al. Practice parameter: Diagnosis of dementia (an evidence-based review). Report of the Quality Standards Subcommittee of the American Academy of Neurology. *Neurology* 2001;56:1143–1153.
Current guidelines for diagnosis of dementia.

Lanska DJ. Dementia mortality in the United States. Results of the 1998 National Mortality Followback Survey. *Neurology* 1998;50:362–367.
Findings that, in the last year of life, most demented patients require assistance with multiple basic activities of daily living, have severe impairments in cognitive functioning, and receive some care in general medical-surgical hospitals.

Lanska DJ. Time is money—or is it? Estimating the costs of informal caregiving. *Neurology* 2002;58:1718–1719. (Erratum *Neurology* 2002;58:1476.)
Estimated costs of informal caregiving are underestimated and depend heavily on the perspective and model used to estimate them.

Lonergan E, Luxemberg J, Colford J. Haloperidol for agitation in dementia. *Cochrane Database Syst Rev* 2002;(2): CD002852.
Systematic review of available evidence concerning use of haloperidol for aggression and agitation in dementia.

Mace NL, Rabins PV. *The 36-hour day: A family guide to caring for persons with Alzheimer's disease, related dementing illnesses, and memory loss in later life.* 3rd ed. New York: Warner Books, 2001.
An excellent resource for families of demented persons.

Mendez MF, Cummings JL, Cummings J. *Dementia: A clinical approach*, 3rd ed. Boston: Butterworth-Heinemann, 2003.
An excellent, practical, and easily readable source of clinical information on dementia and various dementing illnesses.

Peterson RC, Stevens JC, Gangluli M, Tangalos EG, Cummings JL, DeKosky ST. Practice parameter: Early detection of dementia—Mild cognitive impairment (an evidence-based review). Report of the Quality Standards Subcommittee of the American Academy of Neurology. *Neurology* 2001;56: 1133–1142.
Because of their increased risk of developing dementia, people with mild cognitive impairment should be evaluated and monitored.

U.S. Preventive Services Task Force. Screening for dementia: Recommendation and rationale. *Ann Intern Med* 2003;138: 925–926.
Current evidence does not support screening in asymptomatic individuals.

Coma

Joseph R. Berger

Evaluation and management of the comatose patient require the physician to obtain a history, perform and interpret general physical and neurologic examinations, and begin therapy on an emergent basis. This chapter introduces the clinician to fundamental principles about the evaluation and management of the comatose patient. The chapter begins with key definitions and a brief discussion of the neuroanatomic principles underlying coma. Key elements of diagnosis in the comatose patient, dealing with the level of neurologic dysfunction and the most probable etiology of the coma, are presented. This is followed by a discussion of the emergency management of a patient presenting with an altered level of consciousness. The chapter concludes with a discussion of the prognosis of patients presenting with coma, including a discussion of the vegetative state.

Terminology

Consciousness is the state of awareness of oneself and the environment. Consciousness is composed of two elements: arousal and awareness. Coma involves the first of these elements—arousal. Coma is a clinical syndrome in which an altered state of consciousness is characterized by an unresponsive, unarousable patient who typically lies with his eyes closed. The inability to arouse the comatose patient is the key distinguishing feature from sleep, a normal form of altered consciousness. Coma is not an etiologic diagnosis. Evaluation of a comatose patient must include a search for the underlying cause of the patient's condition.

The various levels of consciousness form a spectrum of clinical pictures. At one end of the spectrum is the normal patient who is fully awake and alert. At the other end of the spectrum is the patient who is in a deep coma. This patient lies unresponsive, with eyes closed, and cannot be aroused by any degree of external stimuli, including pain. Between these two end-points is a continuum of patient conditions that have been described using various terms including lethargy, drowsiness, and stupor.

Despite their popularity, these terms should be avoided, or at least, not used without other descriptors in clinical practice. Instead, explicit descriptions of a patient's behavior and response (or lack thereof) to stimuli are preferable for several reasons. First, the terms have a variety of interpretations, and descriptions lessen confusion. Second, specific descriptions facilitate recognition of and communication about small changes in patient behavior. Even small clinical changes can have great meaning in the evaluation and prognosis of the comatose patient. Finally, specific descriptions of patient behavior will lessen the likelihood of misdiagnosing certain clinical conditions as coma.

Neuroanatomic Basis of Consciousness

Many conditions can be associated with coma. Table 13.1 lists various causes. To understand how coma occurs, it is important to review the neuroanatomic basis of arousal. Two major neuroanatomic structures are involved in consciousness. The first is the cerebral cortex. The second is the ascending reticular activating system (ARAS), a dif-

Table 13.1 Causes of coma

I   Symmetric-nonstructural

A   Toxins
   Lead
   Thallium
   Mushrooms
   Cyanide
   Methanol
   Ethylene glycol
   Carbon monoxide

B   Drugs
   Sedatives
   Barbiturates
   Other hypnotics
   Tranquilizers
   Bromides
   Alcohol
   Opiates
   Paraldehyde
   Salicylate
   Psychotropics
   Anticholinergics
   Amphetamines
   Lithium
   Phencyclidine
   Monoamine oxidase inhibitors

C   Metabolic
   Hypoxia
   Hypercapnia
   Hypernatremia
   Hyponatremia*
   Hypoglycemia*
   Hyperglycemic nonketotic coma
   Diabetic ketoacidosis
   Lactic acidosis
   Hypercalcemia
   Hypocalcemia
   Hypermagnesemia
   Hyperthermia
   Hypothermia
   Reye encephalopathy
   Aminoacidemia
   Wernicke encephalopathy
   Porphyria
   Hepatic encephalopathy*
   Uremia
   Dialysis encephalopathy
   Hypothyroidism
   Addisonian crisis

D   Infections
   Bacterial meningitis
   Viral encephalitis
   Postinfectious encephalomyelitis
   Syphilis
   Sepsis
   Typhoid fever
   Malaria
   Waterhouse-Friderichsen syndrome

E   Psychiatric
   Catatonia
   Conversion reaction

F   Other
   Postictal*
   Diffuse ischemia (myocardial infarction,
     cardiac heart failure, arrhythmia)
   Hypotension
   Fat embolism*
   Hypertensive encephalopathy

II   Symmetric-structural

A   Supratentorial
   Bilateral internal carotid occlusion
   Bilateral anterior cerebral artery occlusion

   Subarachnoid hemorrhage
   Thalamic hemorrhage*
   Trauma – contusion, concussion*
   Hydrocephalus

B   Infratentorial
   Basilar occlusion*
   Midline brainstem tumor
   Pontine hemorrhage*

III   Asymmetric-structural

A   Supratentorial
   Thrombotic thrombocytopenic purpura†
   Disseminated intravascular coagulation
   Nonbacterial thrombotic endocarditis
     (marantic endocarditis)
   Subacute bacterial endocarditis
   Fat emboli unilateral hemispheric mass
     (tumor, bleed; with herniation)

   Subdural hemorrhage (bilateral
     subdurals may be symmetric)
   Intracerebral bleed
   Pituitary apoplexy†
   Massive or bilateral supratentorial
     infarction
   Multifocal leukoencephalopathy
   Adrenal leukodystrophy
   Cerebral vasculitis
   Cerebral abscess

   Subdural empyema
   Thrombophlebitis†
   Multiple sclerosis
   Leukoencephalopathy associated
     with chemotherapy
   Acute disseminated
     encephalomyelitis
   Creutzfeldt-Jakob disease

B   Infratentorial
   Brainstem infarction
   Brainstem hemorrhage

---

*Relatively common asymmetric presentation.
†Relatively symmetric.
From Berger J. Coma. In Bradley, Daroff, Fenichel, and Marsden (eds.), *Neurology in Clinical Practice*; incorporating data from Plum and Posner (1980) and Fisher (1969).

fuse but organized system of neurons and neural pathways extending through the brainstem from the caudal medulla to the midbrain. There are many projections between the ARAS and the cerebral cortex.

Coma results from either dysfunction of the ARAS or the diffuse involvement of the cerebral cortex bilaterally. Dysfunction of only a portion of the cerebral cortex, for example, following a focal cerebral vascular accident, does not typically cause coma. Both structural lesions and toxic–metabolic conditions can cause coma. When the cause is a structural lesion, coma occurs either because the structural lesion directly affects the ARAS (e.g., brainstem hemorrhage) or because secondary effects of a structural lesion (e.g., increased intracranial pressure related to a subdural hematoma) impact the ARAS. Unilateral supratentorial structural lesions do not cause coma unless associated with mass effect and compression of brainstem structures. Toxic–metabolic conditions (e.g., poisoning) cause coma via diffuse involvement of the cerebral cortex or by direct effects on the ARAS.

What Coma Is Not

In exploring what coma *is*, it is helpful to recognize what coma is *not*. Coma is not sleep. Sleep is a normal alteration of arousal, experienced by all living creatures. The key distinguishing behavioral feature between sleep and coma is the fact that the sleeping individual can be aroused.

Coma must be distinguished from the *locked-in syndrome*. The unfortunate patient with locked-in syndrome appears to be comatose because he is quadriplegic, unable to speak, and unable to move facial musculature. However, these patients are alert, aware of the environment, able to hear, understand, and feel. Typically, the locked-in patient's voluntary movements are limited to eye blinks and/or vertical eye movements, as these are the only motor pathways spared by the underlying lesion. The locked-in syndrome is usually caused by large pontine lesions that destroy the descending corticospinal and corticobulbar tracts. However, similar clinical situations have been described with bilateral internal capsule lesions, bilateral midbrain peduncular lesions, and severe polyneuropathies, including acute inflammatory demyelinating polyneuropathy. It is critically important that *every* apparently comatose patient be evaluated for the ability to open the eyes and move the eyes in the vertical plane (with the examiner holding the eyelids open) in order to rule out the locked-in syndrome. This should be done in a serial fashion, as patients can improve to a locked-in state during the course of their recovery.

On occasion, patients in a *vegetative state* have been described as comatose. The vegetative state has been called "eyes open unconsciousness," and occurs when there is complete loss of functioning of the cortex but intact functioning of the brainstem. The vegetative state is characterized by a total absence of cognitive functioning, including the abilities to think, feel pain, experience pleasure, communicate, or interact with the environment. However, vegetative functions including respiration and brainstem-mediated reflexes (pupillary, eye movements) remain intact. Sleep–wake cycles are present in the vegetative state. Patients in the vegetative state may also have some spontaneous, although nonpurposeful, movements including vocalizations and eye movements. Patients who survive extensive damage to both cerebral hemispheres (e.g., anoxic encephalopathy) may initially present with coma, but then may enter a vegetative state. The vegetative state may emerge at any time following coma, but usually does so within several weeks. After the vegetative state has been present for 1 month, the clinical condition is referred to as a *persistent vegetative state* (PVS). After 1 year, it is called a *permanent vegetative state*. These conditions are discussed later in the chapter.

On occasion, patients with a new onset of global aphasia have been mislabeled as confused or having an alteration in level of consciousness. This results from the patient's inability to understand, carry out commands, or communicate in any purposeful way. Misdiagnosis can be avoided by noting that the patient frequently appears to be awake and alert, can mimic activities performed by the examiner, and often displays focal findings indicative of left-sided cerebral dysfunction including right hemiplegia.

Finally, it is important to distinguish coma from *pseudocoma*. Pseudocoma is hysterical or deliberate assumed depression of consciousness. It occurs most commonly within the setting of psychiatric illness, but may be a conscious effort on the part of a malingering patient.

▼

Pearls and Perils

Coma

► Trauma is a frequent cause of unexplained coma; keep a high index of suspicion when evaluating the patient with unexplained coma.

► Descriptions of patient behavior are more useful than generic terms.

► Be careful to distinguish those conditions—pseudocoma, locked-in syndrome, etc.—that may look like coma, but are not.

► Patient odor can provide important clues to the etiology of coma, but do not overestimate the importance of alcohol.

► Except in extraordinary circumstances, lumbar puncture should not be done in comatose patients without prior imaging studies to rule out a structural abnormality.

Although physiologically awake, patients in pseudocoma appear to be unresponsive. Characteristics that may be helpful in distinguishing this condition from coma include the following: heart and respiratory rates and patterns are usually normal; muscle tone is frequently normal; there is little or no resistance to passive movement; and unexpected motor responses may be exhibited. Examples of the latter include the patient's hand falling to the side rather than falling on the face when the examiner drops the patient's hand over the patient's face. The patient may forcefully resist eyelid opening with associated movement of the eyeballs upward and outward (Bell phenomenon). Resistance to eyelid opening does not occur in true coma. In addition, the eyes of a comatose patient will close slowly and gradually after being opened passively by the examiner. This is extremely difficult to feign and will not be seen in most patients in pseudocoma. Roving eye movements—slow, random deviations of the eyes—cannot be mimicked and when present, indicate true coma with intact brainstem oculomotor pathways and intact oculomotor nerves. The pupillary light reflex can also be useful in distinguishing pseudocoma from true coma, particularly when pupillary dilation occurs upon passive eye opening. When the eyelids of a normal sleeping patient or of a comatose patient are closed, the pupils constrict. When opened, pupillary dilation occurs. In contrast, when an awake individual closes his eyes, pupillary dilation occurs. When the eyelids are opened, an initial constriction of the pupils occurs. Furthermore, oculocephalic and oculovestibular reflexes are intact in patients in pseudocoma. They will frequently be abnormal or absent in a true coma. Finally, the electroencephalogram (EEG) may provide useful additional indications that an apparently comatose patient is, in fact, awake.

Although pseudocoma may be more common in patients with psychiatric disease, these patients are as susceptible to the usual causes of coma as patients without such a history. Patients with known psychiatric disease must still receive careful attention and evaluation for the possibility of a true coma. It is inappropriate to prejudge a diagnosis, and to do so may prove fatal for the patient.

Finally, it is important to distinguish coma from *brain death*. Brain death is defined as the total and irreversible cessation of total brain (cerebrum and brainstem) function. A diagnosis of brain death should be made only by a clinician who is experienced in diagnosing the condition and only after confounding factors are ruled out. Confounding factors include hypothermia and central nervous system (CNS) depressants (e.g., barbiturate) intoxication, which may mimic the clinical picture of brain death but are reversible states. The total loss of brain function must be demonstrated via a careful neurologic examination, which includes formal tests of cerebral and brainstem function, including apnea testing and brainstem reflexes. The irreversible nature of the condition must be demonstrated by serial tests or by other means (e.g., cerebral blood flow studies). Electroencephalography and cranial imaging tests may also be useful.

Diagnostic Approach to the Comatose Patient

Integration of Diagnosis and Management

Diagnosis in coma is directed toward identifying the level of neurologic dysfunction and the probable etiology of the coma. Diagnosis takes place concurrently with emergent management of the patient. Delay in management can result in the patient's death. The physician must keep an open mind about etiologic possibilities, incorporating the elements of known history but not forgetting that other events may have also supervened.

The diagnostic approach to coma calls upon the physician to combine history, physical examination, and neurologic examination with a sound knowledge of neuroanatomy. Specific questions that the examiner should be considering during the examination include the following: What is the level of the patient's consciousness? What portions of the brain are working, and what portions are not? What are the likely causes for this condition? What laboratory tests are necessary? What emergent and/or empiric therapies should be ordered? Is there evidence of improvement or deterioration over time?

History

A history provides invaluable information about coma. The patient is unable to provide this history, but examination of pocket contents, purse and/or wallet, and the setting where the patient was found may be helpful. The physician must take the time to speak to others who may have witnessed the event leading to coma or have other knowledge of the patient's past history. Knowledge of preexisting medical illness, psychiatric illnesses, medications that the patient was on or had access to, recent behaviors, and other elements of the history can be critically important.

General Physical Examination

The importance of a good general physical examination cannot be overstated. Vital signs provide valuable information. As will be discussed later, the respiratory pattern provides both important data about what portions of the brain are working and a mechanism of identifying progression of the coma. Temperature should be evaluated with a rectal thermometer. Hypothermia can cause alterations in level of consciousness, especially with core body temperatures of less than 32°C. Hypothermic coma occurs with environmental exposures, hypothyroidism, hypopituitarism, hypothalamic lesions, and various toxic–metabolic conditions, including hypoglycemia and overdoses of CNS depressants (e.g., barbiturates, phenothiazines, alcohol). Since hyperthermia does not typically cause alterations in consciousness, any comatose patient with a fever should be considered to have an infectious process until proven otherwise. Certain patients, particularly the elderly and the immunosuppressed, may not have fever despite infection. Noninfectious conditions in which coma is associated with fever include heat stroke, neuroleptic malignant syndrome, malignant hyperthermia, status epilepticus, and anticholinergic intoxication. The heart rate and rhythm may suggest cardiac disease. Hypotension can lead to coma via failure of cerebral perfusion. Hypertension, except in the case of malignant hypertension, does not typically lead to alterations in consciousness.

Odors associated with certain medical conditions (e.g., hepatic coma, diabetic ketoacidosis) and other characteristic odors (e.g., alcohol) may provide diagnostic clues. Take care, however, not to overinterpret the smell of alcohol on a patient's breath. Unfortunate instances have been documented in which treatable causes of alteration in consciousness (e.g., intracranial hemorrhage from head trauma, drug intoxicants) have been missed when a patient's coma was attributed to inebriation. Serum alcohol levels may be difficult to obtain quickly, but serum osmolality may be extremely helpful in interpreting whether or not the patient has enough alcohol on board to account for a significant change in the level of consciousness. Alcohol is an osmotically active particle and will increase the osmolar gap proportional to its blood level. Consequently, the difference between the measured serum osmolality (done by the laboratory) and the calculated serum osmolality (done by the clinician using the formula: $2(Na^+[mEq/L] + K^+[mEq/L] + BUN(mg/dL)/2.8 + glucose (mg/dL)/18)$ represents unmeasured osmotically active particles, and provides an indication of the presence of alcohol.

Examination of the skin may reveal a wide variety of features, including jaundice, petechiae, and unusual hair pattern or body habitus, which suggest addisonian crisis, liver disease, acquired immune deficiency syndrome (AIDS), or some other etiology for the patient's coma. Eye examination may reveal subhyaloid hemorrhages or papilledema, both of which point toward structural etiologies for the patient's condition. Bruising over the mastoid process (Battle sign), periorbital bruising (raccoon eyes), and blood behind the tympanic membrane may indicate basilar skull fracture. A comatose patient's neck should not be manipulated until the possibility of cervical trauma has been ruled out. Once examined, however, increased resistance to passive flexion of the neck may indicate meningeal irritation related to an infectious process or increased intracranial pressure with herniation. The abdominal examination may suggest unexpected trauma.

Neurologic Examination

The neurologic examination is critical for defining the patient's level of neurologic functioning, as well as for suggesting likely causes for the coma. The neurologic evaluation of the comatose individual is directed at five major areas of concern: responsiveness, respiratory pattern, pupillary responses, eye movements, and motor responses. Examination findings frequently fluctuate over time. The level of neurologic dysfunction in coma frequently progresses in a rostrocaudal manner, particularly with increasing intracranial pressure. Careful documentation of the patient's evolving clinical condition provides valuable information about ongoing processes and prognosis. Also, many neurologic abnormalities described in coma present in partial form.

Responsiveness

The patient's responsiveness should be evaluated at rest and with stimulation. Stimuli presented to the patient should be of a variety of types and intensities. Examples include calling the patient's name, shouting, gentle touch, and applying deep painful pressure over the sternum, supraorbital notch, or nail beds. Nail bed pressure is a very effective noxious stimulus, which can be applied unobtrusively to the base of the fingernails or toenails using a pen or penlight. Pinching or twisting of the nipples is unseemly and should be avoided. The examiner is interested not only in what, if any, stimuli provoke a response, but also what that response is.

A patient with a mild alteration in level of consciousness may vocalize or have some purposeful movements at rest or in response to stimuli. For example, the

---

Key Clinical Questions

▶ What are the patient's examination findings with regard to level of responsiveness, respiratory pattern, pupillary responses, eye movements, and motor responses/posturing?

▶ Is there evidence of impending brain herniation?

▶ Is there a medical setting/condition (e.g., hypothermia, hypothyroidism, hypopituitarism, hypoglycemia, overdose of central nervous system depressants) that suggests a likely cause for the patient's coma?

▶ Has cervical trauma been ruled out?

▶ Is there meningeal irritation?

▶ Has the possibility of locked-in syndrome been ruled out?

patient may try to push or move away from, noxious stimuli. Asymmetries in these movements may reflect underlying neurologic disease. With decreasing levels of consciousness, patients will have fewer purposeful movements. In deep coma, the patient will have no vocalizations or movements. Nonetheless, even in deep coma, patients may have spinal reflexes, which should not be misinterpreted as purposeful movements on the patient's part. The most prominent spinal reflex is the triple flexion response, which produces withdrawal of the foot, leg, and thigh and fanning of the toes with noxious stimuli.

Respiratory pattern

Normal breathing occurs when automatic respiratory efforts mediated by the brainstem are modulated by higher cortical functioning. This allows us to breathe without conscious effort, and for higher-level activities—like speech—without conscious interruption of breathing. The major types of respiratory patterns seen in comatose patients are pictured in Figure 13.1. These patterns include Cheyne-Stokes respiration, central neurogenic hyperventilation, apneustic breathing, cluster breathing and ataxic breathing. These patterns cannot be identified when the patient is being mechanically ventilated. The respiratory pattern provides information about the baseline level of brain functioning (or dysfunctioning), gives clues as to the etiology of the coma, provides a means of following the patient's course, and provides early warning of impending brain herniation.

Cheyne-Stokes respirations are seen in situations in which there is bilateral cerebral hemispheric or diencephalic dysfunction, and also in severe congestive heart failure. Cheyne-Stokes respirations are characterized by a period of regular respirations that build in intensity and frequency and then fade in a similar fashion until the patient enters a shorter period of apnea. This pattern is believed to reflect an abnormal response of the respiratory centers to carbon dioxide. A period of apnea leads to high levels of carbon dioxide. The hyperpnea begins in response to this high level. In turn, this leads to the carbon dioxide being blown off, which causes the apneic phase. Then carbon dioxide builds again and the hyperpnea restarts.

Cheyne-Stokes respirations are fairly common in metabolic problems. Although the breathing pattern, by itself, is not of great concern, new Cheyne-Stokes respirations in the clinical context of a known intracranial

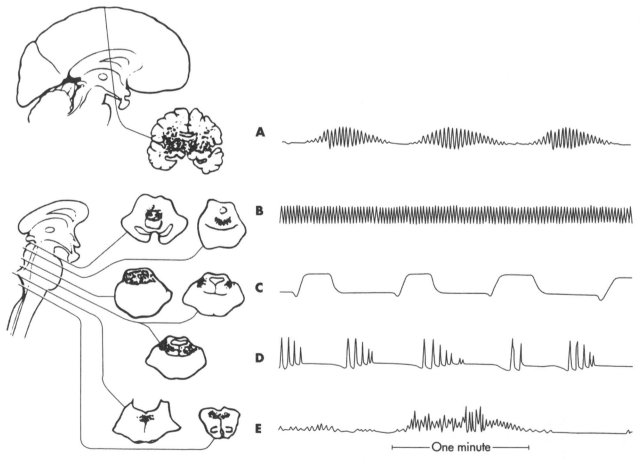

Figure 13.1 Respiratory patterns in coma. A: Cheyne-Stokes respirations. B: Central neurogenic hyperventilation. C: Apneusis. D: Cluster breathing. E: Ataxic breathing. From Plum F, Posner JB. *Diagnosis of stupor and coma*, 3rd ed. Philadelphia: FA Davis, 1980, with permission.

mass lesion should raise suspicion of early herniation. The progression of Cheyne-Stokes respirations to one of the other brainstem patterns of respiration is indicative of neurologic deterioration.

Central neurogenic hyperventilation is a rare respiratory pattern seen in lesions that involve the lower midbrain and upper pons, particularly lesions ventral to the aqueduct or fourth ventricle. Central neurogenic hyperventilation is characterized by rapid, regular respirations with rates of 40–70 breaths/minute. Central neurogenic hyperventilation must be distinguished from hyperventilation related to metabolic and pulmonary causes. In fact, regular deep breathing and hyperventilation are far more commonly related to metabolic or pulmonary causes than to CNS structural lesions. For that reason, hyperpnea should not be attributed to a CNS lesion when the Po_2 is less than 70–80 Hg or the Pco_2 is more than 40 Hg.

Apneustic breathing is seen with dysfunction of the lower pons, usually due to infarction, but it may also be seen either with brainstem compression from mass lesions involving the cerebellum or with rare episodes of upward herniation through the tentorial notch. The pattern consists of a prolonged inspiratory gasp with a pause at full inspiration prior to expiration. *Cluster breathing* occurs with high medullary lesions. It is characterized by disorderly, close groups of respirations followed by periods of

apnea. Finally, *ataxic breathing* is a preterminal breathing pattern characterized by chaotic breaths that lead to agonal gasps and cessation of all respiratory efforts. This form of breathing occurs as the medullary respiratory center becomes involved by the underlying pathology. Patients exhibiting these respirations should be intubated, as should all patients who exhibit progressive levels of respiratory dysfunction.

Pupillary responses

Pupillary light abnormalities provide a wealth of information in coma evaluation, since pupillary light responses are mediated by sympathetic and parasympathetic neural pathways, which traverse much of the brainstem. The light reflex pathway is shown in Figure 13.2. The afferent arm of the pupilloconstrictor portion (parasympathetic) of the pupillary light reflex begins at the optic nerve (cranial nerve II). Some of these fibers cross to the other side via the optic chiasm, while others remain on the same side. The fibers continue through the optic tracts to the midbrain, where they run through the tectum to the Edinger-Westphal nuclei on both sides. The efferent arm of the parasympathetic pupilloconstrictor portion of the reflex begins in the Edinger-Westphal nucleus and travels via the oculomotor nerve (cranial nerve III) to the ciliary ganglion and then to the pupillary constrictor muscles.

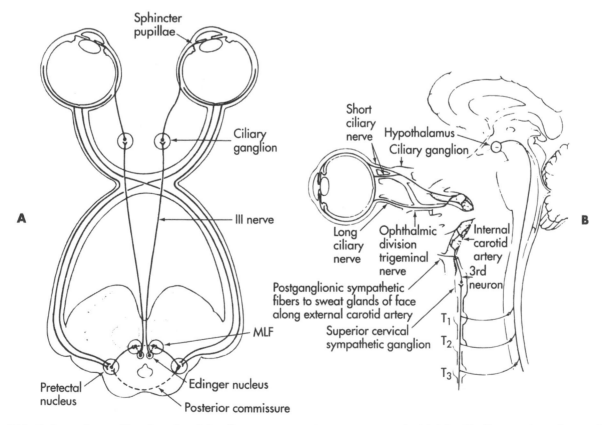

Figure 13.2 Pathways for pupillary function. A: Pupilloconstrictor pathway (parasympathetic). B: Pupillodilator pathway (sympathetic). From Plum F, Posner JB. *Diagnosis of stupor and coma*, 3rd ed. Philadelphia: FA Davis, 1980, with permission.

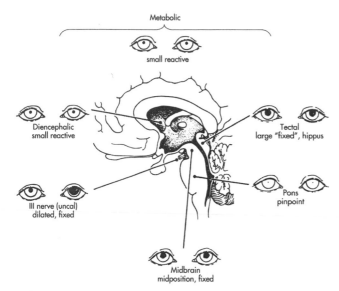

Figure 13.3 Typical pupillary abnormalities in coma. From Plum F, Posner JB. *Diagnosis of stupor and coma*, 3rd ed. Philadelphia: FA Davis, 1980, with permission.

The sympathetic pupillodilator portion of the reflex is a three-neuron pathway. The first-order neuron begins in the hypothalamus, travels through the brainstem, and synapses in the cervical spinal cord at the level of the first thoracic nerve root. The second-order neuron synapses in the superior cervical ganglion from which the third-order neuron travels alongside the carotid artery. Various sympathetic fibers mediate pupillary dilation and motor control of the levator palpebrae superioris muscle, which is responsible for opening the eyelid.

Pupils should be evaluated at rest, and their response to light should be tested using a bright light to provide a maximal stimulus to the pathway. Critical information can be conveyed by extremely small pupillary movements, so examination should include magnification in cases with apparently nonreactive pupils. An otoscope may be useful as it provides both a good light source and magnification. In the absence of intrinsic eye diseases, the pupils are generally symmetric. Typical pupillary abnormalities are outlined in Figure 13.3.

Metabolic coma is frequently associated with symmetric alterations in pupillary size, but pupillary responses are usually retained even in deep metabolic coma. Opiates, for example, cause pinpoint pupils. Anticholinergic agents, such as atropine and tricyclic antidepressants, cause wide pupillary dilation. Avoid medicating patients with agents that may cause pupillary dilation when they are being observed in the hospital setting for neurologic deterioration. When mydriatic agents are necessary, it is important to document their use to avoid misinterpretation of a large pupil.

Other pupillary findings in coma may localize dysfunction to a specific level of the neuraxis. *Diencephalic pupils* are small and reactive to light, and are seen when there is bilateral hemispheric dysfunction or a thalamic lesion. Sympathetic dysfunction at the level of the hypothalamus is the cause of the small pupils. Bilateral midposition, unreactive pupils of 4–7 mm occur in midbrain lesions affecting the tectum. The size and lack of reactivity reflect involvement of both sympathetic and parasympathetic fibers. *Pontine pupils* are small pupils seen with pathology involving the pons. They do react to light, but the reaction is so small that magnification may be necessary in order to identify it.

Special attention must be paid to the presence of asymmetries on examination. Because pupillary reflexes are mediated chiefly by midbrain structures and the oculomotor nerve, unilateral pupillary dysfunction suggests pathology at one of these two sites. Although pupillary asymmetries do occur in normal individuals, any asymmetry in a comatose patient must raise concern about either the presence of a Horner syndrome or of oculomotor nerve involvement. Distinguishing the two causes of pupillary asymmetry is important. Occasionally, an examiner becomes very concerned about a "blown" pupil on one side when, in fact, a Horner syndrome is present on the other side. The major concern with oculomotor nerve dysfunction is whether or not it indicates herniation of the brain.

Horner syndrome is characterized by miosis (a small pupil) caused by unopposed parasympathetic response, ptosis of the ipsilateral eyelid, and possible anhidrosis, depending on what portions of the sympathetic tract are involved. The syndrome is caused by pathology involving the sympathetic fibers on the same side as the abnormal eye. The pupil involved in a Horner syndrome will typically react to light, albeit minimally.

Oculomotor nerve (cranial nerve III) palsies are characterized by an enlarged pupil on the side of the lesion caused by unopposed sympathetic tone and by a loss of eye movements mediated by the third nerve, with resultant deviation of the affected eye outward and downward. Anatomically, the third nerve has the pupilloconstrictor fibers located at the periphery and oculomotor fibers located more toward the center of the nerve. This anatomy is very helpful in analyzing third-nerve lesions. In early third-nerve palsies resulting from pressure on the third nerve, pupillary dilation may be seen without involvement of the oculomotor component of the nerve. In this context, herniation must be strongly considered, as the third nerve is susceptible to compression at the midbrain and at the temporal incisura. On the other hand, structural lesions in the brainstem that compromise the oculomotor nerve tend to cause more complete destruction with earlier involvement of the motor component, as well as the pupillodilator component.

Eye movements

The neural pathways controlling eye movements are extensive throughout the cerebrum and brainstem. Voluntary conjugate eye movements are initiated by the frontal eye fields and coordinated through an extensive neural network that involves the paramedian pontine reticular formations, median longitudinal fasciculi, and oculomotor and abducens nerves. The pathway, with emphasis on those portions related to left conjugate gaze, is outlined in Figure 13.4.

Clues to the level of neural dysfunction and the etiology for the patient's condition may be obtained from careful examination of ocular motility. The resting position of the eyes, and spontaneous eye movements with and without environmental cues, should be documented. Reflex eye movements should be checked.

Normally, the eyes track objects in their visual fields with appropriate conjugate movements. Lateral conjugate eye deviation is most consistent with a cerebral hemispherical process on the side of the direction of deviation, whereas brainstem lesions typically result in gaze deviation away from the side of the lesion. Other features of the examination help differentiate supratentorial from infratentorial lesions. Eye deviation below the horizontal (setting-sun sign) and skew deviation (a supranuclear ocular misalignment in the vertical plane) can be caused by brainstem lesions. Thalamic lesions can cause the patient's eyes to be deviated inward and downward (looking at the patient's nose), or conjugately away from the lesion (so-called "wrong-way eyes"). Conjugate nystagmoid movements at rest, particularly in conjugately deviated eyes, may indicate an irritative cortical focus of seizure activity.

Cranial nerve palsies resulting in dysconjugate resting eye positions can provide valuable information about the location of pathology. Small discrepancies in eye positioning may suggest an incomplete palsy of one of the cranial nerves subserving ocular motility. An abducens nerve palsy results in esotropia and difficulties abducting the affected eye, whereas an oculomotor nerve palsy results in exotropia and difficulty adducting the affected eye. The long course of the abducens nerve often precludes assumptions regarding the specific location of a lesion. Other lesions also cause abnormalities in resting eye position. An internuclear ophthalmoplegia, characterized by impaired adduction of the eye ipsilateral to the lesion, with or without nystagmus of the abducting eye, is the consequence of involvement of the median longitudinal fasciculus.

The awake patient has spontaneous conjugate eye movements and consciously tracks objects in the environment. Spontaneous, nonpurposeful, conjugate roving eye movements are seen with cortical dysfunction in lighter stages of coma, particularly in metabolic coma. A variety of other spontaneous, nonpurposeful, eye movements can be seen and are helpful in localizing the area of dysfunction. These include ocular bobbing, reverse ocular bobbing, and ping-pong eye movements.

Reflex eye movements related to the vestibular system, and its input to the paramedian pontine reticular formation, are pictured in Figure 13.4. Oculocephalic ("doll's eyes") and oculovestibular reflexes ("calorics") provide input about the integrity of these systems and their associated cranial nerves. To perform oculocephalic

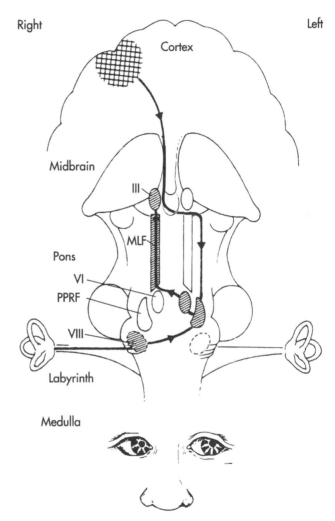

Figure 13.4 Diagram of the conjugate vision pathways. Nuclei and paths are shaded to include those important to left conjugate gaze: fibers from the right frontal cortex descend, then cross the midline, and synapse in the left paramedian pontine reticular formation (PPRF). Fibers then travel to the nearby left abducens (cranial nerve VI) nucleus (to move the left eye laterally) and then cross the midline to rise in the right median longitudinal fasciculus (MLF) to the right oculomotor (cranial nerve III) nucleus (to move the right eye medially).

In addition to the cortical influence on the left PPRF, vestibular influence is also present. With vestibular activation from the right, the left PPRF is stimulated, and the eyes conjugately move to the left. Instillation of ice water into the right ear canal will test the integrity of this vestibular-PPRF-abducens nerve (VI)-oculomotor (III) nerve circuit, and if the eyes move to vestibular stimulation, the brainstem from medulla to midbrain must be functioning. From Lewis S, Topel J. Coma. In Weiner W, Goetz C (eds.), *Neurology for the non-neurologist*. Philadelphia: JB Lippincott, 1994, with permission.

reflex testing, the examiner holds the eyes open and moves the entire head briskly either to one side, forward or backward. Because movement of the head and neck occurs, it is critically important to ensure that there is no neck trauma before attempting this maneuver. Eye movements are evaluated relative to the movement of the head. In the awake patient, fixation usually overrides the reflex. In a comatose patient with an intact, functioning brainstem, the eyes move conjugately in a direction opposite to the direction of head movement. Dysconjugate movements of the eyes imply focal dysfunction of the brainstem or cranial nerves. Failure of the eyes to move with oculocephalic maneuvers in comatose patients implies diffuse dysfunction of these pathways.

Oculovestibular reflex testing evaluates the same brainstem pathway as oculocephalic reflex testing. However, the stimulus used (cold water injected into the ear canal versus head movements) is far stronger. Because of this, the testing may yield a response when oculocephalic testing is negative. The test is also useful if oculocephalics cannot be evaluated because of possible neck trauma. However, if oculocephalic reflexes are intact and normal, there is no need to do oculovestibular testing.

The oculovestibular reflex is elicited by the slow infusion of 10 mL of ice water into the external ear canal with the patient's head elevated to 30 degrees above the horizontal (for optimal positioning of the horizontal semicircular canal). Prior to doing the test, the examiner must ensure that the tympanic membrane is intact and that the external auditory canal is clear of wax. In the awake state, the eyes will conjugately deviate to the side of the cold stimulus and nystagmoid movements away from the stimulus will be seen. The response to stimulation of each side should be documented and compared. With hemispheral dysfunction, ipsilateral conjugate deviation of the eyes to the side of ice water stimulus without any nystagmus will be seen. Dysconjugate eye movements and/or lack of response on one or both sides may be seen with pathologic involvement of the median longitudinal fasciculus or other lesions of the brainstem and cranial nerves.

As part of the eye evaluation, the corneal response should be checked by touching a piece of tissue to the cornea at the limbus. This response evaluates the integrity of the brainstem and the oculomotor, trigeminal, and facial nerves. The stimulus is transmitted via the trigeminal nerve, and the motor response of eyelid blinking is mediated by the facial nerve. To check the oculomotor nerve, the examiner holds the eyelid open and looks for upward movement of the eye (Bell phenomenon) in response to the stimulus.

Motor responses and posturing

In evaluating the motor system, the patient should be observed both at rest and in response to stimuli. The patient's resting position, movements (if any), muscle tone,

and reflexes should be evaluated. The patient's position and behavior at rest may provide evidence of a focal neurologic process, particularly when asymmetric. For example, head and eye deviation to one side with contralateral hemiplegia suggests a supratentorial lesion, whereas hemiplegia on the same side as eye deviation suggests a brainstem lesion. External rotation of the leg may suggest a hemiplegia. Differences in muscle tone from one side to the other may also suggest a focal process; metabolic processes usually reduce tone symmetrically. Bilateral Babinski responses are common in coma; a unilateral response suggests a focal process.

The patient should be observed for any evidence of posturing, as pictured in Figure 13.5. Decorticate posturing indicates hemispheric dysfunction and is characterized by flexion of the wrists and arms and extension of the legs. Decerebrate posturing indicates pathology at midbrain or pontine levels and is characterized by extension of all four extremities and internal rotation of the shoulders. With dysfunction below this level, the limbs will be flaccid. Posturing can occur spontaneously or in response to noxious or other stimuli. Although posturing is usually bilateral, unilateral posturing can occur and suggests focal cerebral dysfunction. A mistake to be avoided is misinterpreting posturing (especially when intermittent) as seizure activity. Posturing often provides early evidence of herniation, and progression of posturing in a rostrocaudal manner (i.e., decorticate followed by decerebrate posturing) is ominous.

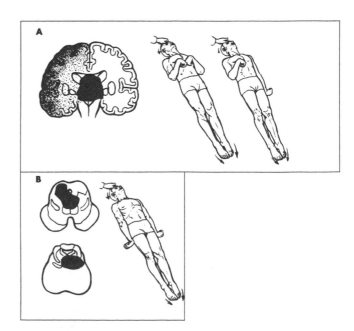

Figure 13.5 A: Decorticate posturing. B: Decerebrate posturing. From Plum F, Posner JB. *Diagnosis of stupor and coma*, 3rd ed. Philadelphia: FA Davis, 1980, with permission.

The Glasgow Coma Scale

The Glasgow Coma Scale (GCS) was initially developed to assess levels of consciousness following traumatic brain injury. Subsequently, it has been widely employed to assess the level of consciousness in patients with other conditions. The GCS provides an objective, reproducible, easily used means of assessing the severity of traumatic brain injury with high inter- and intra-rater reliability. This scale, which is featured in Table 13.2, is based on patient response in three areas: best motor response, best verbal response, and the stimulus necessary to induce patient eye opening. Patients can be repeatedly assessed, and serial scores provide evidence of a patient's improving or worsening condition. The reproducibility and ease of use of the GCS make it a very popular tool in the care of these patients and, despite the promotion of other scales, such as the FOUR score (Wijdicks, 2006), is unlikely to be supplanted. It is important to note that this and other scales of consciousness do not assess all critical neurologic parameters and that there is no substitute for detailed neurologic assessment of the patient with an altered level of consciousness.

Differential Diagnosis

The immediate goals for physicians evaluating patients in coma are to identify the cause of coma and rapidly initiate appropriate therapy. History, physical examination, neurologic examination, and laboratory studies contribute to accomplishing these goals. A first step in making a diagnosis is determining whether the coma is related to a toxic–metabolic or structural cause. The majority of all cases of coma are due to toxic–metabolic causes. In one study (Plum and Posner 1995), 326 out of 500 comatose patients had metabolic brain dysfunction. About half of these patients had drug poisoning.

Toxic–metabolic versus Structural Coma

As suggested in Table 13.3, elements of the history, general and neurologic examinations, and response to initial therapy will assist in distinguishing toxic–metabolic and structural causes of coma. Structural lesions causing coma are more commonly abrupt in onset, whereas toxic–metabolic coma tends to have a gradual onset. However, exceptions to this rule abound. For example, slow-growing brain tumors with associated edema may present in a progressive manner, and hypoglycemic coma may develop abruptly. Patients with metabolic etiologies will often be in lighter stages of coma and may have waxing and waning levels of consciousness. Coma with structural lesions tends to remain constant or progressively deteriorate (Table 13.4).

Generally, the neurologic examination in toxic–metabolic coma is notable for its symmetry. Focal findings, including asymmetries in muscle tone, reflexes, and posturing point toward an underlying structural process. However, focal findings may be seen with toxic–metabolic coma. Their presence should increase suspicion of preexisting neurologic disease (e.g., old stroke), hypoglycemia, hyponatremia, hepatic encephalopathy, and poisoning with barbiturates or lead. On the other hand, certain structural lesions can mimic a toxic–metabolic presentation, including subarachnoid hemorrhage, intracranial venous thrombosis, and chronic subdural hematoma (Table 13.5).

Table 13.2 The Glasgow Coma Scale

Best motor response

Obeys	M6
Localizes	5
Withdraws	4
Abnormal flexion	3
Extensor response	2
Nil	1

Verbal response

Oriented	V5
Confused conversation	4
Inappropriate words	3
Incomprehensible sounds	2
Nil1	1

Eye opening

Spontaneous	E4
To speech	3
To pain	2
Nil	1

Table 3.13 Toxic/metabolic coma

Discriminating features

▶ Symmetric abnormalities on neurologic exam; lack of focal findings

▶ Mental status change precedes motor signs

▶ MRI/CT does not show lesion

▶ EEG shows diffuse slowing

Consistent features

▶ Abnormal respiratory pattern

▶ Pupillary responses intact

▶ Tone is normal or slightly reduced

▶ Waxing and waning level of responsiveness

Variable features

▶ Laboratory studies abnormal

▶ Abnormal movements common

Table 13.4 Coma due to supratentorial structural lesions

Discriminating features
▶ Focal findings in a pattern consistent with a hemispheral process
▶ MRI/CT scan shows lesion
▶ EEG has focal slowing

Consistent features
▶ Asymmetric motor signs (movements, tone, reflexes, posturing)
▶ Abrupt onset of coma
▶ Progressive worsening of condition without intervention

Variable features
▶ Neurologic dysfunction progresses in a rostrocaudal fashion

---

Table 13.5 Coma due to infratentorial structural lesions

Discriminating features
▶ Presents with cranial nerve involvement plus contralateral limb involvement
▶ Intranuclear ophthalmoplegia
▶ MRI/CT shows lesion

Consistent features
▶ Asymmetric pupils
▶ Oculomotor nerve involvement

Variable features
▶ Abnormal respiratory patterns

Papilledema, subhyaloid hemorrhages, and oculomotor nerve lesions suggest a structural process. As already noted, pupil symmetry, pupillary reactivity, and reflex eye movements tend to remain intact in toxic–metabolic coma, although they can be lost with certain drug intoxications (e.g., barbiturates and phenytoin) and in very deep coma. Bilateral asterixis, tremors, myoclonus, and other unusual movements are often seen in toxic-metabolic processes.

Laboratory Studies

Laboratory studies assist in the diagnosis and management of the comatose patient. In general, blood studies should be obtained immediately prior to or concurrent with initial evaluation and management. Blood alcohol levels and toxicology screens should be obtained in any case of coma of unknown etiology. Other laboratory studies include arterial blood gases, complete blood count with differential and platelet count, serum blood glucose, electrolytes, and other chemistry studies including blood urea nitrogen (BUN), creatinine, magnesium, calcium, ammonia, liver and thyroid function studies, and creatine phosphokinase (CK). An elevated CK may suggest previously unrecognized trauma or seizure.

Other laboratory tests should be ordered depending upon the history and clinical presentation. For example, carboxyhemoglobin levels may be helpful if there is clinical suspicion of carbon monoxide poisoning. Toxicology screens of blood, urine, and gastric contents may be warranted. Serum ammonia is not a good predictor of outcome in coma related to liver disease, but is useful in diagnosing hepatic coma in the face of chronic liver disease when liver function tests may remain normal. If addisonian crisis is contemplated, serum electrolytes may be suggestive of the diagnosis, and a serum cortisol should be obtained. A normal or low serum cortisol level should heighten concern, as serum cortisol levels are expected to be high given the stress of coma.

Additional studies that may be of use include an electrocardiogram (EKG), neuroradiologic imaging, and neurophysiologic testing. An EKG may reveal evidence of acute myocardial infarction or arrhythmia, suggest biochemical abnormalities, and provide evidence of preexisting cardiac disease. Neuroradiologic imaging is critical in identifying structural lesions. Scans should be examined for the presence of focal structural lesions, subtle signs of herniation, and isodense subdural hematomas. In general, computed tomography (CT) scanning is preferable to magnetic resonance imaging (MRI) in terms of imaging time, ability to recognize intracranial hemorrhage, difficulties related to movement artifact, and cost. Useful neurophysiologic tests include evoked potentials and EEG. Evoked potentials are helpful to evaluate brainstem integrity and may also be useful in establishing prognosis. An EEG can identify nonconvulsive status epilepticus and partial complex seizures, and may be extremely useful in distinguishing toxic–metabolic coma from coma related to underlying structural abnormalities. The EEG is also used to distinguish coma from other conditions that may be misinterpreted as coma, including pseudocoma, locked-in syndrome, and brain death.

As a general rule, lumbar puncture should not be done in comatose patients unless imaging studies have ruled out the possibility of a mass lesion. This is particularly true if papilledema, focal neurologic findings, or a history suggestive of a focal process is present. Lumbar puncture in the face of increased intracranial pressure, particularly when that increased intracranial pressure is caused by a mass lesion, can result in sudden herniation and death. In situations in which a high level of suspicion of an infectious process exists but neuroimaging cannot be done, empiric antibiotic coverage should be started prior to obtaining cerebrospinal fluid for culture.

Brain Herniation

Brain herniation is one of the most urgent concerns in the evaluation and management of the comatose patient, since failure to recognize or treat this problem results in rapid fatality or severe morbidity. Brain herniation occurs when a focal or generalized brain process causes pressure (either via the process itself or via associated phenomena) which, in turn, leads to abnormal protrusion of parts of the brain outside of their normal boundaries. Once herniation has progressed to the point where midbrain findings are noted, structural injury is likely to have occurred, and the patient's prognosis dims.

Brain herniation due to a supratentorial process usually follows one of two patterns called *uncal* and *central herniation*. Uncal herniation is characterized in its earliest phases by oculomotor nerve compression. The ipsilateral pupil initially dilates due to involvement of the parasympathetic fibers of the third nerve. Afterward, involvement of sympathetic fibers results in the pupil returning to a midposition size. With further progression and compression of the third nerve and midbrain, the motor fibers will be compromised, with resulting deviation of the eye laterally and inferiorly. Unalleviated, increased intracranial pressure will eventually result in compression of key brainstem respiratory centers and the patient's death. In central herniation, the earliest signs tend to be poor concentration and drowsiness. Sometimes patients exhibit agitation. Additional findings may include small but reactive pupils, poor or absent reflex vertical gaze, loss of the fast component of oculocephalic reflexes, and bilateral corticospinal tract signs including increased tone and Babinski signs. Failure to recognize these signs may lead to progression of the clinical syndrome and the patient's death. Increased intracranial pressure invariably accompanies brainstem herniation and may be manifested by bradycardia, hypertension, irregular breathing (Cushing response), and sixth-nerve palsy.

The Therapeutic Approach to the Comatose Patient

Acute Coma Is a Medical Emergency

Management of the comatose patient occurs concurrent with the ongoing evaluation. Coma is a medical emergency and should be treated as such. The initial emergency treatment of a comatose patient is the same as for any other critically ill patient. An adequate airway must be ensured. Endotracheal intubation and ventilatory support may be necessary. Intravenous access is necessary. Support of cardiovascular functioning and blood pressure is critical. As greater information is obtained by the physician, treatment of specific conditions causing the patient's coma will be possible. Serial assessment of these patients is critical.

Treatment of Increased Intracranial Pressure

If increased intracranial pressure is suspected, it must be treated aggressively. Hyperventilation provides the most rapid, albeit short-lasting, mechanism for reliably reducing intracranial pressure. The patient should be hyperventilated to a Pco_2 of 20–25 Hg. Hyperosmolar solutions (e.g., mannitol) should be administered concurrently. Mannitol is given intravenously in a dose of 1–2 g/kg. The value of corticosteroids in the management of elevated intracranial pressure depends upon its etiology. Corticosteroids can be helpful in selected cases, particularly with vasogenic cerebral edema related to a brain tumor. Corticosteroids are not helpful with cytotoxic cerebral edema, as from a stroke, or with osmotic cerebral edema, as sometimes occurs with treatment of diabetic ketoacidosis.

Empiric Therapies

As blood work is obtained, several medications are routinely given on an empiric basis. Fifty milliliters of 50% dextrose in water (D50W) should be given to any patient with coma of unknown cause to treat hypoglycemic coma. Arguments against the routine use of hypertonic dextrose solutions include the worsening of hyperkalemia in some contexts and the potential aggravation of ischemic cerebrovascular lesions. There is no question that empiric use of this therapy results in unnecessary treatment of many patients. Nonetheless, the continued use of this therapy is recommended based upon the incidence of hypoglycemic coma, the potential reversibility of the condition, the low likelihood of harm to patients from its use (patients who present with coma related to a cerebral ischemic event appear to have a grave prognosis with or without the administration of hypertonic dextrose solutions), the low cost of the therapy, and the tremendous personal and financial costs associated with a missed opportunity for treatment.

One hundred milligrams of thiamine should be given intravenously when the D50W is given. D50W should not be withheld if thiamine is not immediately available, however. The purpose of the thiamine is to prevent the onset of acute thiamine deficiency in at-risk patients (e.g., chronic alcoholics) and to treat the rare patient who may be presenting with an alteration in level of consciousness related to Wernicke encephalopathy. Arguments against the use of routine thiamine include possible allergic reactions and the recognition that its empiric use will result in unnecessary overtreatment of many people. These risks are believed to be minimal and dramatically outweighed by the consequences of missing the opportunity to avoid unnecessary morbidity related to thiamine deficiency.

Naloxone is an opioid antagonist used to reverse the effects of acute opioid intoxication. Justification for the empiric use of naloxone is less straightforward than for either dextrose or thiamine. Naloxone use can precipitate acute opioid withdrawal and unmask side effects of other drugs if the patient is a polydrug user. For that reason, care must be taken in deciding which patients should receive this drug. In general, naloxone in an intravenous (IV) dose of 0.4 should be used as empiric therapy for individuals who present with CNS or respiratory depression possibly related to opiates and who are felt to be unlikely candidates for opioid addiction or polydrug intoxication. In patients who are considered at risk for either polydrug intoxication or chronic opioid addiction, Hoffman and Goldfrank suggest using very small doses of naloxone (0.1–0.2) to increase arousal and respiratory effort, and yet minimize the likelihood of either acute withdrawal or the unmasking of other drug effects. Regardless of the treatment approach, it is critically important to remember that naloxone has a very short half-life. Patients who respond to naloxone must be observed carefully in an intensive care setting, and additional doses should be given as appropriate. Continuous IV infusions of naloxone may be used in the appropriate patients.

In recent years, a pure benzodiazepine antagonist, flumazenil, has been used for the reversal of benzodiazepine-induced sedation. This drug is used increasingly in the emergency setting to treat benzodiazepine-induced coma. Like naloxone, there is concern about using this drug because of the potential of sudden benzodiazepine withdrawal, as well as the likelihood of uncovering side effects of other drugs in a polydrug intoxication. The use of flumazenil has also been associated with the occurrence of seizures, particularly in patients who have been on benzodiazepines for a long time, or in polydrug overdose cases involving large doses of cyclic antidepressants. In part because the drug is new, its empiric use is not recommended at this time. However, in those patients with a strong clinical likelihood of benzodiazepine intoxication, its use may be justified. Cautions related to flumazenil are similar to those with naloxone. Unmasked symptoms of other drugs must be treated. The half-life of this drug is significantly shorter than that of the benzodiazepines. Ongoing observation of the patient in an intensive care setting and readministration of the drug may be necessary. Practitioners using flumazenil should also be prepared to manage seizures.

The index of suspicion for trauma must be high in all cases of coma. This trauma may be the cause of the coma or may have been sustained after a patient becomes comatose (e.g., via a fall). In all cases of possible trauma, the comatose patient's neck should be stabilized and not manipulated until the cervical spine can be evaluated radiologically. General surgical consultation should be obtained if trauma is suspected. Peritoneal lavage may yield evidence of previously unsuspected trauma.

Prognosis

The physician is often called upon to offer an opinion regarding the prognosis of a comatose patient. Significant resources are utilized in caring for the patient. Families and other loved ones frequently want to know what to expect. Consequently, it is important to be able to provide information about the likelihood of survival and the anticipated quality of life should the patient survive.

Although there are few definite answers in this area of medical practice, some general statements can be made. Prognosis in coma varies dramatically depending upon the etiology of coma. We will consider nontraumatic coma separately from traumatic coma.

Nontraumatic versus Traumatic Coma

Survival and quality-of-life statistics are highly dependent upon the etiology of nontraumatic coma. Of the nontraumatic types of coma, drug-induced coma has the best prognosis. If the patient can be supported through the acute event, and if other drug-related complications are effectively treated, the patient stands an excellent chance of good-quality recovery. Even barbiturate intoxication, which can render a patient so deeply comatose as to appear brain dead, when diagnosed early and appropriately treated, can result in a good-quality recovery. Some metabolic comas, such as hepatic coma, are associated with relatively good outcomes. Structural lesions resulting from cerebrovascular accidents are typically associated with the worst prognosis.

Neurologic status at the time of presentation appears to be predictive of patient outcome in cases of nontraumatic coma. The poorer the neurologic function, the lower the likelihood of survival or good recovery. The absence of pupillary light response, motor response to pain, and a Glasgow Coma score of less than 5 were predictive of poor neurologic outcome in postcardiac arrest coma-

---

▼

Consider Consultation When...

► The cause of the stupor or coma is not clear after history, physical and neurologic examinations, and appropriate laboratory tests.

► Further expertise or experience is needed to treat the underlying cause.

► The patient does not respond to treatment, or the patient's course is different from expected.

► Technical assistance is needed in interpreting or performing diagnostic or therapeutic procedures.

tose patients. In addition, time spent in coma appears to be predictive of recovery. Patients who remain comatose or in a vegetative state 1 month following the acute event have little or no chance of recovery to independent functioning, and many of these patients will die. Age does not appear to be predictive of recovery in this setting.

Overall, traumatic coma has a better prognosis than nontraumatic coma. A variety of studies looking for predictors of outcome in traumatic coma have identified age and depth of level of unresponsiveness as predictors of survival and quality of life. Young persons do better than old persons, and patients at relatively light levels of unresponsiveness do better than those in deeper levels. In traumatic coma, longer periods of coma do not impact chances of a good recovery to the same degree as it appears to in nontraumatic coma. Even patients who have been in coma for several months have had a good recovery. The cause of the injury, the presence or absence of a skull fracture, and the presence or absence of extracranial injury do not appear to be predictive. Mental disability is more important than physical disability in identifying which patients will be able to be independent after surviving coma.

The Glasgow Outcome Scale was developed to grade patients on the basis of their outcome following coma. This 5-point scale is graded as follows: Grade 1, death without recovery of consciousness; grade 2, persistent vegetative state; grade 3, severely disabled; grade 4, moderately disabled; and grade 5, good recovery. The severely disabled individual (grade 3) is conscious but, because of serious physical and/or mental disability, will need assistance with major aspects of daily life. The moderately disabled patient is physically and/or mentally disabled, but is able to continue working at some form of employment (perhaps not at the job held prior to the coma) and go outside the home. The patient with good recovery is able to perform most normal life functions independently, although he may still display some minor dysfunction of a physical and/or mental nature. This may impact the quality of his life. Good recovery does not imply that the patient has resumed a premorbid lifestyle.

Vegetative States

Although some patients remain comatose for months, most do not. More commonly, patients either die or enter a vegetative state after several weeks. Recovery from vegetative states appears to be more likely in younger patients and in those with traumatic etiologies. It also appears that many patients are misdiagnosed as being vegetative when, in fact, they have a higher level of functioning. In all cases, it is important to serially examine patients and be open to the possibility of improvement.

Traditionally, it has been believed no person in a PVS will ever recover cognitive functioning. However, in recent years, several patients have been described who have had improvement including some return of cognitive functioning. None of these patients has been capable of independent life, however. Nonetheless, Childs' and Mercer's recent description of a 23-year-old PVS patient who, despite continued severe neurologic dysfunction, recovered some cognitive functioning and returned home from an extended care facility, reminds us not to presume for others what constitutes a satisfactory quality of life.

Annotated Bibliography

ANA Committee on Ethical Affairs, Issues in Clinical Neuroscience. Persistent vegetative state: Report of the American Neurological Association Committee on Ethical Affairs. *Ann Neurol* 1993;33(4):386–390.
Reflects the position of the American Neurological Association on diagnostic criteria for the persistent vegetative state and provides useful commentary regarding prognosis.

Berger J. Clinical approach to stupor and coma. In Bradley WG, Daroff RB, Fenichel GM, Jankovic J (eds.), *Neurology in clinical practice*, 4th ed. Boston: Butterworth-Heinemann, 2003;43–64.
Provides a comprehensive and detailed approach to the diagnosis and management of the comatose patient.

Childs NL, Mercer WN, Childs HW. Accuracy of diagnosis of persistent vegetative state. *Neurology* 1993;43:1465–1467.
Excellent discussion of the persistent vegetative state that stresses the importance of accurate diagnosis.

Hoffman RS, Goldfrank, LR. The poison patient with altered consciousness. Controversies in the use of a single "coma cocktail." *JAMA* 1995;274(7):562–569.
This is an excellent review of the emergent management of the patient presenting with poisoning and overdose.

Posner JB, Saper CB, Schiff N, Plum F. *Plum and Posner's Diagnosis of stupor and coma*, 4th ed. New York: Oxford University Press, 2007.
The classic text on coma. Excellent diagrams and comprehensive discussion of all aspects of the examination and the management of the comatose patient are included.

CHAPTER 14

The Epilepsies

Evelyn S. Tecoma and Jody Corey-Bloom

Outline

▶ Definitions
▶ Epidemiology
▶ Classification of seizures
▶ Etiology of seizures and epilepsy
▶ Epileptic syndromes
▶ Differential diagnosis
▶ Diagnosis and evaluation
▶ Treatment
▶ Status epilepticus
▶ Epilepsy in Elderly
▶ Use of antiepileptic drugs in women of childbearing potential and pregnancy
▶ Mortality and morbidity in epilepsy

Seizures are one of the most frequently encountered neurologic disorders. In children, epilepsy accounts for 30% of neurologic visits, whereas among adults, it is exceeded only by vascular disease. Consequently, the epilepsies are a major public health problem. This chapter reviews the diagnosis and treatment of the epilepsies in adults.

Definitions

A seizure is a sudden involuntary alteration in perception or behavior caused by an abnormal synchronized discharge of cortical neurons in the central nervous system. A person may have one or more seizures, or a reactive seizure in the face of a temporary and reversible brain insult (such as severe hypoglycemia, drug intoxication); these are called reactive seizures and do not meet criteria for a diagnosis of epilepsy. Epilepsy, on the other hand, refers to chronic recurrent seizures due to an underlying brain abnormality. There is a trend toward referring to epilepsy as a *seizure disorder*. Although patients may prefer this term, the distinction between repeated reactive seizures (alcohol withdrawal, benign febrile seizures) and epilepsy should be clear, as the former do not require antiepileptic drug (AED) therapy.

The seizure (ictus) should be differentiated from the time immediately after a seizure has terminated, known as the *postictal* period. During that time, baseline neurologic function has not yet returned and transient disturbance of mentation, consciousness, motor, or sensory function may be present. The *interictal* period refers to the time when the individual is at baseline neurologic function.

Epidemiology

The annual incidence of epilepsy ranges from 31 per 100,000 in Norway to 114 per 100,000 in rural Chile. In the United States, the annual incidence of epilepsy is 28.9–53.1 per 100,000, whereas the prevalence of epilepsy is approximately 6 per 1,000. Therefore, prevalence is estimated at approximately 1.8 million individuals in the United States, whereas perhaps 50 million worldwide have epilepsy. The incidence of epilepsy is high in early childhood. It then declines, plateaus from age 15–65 years, and then progressively rises among the elderly to surpass levels seen in childhood (Figure 14.1). One percent of the population will have developed epilepsy by the age of 20, and the cumulative lifetime risk of developing epilepsy ranges from 1.4% to 3.3%. The lifetime risk of a seizure of any kind is about 10%.

Classification of Seizures

Seizures have a myriad of manifestations. They can be simple or complicated, brief or long in duration, may or may not affect consciousness, and may produce motor, or

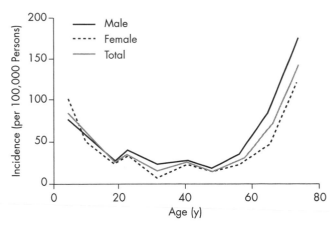

Figure 14.1 A: Age-specific average annual incidence of epilepsy per 100,000 population in Rochester Minnesota. Adapted from Hauser WA, Annegers JF, Kurland LT. B: Incidence of epilepsy and unprovoked seizures in Rochester, Minnesota, 1935–1984. *Epilepsia* 1993;34:453–468, with permission.

sensory, affective, psychic, or autonomic symptoms. This section will review the classification of seizures defined by the International League Against Epilepsy (ILAE) based on their behavioral and electroencephalographic (EEG) features (Box 14.1).

Partial Seizures

Partial seizures begin focally in a restricted area of cortex. In contrast, *generalized seizures* are believed to arise diffusely in deep midline structures or in both hemispheres. Partial seizures may be subdivided into three types:

▸ When consciousness and ability to interact with the external environment are not impaired, the seizure is classified as a *simple partial seizure*.

▸ When consciousness is impaired, the seizure is classified as a *complex partial seizure*. Impaired consciousness is defined as the inability to respond normally to external stimuli because of altered awareness. It is important to note that patients do not appear "unconscious" and often deny losing consciousness. Eyes are typically open; patients may speak and may have partial recall. There may be a continuum of features in a given patient as the seizure spreads from a focal onset to involve both hemispheres. The distinction of simple partial and complex partial seizures is critical for safety and driving issues, and may be difficult to determine without the aid of video EEG ictal recordings.

▸ *Secondarily generalized partial seizures* are those in which consciousness is impaired and tonic–clonic (convulsive) movements occur. A

given patient may experience all three seizure types under different circumstances.

Simple partial seizures

Simple partial seizures, also known as *auras*, are the most spatially restricted of the partial seizures. The discharge is nearly always confined to a single lobe or hemisphere, and the symptoms are specific to the affected brain region. For example, an occipital lobe seizure may produce formed or unformed visual hallucinations, a parietal lobe seizure localized tingling, a frontal lobe seizure either tonic or clonic movement, and a temporal seizure either psychic or emotional symptoms. It is the failure of the cortical discharge to spread throughout the brain that spares consciousness. There are four main types of simple partial seizures: (1) simple partial seizures with motor signs, (2) simple partial seizures with sensory symptoms, (3) simple partial seizures with autonomic symptoms or signs, and (4) simple partial seizures with psychic symptoms (Table 14.1).

Simple partial seizures with motor signs. These typically begin with clonic or tonic movements of a discrete body part. If a seizure discharge spreads in an orderly fashion along the precentral gyrus, a progression of clonic motor symptoms occurs, known as a jacksonian march. More commonly, however, ictal discharges in the frontal cortex activate multiple muscle groups to produce complex versive movements such as turning of the head, eyes, or body to one side and tonic posturing of one or more extremities. Involvement of the supplementary motor cortex classically results in adversive seizures, with turning of the head and eyes and bilateral proximal limb movement. Other manifestations of simple partial seizures include speech arrest or vocalizations when language areas are involved, and eyelid twitching, initiated from frontal or occipital foci.

Sensory simple partial seizures. Sensory simple partial seizures occur when the sensory cortex is involved in an ictal discharge. Thus, localized paresthesias or numbness

---

▼

Pearls and Perils

Simple partial seizures

▸ Simple partial seizures may not have an EEG correlate. Do not be misled when the EEG is normal during a simple partial seizure.

▸ An aura is a simple partial seizure preceding either a complex partial or secondarily generalized seizure, or it may occur in isolation.

▸ Simple partial seizures occur only in partial epilepsies.

Box 14.1 International classification of epileptic seizures

I. Partial seizures
A Simple partial seizures
1 With motor signs
a Focal motor without march
b Focal motor with march (jacksonian)
c Versive
d Postural
e Phonatory
2 With somatosensory or special-sensory symptoms
a Somatosensory
b Visual
c Auditory
d Olfactory
e Gustatory
f Vertiginous
3 With autonomic symptoms or signs
4 With psychic symptoms
a Dysphasia
b Dysmnesic
c Cognitive
d Affective
e Illusions
f Structured hallucinations
B Complex partial seizures
1 Simple partial seizures at onset, followed by impairment of consciousness
a With simple partial features
b With automatisms

2 With impairment of consciousness at onset
a With impairment of consciousness only
b With automatisms
C Partial seizures evolving to secondarily generalized seizures
1 Simple partial seizures evolving to generalized seizures
2 Complex partial seizures evolving to generalized seizures
3 Simple partial seizures evolving to complex partial seizures evolving to generalized seizures

II. Generalized seizures
A Absence seizures
1 Typical absence seizures
a Impairment of consciousness only
b With mild clonic components
c With atonic components
d With tonic components
e With automatisms
f With autonomic components
2 Atypical absence seizures
B Myoclonic seizures
C Clonic seizures
D Tonic seizures
E Tonic–clonic seizures
F Atonic seizures

Adapted from Holmes GL. Classification of seizures and the epilepsies. In: Schachter SC, Schomer DL, eds., *The Comprehensive Evaluation and Treatment of Epilepsy*. San Diego, CA: Academic Press, 1997; 1–36, with permission.

---

arise, with seizures emanating from the parietal lobe, unformed visual imagery occurs with occipital lobe lesions, and unpleasant olfactory and gustatory sensations, vertigo, and sounds result from the temporal or frontal cortex. Formed visual hallucinations can occur with seizures emanating from the occipital or posterior temporal association areas, whereas auditory symptoms (hyperacusis, hypoacusis, paracusis) are associated with lateral temporal lobe seizures. Simple partial seizures limited to the Herschel gyrus of the temporal lobe may produce unformed auditory hallucinations described as white noise, TV static, or helicopter noise.

Autonomic simple partial seizures. These seizures are typically caused by ictal involvement of limbic structures in the mesial temporal and frontal lobes that project to the hypothalamus and brainstem, producing epigastric rising or distress, nausea, or lightheadedness. Other signs and symptoms include pallor, flushing, sweating, thirst, piloerection, pupillary dilation, cardiac arrhythmias (especially tachycardia), urinary or fecal urgency, and rarely incontinence.

Psychic simple partial seizures. Psychic simple partial seizures may arise in limbic and association cortex and sometimes exhibit features of psychiatric disorders. These include feelings of familiarity (*déjà vu*) and unfamiliarity (*jamais vu*), forced thinking, cognitive disturbances such as dreamy states, depersonalization, and time distortion; affective syndromes such as fear and dread, or even euphoria and mystical experiences.

As with all other types of seizures, the diagnosis of simple partial seizures is typically based on the history of stereotyped paroxysmal transient symptoms, and sometimes, an abnormal interictal EEG. The ictal EEG is abnormal in only 25% of simple partial seizures, and a negative EEG does not exclude epilepsy. Reaching a diagnosis may be difficult when simple partial seizures occur as the sole manifestation of epilepsy and the EEG is

Table 14.1 Simple partial seizures

Discriminating features
▶ No impairment of consciousness
▶ Stereotyped
▶ Focal spikes in interictal EEG

Consistent features
▶ Brief duration
▶ Paroxysmal
▶ No impairment of consciousness
▶ No post-ictal period

Variable features
▶ May manifest as abnormal sensations (smells, flashing lights, paresthesias), focal motor activity, or psychic phenomena (déjà vu, fear)
▶ Associated with a focal structural lesion
▶ May occur independent of or prior to a complex partial seizure

Pearls and Perils

Complex partial seizures

▶ These seizures can be mistaken for absence seizures. Patients may refer to them as *petit mal seizures*. However, complex partial seizures, unlike absence seizures, are usually preceded by a well-defined aura. Complex partial seizures last longer and are followed by postictal confusion. Eyewitness observation and EEG helps distinguish between these two seizure types.
▶ Complex partial seizures of frontal origin may lack an EEG correlate and postictal confusion.
▶ Complex partial seizures are not associated with goal-directed violence, but rather defensive behavior perceived as violent by witnesses.

normal. Then, other diagnostic possibilities must be entertained, and these are discussed elsewhere in this text.

Complex partial seizures

Complex partial seizures, formerly called *psychomotor seizures*, are quite common. They most often emanate from a temporal lobe, although frontal, parietal, and occipital lobes can also serve as their source. Complex partial seizures typically last from 30 seconds to several minutes. They can occur in both wakefulness and sleep. Most begin with an aura, or simple partial seizure, which is then followed by impairment of consciousness. *Automatisms*, which are involuntary movements during altered consciousness, are common during complex partial seizures. Examples of automatic behavior include chewing, tongue movements, lip smacking, swallowing, hand gestures, scratching, moaning, laughing, and repeating words or phrases. The activity can be complex and quasi purposeful such as eating, walking, playing cards, or drawing. However, automatic behavior is a relatively nonspecific sign, and may occur in limited form in absence seizures, partial seizures, and in the postictal phase of a generalized tonic–clonic or complex partial seizure. Most patients are at least partially amnesic for their ictal behavior and events that happen while consciousness is impaired. Postictal confusion and tiredness typically follow complex partial seizures, although rare exceptions may be seen, particularly in complex partial seizures from a frontal lobe (Table 14.2).

Secondarily generalized tonic–clonic seizures

These were previously termed *grand mal* or convulsive seizures and are the most dramatic of seizures. Generalized tonic–clonic seizures have a predictable presentation. A secondarily generalized seizure may begin in

several ways. Sometimes, it begins suddenly without warning. Many secondarily generalized tonic–clonic seizures begin with either a simple partial or complex partial seizure that progresses to tonic–clonic activity. The tonic or clonic movements are often asymmetric in secondarily generalized partial seizures, in contrast to the symmetry of primary generalized tonic–clonic seizures. The tonic phase begins with a cry as air is expired forcefully against a closed glottis and tonic spasms occur in truncal muscles. This is followed by a predictable series of motor and autonomic phenomena. After 10–30 seconds of tonic rigidity, the tonic spasm is interrupted by intermittent muscle relaxation of progressively lengthened duration creating the clonic phase. The tonic and clonic phases are associated with in-

Table 14.2 Complex partial seizures

Discriminating features
▶ Consciousness is altered
▶ Stereotyped
▶ Focal spikes in interictal EEG

Consistent features
▶ Approximately 60–180-second duration
▶ Paroxysmal
▶ Post-ictal confusion

Variable features
▶ Presence of aura
▶ Automatisms
▶ Autonomic features
▶ May secondarily generalize to a tonic-clonic seizure
▶ Associated with focal structural lesion
▶ May elevate prolactin level

creases in heart rate and blood pressure, salivary and respiratory secretions, and prolonged apnea leading to cyanosis. Incontinence occurs at the beginning of the postictal period. Respiration returns postictally, but excessive salivation and flaccid pharyngeal musculature can lead to airway obstruction. The tonic–clonic phase typically lasts about 1 minute. The seizure is often followed by postictal stridor, confusion, and a deep sleep, more intense than the postictal fatigue seen after a complex partial seizure. Incomplete secondary generalization may occur in some patients, with lateralized clonic activity and postictal weakness on the side contralateral to the seizure focus (Todd paresis), as well as focal deficits of language, sensation, or vision, depending on the seizure focus. These lateralized deficits may be mistaken for stroke or transient ischemic attack (TIA) in patients without a documented history of seizures.

Generalized Seizures

In generalized seizures, a diffuse disturbance of cortical or thalamocortical function occurs, and seizures begin more or less simultaneously in both hemispheres. Consciousness is usually impaired and motor manifestations are usually bilateral. The interictal and ictal EEG abnormalities are bilateral and reflect a neuronal discharge, which is widespread in both hemispheres. This section will discuss the six types of generalized seizures: tonic–clonic seizures, absence seizures, myoclonic seizures, clonic seizures, tonic seizures, and atonic seizures (Table 14.3).

Tonic–clonic seizures

These seizures are similar in behavior to secondarily generalized seizures, but they begin without an aura or complex partial seizure. Rarely, tonic–clonic seizures begin with myoclonus or absence seizures. Sometimes a nonspecific prodrome occurs, beginning hours before onset. This may consist of headache, insomnia, mood change, and irritability, which occur before the seizure. A loud ictal cry with mouth and eyes open is fairly common at seizure onset. Postictally, stridor, confusion, somnolence are common, and motor weakness should be symmetric.

Absence seizures

These seizures were formerly termed *petit mal* seizures. There are two distinct types of absence seizures: typical and atypical. Typical absences are characteristic of the idiopathic (primary) generalized epilepsies, whereas atypical absences are seen in the symptomatic generalized epilepsies (Table 14.4).

Typical absence seizures are characterized by sudden episodes of unresponsive staring that rarely last longer than 10 seconds. The EEG shows paroxysmal, symmetric regular three-per- second spike-and-wave discharges, with rapid return to normal baseline. The patient

may or may not be aware of the lapse, and typically picks up activity where left off. Postural tone is usually maintained and eyes are open, or flutter slightly. Typical absence seizures may have subtle orofacial automatisms, finger rubbing, and autonomic changes. Autonomic signs associated with absence seizures include pallor, pupil dilatation, flushing, piloerection, tachycardia, salivation. Absence seizures are followed by immediate return of normal mentation without postictal confusion. Typical absence seizures are induced by hyperventilation and photic stimulation in the EEG lab, or during routine activities by flickering lights, certain video games, and repetitive light–dark patterns such as driving past posts on a bridge. Absence seizures associated with juvenile myoclonic epilepsy (JME; see epileptic syndromes in this chapter) may be briefer than typical absence seizures and may not fully impair awareness, with four- or five-per-

---

Table 14.3 Generalized tonic–clonic seizures

Discriminating features
▶ Initial tonic phase followed by clonic activity involving all extremities

Consistent features
▶ Loss of consciousness
▶ Typically 60-second duration
▶ Post-ictal period associated with confusion and drowsiness
▶ Elevation of prolactin

Variable features
▶ Tongue biting or injury
▶ Urinary incontinence
▶ Nonspecific prodrome
▶ Post-ictal paralysis

Table 14.4 Absence seizures

Discriminating features
▶ Very brief duration (5–15 seconds)
▶ Family history of typical absence seizures
▶ Response to ethosuximide and valproate

Consistent features
▶ EEG correlate in typical absence of 3 cycles/sec of generalized spike-and-wave; in atypical absence of 1.5–2.5 generalized spike-and-wave
▶ No aura
▶ Impaired consciousness
▶ No post-ictal state

Variable features
▶ Automatisms
▶ Change in body tone
▶ Precipitation by hyperventilation

Pearls and Perils

Generalized tonic–clonic seizures

▶ This is the most common type of seizure associated with alcohol withdrawal seizures.

    If the onset of a convulsive seizure is not seen, it may be difficult to tell a generalized from a secondarily generalized seizure. Asymmetry of movements, "sign of four" posturing, or postictal Todd paresis suggest a seizure of partial onset.

▶ Be wary of generalized motor seizures with flailing movement of extremities, forced eye closure, pelvic thrusting, and side-to-side rolling, waxing and waning of intensity, and unlabored breathing postictally. These could be nonepileptic episodes.

▶ During a generalized tonic–clonic seizure, make certain that the patient is safe from the surrounding environment. Do not attempt to restrain the patient or place objects in her mouth.

Pearls and Perils

Absence seizures

▶ Atypical absences are often associated with automatisms.

▶ Atypical absence is often a component of Lennox-Gastaut syndrome. Typical absence seizures characterize the benign idiopathic generalized syndromes.

▶ Typical absences are induced by hyperventilation, whereas atypical absences usually are not.

---

second generalized EEG spike-and-wave discharges.

Atypical absences may produce motor signs, especially changes in tone. Postural changes may result from an increase in tone leading to truncal arching, or a decrease in tone that causes head drop. Automatisms can include facial movements or more purposeful behavior such as rocking. They last from 10 to 25 seconds and may be followed by postictal confusion, unlike typical absence seizures. Automatisms, such as walking and other semi-purposeful movements, occur rarely in absence seizures lasting less than 10 seconds, but are not uncommon in those persisting more than 30 seconds. Atypical absences more often occur on awakening and in drowsiness, but are not provoked by hyperventilation. Atypical absence seizures are usually associated with other forms of generalized seizures and are more common in symptomatic generalized epilepsy. During atypical absence seizures, the EEG also shows generalized spike-and-wave bursts, but the frequency of the discharge is irregular and usually slower than three cycles per second (Table 14.4).

Myoclonic seizures

Myoclonus is a sudden, involuntary, brief, shock-like muscle contraction that can result from epileptic and nonepileptic mechanisms. This section will deal with epileptic myoclonus; myoclonus due to spinal cord disease, hypnic jerks, essential myoclonus, and opsoclonus are discussed elsewhere. Myoclonic seizures are unilateral or bilateral synchronous jerks that can be single or repeated arrhythmically in trains. These seizures can involve isolated muscle groups such as facial muscles or can involve the entire body. They occur either spontaneously or

may be provoked by sensory stimulation. Brief myoclonic seizures are believed to occur with preserved consciousness, but detailed testing is not possible because of their short duration. Myoclonic seizures can occur in both primary and secondary generalized epilepsies and are a defining feature of JME. The ictal and interictal EEG show brief bursts of generalized spike-and-wave or polyspike-and-wave discharges at three to five cycles per second (Table 14.5).

Clonic seizures

Clonic seizures usually begin before age 3. They are essentially tonic–clonic seizures without the tonic component. They may be asymmetrical and exhibit loss of consciousness. These seizures are followed by postictal confusion. The ictal EEG during clonic seizures reveals high-amplitude polyspike-and-wave discharges followed by low-amplitude slowing or generalized EEG suppression.

Tonic seizures

Tonic seizures typically begin in the first few years of life, although some start as late as adolescence. They are characterized by tonic spasms of truncal and facial muscles, with associated flexion or extension of the extremities and

---

Table 14.5 Myoclonic seizures

Discriminating features
▶ Shock-like muscle contractions
▶ No impairment of consciousness

Consistent features
▶ Brief duration
▶ No aura
▶ No post-ictal period
▶ Generalized spike wave in the interictal EEG

Variable features
▶ Specific muscle groups involved (isolated or whole body, unilateral or bilateral)
▶ Association with a progressive neurologic syndrome
▶ Occur spontaneously or may be provoked by sensory stimulation

▼

Pearls and Perils

Myoclonic seizures

▶ Nonepileptic myoclonus does not respond to most antiepileptic medication, although benzodiazepines may be helpful.

▶ The myoclonic seizures of juvenile myoclonic epilepsy (JME) generally occur during the first several hours after awakening from a night's sleep or a nap.

　Patients may not recognize jerks as seizures and may not report these unless specifically asked.

　Certain antiepileptic medications may reduce generalized tonic–clonic seizures but may worsen myoclonic jerks.

▶ The EEG in JME may be diagnostic if jerks are associated with polyspikes or four- to five-per-second generalized epileptiform discharges.

impairment of consciousness. Bilateral arm elevation ("touchdown sign") and brief gasp or cry may occur. They usually last 5–20 seconds. The EEG during tonic seizures reveals generalized low-voltage fast activity followed by semi-rhythmic delta activity. Seizures may cluster during sleep, drowsiness, or arousal. If standing, the patient may fall without warning. Thus, they may be difficult to distinguish from atonic drop attacks and also predispose the patient to bodily injury.

Atonic seizures

Atonic seizures, or *drop attacks*, consist of a sudden loss of tone in postural muscles. Generally, these seizures also begin in childhood. When mild, they may cause a brief head drop. When more severe, they lead to sudden collapse, with the potential for lacerations and fractures. These seizures typically last less than 5 seconds. Although associated with change of consciousness, usually no noticeable postictal symptoms occur. Atonic seizures typically occur in the symptomatic generalized epilepsies. The ictal EEG shows a suppression of electrical activity that is usually preceded by a spike-and-wave discharge or slow wave.

▼

Pearls and Perils

Atonic seizures

▶ Atonic seizures are a major cause of injury in the Lennox-Gastaut syndrome.

▶ Atonic seizures are frequently refractory to medications, but may respond to corpus callosotomy or vagus nerve stimulation.

Etiology of Seizures and Epilepsy

Table 14.6 outlines the causes of the epilepsies according to age group. Childhood-onset epilepsy is most often caused by birth and neonatal injuries (58%), followed by central nervous system (CNS) infections (15%), head trauma (12%) and less often by metabolic derangements, tumors, vascular insults, and genetic predisposition. Adult-onset epilepsy is most commonly caused by vascular lesions such as infarcts or hemorrhage (60%), metastatic tumors (10%), and CNS infections (9%), and less often caused by toxic or metabolic abnormalities such as toxin ingestion or drug withdrawal. Despite investigation, epidemiologic studies have shown that the etiology remains unknown in up to 65% of affected individuals. However, many of these studies were done prior to modern neuroimaging. As magnetic resonance imaging (MRI) and laboratory testing improve, the percentage of patients with unknown etiologies should continue to decline.

Genetic Factors in Epilepsy

Considerable evidence supports a genetic contribution to the etiology of the epilepsies. The hereditary causes of epilepsy may manifest in three ways: (a) a specific inherited trait in which the epileptic seizures are the principal phenotypic expression of the genetic defect (i.e., childhood absence epilepsy, JME); (b) an inherited trait in which the phenotypic expression is a neurologic or systemic disorder that is associated with seizures (i.e., neurofibromatosis, tuberous sclerosis); or (c) a trait that alters the seizure threshold, so that some individuals may be more susceptible to the development of seizures in the setting of a nonspecific neurologic insult, such as trauma. Additional genetic factors may influence treatment response, including drug absorption, transport, metabolism, receptor binding, and tolerance.

The list of specific genes linked to epilepsy is growing quickly, revealing diverse targets for gene alterations in both generalized and focal epilepsies. *Channelopathies* are a target of intensive research. Ion channel gene mutations are being found in many types of familial idiopathic epilepsies. At this time, epileptic disorders have been mapped to specific mutations in the voltage-gated sodium channel (SCN1A, SCN2A, and SCN1B for GEFS+, a syndrome of generalized epilepsy with febrile seizures plus other seizures including partial seizures), or to γ-aminobutyric acid (GABA)$_A$ receptor subunit 2 (GABRG2, another mutation causing GEFS+). A familial form of partial seizures (ADFLE, autosomal dominant frontal lobe epilepsy) has been linked to at least two different subunits of the ligand-gated nicotinic acetylcholine receptors (CHRNA4 and CHRNB4). Mutations in ligand-gated GABA receptors (GABRA1 and GABRG2) are linked to JME. Mutations in voltage-

Table 14.6 Etiology of the epilepsies by age group

0–14 years	15–34 years	35–64 years	Over 65 years
Birth trauma	CNS infection	Vascular disease	Vascular disease
CNS infections	Trauma	CNS tumors	CNS tumors
CNS hemorrhage	CNS tumors	CNS infections	Degenerative
Congenital malformations	Vascular disease	Trauma	CNS infections
Genetic predisposition			Trauma
Metabolic defects			
Tumors			

gated potassium channels (KCNQ2 and KCNQ3) are associated with benign familial neonatal convulsions. Mutations in CLCN2, a chloride-transporting protein, have been linked to various forms of generalized epilepsies. Mutations in voltage-gated calcium channels are linked to other paroxysmal neurologic disorders and may also predispose to childhood absence and other forms of generalized epilepsies. Further progress in this active field is likely to contribute valuable information to understanding the mechanisms underlying idiopathic epilepsies, and, hopefully new avenues to treatment.

More than 200 inherited disorders associated with the epilepsies, ranging from inherited metabolic derangements to dysplastic syndromes. Many mutations affect gene products whose function is not well understood. Several lissencephaly syndromes are associated with failure of neuronal migration during embryonic development, resulting in neocortical disorganization. Mitochondrial encephalopathies may occur with nuclear or mitochondrial mutations, inherited maternally. Familial disorders causing cerebral lesions that give rise to seizures are symptomatic syndromes because the seizures are a consequence of more widespread pathology. In these disorders, the seizures occur in only some patients, and other neurologic and systemic disturbances coexist.

The *seizure threshold* is a concept that embodies an individual's underlying genetic resistance to seizures. For example, only some people with head injuries of similar severity develop epilepsy. Investigators are currently exploring genetic susceptibility and the factors that contribute to this entity.

Epileptic Syndromes

The ILAE has proposed a classification of the epilepsies to better characterize them (Box 14.2). This syndromic classification is based on the history, seizure type, neurologic examination, and laboratory findings, including EEG and neuroimaging. Two broad distinguishing features are used in the classification scheme. One distinction is between localization-related epilepsies and the generalized epilepsies. *Localization-related epilepsies* are characterized by seizures that have a focal or partial onset. The generalized epilepsies are characterized by seizures with diffuse cortical origin. The second main distinction is between the idiopathic and symptomatic epilepsies. Epilepsies associated with known or demonstrable brain diseases or lesions are labeled *symptomatic*. Disorders that are likely secondary to an insult where the lesion or pathology cannot be revealed by current diagnostic techniques are termed *cryptogenic* and are included in the symptomatic grouping. Epilepsies that are inherited or lack identifiable brain pathology are labeled *idiopathic*. The idiopathic epilepsies often carry a better prognosis than symptomatic disorders.

Localization-related (Partial) Epilepsy Syndromes

Idiopathic

Four idiopathic localization-related epilepsies all begin in childhood and remit by late adolescence. These syndromes include: benign focal epilepsy of childhood with centro-temporal sharp waves, benign partial epilepsy with occipital spike waves, benign epilepsy with affective symptoms, and benign frontal epilepsy of childhood. Since all of these syndromes remit by adolescence, the reader is referred to the pediatric neurology text in this series for a detailed discussion of these.

Symptomatic (secondary)

Mesial temporal lobe epilepsy. Mesial temporal lobe epilepsy is a condition characterized by seizures originating from mesial temporal limbic structures, mainly hippocampus and amygdala. This syndrome is the most frequently encountered chronic partial epilepsy, accounting for 60–75% of patients with symptomatic partial epilepsy.

Mesial temporal lobe epilepsy most often begins in childhood, although it can appear at any age. Almost all patients experience complex partial seizures and most report simple partial seizures too. Some present with secondarily generalized convulsions, which become less common once a patient is started on AED therapy. Although 25% deny simple partial seizures, this could be due to retrograde amnesia for the aura.

▼

Box 14.2 International classification of the epilepsies and epileptic syndromes

1 Localization-related (focal, local, partial) epilepsies and syndromes
  1.1 Idiopathic with age-related onset
    a Benign childhood epilepsy with centro-temporal spikes
    b Childhood epilepsy with occipital paroxysms
  1.2 Symptomatic
2 Generalized epilepsies and syndromes
  2.1 Idiopathic, with age-related onset (listed in order of age)
    a Benign neonatal familial convulsions
    b Benign neonatal convulsions
    c Benign myoclonic epilepsy in infancy
    d Childhood absence epilepsy (pyknolepsy)
    e Juvenile absence epilepsy
    f Juvenile myoclonic epilepsy (impulsive petit mal)
    g Epilepsy with grand mal seizures on awakening
  2.2 Idiopathic and/or symptomatic (listed in order of age)
    a West syndrome (infantile spasms)
    b Lennox-Gastaut syndrome
    c Epilepsy with myoclonic-astatic seizures
    d Epilepsy with myoclonic absences
  2.3 Symptomatic
    a Nonspecific etiology
      • Early myoclonic encephalopathy

  b Specific etiology
    • Epileptic seizures may complicate many disease states
3 Epilepsies and syndromes undetermined as to whether they are focal or generalized
  3.1 With both generalized and focal seizures
    a Neonatal seizures
    b Severe myoclonic epilepsy in infancy
    c Epilepsy with continuous spike waves during slow-wave sleep
    d Acquired epileptic aphasia (Landau-Kleffner syndrome)
  3.2 Without unequivocal generalized or focal features
4 Special syndromes
  4.1 Situation-related seizures
    a Febrile convulsions
    b Seizures related to other identifiable situations such as stress, hormonal changes, drugs, alcohol, or sleep deprivation
  4.2 Isolated, apparently unprovoked epileptic events
  4.3 Epilepsies characterized by specific modes of seizure precipitation

Adapted from Holmes GL. Classification of seizures and the epilepsies. In: Schachter SC, Schomer DL, eds., *The Comprehensive Evaluation and Treatment of Epilepsy*. San Diego, CA: Academic Press, 1997; 1–36, with permission.

Complex partial seizures typically begin with an aura, and several types have been reported. Among the most common are an epigastric rising sensation, dizziness, *déjà vu*, fear, or indescribable feelings. The unresponsiveness phase often begins with a stare, and automatisms, particularly chewing and lip smacking often are seen. Seizures last from 1–3 minutes and are followed by several minutes of postictal confusion. They are commonly exacerbated by stress, sleep deprivation, and in approximately one-third of women correlate with the menstrual cycle (Table 14.7).

Patients with temporal lobe epilepsy usually have a normal neurologic examination except for short-term memory deficits and an asymmetry of the nasolabial folds. The interictal EEG shows either unilateral or bilateral asynchronous temporal spikes or sharp waves, usually with maximal amplitude in basal temporal leads (sphenoidal). When recorded, seizures usually begin in one of the temporal regions. The MRI reveals mesial temporal sclerosis characterized by unilateral hippocampal atrophy with increased T2 or fluid-attenuating inversion recovery (FLAIR) signal and enlargement of the temporal horn of the lateral ventricle. Positron emission tomogra-

phy (PET) scans shows interictal unilateral temporal lobe hypometabolism in 70–90% of patients and hypoperfusion with single positron emission computed tomography (SPECT) in 45–60% of patients. Magnetic resonance spectroscopy (MRS) may reveal decreased neuronal biochemical markers in relation to general cell markers in the affected hippocampus.

The etiology of mesial temporal lobe epilepsy is unknown. Patients often have a history of febrile convulsions, but whether these are incidental or causal is not certain. The hippocampus is vulnerable to injury in early childhood, and it is assumed that the lesions are produced early in life. Subtle dysplasia or microdysgenesis of the hippocampal layers may predispose a patient to prolonged febrile seizures and later temporal epilepsy.

The prognosis of temporal lobe epilepsy is not known. Although many patients with mesial temporal lobe epilepsy are refractory to AEDs, no good population-based studies examine therapeutic response rates to medication. Temporal lobe epilepsy, however, often responds favorably to surgical therapy (see later discussion under the heading Surgical Intervention).

Table 14.7 Mesial temporal lobe epilepsy

Discriminating features
▶ Unitemporal or bitemporal spikes in the interictal EEG
▶ Hippocampal sclerosis

Consistent features
▶ Simple partial and/or complex partial seizures
▶ Impaired memory

Variable features
▶ MRI demonstrating hippocampal atrophy or a focal temporal structural lesion
▶ History of febrile convulsions at an early age
▶ Psychic or emotional auras

Neocortical temporal lobe epilepsy. This syndrome is less well defined than mesial temporal lobe epilepsy and is more heterogeneous in its manifestations. This is more often a syndrome of adolescence or adulthood. Seizures often begin with auras and have automatisms, and secondary generalization may be more common than in mesial temporal lobe epilepsy. The interictal EEG is similar to that in mesial temporal lobe epilepsy, with unilateral or bilateral asynchronous spike waves. Similarly, the ictal EEG will show seizure onset in either temporal lobe. The MRI may or may not demonstrate a structural lesion in the lateral temporal lobe, and mesial temporal structures are normal. Advanced neuroimaging with 3 Tesla MRI, magnetoencephalography, ictal SPECT, or MRS are useful in these cases to detect focal pathology. Phase II video EEG monitoring with intracranial electrodes may be necessary to identify potential surgical candidates in nonlesional cases. The same is true in other types of non-lesional epilepsy originating outside the temporal lobe (see later discussion under the heading Surgical Intervention). The remission rate is not known.

Frontal lobe epilepsy. Frontal, parietal, and occipital lobe epilepsies remain ill-defined. Much of the information is based on surgical series. Patients with frontal lobe epilepsy comprise perhaps 5–15% of those with symptomatic partial epilepsy. Frontal lobe epilepsy produces a wide variety of seizure types, depending on seizure onset and propagation. Seizures beginning in the primary motor cortex start with localized contralateral clonic activity. Supplementary motor seizures begin with bilateral proximal limb movement and turning of the head. Orbitofrontal or cingulate seizures may begin with olfactory, psychic, or emotional auras and are followed by complex automatisms. Prefrontal seizures usually have no warning and simply lead to bilateral tonic–clonic activity. Frontal lobe seizures often have prominent motor manifestations, which at times can be mistaken for nonepileptic episodes. Complex partial seizures are often brief, less than 60 seconds in du-

ration, frequent, and lack postictal confusion. Nocturnal onset and seizure clustering are common.

The EEG often shows interictal spikes in one or both frontal lobes, although temporal lobe spikes may also be seen. Some patients have no interictal spikes. Neuroimaging is usually negative, although focal lesions such as tumors, vascular malformations, or heterotopias are seen in patients with lesional epilepsy.

The prognosis of frontal lobe epilepsy is not yet known, and epidemiologic studies are needed.

Parietal lobe epilepsy. This syndrome is less common than frontal lobe epilepsy. Parietal lobe seizures usually begin with positive or negative sensory symptoms such as numbness, tingling, or even pain. Nausea, abdominal sensations, vertigo, and language disturbances may also occur. Simple partial, complex partial, and secondary generalized tonic–clonic seizures occur. These may be clinically similar to seizures of temporal lobe origin, especially if the ictal activity spreads to the temporal lobe(s). The interictal EEG shows unilateral or bilateral parietal spikes, and neuroimaging may be normal or show a structural lesion. Prognosis is not known.

Occipital lobe epilepsy. This is also an uncommon localization-related epilepsy. The clinical features of occipital lobe epilepsy can be grouped according to location. Symptoms from primary visual cortex (area 17) include unformed visual hallucinations (sparks, flashes), as well as blurring or extinction of vision. Complex visual hallucinations result from seizures beginning in occipital association area cortex (areas 18, 19). Contralateral tonic–clonic, nystagmoid eye movements and blinking can also occur. Spread of the ictal discharge may lead to complex partial or secondarily generalized tonic–clonic seizures.

The neurologic examination discloses visual field defects in up to 60% of patients with occipital lobe epilepsy. The interictal EEG reveals posterior temporal or occipital spike discharges. Bitemporal interictal spikes are seen in up to 25% of patients as well. The EEG ictal onset can be misleading.

Seizures are controlled in perhaps 60% of patients with occipital epilepsy using traditional anticonvulsants. The natural history of this condition is not definitively known.

Epilepsia partialis continua. Epilepsia partialis continua is a form of simple partial status epilepticus, a partial epilepsy that involves the motor cortex. Patients have continuous arrhythmic myoclonic jerking of one or more muscle regions. Epilepsia partialis continua is caused either by a unilateral chronic encephalitic process that may ultimately involve an entire hemisphere or by a more discrete lesion.

The chronic encephalitic form of epilepsia partialis continua, Rasmussen syndrome, begins between 4 and 8 years. One hemisphere is progressively involved. It is characterized by unilateral continuous or frequent intermittent partial seizures that either remain confined or evolve into complex partial or secondarily generalized seizures. The EEG can show either focal spikes in the affected cortex or irregular focal slow-wave activity. Magnetic resonance imaging typically reveals nonspecific changes. Serial imaging may demonstrate progressive hemispheric atrophy. The seizures are resistant to medications, and progressive focal motor deficits and mental deterioration usually occur. These patients should be evaluated in a specialized center and may be candidates for surgery, including subpial transection or modified hemispherectomy (see later discussion under the heading Surgical Intervention).

A more focal form of epilepsia partialis continua begins at any age. The seizures are discrete, focal motor seizures without other types or progression of symptoms. The EEG shows a normal background with focal spikes in the contralateral rolandic region. The MRI will usually demonstrate a discrete lesion such as a scar, tumor, vascular malformation, or dysplasia adjacent to the precentral gyrus. This type of epilepsia partialis continua is not progressive, and prognosis depends on the etiology of the lesion.

Generalized Epilepsy Syndromes

Many well-characterized generalized epilepsy syndromes begin in childhood or adolescence. Since they can persist to adulthood, they are discussed briefly. It is not unusual to see patients in their 20s and 30s presenting with new-onset generalized seizures, comprising less well- characterized idiopathic generalized epilepsy syndromes.

Idiopathic (primary)

Childhood absence epilepsy. This autosomal dominant disorder with incomplete penetrance is characterized by the appearance of typical absence seizures in otherwise normal children. It begins between the ages of 4 and 8 years. The seizures often occur very frequently, with dozens to hundreds per day.

The EEG shows stereotyped paroxysmal generalized three to four cycle per second spike-and-wave discharges. The prognosis for this epilepsy syndrome is reasonably good. The absence seizures tend to remit in adolescence, although generalized tonic–clonic seizures appear then in up to 40% and may persist if untreated. Seizures are more likely to continue in adulthood if tonic-clonic seizures preceded absence seizures, the absences have myoclonic or atonic components, or if the neurologic examination is abnormal.

Juvenile absence epilepsy. This syndrome is much less common than childhood epilepsy, and its inheritance pattern is not clearly elucidated. Seizures begin later than in childhood absence epilepsy, at age 10–12. The absence seizures occur less frequently, typically only several times per day, and tonic–clonic seizures more often develop. The interictal EEG shows spike-and-wave discharges at four to six cycles per second. The prognosis for remission is not as good as with childhood epilepsy.

Juvenile myoclonic epilepsy. This syndrome is characterized by myoclonus, absence seizures, and tonic–clonic seizures, although not all seizure types must be present in an affected individual. Seizures begin in adolescence, usually at age 13–14, although some experience their first seizure as late as age 19. The myoclonus is brief (less than 1 second), tends to involve the arms, commonly resulting in dropping objects, and most commonly occurs within an hour of awakening in the morning. Ninety percent of people with JME experience at least one generalized tonic–clonic seizure and 15% have absence seizures as well (Table 14.8).

The neurologic examination is normal. The EEG shows frontally predominant four- to six-cycle/second bilaterally synchronous spike-and-wave or polyspike-and-wave discharge. The inheritance pattern for this syndrome appears autosomal dominant in many families. Approximately 80% of patients respond to therapy. Since few individuals (<15%) remit, treatment must be lifelong.

Epilepsy with generalized tonic–clonic seizures on awakening. This rare syndrome is characterized by generalized tonic–clonic seizures that occur on awakening from sleep at any time during drowsiness. Absence seizures and myoclonus can also occur. Seizures begin in the second decade of life and persist to adulthood. This syndrome is probably due to a genetic predisposition. The interictal EEG is similar to other idiopathic generalized epilepsies with four to six cycles per second spike-and-wave discharges and often shows a photoparoxysmal response. Most patients respond completely to medication, but 40% relapse if it is discontinued.

Table 14.8 Juvenile myoclonic epilepsy

Discriminating features
▶ Multiple seizure types including myoclonic seizures, absence seizures, and generalized tonic–clonic seizures
▶ Presence of myoclonus

Consistent features
▶ Onset at puberty
▶ Seizures often occur shortly after awakening
▶ 4–6·Hz generalized polyspike and slow wave on EEG
▶ Good response to ethosuximide, valproic acid, or levetiracetam

Variable features
▶ Concurrent absence seizures
▶ Seizures precipitated by sleep deprivation or alcohol
▶ Normal neurologic examination

Symptomatic generalized epilepsy

The symptomatic generalized epilepsies have their onset in childhood but are generally lifelong. For a discussion of the other syndromes under this heading that do not persist to adulthood (i.e., infantile spasms and early myoclonic encephalopathy), please refer to the pediatric neurology text in this series.

Lennox-Gastaut syndrome. The Lennox-Gastaut syndrome (Table 14.9) has three characteristic features: (1) the occurrence of multiple seizure types that are refractory to medications, including atonic seizures, tonic seizures, atypical absence, myoclonic, and tonic–clonic seizures; (2) cognitive impairment with mental retardation; and (3) interictal slow spike-and-wave discharge (<2.5 cycles per second). Trauma, intracranial hemorrhage, cerebral infections, and tuberous sclerosis can all cause Lennox-Gastaut. This syndrome usually begins between the ages of 1 and 6 years, and it tends to affect males more often than females.

 The prognosis for Lennox-Gastaut syndrome is poor. Fewer than 33% of patients respond well to antiepileptic medication. Tonic and atonic seizures increase morbidity substantially. Ambulatory patients may require helmets and other protective gear to avoid injury from sudden falls without warning. As discussed in the section on epilepsy surgery, vagus nerve stimulation or corpus callosotomy may be effective, but rarely renders patients seizure free.

Differential Diagnosis

Any paroxysmal event associated with transient alteration in neurologic function can be mistaken for an epileptic seizure. This section will briefly explore the more common organic or psychogenic entities mistaken for epilepsy. Most of these topics are discussed in detail in other chapters.

Pearls and Perils

Lennox-Gastaut syndrome

▸ Lamotrigine, topiramate, and felbamate are newer antiepileptic drugs (AEDs) effective for this syndrome.
▸ Felbamate is the only AED with proven efficacy against drop attacks.
▸ The ketogenic diet, corpus callosotomy, and vagus nerve stimulation (VNS) may have some efficacy in this syndrome.
▸ Behavioral problems are common and should be managed in consultation with an experienced psychiatrist.

Table 14.9 Lennox-Gastaut syndrome

Discriminating features
▸ Triad of: (1) mental retardation, (2) generalized slow spike-and-wave on EEG, (3) multiple seizure types—atonic, atypical absence, myoclonic, partial, and tonic–clonic seizures

Consistent features
▸ Atonic seizures
▸ Onset before age 8
▸ Seizures are refractory to treatment
▸ Poor prognosis

Variable features
▸ Association with symptomatic early brain insults
▸ Cryptogenic onset in 30% of cases
▸ Behavioral disturbances

Syncope

This is the most common paroxysmal event confused with seizures, especially in the elderly. A prodrome of lightheadedness and dimming of vision sometimes precedes syncope. Syncope may be accompanied by tonic rigidity and brief symmetric jerking of the limbs, resembling a tonic–clonic seizure (convulsive syncope). Urinary incontinence may occur. Syncope typically lasts a few seconds and, if a brief postictal period of confusion occurs, recovery is quick. If the history is unhelpful, prolonged electrocardiogram (EKG) or EEG monitoring may be needed for diagnosis. Syncope may be vasovagal, cardiogenic, or due to carotid sinus hypersensitivity. The authors have seen patients with cardiogenic syncope (bradycardia, progressing to asystole, followed by tachycardia and recovery of awareness) in which patients demonstrate fear and confusion postictally, likely due to autonomic changes.

Transient Ischemic Attacks

Transient ischemic attacks cause negative phenomenon, in contrast to seizures, which usually produce positive behaviors. However, aphasia, for example, is a symptom of both. Generally, the positive motor phenomena of seizures are helpful distinguishing features, and the two discrete ictal and postictal phases of seizures help distinguish these from TIAs. The EEG is usually helpful, but is generally not definitive. Magnetic resonance imaging is not specific, since it may disclose an underlying infarction that could serve as a nidus for seizures or as a marker for TIAs.

Narcolepsy and Other Sleep Disorders

Narcolepsy refers to excessive daytime sleepiness in association with cataplexy, sleep paralysis, automatic behavior, and hypnagogic hallucinations. Most of these symptoms, particularly cataplexy and automatic behavior, could be mistaken for seizures. They can be differentiated from seizures by the EEG and the presence of triggers (for cataplexy) or the symptom complex.

Parasomnias, paroxysmal slow-wave sleep arousal disorders, night terrors, rapid eye movement (REM) behavioral disorders, and somnambulism can be mistaken for seizures. Although these can resemble complex partial seizures, the parasomnias lack synchronized motor behavior and a postictal confusional state.

Movement Disorders

Some paroxysmal motor disturbances can be confused with epilepsy. Hemifacial spasms consist of rhythmic twitching of facial muscles, including blinking and a characteristic electromyograph (EMG) with a normal EEG. This condition differs from epilepsy in the irregularity of the jerks and in their frequency. Paroxysmal dyskinesias include familial kinesogenic, familial nonkinesigenic, and acquired nonkinesigenic dyskinesias. The kinesogenic form is characterized by episodes of tonic, choreiform, or athetoid movements or posturing lasting 4–5 minutes that occur several times per day. They are elicited by a startle reaction or a brief sudden movement. The nonkinesigenic paroxysmal dyskinesias occur less often, sometimes only one per month, but last longer than 5 minutes. The movements are either choreoathetotic or dystonic. Both familial kinesogenic and nonkinesigenic dyskinesias are preceded by a prodrome of paresthesias in the affected extremity. The acquired form is often associated with metabolic diseases such as hypoparathyroidism and thyrotoxicosis.

The dyskinesias differ from seizures in that consciousness is not affected, and the EEG remains normal. Antiepileptic drugs treat the kinesogenic form of paroxysmal dyskinesia, and clonazepam may reduce the frequency of nonkinesigenic episodes.

Psychogenic Nonepileptic Episodes (Psychogenic Seizures, Nonepileptic Seizures, or Pseudoseizures)

These may superficially resemble epileptic seizures. Nonepileptic episodes of psychogenic origin are manifestations of conversion disorder, somatoform disorders or, rarely, malingering. They occur in perhaps 5–20% of people with epilepsy and 10–40% of patients presenting to tertiary epilepsy centers for uncontrolled seizures. Nonepileptic episodes are more often diagnosed in women than men, particularly if there is a history of physical or sexual abuse (Table 14.10).

Certain features distinguish psychogenic from epileptic seizures, but no feature is pathognomonic. Thrashing, flailing, nonsynchronous movements that are discontinuous and lack orderly progression are common

in nonepileptic episodes. Epileptic tonic–clonic seizures rarely last more than 1 minute, whereas nonepileptic episodes tend to last longer. Nonepileptic episodes can be associated with urinary incontinence and occasionally result in injury, so these cannot be used as distinguishing features. Some epilepsy syndromes, especially frontal lobe epilepsy, cause peculiar hypermotor activity or thrashing behaviors that resemble nonepileptic episodes. Nonepileptic seizures should be suspected when the ictal behavior is unusual and lacks stereotypy, when seizures fail to respond to anticonvulsants, and when the interictal EEG is persistently normal.

Nonepileptic episodes are best diagnosed by direct observation with simultaneous EEG and ECG recording. Demonstration of a normal ictal EEG in the face of impaired consciousness strongly suggests a nonepileptic nature of the seizure. Also, obtaining serum prolactin levels 15–20 minutes after seizure onset may be helpful, since prolactin levels rise after tonic–clonic seizures and most complex partial seizures, but not after pseudoseizures. Induction of a nonepileptic episode by suggestion may also aid in making the diagnosis.

The diagnosis of nonepileptic psychogenic episodes should be presented to the patient carefully, by an experienced physician. Malingering is difficult to prove, and patients should be given the benefit of the doubt. The patient should never be told they are "faking" seizures, or are "hysterical." We have adopted a positive approach, emphasizing the "good news" that the patient does not have epilepsy and may not need to take epilepsy medication. We are moving away from the term nonepileptic "seizures," as this may confuse the patient or family. "Spells" or "episodes" are a better term. Patients are informed that their diagnosis is real, but does not usually respond to AEDs. They are advised to seek evaluation by a social worker or mental health professional. Literature in lay language is provided. The prognosis can be very good in pa-

---

Table 14.10 Nonepileptic episodes

Discriminating features
▶ Variability in duration of episodes
▶ No increase in serum prolactin
▶ Induced by suggestion

Consistent features
▶ Normal EEG during seizures and in the interictal state
▶ Never occur during sleep

Variable features
▶ Manifestations of episodes (altered responsiveness, motor activity, vocalizations)
▶ Asynchronous extremity movements
▶ Forced eye closure
▶ MMPI suggestive of conversion

Pearls and Perils

Nonepileptic episodes

▶ If nonepileptic episodes are suspected, refer for video EEG monitoring to ascertain the diagnosis.

▶ A clinical seizure without EEG correlate does not always connote nonepileptic episodes. Complex partial seizures of frontal lobe origin as well as simple partial seizures may lack an EEG correlate.

    Limp unresponsiveness and pseudo-convulsions are common phenotypes.

    Look for forced eye closure (psychogenic) versus eyes open with dilated pupils (epileptic) during seizure.

▶ Nonepileptic episodes can be associated with self-injury and urinary incontinence.

▶ Nonepileptic patients may have a remote history of physical or sexual abuse.

    Not all nonepileptic episodes are psychogenic in nature. Organic nonepileptic disorders include TIAs, complicated migraine, hypoglycemic spells, parasomnias (night terrors, REM behavior disorder, nightmares, sleepwalking), convulsive syncope, and paroxysmal movement disorders such as kinesigenic dystonia. The value of video EEG monitoring cannot be overemphasized.

---

tients who are receptive to the diagnosis. Driving should be restricted until the spells are clearly in remission. Those with important secondary gain may be more intractable.

Diagnosis and Evaluation

The office interview is the means by which epilepsy is diagnosed. Few patients have seizures witnessed by physicians, who must instead rely on history provided by either the patient or family members. The diagnosis is therefore made by inference. The only way to positively diagnose epilepsy is to record the EEG during a seizure, a procedure too inconvenient and expensive (and usually unnecessary) to perform on a routine basis.

The neurologic examination is often normal in patients with epilepsy, but diagnosis is aided when focal or generalized neurologic deficits can be demonstrated to suggest a symptomatic epilepsy syndrome. Focal or lateralized features can help distinguish partial from generalized epilepsies. Examination during the immediate postictal period, too, can reveal lateralized neurologic dysfunction that otherwise is not apparent.

The neurologic examination often shows impairment of memory in the symptomatic epilepsies. Memory disturbances can result from the underlying lesion, can be due to AED effects, or can reflect reversible dysfunction induced by seizures.

A number of procedures are used in evaluating people with epilepsy. The purpose of these tests is to help classify the epilepsy syndrome and seek remediable causes (i.e., tumors). This section will review EEG and neuroimaging. A more lengthy review of these topics is found in other chapters.

Electroencephalography

The EEG is the single most informative diagnostic test. It should nearly always be performed. The EEG greatly aids in classifying the seizure type, helps distinguish between the localization-related and generalized syndromes, and is used to define some of the inherited syndromes.

The characteristic interictal abnormality in epilepsy is the spike or sharp wave. Focal, or localized, spikes are seen in partial epilepsy, whereas generalized spikes (or spike wave) typically occur in the generalized epilepsies. The interictal EEG shows a spike in approximately 90–95% of patients with epilepsy, although up to three recordings may be needed to demonstrate the spike. Recording the EEG during sleep in the laboratory or overnight recording with an ambulatory EEG device increases the yield of this procedure.

It is important to note that "interictal" spikes are seen in a small percentage of normal individuals (<2%). Therefore, finding a spike in the EEG does not establish the diagnosis of epilepsy. The diagnosis can only be absolutely confirmed with EEG if a seizure is recorded. Otherwise, the clinical history is ultimately the major factor in determining the diagnosis. For further details regarding EEG, the reader is referred to Chapter 2 of this text.

Neuroimaging

Magnetic resonance imaging

Magnetic resonance imaging is the preferred imaging modality for evaluating a patient with epilepsy. It is highly sensitive and identifies nearly all macroscopic lesions, in-

---

Pearls and Perils

EEG in epilepsy

▶ A normal single electroencephalogram (EEG) does not exclude the diagnosis of epilepsy.

▶ If a normal awake EEG is obtained in an individual with the clinical suspicion of seizures, one should repeat the EEG capturing sleep because many epileptic abnormalities appear only in sleep.

▶ Interictal findings in the EEG are invaluable aids for classifying seizures and epilepsy syndromes.

cluding tumors, dysplasias, vascular malformations, encephalomalacia, and atrophy. Finding a focal disturbance leads one toward a diagnosis of partial epilepsy, provided the history is consonant. Magnetic resonance imaging should be performed in all individuals who do not have an inherited epilepsy syndrome. Patients whose seizure types change or who are refractory to medication often merit a repeat study. Epilepsy centers often have specialized MR protocols, and if referral to such a center is contemplated, it may be appropriate to defer the MRI until it can be performed there.

Computed tomography

Although MRI is clearly superior, computed tomography (CT) is still useful. Tumors more than 1 or 2 cm in size can usually be identified. However, lesions in the temporal lobe can be missed with CT because of bony artifact. The CT scan is better at identifying calcifications than the MR scan. However, if normal, a CT scan cannot be considered adequate, and an MRI should be performed. Consequently, CT is useful only if MR is not available and imaging needs to be performed immediately.

Positron emission tomography

Positron emission tomography is used in epilepsy mainly for evaluating patients for epilepsy surgery. The interictal PET usually shows a hypometabolic region that correlates with the source of seizures. At present, PET has no role in routine evaluation.

Single photon emission computed tomography (SPECT)

Single photon emission computed tomography, like PET, is mainly used in epilepsy surgery, and has little practical value in routine diagnosis. See Chapter 4 for information on neuroimaging.

Treatment

The main goal of epilepsy treatment is to enable affected individuals to live as normal a life as possible. Hence, therapy is directed not only at seizures, but should also remediate any psychosocial impairment as well. This section will review the medical treatment of epilepsy.

Antiepileptic Drugs

Antiepileptic drugs are given to prevent seizures, the primary symptom of epilepsy. Although they are not cures for the epilepsies, it is possible that seizure prophylaxis favorably alters the natural history of the syndrome in some people. When choosing an AED, one should select an effective agent for the epilepsy syndrome. The efficacy and side-effect profile of the AED, age, response to previous AEDs, concomitant medications, frequency of ad-

ministration, and cost should all be factored into the decision. Drug interactions are perhaps the most challenging aspect of epilepsy treatment in patients on multiple drugs. The AEDs often alter serum concentrations, protein binding, and metabolism of other drugs. Side effects are quite common. Therefore, patients should be carefully monitored after initiation of therapy to ensure that the treatment remains more benign than the underlying disorder. Prior to 1993, six major AEDs (carbamazepine, phenobarbital, phenytoin, primidone, valproic acid and, for absence seizures, ethosuximide) were available for the treatment of all forms of epilepsy. In the last 15 years, nine new AEDs (felbamate, gabapentin, lamotrigine, levetiracetam, oxcarbazepine, tiagabine, topiramate, zonisamide, and pregabalin) have been approved by the U.S. Food and Drug Administration (FDA). Although the older drugs are effective in patients with newly diagnosed epilepsy and have the advantage of familiarity, wider availability, and lower cost, many clinicians have expressed concern about their drug–drug interactions, side effects, and overall impact on quality of life. Some of the second-generation AEDs are coming off patent protection, so that less expensive generic forms are available, thus increasing their accessibility. New parenteral preparations and slow-release oral forms of AEDs make more options available to patients and clinicians.

Medical treatment should always begin with the use of a single AED. A treatment is deemed adequate provided there is a favorable response and tolerable side effects. Many of the newer AEDs do not have target therapeutic drug levels, and routine monitoring is not indicated. When drug levels are indicated, therapeutic serum drug levels should be targeted when starting therapy, and these help to assess medication compliance and to gauge dosage. However, the suggested therapeutic levels are only guidelines, and do not represent absolute ranges. Some patients need low serum concentrations of AEDs for benefit, whereas others require higher than usual levels and still remain free from side effects. Individuals with preexisting neurologic damage and the eld-

---

Pearls and Perils

Antiepileptic drugs

▶ Monotherapy should be the goal of initial AED therapy. If an AED is not working, one should plan to taper this medication and substitute a new AED.
▶ Avoid the temptation to continue AEDs that have not helped control seizures.
▶ Always check for potential drug interactions when using AEDs with other prescription and nonprescription drugs.

erly are particularly susceptible to side effects at low concentrations. Pharmacokinetic data on commonly used AEDs are summarized in Table 14.11.

Some patients have persistent seizures despite a satisfactory AED concentration. In this circumstance, a second drug may be tried. It is added to the first, which is then tapered and discontinued. Several agents may be tried sequentially in this way. The use of two medications simultaneously is reserved for difficult-to-control patients, and is best left to a specialist. Typically, agents with different mechanisms of action should be used in combination therapy (*rational polytherapy*). Be sure that the diagnosis is secure, as some agents effective in partial epilepsies are less effective in generalized syndromes and can potentially exacerbate certain types of generalized seizures. For example, pure GABAergic drugs, such as tiagabine, or narrow-spectrum agents, such as carbamazepine and gabapentin, may occasionally worsen generalized spike-and-wave in generalized seizure disorders, thus leading to increased absence or myoclonic seizures in mixed generalized epilepsies. Excessive GABA activation may also contribute to spike-and-wave stupor, a subtle form of absence status epilepticus.

Carbamazepine

Carbamazepine (Tegretol, Tegretol XR, Carbatrol, generic preparations) is indicated for partial seizures in monotherapy or combination therapy. Carbamazepine acts on voltage-gated sodium channels to decrease repetitive neuronal firing, and thus has a similar mechanism of action and spectrum as phenytoin. Rarely, it may precipitate absence or myoclonic seizures. Immediate-release (2–4 daily doses) and twice-a-day extended-release formulations are available. Treatment with carbamazepine should be initiated at 200–400 mg daily. The dose is then gradually increased at a rate of 200 mg every 3–4 days to minimize side effects until maintenance dosage is reached (10–20 mg/kg/day). Carbamazepine induces microsomal enzymes and its own metabolism. It induces the metabolism of oral contraceptives, Coumadin, tricyclic antidepressants, and cyclosporine. It has significant potential for drug interaction with other drugs that induce (phenobarbital, primidone, phenytoin, felbamate) or inhibit (erythromycin, isoniazid, chloramphenicol, propoxyphene) microsomal enzymes, as well as nonprescription enzyme inhibitors like grapefruit juice and St. John's wort.

Common dose-related side effects include nausea, diplopia, headache, dizziness, and, at high levels, drowsiness and ataxia. Idiosyncratic adverse effects include skin rash, leukopenia, thrombocytopenia, aplastic anemia, toxic hepatitis, and pancreatitis, although serious side effects are quite rare (aplastic anemia has an incidence of 0.002%). Because of the seriousness of blood dyscrasias, it is recommended that a complete blood count be obtained prior to initiating therapy, at 1 month, and then periodically (at least yearly) thereafter. If abnormalities are noted, more frequent testing is recommended. Carbamazepine is also associated with an antidiuretic hormone-like action resulting in modest hyponatremia, with serum sodium rarely falling below 128 mEq/L.

Table 14.11 Pharmacokinetic data on common antiepileptic drugs

Antiepileptic drug	Maintenance daily dose (mg/day)	Half-life (hours)	Daily doses	Therapeutic serum levels(µg/mL)
Carbamazepine**	400–2,400	8–40	2–4	4–12
Clonazepam	1–6	20–50	2–3	N/A
Ethosuximide*	500–2,000	30–60	2–3	40–100
Felbamate#	2,400–3,600	20–23	3–4	22–137
Gabapentin	900–3,600	4–6	3–4	N/A
Lamotrigine	200–500	15–30	2	3–15
Levetiracetam	1,000–3,000	6–8	2	N/A
Oxcarbazepine*	600–2,400	4–9	2	10–30
Phenobarbital**	90–300	72–96	1–2	15–40
Phenytoin**	300–600	12–24	1–3	10–25
Pregabalin	150-600	5-7	2-3	N/A
Primidone**	750–2,000	4–12	3–4	5–12
Tiagabine	16–56	4–8	2–4	N/A
Topiramate*	200–400	15–23	2	N/A
Valproic acid##	750–3,000	7–17	1–4	50–150
Zonisamide	100–400	24–60	1–2	10–40

Effects on hepatic microsomal enzymes: *weak or partial inducer, **potent inducer, #weak or variable inhibitor, ##potent inhibitor

▼

Pearls and Perils

Standard antiepileptic drugs

▶ Never taper phenobarbital quickly, since this may precipitate withdrawal seizures.

▶ When measuring serum primidone levels, one should also check the phenobarbital level, since this is a product of primidone metabolism.

▶ Carbamazepine should be initiated slowly to avoid side effects.

▶ Enzyme-inducing drugs such as carbamazepine, phenytoin, phenobarbital, and primidone will alter levels of other concomitantly administered medications that are metabolized by the liver.

▶ Ethosuximide should be administered with extreme caution to patients with known liver or kidney disease.

▶ Patients taking enzyme-inducing AEDs chronically should have bone density scans because of the risk of osteomalacia. Use calcium and vitamin D supplementation for patients at risk.

Clonazepam

Clonazepam (Klonopin, generic preparations) is a benzodiazepine that is useful in absence, myoclonic, tonic–clonic seizures refractory to other AEDs, and Lennox-Gastaut syndrome. Benzodiazepines bind to a specific site in the $GABA_A$ receptor, enhancing the effects of GABA on postsynaptic inhibition of neuronal firing. The starting dose is 0.5–1 mg per day, divided two or three times daily, with the largest amount at bedtime. Dosage may be progressively increased in 0.5–1 mg increments every 5–7 days until a therapeutic effect or side effects occur. Typical adult therapeutic doses should not exceed 8 mg daily. The most common side effects include drowsiness, ataxia, and behavioral changes. Like other benzodiazepines, clonazepam may cause physical and psychological dependence. Additionally, one-third of patients who initially respond to clonazepam develop tolerance, with loss of seizure control. Clonazepam should not be used in patients with significant liver dysfunction or in patients with acute narrow-angle glaucoma. It is unusual to use clonazepam as initial monotherapy, for partial seizures, or as drug of choice. Patients specifically seeking clonazepam for epilepsy and refusing all alternatives should be carefully evaluated for possible drug dependence.

Ethosuximide

Ethosuximide (Zarontin) affects T-type calcium channels and is used almost exclusively for absence seizures. It is dosed two or three times per day and does not induce hepatic enzymes. Five hundred milligrams per day is the usual starting dose, with 250-mg increases every 4–5 days to a total of 1–2 g/day as needed. The side effects are generally mild and most often involve the gastrointestinal system, although anorexia, dizziness, headaches, and hiccups also may occur. In rare instances, ethosuximide has been linked to rash, blood dyscrasias, a lupus-like syndrome, and behavioral changes. It should be administered with extreme caution to patients with known liver or kidney disease.

Felbamate

Felbamate (Felbatol) is a broad-spectrum drug that has been shown to be effective for partial seizures and in the treatment of Lennox-Gastaut syndrome. It has multiple mechanisms of action, including modulation of sodium channels, blockade of N-methyl-D-aspartate (NMDA) receptors and voltage-gated calcium channels. It is one of the few AEDs with reported efficacy against atonic seizures (drop attacks). The special risks of felbamate should probably limit its use to an epilepsy expert. The starting dose of felbamate is 400 mg 2–3 times daily with the dose increased by 600–1,200 mg every week. Felbamate has complex interactions with other AEDs. When added to either, phenytoin, carbamazepine, or valproic acid, their serum levels rise. Thus, the dose of these agents should be reduced by 20–30% on initiation of felbamate therapy.

Adverse effects are a major limitation in the use of felbamate. Aplastic anemia has been reported at a rate of 1 per 5,000. Hepatic failure has also been reported, with a lower incidence. Less serious but common side effects include nausea, vomiting, weight loss, headache, and insomnia. Thus, felbamate is limited to those patients with injurious seizures in whom other treatments have failed. Complete blood counts and liver enzymes need to be checked monthly for at least the first year, and then frequently thereafter.

Gabapentin (Neurontin, generic preparations) increases brain GABA levels by an unknown mechanism, and also affects calcium and potassium currents; its efficacy in pain modulation may result from binding to the $\alpha_2\alpha$ subunit of calcium channels. Gabapentin is indicated as add-on therapy in adults and children with refractory partial seizures. However, it may worsen absence and myoclonic seizures, so caution should be observed with these seizure types. Since it has a short half-life, it is dosed three or four times daily. The initial starting dose is 300 mg/day, with the dose increased by 300 mg (in three or four divided doses) every 1–3 days to the maximum tolerated dose. Efficacy is dose-dependent, and maintenance doses may range from 900 to 3,600 mg/day. It does not affect hepatic microsomal enzymes, and it is excreted by the kidneys.

Gabapentin is usually well tolerated, but may cause sedation, ataxia, mild gastrointestinal upset, weight gain, peripheral edema, and behavioral changes (especially in children). Its lack of drug interaction and relatively low side-effect profile make gabapentin a good choice in elderly individuals and those who take several medications

---

▼ Pearls and Perils

New antiepileptic drugs

▶ Gabapentin and pregabalin may be useful in patients on multiple medications because of their lack of drug interactions. Consider these for patients with hepatic disease or concurrent chronic or neuropathic pain.

▶ Lamotrigine half-life varies greatly with concomitant AEDs. Initiation protocols are extremely slow in the face of valproic acid, which inhibits its metabolism, moderate in the face of no AED, and more rapid in the face of enzyme-inducing AEDs.
Lamotrigine is indicated for bipolar affective disorder, and thus may be useful in patients with dual diagnosis.

▶ Felbamate should be reserved for severely affected intractable patients because of its relatively high risk of aplastic anemia and hepatic failure.

▶ Levetiracetam lacks drug interactions and is well tolerated at initial therapeutic dose. Reduce by 50% in patients with renal insufficiency. Monitor patient for mood alterations.

▶ Patients with absence seizures or spike-and-wave patterns on their electroencephalogram should not be prescribed tiagabine.

▶ Monitor patients on topiramate for metabolic acidosis, weight loss, cognitive changes. Use with caution in patients with a history of kidney stones or those taking acetazolamide, high-dose vitamin C, or calcium supplementation because of the increased risk of kidney stones. Topiramate, like valproic acid, is indicated for prophylaxis of chronic migraine and may benefit patients with comorbid epilepsy and migraine.

---

that are metabolized by the liver. It is useful in postherpetic neuralgia and neuropathic pain in general; thus, patients with comorbid pain syndromes may benefit.

Lamotrigine

Lamotrigine (Lamictal) is a broad-spectrum AED that acts via voltage- and use-dependent blockade of sodium channels, and may have other effects on calcium channels. Lamotrigine may be used as monotherapy for newly diagnosed adolescents and adults with either partial or mixed seizures. It may also be an option for children with newly diagnosed absence seizures and in the treatment of Lennox-Gastaut syndrome. Lamotrigine is appropriate as add-on therapy in adults and children with refractory partial seizures. Dosing and titration of lamotrigine depends on whether the patient is taking additional AEDs. If lamotrigine is used as monotherapy for young adults, the starting dose is 25 mg/day, increased every 2 weeks by 25 mg daily as needed, usually to 100–200 mg a day. For

young adults who are taking hepatic enzyme–inducing AEDs, however, lamotrigine is usually started at 25 mg twice a day. This can be increased by 50 mg per day every 1–2 weeks as required to a target dose of 300–500 mg/day. The AEDs that require these higher dosages of lamotrigine are carbamazepine, phenytoin, phenobarbital, and primidone. For adults taking valproate, the initial dose is 12.5–25 mg every other day, with increases of 25 mg per day every 2 weeks as needed and tolerated, usually to 150–200 mg/day.

Side effects of lamotrigine include dizziness, blurred vision, ataxia, and sedation, especially when lamotrigine is combined with other AEDs. In addition, tics (especially in children) and insomnia have been described. Lamotrigine may increase myoclonic seizures in patients with JME, or other mixed generalized syndromes with myoclonic seizures. The major idiosyncratic reactions are Stevens-Johnson and Lyell syndromes. The risk of an allergic skin reaction diminishes when lamotrigine is begun at a low dose and slowly increased. Severe rash is more common in individuals receiving valproate. Other serious adverse events include hepatic and renal failure, disseminated intravascular coagulation (DIC), and arthritis. Its FDA approval for use in bipolar affective disorder offers a convenient option for patients with dual diagnosis of epilepsy and mood disorder.

Levetiracetam

Levetiracetam (Keppra) has a unique mechanism of action, not entirely defined, but it is the only approved AED with widespread binding to the SV2 protein of brain synaptic vesicles. Levetiracetam was initially approved for add-on therapy in patients of 4 years and older with refractory partial seizures. It has subsequently been approved for adjunctive therapy in primary generalized epilepsy in patients of 5 years and older, and in JME patients of 12 years and older. There are no known interactions with other AEDs. Treatment in adults can be initiated at 500 mg twice daily. The dosage can be titrated by 1,000 mg every 2 weeks, up to 3,000 mg/day as needed for seizure control. The half-life of levetiracetam is 6–8 hours, and elimination occurs in the kidney and by hydrolysis of an acetamide group. Doses in patients with renal insufficiency should be reduced by 50%. An intravenous (IV) formulation is available, with dose equivalence to oral levetiracetam. Its use in serial seizures, status epilepticus, and nonconvulsive status epilepticus has not been established, but its nonhepatic clearance and lack of drug interactions make it a useful option in intensive care unit patients requiring rapid seizure management. Side effects include irritability and other behavioral changes, including anxiety and agitation.

Oxcarbazepine

Oxcarbazepine (Trileptal, generic preparations) is structurally related to, and has actions similar to carbamazepine, but the metabolism avoids the toxic intermediate 10-11-epoxide of carbamazepine. Direct comparator studies performed in Europe suggest that oxcarbazepine is modestly better tolerated than carbamazepine, with similar efficacy. Oxcarbazepine is recommended for newly diagnosed adolescents and adults with either partial or mixed partial and secondarily generalized seizures. It is considered a narrow-spectrum drug, and should be used with caution in patients with suspected primary generalized epilepsy, as it may worsen spike-and-wave activity. It can be used as monotherapy and adjunctive therapy in patients with refractory partial epilepsy. Oxcarbazepine is begun at a dose of 300 mg twice daily and increased by 300 mg/day every 3 days to a maximum of 2,400 mg/day. Its half-life is 4–9 hours, and it is eliminated by the liver, but is not considered a strong enzyme-inducing AED. Patients who respond to carbamazepine, but are troubled by side effects, may be converted quickly to oxcarbazepine. The conversion factor is roughly 200 mg carbamazepine to 300 mg oxcarbazepine, and the tablets are conveniently provided to reflect this ratio. Side effects include sedation, dizziness, double vision, nausea, and rash. Hyponatremia (and isolated cases of hyponatremic coma) may occur, more commonly in the elderly. Patients demonstrating hyponatremia on carbamazepine are likely to develop similar or more severe hyponatremia on oxcarbazepine. This hypotonic hyponatremia appears not to be due to the syndrome of inappropriate antidiuretic hormone (SIADH), but may occur as a result of altered sensitivity to circulating antidiuretic hormone (ADH), or changes in the properties of renal collecting tubules. Symptomatic patients should be taken off the drug, but milder cases may respond to fluid restriction or observation with serial serum chemistry monitoring.

Phenobarbital

Phenobarbital (generic preparations, oral and parental) acts at the $GABA_A$ receptor at a site separate from the benzodiazepine binding site, to prolong the duration of chloride channel opening and thus inhibit neuronal firing. This is the oldest and least expensive of the commonly used AEDs. It treats partial seizures and generalized tonic–clonic seizures. The oral maintenance dose ranges from 1.0 to 4.5 mg/kg/day. It is initiated at 60 mg, and increased gradually according to response. Since phenobarbital has a long half-life (72–96 hours), once-daily dosing at bedtime generally suffices. Unlike phenytoin, serum levels are typically linear with dose in monotherapy. It induces hepatic microsomal enzymes, thus caution is advised with oral contraceptives and other drugs with hepatic metabolism. Its metabolism is significantly slowed with co-administration of valproic acid. Most clinicians monitor complete blood count (CBC), liver panel, and drug levels with decreasing frequency over years of therapy. Bone health should be monitored with long-term use.

The most common side effect in adults is sedation. However, tolerance usually develops. Paradoxical hyperactivity may occur in younger patients or those with mental deficiencies. Other side effects include personality change, depression, nausea, diplopia, ataxia, and dizziness. Idiosyncratic reactions include Dupuytren contractures, shoulder–hand syndrome, hepatitis, Stevens-Johnson syndrome, and anemia.

Phenytoin

Phenytoin (Phenytek, Dilantin, Fosphenytoin, generic preparations) acts on voltage-gated sodium channels to decrease repetitive firing. It is among the most commonly prescribed, inexpensive, and effective medications. Oral and parenteral formulations are available. Phenytoin is useful for the treatment of all partial seizures, generalized tonic–clonic seizures, and occasionally tonic and atonic seizures. Parenteral phenytoin, some chewable oral preparations, and rapid-release generic forms should be administered two to three times daily, although many tolerate once-daily dosing of extended release formulations. Phenytoin is typically dosed at 3–6 mg/kg/day, and can be begun at the maintenance dose. It has zero-order kinetics. Once hepatic enzymes are saturated, its half-life progressively increases with increasing serum levels. Monitoring of serum levels is important because of metabolic properties. Phenytoin induces hepatic microsomal enzymes.

The related prodrug fosphenytoin is a more expensive alternative parenteral preparation when rapid drug delivery is essential, as it can be given intravenously at three times the rate of phenytoin, and it can be given intramuscularly. It has a much lower risk of phlebitis after rapid IV infusion, and cost is the limiting factor in most U.S. institutions. Fosphenytoin is rapidly converted to phenytoin, and has the same efficacy and metabolism. In order to avoid confusion, it is ordered in phenytoin-equivalent units.

Side effects include gingival hypertrophy and hirsutism, which resolve when phenytoin is discontinued. At higher doses, ataxia, cognitive impairment, and lethargy are seen. Liver enzymes and a CBC should be checked periodically after starting therapy (1 month after and then as indicated). Phenytoin may cause a mild elevation of liver enzymes (SGOT, SGPT), which is not a reason for discontinuation, provided enzyme levels are less than 2–3 times normal. GGT, an induction enzyme, may be more markedly increased. Long-term use of phenytoin has been associated with osteomalacia, and bone density studies are recommended for patients taking phenytoin. Some evidence suggests cerebellar atrophy in long-term use, particularly if begun at an early age, but prospective studies are lacking. Idiosyncratic reactions include Stevens-Johnson syndrome, lymphadenopathy, thrombocytopenia, megaloblastic anemia, and leukopenia.

Pregabalin

Pregabalin (Lyrica) is the most recently approved AED. It is structurally related to gabapentin, with similar mechanisms of action. It is more potent, and lower doses appear effective as adjunctive therapy in adults with partial seizures with or without secondary generalization. The starting dose is typically 50–75 mg twice daily, increasing to therapeutic benefit to a maximum of 600 mg daily in two or three divided doses. The side-effect profile is similar to gabapentin, with sedation being a major feature. Like gabapentin, it lacks significant drug interactions and is a valuable agent for patients with hepatic failure or those on many other medications. It is also indicated for several pain syndromes, including fibromyalgia, postherpetic neuralgia, and diabetic neuropathy. Thus, it may benefit patients with comorbid chronic pain disorders.

Primidone

Primidone (Mysoline) is an older AED used to treat generalized tonic–clonic and partial seizures. It is metabolized by the liver to phenylethylmalonamide (PEMA) and phenobarbital, both of which have anticonvulsant properties. The mechanism of antiepileptic action of PEMA remains unknown. Primidone is an inducer of hepatic microsomal enzymes, and has drug interactions similar to phenobarbital. The adult daily dose of primidone is 750–1,500 mg dosed three or four times per day. A slow titration to therapeutic response is recommended. The side effects of primidone are similar to phenobarbital. Lower doses (50–500 mg/day) are useful in treating essential tremor.

Tiagabine

Tiagabine (Gabitril) has a "pure" mechanism of action, irreversibly blocking glial and neuronal GABA reuptake by the transporter GAT-1, thus increasing local inhibitory effects of GABA at the postsynaptic membrane. Tiagabine may be considered as add-on therapy in patients with refractory epilepsy. The starting dose of tiagabine is 4 mg/day. It can be increased by 8–16 mg per day each month, to a maximum of 32–56 mg/day, divided into two to four doses. Tiagabine is rapidly metabolized by the liver, and has a half-life of 6 hours. This half-life is shortened when co-administered with enzyme-inducing drugs. Thus, three to four daily doses are required to maintain a steady-state serum level. It has no clinically significant effects on other AEDs, and does not itself induce or inhibit liver enzymes.

Side effects include weakness, fatigue, dizziness, tremor, and gastrointestinal upset. Rapid increases in dose may lead to stupor, spike-and-wave stupor, or transient cognitive disturbances, so slow increases are advised. Patients with absence seizures or general spike-and-wave patterns on their EEG should not be prescribed tiagabine. Some anecdotal evidence suggests that patients with spasticity or anxiety disorders may be good candidates for tiagabine therapy, but the drug is not specifically indicated for these conditions.

Topiramate

Topiramate (Topamax, generic preparations) has a mixed mechanism of action, including blocking of kainate/α–amino-3-hydroxy-5-methyl-4-isoxazopropionic acid (AMPA) subtypes of glutamate receptors and voltage-gated sodium and calcium channels, while enhancing GABA-mediated chloride conductance and potassium conductance. It is also a weak inhibitor of carbonic anhydrase. Topiramate may be used as monotherapy for newly diagnosed adolescents and adults with either partial or mixed seizures. It can be used as monotherapy and adjunctive therapy in patients with refractory partial epilepsy, and for the treatment of refractory generalized tonic–clonic seizures in adults and children. Topiramate may be used to treat drop attacks associated with the Lennox-Gastaut syndrome in adults and children. The initial adult dosage is 25–50 mg/day in two divided doses. The daily dose is increased by 25–50 mg on a weekly basis. Many patients respond at less than 200 mg/day, but the dose may be titrated to 400 mg/day, as tolerated. It is excreted by the kidney and does not affect hepatic microsomal enzymes. The half-life of topiramate is 15–23 hours.

Side effects include dizziness, insomnia, confusion (especially at the onset of therapy or with rapid dose escalation), weight loss, and language dysfunction. Serious adverse events include metabolic acidosis, open-angle glaucoma, and hypohidrosis (especially children). Patients with a history of kidney stones or those taking high-dose vitamin C or calcium supplementation should not take topiramate because of the increased risk of kidney stones. It should be used with caution in patients on zonisamide or acetazolamide due to combined effects on carbonic anhydrase.

Valproic acid

The antiepileptic mechanism of action of valproic acid (Depakene, Depakote, Depakote ER, Depacon, generic formulations) is not well established, but it has been shown to potentiate GABA inhibition, and has activity at glutamate receptors, T-type calcium channels, and voltage-gated sodium channels. It is considered a broad-spectrum AED. Valproic acid is most effective for the seizures of idiopathic generalized epilepsy, particularly absence seizures, tonic–clonic seizures, and myoclonus. Although less effective than carbamazepine or phenytoin for complex partial seizures, it has some benefit for these as well. In addition to the seizures mentioned, it is used for tonic and atonic seizures. Immediate-release, extended-release, and parenteral formulations are available. The starting dose for adults is 500 mg/day, with subsequent increases based on toxicity or clinical response. Intravenous loading is well tolerated, with dosing equivalent to oral preparations. The role of IV valproic acid in status epilepticus is not established.

Clinically significant interactions occur with other AEDs. This agent inhibits hepatic enzymes, although it is metabolized by the liver. In monotherapy, typical doses range from 10 to 20 mg/kg/day. In patients on other AEDs that induce enzymes, up to 60 mg/kg/day may be needed. Valproic acid prolongs the serum half-life of lamotrigine, phenobarbital, and sometimes ethosuximide. It may increase the toxicity of carbamazepine by increasing the 10,11-epoxide intermediate, and may increase the free fraction of phenytoin, causing increased toxicity at typical therapeutic levels. Valproic acid levels are increased by concomitant use of felbamate.

Common side effects of valproic acid are tremor, nausea, weight gain, alopecia, and menstrual irregularities including amenorrhea. Idiosyncratic reactions include hepatic failure, seen mainly in children on multiple anticonvulsants, encephalopathy secondary to hyperammonemia, pancreatitis, and thrombocytopenia. Valproic acid should not be used in children under the age of 2 years. It should be used with caution in women of childbearing potential, as data from pregnancy registries worldwide have shown an increased risk of fetal malformation compared with other AEDs. Valproic acid is also indicated for treatment of bipolar affective disorder and prevention of migraine headaches; it may be useful in patients with these comorbidities.

Zonisamide

Zonisamide (Zonegran) was studied and introduced in Japan, over a decade before its approval in the United States. It has multiple actions that may contribute to its efficacy as a broad-spectrum AED. It blocks T-type calcium channels, inhibits slow sodium channels, and may inhibit release of glutamate. Zonisamide may be used as adjunctive treatment in patients with refractory partial seizures. It is promising, but not yet indicated, in the treatment of absence seizures and other generalized epilepsies. Zonisamide is metabolized by the liver and excreted renally. It is not a hepatic inducer and does not appear to have clinically significant drug interactions with other AEDs, although patients receiving inhibitors of hepatic microsomal metabolism (CYP3A) may need lower doses of zonisamide. The starting dose is 100 mg orally once per day and upward titration should be slow, with at least 2 weeks between increases. Efficacy is usually seen at 200–400 mg/day, but doses as high as 600 mg/day may be needed. The long half-life allows once-daily dosing in many patients, usually at night to minimize daytime sedation. Side effects include dizziness somnolence, irritability, photosensitivity, and weight loss, in addition to rash, renal calculi, and hypohidrosis (especially in children, likely due to a carbonic anhydrase effect).

Antiepileptic Drug Selection

First, proper selection of AED by epilepsy syndrome is essential. Next, the physician should attempt to match the drug profile to the patient in terms of side effects, cost, frequency of dosing, and comorbid disorders. Broad-spectrum drugs should be considered when the distinction of partial versus generalized epilepsy is in doubt. Narrow-spectrum drugs—considered effective for all types of partial seizures and secondarily generalized convulsions—may be ineffective or may worsen generalized syndromes such as absence, myoclonic, and idiopathic generalized epilepsies. Narrow-spectrum drugs include tiagabine, oxcarbazepine, gabapentin, pregabalin, and to some extent carbamazepine and phenytoin. Ethosuximide is unique in its efficacy for absence seizures. Current recommendations derive from FDA indications for these drugs and 2004 guidelines from the American Association of Neurology and the American Epilepsy Society.

Table 14.12 summarizes the various treatment options. For newly diagnosed epilepsy, carbamazepine, gabapentin, lamotrigine, oxcarbazepine, phenobarbital, phenytoin, and topiramate are recommended as monotherapy for partial/mixed seizures. Ethosuximide, lamotrigine, and valproic acid are recommended as monotherapy for absence seizures. For refractory partial epilepsy, felbamate, lamotrigine, oxcarbazepine, and topiramate may be used as monotherapy. Felbamate, gabapentin, lamotrigine, levetiracetam, oxcarbazepine, tiagabine, topiramate, and zonisamide are recommended as adjunctive therapy. Idiopathic generalized epilepsies, especially those with prominent generalized spike-and-wave discharges, are best treated with valproic acid (avoid during pregnancy), lamotrigine, levetiracetam, and topiramate. Felbamate and clonazepam are useful in refractory cases.

Monitoring of Antiepileptic Drug Serum Concentrations

For the older AEDs, measurement of AED concentrations in serum aids in managing seizures. Serum levels should be checked after reaching targeted dosage to ensure that the desired targeted level has been reached. Levels help assess efficacy and drug compliance, but are not a primary therapeutic measure. Once a stable dose is achieved in a well-controlled patient, levels can be infrequently checked (every 6 months to a year). Newer AEDs require less drug level monitoring, but safety monitoring may be indicated (see earlier sections on individual drugs).

Initiation and Discontinuation of Treatment

Initiation

Not all seizures require AED therapy. Treatment should be started only if there is an unacceptable chance of seizure recurrence, and the patient ultimately has responsibility for deciding what constitutes an unacceptable risk.

Table 14.12 Recommendations for antiepileptic drug selection

AED	Convulsive seizures—unclear if primarily or secondarily generalized, monotherapy	Partial seizures, ± GTC: initial therapy or alternate monotherapy	Partial seizures, ± GTC, second line or adjunctive therapy	Generalized epilepsy with mixed seizure types (GTC, absence, myoclonic, atonic), generalized spike and wave on EEG	Absence seizures only, generalized spike and wave on EEG
Carbamazepine	X*	X	X	X*	
Phenytoin	X	X	X	X	
Valproate	X	X	X	X	X
Phenobarbital	X	X	X	X	
Primidone	X	X	X	X	
Ethosuximide				X@(absence)	X
Clonazepam			X	X	X#
Felbamate			X	X	
Gabapentin		X#	X		
Topiramate	X	X	X	X	
Tiagabine			X		
Lamotrigine	X	X	X	X*	X#
Levetiracetam	X#	X#	X	X@	
Oxcarbazepine	X*	X	X		
Zonisamide			X	X@#	
Pregabalin			X		
Acetazolamide				X@#	X@#

GTC, generalized tonic–clonic; EEG, electroencephalogram
Not FDA approved for this indication
@Adjunctive therapy
*May exacerbate some seizure types
Based on 2004 AAN and AES newer AED guidelines, 2001 Felbamate guidelines, common usage in referral centers, and authors' experience for use in adults

Knowing the epilepsy syndrome is key to offering sensible guidelines to a patient.

Recurrence rates range from 34% to 71% after a first seizure in adults, depending upon risk factors. The risk of recurrence is increased in patients with structural lesions, a family history of epilepsy, a history of prior seizures, significant head trauma, stroke, prior CNS infection, or a history of cerebral palsy. An abnormal neurologic examination or a history of a postictal Todd paresis indicates a higher risk of a seizure recurrence as well. The EEG also offers prognostic information. Patients with generalized spike-and-wave activity have higher seizure recurrence rates than those with normal or nonspecific EEG findings.

The decision to treat is based on perceived risk and benefit. The impact of a second seizure depends on a variety of subjective factors, as well as driving status, occupation, lifestyle, and medical risk of a second seizure. Untreated patients with partial seizures are subject to secondarily generalized convulsions and similar risk of bodily injury as those with seizures that are generalized from onset. In some patients, proposing treatment of a comorbid illness (such as migraine, chronic pain, bipolar affective disorder) with an AED may make the decision easier.

Discontinuation

Treatment is stopped when the probability of additional recurrences is acceptably small. As with initiation of therapy, what constitutes an "acceptable" risk is ultimately left to the patient's judgment. Since the chance of a major medical complication from the first recurrent seizure is variable, the psychosocial ramifications and the patient's willingness to accept risk are the major determining factors in making the decision. The natural history of the epilepsy syndrome largely determines the probability of remission. Syndromes with low remission rates, such as JME, are treated differently than are syndromes with high remission rates, such as childhood absence epilepsy. A 1991 British study evaluated 1,013 patients who were randomized to withdrawal or continuation of antiepileptic therapy after a 2-year or longer seizure-free period. Twenty-five percent of patients who continued medication experienced seizure recurrence

▼

Pearls and Perils

Monitoring antiepileptic drug levels and more

▶ Check serum levels of antiepileptic drugs (AEDs) at target steady-state level, when side effects occur, or with breakthrough seizures to assess compliance. Note time since last dose.

▶ Check complete blood counts (CBCs) and liver enzymes at baseline and at least once during the initial months of therapy with all AEDs.

▶ Check liver enzymes and CBCs twice a month with felbamate therapy for the first 3 months, and periodically thereafter.

▶ Check sodium level periodically with carbamazepine and oxcarbazepine therapy.

▶ Monitor patients on topiramate for metabolic acidosis.

▶ Monitor bone health with dual-energy X-ray absorptiometry (DEXA) scans in patients on chronic therapy, especially hepatic-inducing AEDs.

▶ When carbamazepine toxicity is suspected but the therapeutic level is normal, consider carbamazepine epoxide level.

▶ When a primidone level is monitored, be certain to check the phenobarbital level as well.

within 5 years, whereas 45% of those who stopped medication had recurrence. The factors associated with successful withdrawal included a normal neurologic examination, normal IQ, normal EEG, and single type of seizure.

Ketogenic Diet

The ketogenic diet provides a nonpharmacologic therapy reserved mainly for severe pediatric epilepsy. It was developed in the 1920s from early observations that fasting was beneficial in reducing seizures. The mechanism of action remains unknown, but ketosis may affect intermediary metabolism to influence the dynamics of excitatory and inhibitory neurotransmitters. To be effective, a state of continuous ketosis must be maintained. This is beyond the typical Atkins diet or low-carbohydrate diet. To maintain severe ketosis, typical calories from fat are in the 80–90% range. Protein intake is liberal, but carbohydrates are severely restricted. Even minor deviations from the ketotic state may result in seizure flurry or even status epilepticus. The diet should be attempted only with the supervision of a nutritionist and experienced neurologist. Adults are unlikely to maintain the diet voluntarily for extended periods. Those who are not self-sufficient may adhere well if a consistent, trained caregiver is involved. Long-term effects are unknown. Small series and anecdotal reports suggest that adults may benefit, but few are able to use the ketogenic diet as the mainstay of therapy.

Surgical Intervention

Surgery has become widely accepted as a safe and effective treatment for patients with medically refractory seizures. It is not a treatment of last resort. Surgery allows permanent remission in some patients, and ameliorates seizures in others. It reduces the medical morbidity and mortality of epilepsy and improves psychosocial status in some individuals. Most patients remain on AEDs after surgery, but seizure-free patients may tolerate reduction or even discontinuation of AEDs after several years.

Patients are candidates for surgery if they experience recurrent seizures despite adequate treatment with at least three appropriate AEDs. Patients should have seizures that either cause impaired consciousness (i.e., complex partial, tonic–clonic seizures) or produce injury (i.e., tonic–clonic, tonic, atonic seizures). Surgical candidates typically have seizures at least once every 1 or 2 months, and on occasion, disabling or unpleasant simple partial seizures may lead to surgical consideration. Epilepsy surgery is practiced by specialized multidisciplinary comprehensive epilepsy centers; most are registered with the National Association of Epilepsy Centers as Level 1–4, depending on their range of services and experience.

Two types of procedures can be performed, localized (focal) resection and corpus callosotomy. In focal resection, the pathologic cortex responsible for seizures is excised. Patients must demonstrate on video EEG ictal recordings a single localized onset of habitual seizures in an area of the brain that will tolerate tailored resection. Because the majority of operable patients have seizures from a temporal lobe, the most common operation performed is anterior temporal lobectomy. Class I evidence from a randomized controlled clinical trial supports the superiority of temporal lobectomy over best medical management in surgical candidates with appropriate presurgical evaluation (Weibe et al., 2001). However, cortical excision can be performed anywhere in the cerebral hemispheres. Results vary depending on the area of brain resected, with postoperative improvement rates ranging from 60–90%, depending upon the procedure. Complications resulting in permanent serious neurologic deficits average fewer than 2%. A nonresective procedure, subpial transection, is sometimes performed instead of resection when epileptic tissue is in eloquent neocortex. Practiced in a relatively small number of centers, the procedure is appropriate in Landau-Kleffner syndrome, Rasmussen encephalitis, and other epilepsies with broad regional or multilobar seizure onset. The success rate is yet to be defined.

In a corpus callosotomy, the corpus callosum is divided to interrupt the interhemispheric pathways required for generalization of seizures. A partial division of the corpus callosum involving the anterior 66–80% is usually sufficient for clinical effect. This palliative procedure reduces seizure frequency and severity in 50–80% of individuals, but rarely results in seizure-free patients. This procedure is indicated for atonic, tonic, and tonic–clonic seizures when resection cannot be done. The frequency of this procedure has declined in the last decade since the introduction of vagus nerve stimulation.

Vagus nerve stimulation

Neurostimulation is a new avenue of treatment for epilepsy. Vagus nerve stimulation provides intermittent extracranial stimulation via an implantable device approved in the United States, in 1997. A battery-powered generator is implanted in the chest, and a subcutaneous lead applied to the left vagus nerve. The left nerve is chosen because vagal fibers supplying the sinoatrial node are generally found in the right vagus nerve. The stimulation parameters are programmed via an external programming wand. Typical duty cycle is 10%, with 30 seconds stimulation alternating with 5 minutes off. The patient is provided with a magnet to turn the device off (when the magnet is in contact with the generator) or to advance the cycle (when swiped over the generator) to stimulate at the time of an aura or seizure. The exact mechanism of action is not fully understood, but is felt to involve brainstem connections via the nucleus solitarius with higher limbic and cortical centers bilaterally. In two randomized double-blind trials, partial-onset seizure frequency declined about 30% after VNS treatment for 3 months. In long-term observation studies, efficacy is sustained or even improved. The efficacy is comparable to that of the newer AEDs, but it has certain advantages in terms of tolerability, since no CNS adverse effects are noted. Local adverse effects include tingling and hoarseness during stimulation. Rare device complications may occur. The generator is replaced every 5–10 years, depending on model and stimulus parameters.

Vagus nerve stimulation is generally viewed as an option for patients with medically refractory epilepsy who are not candidates for surgery. Although tested and indicated for refractory partial seizures, experience worldwide has shown favorable efficacy in a broad range of epilepsy syndromes, including generalized epilepsies. Prior to implantation with VNS, most patients should be monitored with video EEG to verify the diagnosis, determine if they are candidates for epilepsy surgery, and to exclude those with nonepileptic spells and mixed disorders.

Status Epilepticus

Status epilepticus (SE) is among the most frequent and serious neurologic emergencies encountered by the neurologist.

Both clinical and experimental evidence show that status epilepticus causes brain damage independent of systemic metabolic derangements. For epidemiologic purposes, SE is defined as clinical or electrographic seizures lasting at least 30 minutes or serial seizures in which consciousness is not regained between seizures. However, for practical purposes, seizures that last long enough to raise concern about an altered physiologic state (e.g., tonic–clonic seizures lasting more than 5 minutes) should be treated as SE. Although any seizure type can develop into SE, tonic–clonic (convulsive) SE is the most severe type and constitutes a neurological emergency.

Status epilepticus is caused by acute CNS insults such as stroke, infection, hemorrhage, and traumatic brain injury, and systemic derangements from intoxications and metabolic abnormalities. Morbidity and mortality chiefly depend upon the underlying cause of the SE. For example, SE caused by AED withdrawal has a more benign prognosis than SE due to anoxic injury.

Time is crucial in the management of SE. Although etiology must be determined, treatment should begin immediately. Adequate ventilation, cardiac output, and cerebral perfusion should be maintained. Laboratory testing will look for metabolic causes of seizures. Hyponatremia, hypoglycemia, hypocalcemia, and other metabolic derangements should be promptly reversed. Fifty percent glucose with 100 mg thiamine should be given intravenously in a bolus if seizures might be due to hypoglycemia. Maintenance fluids should be started using 5% dextrose in half normal or normal saline unless there is fluid overload or suggestion of increased intracranial pressure. Urine output and renal function must be monitored, since rhabdomyolysis from excessive muscle activity can occur. It is preferable to support respiration and blood pressure by artificial

---

Pearls and Perils

Nonconvulsive status epilepticus

▶ Suspect nonconvulsive status epilepticus (NCSE) in a confused or unconscious patient if there is no obvious cause for the change. Obtain an electroencephalogram (EEG) urgently for confirmation and treatment.

▶ Complex partial and absence status epilepticus may result in a dreamy or twilight state in an ambulatory patient.

▶ NCSE may occur in a patient with epilepsy treated with excessive GABAergic drugs or narrow-spectrum drugs (tiagabine).

▶ Management is usually not as aggressive as for tonic–clonic status if the patient is conscious and interactive.

▶ An unconscious patient found to be in electrographic NCSE should be treated aggressively, as for status epilepticus.

means than to allow seizures to continue. A common treatment algorithm is summarized in Box 14.3. It is most important for physicians to use a consistent treatment regimen, for familiarity leads to greater success.

Epilepsy in the Elderly

The incidence of epilepsy is bimodal, with a rise in infancy and early childhood, and a second rise in the older adult population (Figure 14.1). The etiologies for the condition are quite different in the two populations. Idiopathic and genetic syndromes are rare in the older age group, while symptomatic partial epilepsies are the norm. The cause should be diligently sought. The most common causes are cerebrovascular disease, tumors, trauma, degenerative, and toxic-metabolic.

Presentation.

The recognition of epilepsy in an older adult may be delayed, overlooked, or misinterpreted. It is common to have bland nonconvulsive seizures, usually partial onset, related to a structural lesion. Post-stroke patients may have a transient focal seizure in the area affected by the stroke, followed by exacerbation of the neurologic deficit. This Todd's paresis, superimposed upon a pre-existing deficit, may last for hours and can confuse the patient as well as the caregiver. If unwitnessed, this may resemble an extension of the original stroke.

Partial seizures with speech disturbance are frequently interpreted as TIAs in the elderly. This may prompt a stroke workup and divert attention away from the electrical nature of the disorder. Recurrent stereotyped episodes with altered awareness and amnesia for the event, especially in the absence of a motor deficit, should trigger a search for partial seizures.

Some elderly patients with cognitive and memory impairment cannot recognize or report episodic disturbances caused by partial seizures. They may appear to others to have "good days" and "bad days" based on seizure activity and postictal confusion. It is estimated that 9-16% of patients with Alzheimer's disease have partial seizures, and this may be an underestimate. There is a need for increased surveillance and more data from prolonged EEG monitoring in elderly patients showing fluctuating levels of cognition and memory.

Seizures and falls create a vicious circle. Seizures beget falls; falls beget seizures. Even modest head injury may produce intracranial bleeding in elderly persons with diffuse brain volume loss. New subdural hematomas and parenchymal contusions bring new epileptogenic potential, may create new deficits, and may hasten decline.

Seizures due to toxic-metabolic causes are more likely to present as generalized tonic clonic seizures. If a

---

Box 14.3 Treatment protocol for convulsive status epilepticus

Time: 0 minutes (Airway, Breathing, Circulation)

▶ Initiate general systemic support of the airway (insert nasal airway or intubate if needed) and blood pressure; begin nasal oxygen; monitor electrocardiogram (EKG) and respiration, pulse oximetry; check temperature frequently; obtain history; perform neurologic examination.

▶ Start intravenous line containing isotonic saline at a low infusion rate.

▶ Check Dextrostix, send serum samples for electrolyte, blood urea nitrogen, glucose, complete blood count, drug screen, and anticonvulsant levels; check arterial blood gas values.

▶ Inject 50 ml of 50% glucose intravenous (IV) and 100 mg of thiamine IV or intramuscular (IM).

▶ Call electroencephalograph (EEG) laboratory to start recording as soon as feasible.

▶ Administer lorazepam 0.1–0.15 mg/kg IV (2 mg/min) up to 8 mg; if seizures persist, administer phenytoin (or preferably fosphenytoin), 20 mg/kg IV (50 mg/min or 150 mg/min if fosphenytoin).

▶ If seizures persist, give additional 10 mg/kg phenytoin IV.

▶ If febrile, consider lumbar puncture; if focally abnormal, obtain head computed tomography (CT) scan first.

Time: 30–40 minutes

▶ If seizures persist, intubate; insert bladder catheter; start EEG recording; check temperature.

▶ Administer phenobarbital, loading dose of 20 mg/kg IV (100·mg/min).

▶ If seizures persist, give additional 10 mg/kg phenobarbital IV.

Time: 45–60 minutes

▶ If seizures persist, begin pentobarbital infusion, 5 mg/kg IV initial dose, and then push until seizures have stopped using EEG monitoring. Continue pentobarbital infusion at 1–5 mg/kg/hr; slow infusion rate every 4–6 hours to determine if seizures have stopped, with EEG guidance. Monitor blood pressure and respiration carefully; support blood pressure with pressors if needed.

Or

▶ Administer midazolam loading dose of 200 μg/kg followed by 1–3 μg/kg/min continuous IV infusion. Increase maintenance dose to stop electrographic seizures based on EEG monitoring. If this fails, use pentobarbital as noted above.

Or

▶ Administer propofol 1–2 mg/kg loading dose followed by IV infusion, not to exceed 67 μg/kg/min and for short duration to avoid metabolic acidosis and other complications.

treatable cause is found, the patient may be spared treatment with AEDs. Medications, missed medications (especially benzodiazepines), hyponatremia, hypoglycemia, and hypothyroidism, are frequent reversible causes of new onset convulsive seizures in the elderly. Nonketotic hyperglycemia may produce focal deficits and focal seizures.

Cardiogenic syncope can be mistaken for a convulsive seizure, especially if a few clonic jerks are noted by the observer. Look for rapid recovery and absence of prolonged postictal confusion to help distinguish syncope from epileptic spells with sudden loss of consciousness. Prompt diagnosis of a cardiac dysrhythmia can be lifesaving in this setting.

Prolonged confusional state in the elderly should trigger consideration of nonconvulsive status epilepticus. This "twilight state" is associated with continuous epileptiform abnormality on EEG. Untreated or undertreated patients with partial seizures may experience bland seizures followed by a prolonged postictal encephalopathy lasting hours or days. In these cases the EEG reveals profound polymorphic slow waves typical of the postictal state. Nocturnal partial seizures may mimic sleep disorders, such as sleepwalking and REM behavior disorder. These conditions are easily clarified with video-EEG monitoring.

In summary, the diagnosis of epilepsy in the elderly requires a high level of suspicion, and awareness of the common and uncommon presentation of seizures in this group. Fortunately, most seizures in this age group are responsive to well-chosen AEDs.

Treatment.

The same rules of AED selection by seizure type apply to the elderly. However, the selection based on side effect profile is especially important. As most elderly patients are on multiple medications, choose a drug with low potential for drug interactions. Avoid drugs with high potential for sedation, such as phenobarbital, primidone, and benzodiazepines. Several newer AEDs such as gabapentin, pregabalin and zonisamide may be sedating initially, but most patients accommodate if titrated slowly. Absence of drug interactions and renal elimination make gabapentin, pregabalin and levetiracetam attractive choices. Drugs associated with bone loss (phenobarbital, phenytoin, carbamazepine, primidone, valproate) should be used with caution, especially in patients with preexisting osteopenia or osteoporosis. Routine calcium and vitamin D supplementation is recommended.

A double blind, randomized 2005 VA Cooperative study of newly diagnosed partial epilepsy in patients 60 and older compared carbamazepine, lamotrigine and gabapentin as initial monotherapy. All were found effective, but lamotrigine was significantly better tolerated, followed by gabapentin. Lamotrigine also proved more tolerable than carbamazepine in a 1999 United Kingdom study comparing the two drugs in an elderly population. However, a 2007 multinational double blind trial comparing slow release carbamazepine with lamotrigine found no significant differences in efficacy or tolerability.

Pharmacokinetic differences in the elderly include reduced hepatic metabolism and less enzyme inducibility. After age 40, renal elimination declines by 10 percent per decade. Highly protein bound drugs (such as phenytoin, carbamazepine, and valproate) are affected by lower concentrations of plasma binding proteins with age, increasing the chance of toxic symptoms at "therapeutic levels" or at common doses. Other factors include changes in volume of drug distribution, decreased gastric motility and increased gastric pH, altering drug absorption. Older patients may be more susceptible to adverse effects from generic drug substitution due to these pharmacokinetic variables. However, patients on a fixed income may find brand name drugs unaffordable. Regardless of the drug, "start low, go slow" and minimize switching manufacturer for best results.

Finally, compliance should be confirmed, if possible, from a third party or family member. Use of pill boxes, medication reminders, or automated refills may be necessary in patients with cognitive impairment. Swallowing difficulties should be kept in mind when prescribing large tablets, or half tablets that may produce rough edges. Consider liquid or "sprinkle" formulations where available.

Use of Antiepileptic Drugs in Women of Childbearing Potential and Pregnancy

Women of Childbearing Potential

Women of childbearing potential should be counseled about the possible interactions between oral contraceptives and AEDs. Oral contraceptives usually do not exacerbate seizures, but AEDs that induce hepatic metabolism—such as phenytoin, phenobarbital, primidone, carbamazepine, and possibly high-dose topiramate—diminish the effectiveness of oral contraceptives, increasing the likelihood of pregnancy. Therefore, medium- to high-dose estrogen should be given in oral contraceptives, and pills should be supplemented by a barrier method if pregnancy is to be avoided. Some AEDs, notably lamotrigine, are metabolized more quickly when co-administered with oral contraceptives or other hormone therapies. Thus, stopping or starting hormones during lamotrigine therapy may significantly affect the level and seizure control. Since AEDs are teratogenic, their use should be discussed in women of childbearing age, and specific measures should be planned. When possible, women who plan to become pregnant should be treated with a single agent at the lowest effective dose.

Pearls and Perils

Antiepileptic drugs in women of childbearing age and pregnancy

▶ Of the older AEDs, phenobarbital, primidone, and valproic acid appear most, and carbamazepine least, teratogenic in registry data. The safety of the newer drugs is under study, with low malformation rates found for lamotrigine in several studies.

▶ Aim for monotherapy in pregnant women at the lowest effective dose.

▶ Enzyme-inducing AEDs (carbamazepine, phenytoin, phenobarbital, primidone) may diminish the effectiveness of oral contraceptives, and a medium- to high-dose estrogen oral contraceptive should be used. One should use 50 μg estrogen pills if tolerated, and consider an additional barrier method.

▶ Consider multivitamin–folate supplementation in all women of childbearing potential.

▶ In pregnant women, 10 mg daily vitamin K should be administered at 4 weeks before delivery to counteract vitamin K clotting factor deficiencies associated with neonatal exposure to AEDs.

▶ Any woman on AEDs complaining of sexual dysfunction, menstrual irregularities, or difficulty becoming pregnant should have a full reproductive endocrine evaluation.

▶ Bone health may be affected in all patients on AEDs, especially hepatic inducers. Calcium–vitamin D supplementation is advised.

Pregnancy

Children of women with epilepsy have elevated rates of congenital anomalies and major malformations. Exposure of the developing fetus to AEDs taken by the mother appears to be responsible for the increase. The commonly used older AEDs (phenytoin, carbamazepine, valproic acid, primidone, and phenobarbital) have variously been shown to increase the baseline risk of major fetal malformation about two- to threefold, that is, from 1–3% to 3–9%. Polytherapy further increases the risk. Most major malformations are due to early exposure, in the first 6–8 weeks of pregnancy. Midline malformations, cleft lip and cleft palate, and cardiac and urogenital malformations are among the major malformations noted. Valproic acid and carbamazepine have been associated more specifically with neural tube defects: spina bifida, meningomyelocele, and hydrocephalus (1–2%).

Following the introduction of newer AEDs, pregnancy registries have been established in North America, a consortium of European countries, the United Kingdom, and Australia. Some pharmaceutical companies also have individual pregnancy registries regarding the terato-genicity of AEDs. These databases have provided consistent evidence of substantial increased risk of major congenital malformations for valproic acid used in mono- or polytherapy. The risk appears dose-dependent, higher with doses of greater than 1,000 mg/day. An ongoing U.S. evaluation of infants born to mothers with epilepsy suggests that valproic acid may be associated with a higher risk of developmental delay in the offspring. One report from the North American registry also indicated a higher malformation risk with phenobarbital. Of the newer AEDs, the largest data set exists for lamotrigine. In most studies, lamotrigine shows a favorable overall risk profile, but a U.K. study suggested a dose-dependent risk of increased malformations in women taking more than 200 mg/day. Based on very few cases, the North American registry reported an increased specific incidence of oral clefts with lamotrigine exposure, although the overall risk of malformations remained low. Additional studies are needed to fully delineate these findings, and to provide data for other AEDs. The teratogenic effects of the most of the newer AEDs (gabapentin, felbamate, Topamax, pregabalin, levetiracetam, zonisamide) are unknown.

Most experts recommend AED monotherapy at the lowest possible effective dose, based on epilepsy syndrome and side effects for the individual. This is essentially the goal in all patients, but it is especially important to reassess prior to conception. Patients should not "take their chances" and go drug-free during pregnancy, as seizures may recur with greater frequency and severity off medication, potentially harming the fetus. It is advisable to begin prenatal vitamin supplementation, including 1–4 mg of folate prior to conception in all women who are planning a pregnancy or who do not use adequate contraceptive methods, as many pregnancies are unplanned. Perhaps one-third of women with epilepsy have an increase in seizures while pregnant, particularly in the first and third trimesters. Tonic–clonic seizures particularly increase fetus risk due to possible trauma and hypoxia. Some women with hormone-sensitive epilepsy enjoy a remission of seizures during pregnancy, possibly due to the antiseizure effects of progesterone. Drug metabolism may

Key Clinical Questions

▶ Has the patient had only one seizure or recurrent unprovoked seizures?

▶ Does the patient have a known or suspected brain lesion, or is the seizure without identifiable pathologic cause?

▶ Is the patient's seizure of focal onset or generalized from the start?

▶ Are there special conditions or comorbidities to consider when selecting an antiepileptic treatment?

▼

Consider Consultation When...

Consider consultation with a neurologist in:

▶ individuals with new onset epilepsy;

▶ patients in whom seizures are suspected but diagnosis is not clear;

▶ women with epilepsy who are planning a family;

▶ patients in status epilepticus or suspected status epilepticus;

▶ patients who have an inherited epilepsy syndrome and require genetic counseling.

▶ patients whose seizures fail to respond completely to each of two drugs;

▶ patients with suspected nonepileptic episodes; and

▶ patients who may benefit from surgical intervention.

change significantly during pregnancy, and levels should be monitored where appropriate. Of the newer AEDs, lamotrigine metabolism may be affected by hormonal changes, and dosing should be adjusted throughout the pregnancy and postpartum.

A vitamin K–dependent clotting deficiency that can result in neonatal bleeding has been linked to phenobarbital, phenytoin, carbamazepine, primidone, and ethosuximide. This may occur in up to 7% of women. Vitamin K should be administered to the mother in the last month of pregnancy to prevent neonatal hemorrhage, and vitamin K should be given to the neonate after birth as well.

There is no general contraindication for women with epilepsy to breast-feed their infants. The risks and benefits should be evaluated in each individual case and discussed with the pediatrician. The drug concentration in breast milk is usually smaller than that in plasma. Highly protein-bound drugs are less easily transferred to breast milk. However, since drug elimination mechanisms in the neonate are immature, some drugs like lamotrigine may result in accumulation in the infant. Careful observation for signs of infant toxicity is recommended.

Mortality and Morbidity in Epilepsy

People with epilepsy have a higher death rate than the population at large, and this is only partially accounted for by epilepsy-related accidents or SE. At least 30% of the deaths have no identifiable cause. Those at greatest risk for sudden death are between 20 and 40 years old, with a history of seizures for at least 1 year. In medically refractory patients, such as those in clinical trials, sudden unexplained death in epilepsy (SUDEP) occurs in an average of 3.7 per 1,000 patients yearly, and appears even higher in patients with recurrent seizures after epilepsy surgery. Typical SUDEP deaths are unwitnessed and do not necessarily involve a seizure/aspiration/asphyxia as

the proximate cause of death. A patient is often found lifeless in bed. They are more likely than the average patient to have long duration of epilepsy, increased number of medications, frequent dose changes, and history of tonic–clonic seizures. The mechanism of death is not known and is likely related either to cardiac arrhythmias or respiratory derangements. There is controversy among epileptologists about the need to counsel patients about this risk, as there is no known risk-reduction protocol.

People with epilepsy are also at greater risk for accidents and injuries. Lacerations, fractures, and burns may be caused by seizures, and precautions must be taken at work and play to enhance safety. Swimming should only be done in the presence of a certified lifeguard, and heights, moving machinery, and dangerous equipment (e.g., hedge trimmers, chain saws, lawn mowers, etc.) should be avoided. Occupations should be carefully chosen so that the occurrence of a seizure is not disabling to self or others. Patients with well-controlled seizures may drive with proper clearance from the department of motor vehicles, but commercial driving or piloting is usually contraindicated. A balance needs to be struck in recreational activity, using common sense and reasonable precautions.

Annotated Bibliography

Brodie M, Schachter S, Kwan P. *Fast facts: Epilepsy*, 3rd ed. Oxford: Health Press, 2005.
  Pocket-sized and very readable reference guide for residents or general practitioners with excellent chapters on practical management of epilepsy and use of the newer AEDs.
Engel J, Pedley TA, editors. *Epilepsy: A comprehensive textbook*, Vols. 1, 2 and 3. Philadelphia: Lippincott-Raven, 1997.
  An authoritative and comprehensive reference text on all aspects of epilepsy. A second edition is expected.
Engel J, ed. *Surgical treatment of the epilepsies*, 2nd ed. New York: Raven Press, 1993.
  Considers all issues in the surgical treatment of the epilepsies that would be of interest to those working in an epilepsy center; generated by the second Palm Desert Conference on Surgical Treatment of the Epilepsies.
Hauser WA, Hesdorffer DC. *Epilepsy: Frequency, causes and consequences.* New York: Demos, 1990.
  An excellent text detailing the epidemiology and etiology of the epilepsies.
Levy RH, Mattson RH, Meldrum BS, Perucca E, eds. *Antiepileptic drugs*, 5th ed. Philadelphia: Lippincott Williams & Wilkins, 2002.
  A valuable compendium and reference on all anticonvulsants available today.
Miller JW, Silbergeld DL. *Epilepsy surgery: Principles and controversies.* New York: Taylor & Francis, 2006.
  A comprehensive treatise on surgical aspects of epilepsy.
Wyllie E, Gupta A, Lachhwani K, eds. *The treatment of epilepsy: Principles and practice*, 4th ed. Philadelphia: Lippincott Williams & Wilkins, 2006.
  A comprehensive and authoritative text that explores the pathophysiology, etiologies, diagnosis, and treatment of epilepsy.

SECTION 3

NEUROLOGIC DISEASES AND DISORDERS

CHAPTER **15**

Vascular Disease

Richard M. Zweifler and John F. Rothrock

Outline

▶ Epidemiology
▶ Risk factors
▶ Clinical diagnosis
▶ Diagnostic testing
▶ Transient ischemic attack
▶ Relevance of diagnosis to management
▶ Summary

Epidemiology

Stroke ranks as the third leading cause of death and the most common cause of permanent disability in adults. More than 750,000 new strokes and 300,000 transient ischemic attacks (TIAs) occur in the United States each year. At any given time, there are approximately 4.7 million survivors of stroke, and 150,000 individuals die each year in this country as a direct or indirect consequence of stroke. Most recent estimates place the cost of stroke in the United States in excess of $65 billion per year.

Efforts in research over the past decade have yielded treatments that may reduce stroke incidence significantly in certain high-risk populations. These advances in stroke prevention are now being complemented by breakthroughs in the acute treatment of stroke. Coupled with stroke's ubiquity and devastating consequences, this increasing ability to prevent and treat stroke mandates that virtually all clinicians possess the means to diagnose accurately the more common clinical manifestations of cerebrovascular disease.

Risk Factors

Several factors have been associated with an increased risk of stroke, many of which are modifiable (Table 15.1). Age is the single most important stroke risk factor, with incidence doubling each decade after age 55. Stroke incidence is higher in males and in African Americans, East Asians, and some Hispanics. A history of a prior stroke or TIA is a powerful stroke risk factor, and the degree of risk varies according to the etiology of the previous stroke/TIA.

Hypertension is the most prevalent and treatable stroke risk factor, carrying a relative risk on the order of 4. Atrial fibrillation increases stroke risk by 2–3, whereas diabetes, whether insulin-dependent or noninsulin-dependent, and cigarette smoking carry relative risks of 1.5–2. Other well-documented risk factors include sickle cell disease, carotid stenosis, hyperlipidemia, hyperhomocysteinemia, alcohol abuse, and other cardiac diseases (e.g., coronary artery disease, congestive heart failure, and a variety of valvular disorders). Less well-documented stroke risk factors include obesity and physical inactivity.

Key Clinical Questions

▶ Is this a stroke?
▶ If it is a stroke, what stroke subtype am I dealing with?
▶ What specific etiology is most likely to have caused this?
▶ What testing will enable me to confirm my clinical impression?
▶ What treatment(s) is most appropriate?

Table 15.1 Stroke risk factors

Nonmodifiable	Modifiable
Age	Prior stroke/TIA
Sex	Hypertension
Race/ethnicity	Diabetes
Family history	Hyperlipidemia
	Atrial fibrillation
	Homocystinemia
	Carotid stenosis
	Smoking
	Alcohol abuse
	Obesity
	Physical inactivity

Clinical Diagnosis

By and large, the diagnosis of stroke is not difficult. Symptoms typically begin suddenly and are referable to the region of brain that is ischemic or afflicted by hemorrhage. Historically, TIA has been defined as a sudden, focal neurologic deficit that lasts for less than 24 hours, is presumed to be of vascular origin, and is confined to an area of the brain or eye perfused by a specific artery. A new definition for TIA recently has been proposed: a brief episode of neurologic dysfunction caused by focal brain or retinal ischemia, with clinical symptoms typically lasting less than 1 hour and without evidence of acute infarction.

Internal carotid artery distribution strokes often produce unilateral numbness and/or weakness, aphasia, apraxia, agnosia, and visual field defects (Table 15.2). Vertebrobasilar distribution strokes can produce unilateral or bilateral sensorimotor deficits, often accompanied by signs and symptoms more specific for brainstem or cerebellar dysfunction: vertigo, diplopia, disequilibrium, ataxia, and cranial nerve palsies (Table 15.3). As the posterior circulation also supplies parts of the thalamus, internal capsule, and temporal and occipital lobes via the posterior cerebral artery, strokes in this distribution may present with some combination of sensorimotor symp-

Table 15.2 Anterior circulation stroke symptoms and signs

More specific	Less specific	Uncommon
Aphasia	Dysarthria	Ataxia
Apraxia	Headache	Vertigo/disequilibrium
Agnosia	Unilateral numbness or weakness	Nausea/vomiting
	Visual field deficit	

Table 15.3 Posterior circulation stroke symptoms and signs

More specific	Less specific
Ataxia	Dysarthria
Diplopia	Headache
Vertigo or disequilibrium	Nausea or vomiting
Bilateral numbness or weakness	Unilateral numbness or weakness
	Visual field deficit

toms, memory disturbance, and homonymous visual field impairment. Dysarthria is a nonspecific symptom/sign that may occur with stroke in either the carotid or vertebrobasilar distribution.

Stroke Mimickers

A number of disorders may mimic stroke and thus confound diagnosis (Box 15.1). Patients experiencing seizures can present with focal neurologic deficits, especially in the immediate postictal period, when there may be unilateral weakness (Todd paralysis) or other signs also commonly associated with stroke. Such deficits usually resolve over several hours but may persist as long as a day or more. There may or may not be a history of an established seizure disorder. The patient or an observer may relate the occurrence of involuntary, rhythmic movements, but frequently the patient cannot recall the seizure itself, the seizure is unobserved, or the seizure is nonconvulsive and thus unapparent.

Although brain neoplasms more commonly cause gradually progressive symptomatology and signs, tumors—primary or metastatic—also may mimic stroke. Acute, stroke-like deterioration occurs most often when there is hemorrhage within the tumor or tumor-associated seizure activity, but at times symptoms related to tumors may resemble those from stroke or TIA for no discernible reason. Systemic infections and toxic–metabolic disturbances may mimic stroke, especially in patients with preexisting focal brain injury. The acute systemic illness can bring to light old, previously subclinical neurologic deficits. Migrainous aura may be confused with TIA or stroke, especially when it is prolonged and, on rare occasions, ischemic stroke can complicate migraine. With migrainous aura, there is typically a history of prior similar symptoms that have been associated with headache, and the symptoms themselves have "positive" features (e.g., geometric hallucinations of vision, flashes of light) as well as "negative" (e.g., loss of vision). Nausea, vomiting, photophobia, and phonophobia often accompany the aura. Hypoglycemia acutely can produce focal neurologic symptoms and signs that will resolve rap-

---

Box 8.1 Stroke mimickers

▶ Seizure
▶ Mass lesion (e.g., tumor, subdural hematoma)
▶ Systemic infection
▶ Toxic–metabolic encephalopathy
▶ Migraine
▶ Hypoglycemia
▶ Multiple sclerosis
▶ Encephalitis

---

idly following administration of glucose or dextrose. Multiple sclerosis may present acutely with signs and symptoms indistinguishable from stroke on clinical grounds, but a careful history and selective diagnostic testing generally will serve to establish the correct diagnosis. Intracranial hematomas (subdural and epidural) also may present in a stroke-like fashion. With chronic subdural hematoma, a history of recent trauma is far from invariable, and this is especially true in cases involving the elderly or individuals who are receiving warfarin or are otherwise at risk for spontaneous bleeding. Even so, in the absence of antecedent severe trauma, patients with subdural hematomas most often present with headache, fluctuating depression of consciousness, and no or minimal focal neurologic deficit. At times, infectious encephalitis may mimic acute stroke, but fever, seizure activity, alteration of consciousness, and abnormal cerebrospinal fluid findings are likely to be present.

Determining Stroke Subtype

Stroke mechanism

Once the clinician is reasonably certain that the brain event under investigation is vascular in origin, he should seek to determine what pathophysiologic process has generated the stroke and the specific etiology that underlies that process. With regard to pathophysiology, all stroke is divided into two basic categories: ischemic and hemorrhagic. Approximately 80–85% of all strokes are ischemic. These two categories can be divided further into more specific pathophysiologic subtypes according to the basic cause of vascular occlusion and ischemia (e.g., thrombosis versus embolism) or the primary location of the brain hemorrhage (e.g., subarachnoid versus intracerebral). For thrombotic ischemic stroke, it also is useful to distinguish between a primary occlusive process involving small end-vessels (e.g. the penetrating lenticulostriate arteries that supply deep white and gray matter of the cerebral hemispheres) and a primary occlusive process involving a larger artery (e.g., the middle cerebral artery or any of its main cortical branches). Most stroke, then,

can be considered to result from one of these five primary causes: embolism, primary large vessel occlusion, primary small vessel occlusion, intracerebral hemorrhage (ICH), and subarachnoid hemorrhage (SAH). See Table 15.4.

The initial bedside evaluation of the patient and subsequent observation may be useful in determining the mechanism of stroke. For example, antecedent TIA is fairly common in thrombotic stroke, occurring in an estimated 25% of cases, but is unusual in cardioembolism. Furthermore, although all stroke is acute in onset, the subsequent clinical course may differ according to subtype. Embolic stroke tends to inflict maximum neurologic deficit at the time of onset. If anything, the patient may improve over the hours that follow—a phenomenon that has been attributed to spontaneous lysis and fragmentation of the occluding embolus with early reperfusion of the ischemic region. Similarly, thrombotic strokes may be "maximal at onset," but they produce an early clinical course notable for fluctuation in signs and symptoms or for stepwise neurologic deterioration significantly more often than do embolic strokes. Patients with ICH tend to exhibit a clinical course characterized by smoothly progressive neurologic decline over the initial hours. They also will complain of acute headache and suffer early impairment of consciousness more often than patients with ischemic stroke. Aside from this last feature, nothing on physical examination will reliably enable the clinician to distinguish between ischemic stroke and ICH. Brain computed tomography (CT) is frequently unrevealing when performed within the first 24 hours following acute ischemic stroke, even when the stroke is clinically severe. Noncontrasted CT, however, invariably demonstrates evidence of parenchymal hemorrhage in patients with acute ICH exceeding more than a few millimeters in diameter.

Historical evidence of antecedent TIA or the observation of a fluctuating or stepwise/progressive course is not helpful in differentiating between small- and large-vessel thrombosis, as these are elements common to all thrombotic stroke whatever the size of the involved vessel. Given the restricted subcortical or brainstem territory supplied by small penetrating end-arteries, however, as opposed to the often larger cortical regions supplied by the large cervical and intracranial cerebral arteries, the patient's symptoms and signs often point to the size and location of the occluded vessel. For example, the small penetrating branches of the middle cerebral, posterior cerebral, and basilar arteries supply the internal capsule, basal ganglia, and medial pons—regions where neurons and white matter tracts are tightly compacted and where even a small focus of acute ischemia may yield surprisingly extensive clinical deficit. Clinical syndromes traditionally associated with small-vessel occlusive stroke of one of these areas include "pure" sensory; "pure" motor or sensorimotor stroke involving the face, arm, and leg (or arm and leg); dysarthria/"clumsy hand"; and ataxic

Table 15.4 Stroke subtypes

		Discriminating features	Consistent features	Variable features
Ischemic	Small-artery occlusion (lacune)	1. <1.5cm subcortical or brainstem lesion by CT or MRI 2. No large artery or cardioembolic source	1. History of diabetes mellitus or hypertension 2. No cortical signs/symptoms	1. MRI or CT may be normal 2. Waxing and waning course
	Large-artery atherosclerosis (embolus/thrombosis)	1. >50% stenosis of proximal artery 2. No cardioembolic source	1. Cortical, cerebellar, brainstem, or subcortical infarct >1.5cm	1. Cortical or cerebellar signs/symptoms 2. History of TIAs 3. Waxing and waning course
	Cardioembolism (high-risk/medium-risk)	1. High- or medium-risk source (see Table 15.5) 2. No large artery source	1. Cortical, cerebellar, brainstem, or subcortical infarct >1.5cm	1. Cortical or cerebellar signs/symptoms 2. Maximal deficit at onset
	Stroke of other determined etiology	1. Supported by ancillary studies		
	Stroke of undetermined etiology	1. 2 or more causes identified, or 2. Negative evaluation, or 3. Incomplete evaluation		
Hemorrhagic	Intracerebral hemorrhage	1. Evidence of parenchymal bleeding on CT or MRI	1. Smoothly progressive deterioration	1. Headache (1/3) 2. Altered consciousness 3. Seizures
	Subarachnoid hemorrhage	1. Subarachnoid blood on CT/MRI or bloody cerebrospinal fluid	1. Sudden severe headache	1. Altered consciousness 2. Neck pain 3. Seizures

hemiparesis (implying incoordination disproportionately prominent relative to the degree of ipsilateral weakness present). Acute seizure activity, aphasia, gaze palsy, homonymous visual field deficits, inattention, agnosias, and apraxias (all features more commonly associated with lesions involving brain cortex or immediately adjacent subcortical areas) are relatively uncommon in small-vessel stroke. Such cortical signs and symptoms frequently accompany large-vessel stroke but, like the small-vessel stroke syndromes described previously, they are not specific for that subtype and often occur with embolic stroke or ICH as well.

The clinical presentation associated with "spontaneous" (i.e., nontraumatic) SAH typically serves to distinguish this stroke subtype from all others. If a history can be obtained, acute "thunderclap" headache almost invariably is reported. When the hemorrhage is extensive, impaired consciousness will be present on initial examination, and acute seizure activity may occur. Focal neurologic deficits are absent unless there is secondary extension of hemorrhage into the brain parenchyma or ischemia from vasospasm. The latter is rarely seen in the acute setting.

Determining Stroke Etiology

Identification of the pathophysiologic mechanism that has generated the stroke under evaluation is not synonymous with identification of that stroke's specific etiology. For example, one may conclude from bedside evaluation that a patient presenting with "pure" motor stroke involving the right face, arm, and leg has suffered thrombotic occlusion of a small lenticulostriate artery, and subsequent brain imaging and cerebral angiography may confirm that impression. However, even then, there are many different etiologic paths that lead to the common end-point of small-vessel occlusive stroke. Chief among these is so-called *lacunar* stroke, implying infarction less than 1.5–2 cm in diameter due to primary occlusion of a penetrating vessel already narrowed by lipohyalinosis or microatherosclerosis, often in association with chronic hypertension, diabetes, or both. Even so, lupus vasculopathy, amphetamine-induced vasculitis, polycythemia, antiphospholipid antibody-related prothrombosis, eclampsia, and a variety of other disparate conditions and diseases that in one way or another promote arterial thrombosis can produce an identical clinical presentation and pattern of infarction on brain CT or magnetic resonance imaging (MRI).

The most widely accepted classification scheme for ischemic stroke etiology is the Trial of ORG 10172 in Acute Stroke Treatment (TOAST) classification system that delineates the following subtypes: large artery atherosclerosis, small-vessel occlusion, cardioembolism, stroke of undetermined etiology (i.e., cryptogenic), and stroke of other determined etiology. Intracerebral hemorrhage is most often a direct complication of chronic hypertension through rupture of a Charcot-Bouchard microaneurysm. Other etiologies of ICH include rupture of an arteriovenous malformation (AVM), coagulopathy, amyloid angiopathy, drugs, vasculitis, idiopathic thrombocytopenic purpura (ITP), cavernous angioma, dural venous sinus thrombosis, brain neoplasm, cocaine and alcohol use, intracranial aneurysm, hemorrhagic ischemic stroke, and trauma. Subarachnoid hemorrhage is most often secondary to head trauma, with the most common nontraumatic etiology being rupture of a saccular aneurysm. Spontaneous SAH has also been associated with sickle cell anemia, certain drugs of abuse, and coagulopathy.

To determine stroke etiology with any accuracy (and without undue expense), one must consider the age and health history of the patient, details of events surrounding the acute stroke, and findings from the bedside evaluation. Using these data, the clinician can address those questions that direct diagnostic management: What stroke subtype am I dealing with? Which specific etiologies are more likely to have caused this pathophysiologic process? And, what testing will enable me to confirm my clinical impression?

Stroke of Unknown Cause

Even with intensive neurodiagnostic intervention, a specific etiology for ischemic stroke will not be identified in a sizable proportion of patients. This is especially true when it is a young person who has suffered stroke, and the cause is not immediately apparent from the initial bedside evaluation. In several recent studies of large patient groups with acute ischemic stroke, the incidence of "stroke of unknown cause" ranged from 23% to 40%. Whether such cases will exhibit a response to acute or chronic stroke therapy similar to that observed in patients with stroke from an identifiable cause is presently unclear.

Pearls and Perils

Stroke

▶ A negative computed tomography (CT) or magnetic resonance imaging (MRI) does not exclude ischemic stroke (especially when performed acutely).

▶ Hypoglycemia may cause focal neurologic deficit indistinguishable from stroke.

▶ Vasculitis is a rare cause of stroke at any age.

▶ Intracerebral hemorrhage cannot be distinguished reliably from infarction on the basis of bedside evaluation alone.

Diagnostic Testing

Brain Imaging

In the setting of acute stroke, brain imaging is helpful mostly in distinguishing between cerebral hemorrhage and ischemia. Although MRI is more sensitive than CT in most neurologic settings (infarction, central demyelination, neoplasm, etc.), it may fail to demonstrate very early hemorrhage that can be detected by CT. Noncontrasted CT is the neurodiagnostic procedure of choice for excluding hyperacute ICH (Figure 15.1) and, given our inability to distinguish reliably between ischemia and ICH on clinical grounds alone, this procedure is absolutely required in cases of suspected ischemic stroke when thrombolytic therapy is contemplated. A CT or MRI is useful when the diagnosis of stroke is in question and the clinician wishes to rule out "stroke mimickers" (tumor, subdural hematoma, multiple sclerosis, etc.). In studies evaluating routine use of CT for suspected stroke, however, very few noncerebrovascular etiologies were identified, and the diagnostic yield was even lower in patients with suspected TIA. Again, the greatest value of CT for suspected acute stroke lies in its ability to identify patients with parenchymal hemorrhage.

Brain MRI is superior to CT in detecting infarction from small-vessel occlusion at all stages: acute, subacute, and chronic. In cases of acute stroke involving posterior

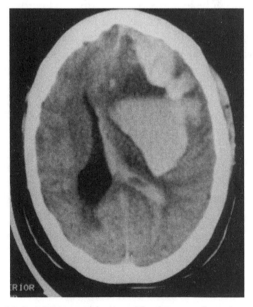

Figure 15.1 A 56-year-old man with a history of poorly controlled hypertension presents with acute right body weakness and slurred speech. Over the 3 hours following presentation, his weakness worsens, and his level of consciousness progressively decreases. Noncontrasted brain computed tomography demonstrates evidence of intracerebral hemorrhage with extension into the lateral ventricle.

fossa structures (i.e., the brainstem and/or cerebellum), artifact from adjacent bone may impair the sensitivity and the specificity of CT. A MRI will provide clearer images of this region. For all ischemic stroke subtypes, MRI will demonstrate evidence of ischemic injury to the brain earlier than will CT, and newer MRI techniques (such as diffusion-weighted imaging) have further increased its sensitivity. The clinical implications of "early positive MRI" or of "diffusion–perfusion mismatch" are as yet unclear, but it is conceivable that this or another noninvasive means of assessing ischemic injury may serve to indicate whether hyperacute interventional therapy is likely to be of benefit.

Neurosonology

Carotid "duplex" testing, implying a combination of Doppler blood flow analysis and ultrasonography, is invaluable in noninvasively evaluating the extracranial internal carotid artery. Although differentiation between very high-grade stenosis and occlusion is difficult, duplex imaging can be effective in supplying information as to vascular patency and the nature of any obstructive lesion, including the specific composition and morphology of atherosclerotic plaque. Duplex imaging is of less value in the evaluation of the vertebrobasilar circulation, and duplex criteria for pathologic conditions affecting this circulation are not well established. The accuracy of carotid duplex imaging varies significantly from center to center, largely according to the expertise of the individual who performs the test and interprets the results. Whenever possible, the responsible clinician should confirm the reliability of the noninvasive vascular laboratory he utilizes.

Transcranial Doppler (TCD) permits noninvasive evaluation of the intracranial vasculature; TCD can detect large-vessel intracranial stenosis or occlusion and is remarkably sensitive in detecting evidence of active embolism to those vessels. Although the clinical utility of TCD largely remains to be established, its ability to demonstrate flow abnormalities in large intracranial arteries can complement bedside clinical diagnosis and may at some future date assist in directing preventative therapy or acute therapeutic intervention.

Cerebral Angiography

Although routine brain imaging, carotid noninvasive testing, or TCD may provide at least indirect evidence of vascular patency or occlusion, cerebral angiography remains the most reliable means of assessing the cerebrovascular system (Figure 15.2). When performed within the first hours following onset of ischemic stroke, selective cerebral arteriography will demonstrate evidence of occlusion in the symptomatic blood vessel in approximately 80% of cases. Unfortunately, arteriography conveys a small but

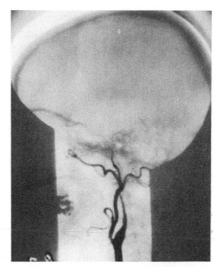

Figure 15.2 Selective right common carotid arteriography of a 25-year-old woman with acute left body weakness demonstrates findings consistent with arterial dissection/thrombosis.

discernible risk of significant morbidity. In one study involving patients with asymptomatic carotid artery stenosis, the stroke risk from arteriography approached that associated with the endarterectomy that was to follow.

Magnetic resonance angiography (MRA) offers a safe, noninvasive alternative to conventional arteriography for evaluation of the cerebral vasculature. Although MRA may overestimate the degree of stenosis present in the larger vessels and as yet cannot equal conventional arteriography in demonstrating with high resolution the intracranial arterial system distal to the circle of Willis, it is rapidly supplanting catheter-dependent arteriography as the angiographic procedure of choice for a variety of cerebrovascular indications. Although this technique is not as widely utilized as MRA, CT angiography (CTA) also can demonstrate both intracranial and extracranial occlusive disease more safely than selective catheter arteriography. Especially when combined with carotid duplex examination, MRA or CTA may obviate the need for conventional arteriography in cases of suspected carotid artery stenosis, be the stenosis symptomatic or asymptomatic. Whether any angiographic procedure will be required to facilitate the management of patients who are to receive interventional therapy for acute stroke remains uncertain.

Echocardiography

The most common sources of cardioembolic stroke are listed in Table 15.5. Echocardiography may be of value diagnostically when the history, physical examination, or electrocardiogram (EKG) suggests one of these conditions or, especially in the younger patient, when the clinical presentation is consistent with embolic stroke, but the specific cause of the stroke is inapparent. Routine use of echocardiography in stroke, however, is not cost-effective.

Table 15.5 Cardiac sources of cerebral emboli

High risk	Low risk
Mechanical prosthetic heart valve	Bioprosthetic heart valve
Atrial fibrillation	Atrial flutter
Myocardial infarction within 4 weeks	Mitral stenosis without atrial fibrillation
Left ventricular thrombus	Myocardial infarction >4 weeks in past
Dilated cardiomyopathy	Left ventricular aneurysm
Akinetic left ventricular segment	Congestive heart failure
Left atrial thrombus	Hypokinetic left ventricular segment
Atrial myxoma	Interatrial septal aneurysm
Infective endocarditis	Patent foramen ovale
	Nonbacterial endocarditis
	Mitral annular calcification

Even when its use is restricted to subpopulations in which diagnostic yield would be expected to be highest, the findings from echocardiography often are simply corroborative and may not alter management. In other cases, the procedure will identify an abnormality that is associated with increased stroke risk but which may not have played any part in causing the stroke under investigation (e.g., patent foramen ovale). Transesophageal echocardiography (TEE) provides better image quality than transthoracic echocardiography (TTE) and can image regions not seen well by TTE, including the aortic arch and the left atrium and its appendage.

Blood Testing

Evidence is accumulating to suggest that prothrombotic states may act in concert with other predisposing factors to produce ischemic stroke and may, in some cases, even represent the sole identifiable cause of the stroke process. Recent studies have demonstrated that otherwise mundane systemic viral infections can be complicated subacutely by brain infarction, and investigators have linked such cases to the occurrence of a transient prothrombotic state presumably triggered by the acute viral illness. An acute or chronic prothrombotic state may accompany a deficiency of protein C or S, elevated titers of antiphospholipid antibodies (anticardiolipin antibodies or the "lupus anticoagulant"), deficiency of antithrombin III, presence of prothrombin gene G20210A mutation or factor V Leiden, or elevated serum levels of homocysteine. Stroke has been a reported complication of all of these disorders, whether they are hereditary or acquired. Acquired deficiency of antithrombin III and protein C and S may occur with a variety of diseases and conditions, including nephrotic syndrome, malignancy, disseminated in-

travascular coagulation, and inflammatory bowel disease. Antiphospholipid antibodies are often present in patients with collagen vascular disease, but may also occur in the absence of any documented autoimmune disorder. Elevated concentrations of fibrinogen and other clotting factors predispose to stroke, as do excessive platelet reactivity, marked thrombocythemia, heparin-induced thrombocytopenia, and sickle cell disease. Thrombotic thrombocytopenic purpura (TTP) may cause cerebral ischemia via microvascular thrombosis, and intracerebral hemorrhage may occur as a consequence of idiopathic thrombocytopenic purpura (ITP). Intravascular sludging associated with polycythemia may induce infarction of territories supplied by small vessels.

Baseline blood studies for patients with acute stroke should typically include a complete blood count (including platelets), prothrombin time (PT) with International Normalized Ratio (INR), partial thromboplastin time (PTT), and basic chemistries including glucose level and a fasting lipid profile (Table 15.6). One may consider obtaining a fasting homocysteine level, but the results from a large multicenter clinical trial indicated no significant reduction in the risk of recurrent stroke when patients with recent stroke and a normal or elevated homocysteine level were treated with vitamin therapy intended to lower that level. An erythrocyte sedimentation rate is frequently obtained as part of the initial panel, but the results rarely lead to a previously unsuspected diagnosis. Although vasculitis from any cause may lead to stroke, it is an uncommon cause of cerebrovascular disease at any age, and rarely will stroke represent the initial or sole manifestation of systemic vasculitis. In selected cases, more sophis-

Table 15.6 Tests commonly performed in the evaluation of suspected stroke

Routine	Variable
Brain CT without contrast	Brain MRI
Electrocardiogram	Carotid duplex
Complete blood count, platelet count, prothrombin time/International Normalized Ratio (INR), partial thromboplastin time	Cerebral angiography
	Echocardiography
	Transcranial Doppler
	Chest x-ray
Blood chemistries	More extensive blood testing: erythrocyte sedimentation rate, fasting homocysteine, antiphospholipid antibody screen, protein C & S levels, etc.
Fasting lipid profile	
	Arterial blood gas levels
	Lumbar puncture
	Electroencephalography

ticated serologic studies (antiphospholipid antibody screen, fibrinogen level, platelet function studies, etc.) may assist in identifying a coagulopathy known to be associated with stroke, but even then, the information obtained may not assist in diagnosis and often fails to alter patient management or outcome in any discernible manner. To confound matters further, stroke itself can result in an elevation of serum fibrinogen or measurable inhibition of endogenous fibrinolytic activity and, to date, no treatment has been identified that will affect positively the long-term prognosis of patients with stroke and an antiphospholipid antibody.

Other Procedures

An EKG should be performed in all patients presenting with acute stroke. Most specific to this clinical setting, EKG will assist in confirming or excluding atrial fibrillation or ischemic injury to myocardium (the latter representing a potential cause or *consequence* of acute stroke). As regards stroke diagnosis specifically, what little usefulness extended cardiac monitoring may have is restricted largely to cases in which there is a strong clinical suspicion of paroxysmal atrial fibrillation.

Brain CT and MRI have greatly reduced the utility of lumbar puncture in the diagnosis of acute stroke. Except in the circumstance when SAH is suspected on clinical grounds and noncontrasted brain CT has shown no evidence of bleeding, lumbar puncture is indicated only in cases of stroke where there is a reasonable suspicion of underlying meningitis or when encephalitis may be mimicking primary cerebrovascular occlusion or hemorrhage. In those rare instances when stroke is caused by arteritis, lumbar puncture may demonstrate a white cell pleocytosis or elevated protein, but these findings are nonspecific, inconstant, and may accompany large ischemic strokes from any cause. Some arteritides (most notably, isolated central nervous system granulomatous angiitis) may produce no such abnormality of the cerebrospinal fluid.

Electroencephalography rarely has a place in the diagnosis of acute stroke and, as a rule, should be used only when a patient exhibits suspected seizure activity or when nonconvulsive seizures are suspected. Use of sophisticated studies to measure cerebral blood flow and metabolism (xenon CT blood flow imaging, single photon emission computed tomography [SPECT], or positron emission tomography [PET]) should generally be restricted to the research setting.

Transient Ischemic Attack

What causes or mimics stroke also may cause or mimic TIA, but identification of the pathophysiologic process and etiology underlying TIA is more difficult than is the case for cerebral infarction. With rare exception, the diagnosis of TIA is based on history obtained from patient or observer, and even when this history is clear, TIA symptoms are not absolutely specific for cerebrovascular disease. Many episodes diagnosed as representing a "TIA" appear to have no prognostic significance whatsoever, and distinguishing these "brain spells" from more ominous events can be a frustrating and even impossible task. Nonetheless, a recent study revealed that the short-term prognosis following TIA was poor, with 25% of patients experiencing a stroke or other adverse event (TIA, death, or hospitalization for a cardiovascular event) within 90 days. Of the 10.5% of patients who experienced a subsequent stroke, half had their event within 2 days of the TIA. These data highlight the importance of rapid evaluation and treatment of patients with TIA.

As indicated previously, brain imaging rarely will demonstrate a symptomatic abnormality when TIA is the likely diagnosis by history and the physical examination is normal. On occasion, CT or MRI will reveal findings suggestive of acute infarction (or, much more rarely, hemorrhage) even when TIA is the correct clinical diagnosis. More commonly, in this setting, the imaging study may demonstrate evidence of prior stroke or chronic ischemic injury, thus indirectly reinforcing the clinical impression of acute TIA.

If the TIA symptoms are referable to the carotid artery system, evaluation of the cervical portion of the symptomatic vessel is of far more clinical relevance than imaging of the brain itself. When the sensitivity and specificity of the unit and operator involved have been established and are acceptable, carotid duplex testing represents an excellent, noninvasive means of screening for the presence of anatomically significant stenosis or occlusion of the distal common carotid and proximal internal carotid arteries. Given the high risk of stroke associated with *symptomatic* high-grade carotid stenosis, along with the documented ability of endarterectomy to reduce that risk substantially, an urgent carotid study should be considered for all patients presenting with recent TIA or minor stroke in the carotid distribution.

Relevance of Diagnosis to Management

Although diagnosis may possess some intrinsic value in and of itself, it is the impact of diagnosis on treatment and outcome that is of greater clinical relevance. New advances in the prevention and acute treatment of stroke have focused attention on the importance of achieving an accurate and specific diagnosis. Although it is gratifying at long last to have therapies that clearly reduce stroke incidence and morbidity, indiscriminate application of those therapies may impose an excessive financial burden and even be harmful to some patients. With further research and more careful efforts at diagnosis, it may become possible to identify prospectively those subpopulations of patients with threatened or acute stroke who will respond positively to treatment and who would otherwise be destined for a poor clinical outcome.

Stroke Prevention

Risk factor reduction

Identification and treatment of modifiable stroke risk factors (Table 15.1) is the cornerstone of stroke prevention. For example, although the optimal blood pressure target remains unknown, it has been estimated that nearly half of all strokes in the United States could be prevented if hypertension was optimally diagnosed and treated. Although previous studies suggested that angiotensin-converting enzyme (ACE) inhibitors and angiotensin receptor blockers (ARBs) may promote a reduction in stroke risk that exceeds the benefit to be expected from their antihypertensive effect. The recently published PRoFESS trial found that therapy with telmisarton did not significantly lower the rate of recurrent stroke, major cardiovascular events, or diabetes. The use of statins has been supported by the Stroke Prevention by Aggressive Reduction in Cholesterol Levels (SPARCL) Study, which reported a benefit of atorvastatin 80 mg/day following stroke or TIA in patients with no known coronary artery disease and LDL cholesterol levels between 100 and 190 mg/dL. Smoking cessation, 30 minutes of moderate-intensity exercise on most days, and maintenance of body mass index (BMI) of less than 25 kg/m^2 is also recommended. Currently in progress are large randomized clinical trials to investigate the value of an ARB in stroke patients and the value of homocysteine modification in stroke/TIA patients with hyperhomocysteinemia.

Antithrombotic therapy

Antiplatelet agents. Platelet antiaggregants prevent stroke, and every patient who has suffered a noncardioembolic ischemic stroke or TIA and lacks a contraindication should be treated with an antiplatelet agent. Currently available agents in the United States are aspirin, ticlopidine, clopidogrel, and the combination of aspirin and extended-release dipyridamole (ASA/ER-DP). The optimal dosage of aspirin is unknown, but the current FDA-approved dosage is 50–325 mg/day. In light of potential toxicity, which includes neutropenia and TTP, the use of ticlopidine 250 mg twice daily has declined significantly following the approval of clopidogrel. Clopidogrel is administered as a single daily dose of 75 mg. The combination of clopidogrel and ASA 75 mg has recently been shown to increase bleeding complications without a reduction in ischemic events. The approved dosage of ASA 25 mg/ER-DP 200 mg is one capsule twice daily. The PRoFESS trial found no evidence that either clopidogrel or ASA/ER-DP was superior to the other in the prevention of recurrent ischemic stroke.

Oral anticoagulants. Warfarin (INR 2–3) is indicated for high-risk patients with nonvalvular atrial fibrillation (Table 15.7) and for patients with prosthetic heart valves. Despite a lack of supportive prospective randomized data, warfarin is also commonly administered following cervicocephalic dissection, cerebral sinus thrombosis, myocardial infarction, and in the presence of intracardiac thrombus. A recent study revealed no apparent benefit of warfarin (compared to aspirin or clopidogrel) in the presence of a markedly reduced ejection fraction, although another study evaluating warfarin versus aspirin in this setting is ongoing. The WASID (Warfarin–Aspirin Symptomatic Intracranial Disease) study, comparing warfarin to aspirin for symptomatic intracranial atherosclerosis, found warfarin to be more hazardous with no significant difference regarding ischemic event prevention. A large, multicenter, randomized trial comparing warfarin to aspirin 325 mg/day for secondary stroke prevention in patients with noncardioembolic stroke (Warfarin—Aspirin Recurrent Stroke Study [WARSS]) found no benefit from warfarin relative to aspirin. Substudies of WARSS likewise found no benefit of warfarin over aspirin in stroke patients with evidence of an antiphospholipid antibody, PFO, or atrial septal aneurysm. Oral thrombin inhibitors and factor Xa antagonists are being evaluated in patients with nonvalvular atrial fibrillation, and one or more of these agents will likely replace warfarin as the anticoagulant of choice in the near future.

Management of carotid atherosclerosis

As mentioned previously, the high risk of stroke associated with symptomatic high-grade carotid stenosis and the documented ability of endarterectomy to reduce that risk establish that an urgent carotid imaging study should be considered for all patients presenting with recent TIA or minor stroke in the carotid distribution. Unless surgi-

---

Table 15.7 High risk factors for thromboembolism in patients with atrial fibrillation

Prior stroke/TIA or systemic embolus

Mitral stenosis

Prosthetic heart valve

More than 1 of the following:

    Age ≥75 years

    Hypertension

    Heart failure

    LV ejection fraction ≤35%

    Diabetes mellitus

cal contraindications exist, patients with symptomatic stenosis of 70% or more should be referred for potential endarterectomy. Angioplasty and stenting with distal protection devices hold promise as an alternative treatment, and the results of a large, randomized trial (CREST) comparing this procedure to endarterectomy are pending at this time. Given the currently available evidence, angioplasty and stenting should generally be reserved for patients who are poor surgical candidates.

The value of endarterectomy for moderate (50–69%) symptomatic carotid disease is less robust than that for more severe anatomic disease. Even so, several risk factors have been identified that may assist in singling out patients who are at higher risk if treated with medical therapy alone: stenosis at the higher end of the 50–69% range, age 75 years or older, male gender, recent (within 3 months) stroke (as opposed to TIA), hemispheric symptoms (as opposed to retinal), and concomitant intracranial stenosis. Surgery is of no benefit in the setting of symptomatic linear stenosis of less than 50%.

Although surgery also reduces stroke risk in patients with 60% or greater asymptomatic carotid artery stenosis, the natural history of that condition is more favorable, and the utility of noninvasive vascular screening examinations and prophylactic surgical intervention is thus more controversial. Endarterectomy should be deferred if the surgical risk (including angiography, if performed) at a given facility is 3% or greater.

The treatment of patients with carotid atherosclerosis should not end with a decision regarding endarterectomy or angioplasty. Medical management of these patients should include risk factor modification, an antiplatelet agent, and consideration of treatment with an ACE inhibitor/ARB, statin, and homocysteine modification with folate-based therapy. ACE inhibitors and statins have been shown to reduce the anatomic progression of carotid artery disease. Reduction of serum homocysteine levels has been demonstrated to cause plaque regression, but evidence of an accompanying clinical benefit has yet to be established. Finally, because of the high prevalence of concomitant, unrecognized coronary artery disease (CAD), patients with carotid artery (and/or other large vessel) atherosclerosis should be considered for noninvasive testing to exclude anatomically significant CAD.

Acute Stroke Treatment

The region of acute ischemic stroke can be divided into two main zones: a *core*, within which cerebral blood flow (CBF) is extremely low, and a surrounding *penumbra*, within which CBF is less severely reduced. Neurons within the core are destined to die, but the penumbral neurons, while inactive acutely, may be viable. Acute stroke therapy is intended to salvage this penumbra. Experimental studies have shown that the fate of penumbral neurons is a function not only of absolute blood flow but also of time. It is generally accepted that the "therapeutic window" following onset of ischemic stroke is on the order of minutes to hours, with 6 hours probably representing the upper limit for the majority of patients. Thus, rapid recognition, evaluation, and treatment of the stroke patient are critical.

Initial management

Once the diagnosis of acute stroke is suspected, symptom onset must be determined. The time elapsed following stroke onset remains the single most important determinant of therapeutic options. Patients with symptom onset of less than 3 hours should be evaluated for potential treatment with intravenous (IV) tissue plasminogen activator (t-PA) (see later discussion).

All acute ischemic stroke patients should receive IV hydration with normal saline, hypoxia should be corrected with supplemental oxygen, hyperglycemia should be treated with insulin, and fever should be treated with antipyretics. An electrocardiogram (EKG) should be performed, and patients should receive continuous cardiac monitoring. Blood should be drawn for a complete blood count (CBC) with platelet count, prothrombin time (PT) with international normalized ratio (INR), partial thromboplastin time (PTT), basic chemistries, and cardiac markers, when appropriate. As discussed previously, additional blood testing may be indicated on a case-by-case basis. Oral intake should be withheld until the patient passes a screening swallow evaluation.

Patients with hyperacute stroke should undergo emergent brain CT. As indicated earlier, the major value of acute CT scanning is in differentiating intracerebral hemorrhage from ischemic stroke and, to a lesser extent, excluding stroke mimickers such as subdural hematoma, tumor, and abscess. By demonstrating a well-established infarct, CT also may delineate the extent of ischemia and/or assist in correcting an inaccurate historical estimate of stroke onset time.

Management of blood pressure

During brain ischemia, cerebral autoregulation is impaired and cerebral blood flow becomes dependent upon systemic blood pressure. Blood flow to ischemic neurons declines in concert with systemic pressure. Blood pressure therefore should not be treated unless one of the following exists: (a) systolic blood pressure (SBP) exceeds 220 mm Hg, or diastolic blood pressure (DBP) exceeds 120 mm Hg via repeated measurements; (b) cardiac ischemia, heart failure, or aortic dissection are present; (c) thrombolytic therapy is planned; or (d) ICH is identified. In the last situation, blood pressure should be maintained below 180/105 mm Hg. Management of blood pressure in the setting of IV thrombolysis is discussed below.

Intravenous thrombolysis

Intravenous thrombolysis with t-PA is indicated for selected patients who present within 3 hours of ischemic stroke onset. It is important to bear in mind that when stroke onset time is unclear (e.g., patient awakens with a deficit), onset time is considered to be the time when a patient was last known to be in their usual state of health. Inclusion and exclusion criteria for t-PA administration are listed in Table 15.8. If blood pressure exceeds 185/110 mm Hg, a single dose of an antihypertensive can be administered, and t-PA therapy is appropriate if the blood pressure declines below this level. Blood pressure should be monitored every 15 minutes for 2 hours following the start of infusion, then every 30 minutes for 6 hours, and then every 60 minutes for 16 hours. For the first 24 hours post-thrombolysis, the blood pressure must be maintained below 180/105 mm Hg and antithrombotic agents must be avoided.

Other considerations

As such treatment has been shown to (modestly) reduce the risk of recurrent stroke and death when administered within the first 48 hours poststroke, patients with ischemic stroke who do not qualify for IV t-PA should be given aspirin. If t-PA is administered, aspirin (or any other antithrombotic agent) should be delayed for 24 hours post-infusion. Neurosurgical consultation should be sought for patients with cerebellar hemorrhage or large cerebellar ischemic infarctions. Nonambulatory patients must receive deep vein thrombosis prophylaxis, preferably with enoxaparin. For those who cannot receive anticoagulation, intermittent external compression stockings should be utilized. Although anticoagulation has never been shown to impact neurologic recovery following arterial stroke, patients with basilar artery thrombosis or dissection of the extracranial carotid or vertebral artery who do not received t-PA often are treated with IV heparin. Early mobilization of stroke patients is recommended, and the use of an indwelling catheter should be avoided, whenever possible. Fever should be treated aggressively with antipyretics, and antibiotics should be administered for infectious causes. Fasting lipid profile should be obtained and a statin administered to most patients with low-density lipoprotein (LDL) cholesterol of 100 mg/dL or greater with consideration of a 70 mg/dL target in patients at very high risk (e.g., diabetic). Physical, occupational, and speech therapy should be ordered when indicated.

Will careful diagnosis of stroke and determination of the specific stroke process or etiology be required for optimal implementation of t-PA or new acute therapies to come? Clearly, physicians should not administer treatment intended for acute ischemic stroke if they are not convinced of that diagnosis and assured via an imaging study as to the absence of brain hemorrhage. Diffusion and perfusion MRI and CT profusion hold promise for selecting patients with stroke onset of greater than 3 hours who may benefit from acute intervention. It remains uncertain whether acute treatment will be more or less effective or safe for a particular ischemic stroke subtype, or whether physicians can predict therapeutic response prospectively on the basis of any clinical parameter.

Complications of Stroke

Neurologic complications of stroke include stroke progression (seen in over 25% of patients) or recurrence (less common, with the rate dependent on the mechanism of the index event). Seizures can occur in up to 10% of pa-

---

Table 15.8 Inclusion and exclusion criteria for intravenous tissue plasminogen activator (t-PA) for acute stroke

Inclusion

▶ Ischemic stroke causing measurable neurologic deficit
▶ Cranial computed tomography (CT) negative for hemorrhage
▶ Onset of symptoms <3 hours before beginning treatment
▶ Patient or family understands the potential risks and benefits from treatment

Exclusion

▶ Minor and isolated neurologic signs
▶ Neurologic deficit that is clearing spontaneously
▶ CT evidence of multilobar infarction (e.g., hypodensity >1/3 cerebral hemisphere)
▶ INR >1.7
▶ Patient receiving heparin within the preceding 48 hours who has a prolonged PTT
▶ Platelet count <100,000/mm³
▶ Pretreatment systolic blood pressure >185 mm Hg or diastolic pressure >110 mm Hg or if aggressive treatment is required to reduce blood pressure to the specified limits prior to thrombolytic therapy
▶ Prior stroke or any serious head trauma in the preceding 3 months
▶ Major surgery within the preceding 14 days
▶ Prior intracranial hemorrhage
▶ Symptoms of stroke suggestive of subarachnoid hemorrhage
▶ Gastrointestinal or urinary tract hemorrhage within the preceding 21 days
▶ Seizure with postictal residual neurologic impairments
▶ Evidence of active bleeding or acute trauma (fracture) on examination
▶ Arterial puncture at a noncompressible site within the previous 7 days
▶ Myocardial infarction in the previous 3 months
▶ Blood glucose <50 mg/dL

tients at some point following stroke and are more common following SAH or ICH and large ischemic lesions involving the cerebral cortex. Stroke-related seizures usually can be controlled with a single anticonvulsant. Increased intracranial pressure (ICP) is the most lethal poststroke complication and may be a direct effect of a hematoma or occur consequent to subacutely developing brain edema. Brain edema following ischemic stroke (usually cytotoxic) typically becomes symptomatic after 1–4 days. Signs and symptoms of raised ICP include depressed level of consciousness, pupillary asymmetry, cranial nerve VI palsy, papilledema, and periodic breathing. Treatment of raised ICP should include fluid restriction, elevation of the head of the bed, administration of osmotic diuretics, and hyperventilation. Hemicraniectomy may be considered for patients with massive hemispheric ischemia and malignant edema. Some degree of cognitive impairment or frank dementia can occur in up to one-third to one-half of patients, and recent evidence suggests that acetylcholinesterase inhibitors may be of value in these patients. Patients should be monitored for poststroke depression, a complication that occurs in up to 60% of patients and is treatable with antidepressants and/or psychotherapy. Acute or subacute medical complications following stroke also include cardiac abnormalities (e.g., arrhythmia, myocardial infarction), pulmonary embolism, infection (e.g., urinary tract, pneumonia), and gastrointestinal bleeding.

Patient and Caregiver Education

Patients and caregivers should be educated regarding both short- and long-term clinical expectations. Symptoms of poststroke depression should be reviewed and patients instructed to seek treatment, if appropriate. Applicable secondary stroke preventive strategies should be discussed, and the symptoms suggestive of recurrent stroke or TIA should be reviewed. The use of emergency medical services (EMS) should be encouraged should the patient experience such recurrent symptoms.

Summary

To diagnose stroke accurately and then apply the diagnostic findings to patient management, the physician must answer a sequence of questions: Is stroke the correct diagnosis? If so, what is the pathophysiologic mechanism of the stroke? What is the specific etiology? And, finally, how should identification of etiology guide management

▼

Consider Consultation When...

▶ The patient with acute ischemic stroke is eligible for treatment with tissue plasminogen activator (t-PA).

▶ The patient with presumed stroke exhibits worsening neurologic deficit.

▶ The patient with presumed stroke exhibits "waxing and waning" neurologic deficit.

▶ Stroke occurs in the setting of head and/or neck injury.

▶ The stroke patient is under the age of 45.

of the patient? With this approach, the clinician can hope to avoid the pitfalls of erroneous diagnosis, fruitless expenditure of resources, and ill-advised application of potentially harmful therapy.

Annotated Bibliography

Adams HP, del Zoppo G, Alberts MJ, et al. Guidelines for the early management of adults with ischemic stroke: A guideline from the American Heart Association/American Stroke Association Stroke Council, Clinical Cardiology Council, Cardiovascular Radiology and Intervention Council, and the Atherosclerotic Peripheral Vascular Disease and Quality of Care Outcomes in Research Interdisciplinary Working Groups. *Stroke* 2007;38:1655.
This consensus paper provides an overview of the basic principles involved in recognition, diagnosis, and management of acute ischemic stroke.

Mohr JP, Choi DW, Grotta JC, et al., eds. *Stroke: Pathophysiology, diagnosis, and management,* 4th ed. Philadelphia: Churchill Livingstone, 2004.
This detailed analysis of cerebrovascular disease is currently regarded as the preeminent reference text on this subject.

Caplan LR. *Stroke: A clinical approach,* 3rd ed. Boston: Butterworth-Heinemann, 2000.
A less detailed but still comprehensive summary of the current body of knowledge regarding stroke. Clinical diagnosis receives particular emphasis.

Sacco RL, Adams R, Albers G, et al. Guidelines for prevention of stroke in patients with ischemic stroke or transient ischemic attack: A statement for healthcare professionals from the American Heart Association/American Stroke Association Council on Stroke: Co-sponsored by the Council on Cardiovascular Radiology and Intervention: The American Academy of Neurology affirms the value of this guideline. *Stroke* 2006;37:577–617.
This comprehensive review provides evidence-based recommendations for the secondary prevention of stroke.

CHAPTER 16

Traumatic Injuries of the Central Nervous System

Lawrence F. Marshall

▼

Outline

- ▶ The classification of head injury
- ▶ The evaluation of the head-injured patient
- ▶ The pathophysiology of head injury
- ▶ The management of head injury
- ▶ Spinal injury
- ▶ The evaluation of the spine-injured patient
- ▶ The mechanisms of spinal column injury
- ▶ Patterns of spinal cord injury
- ▶ The management of spinal injury
- ▶ Summary

Early documents cite Hippocrates as an advocate for trephination in the treatment of certain head injuries, a practice also traced back to the Incas of Central America. The modern practice of this discipline begins with Harvey Cushing, who made tremendous strides in surgical treatment of head injuries during World War I. Despite intensive preventive efforts by social and governmental agencies, traumatic brain injuries (TBI) account for a remarkable number of physician visits and hospital admissions every year, with a comparable cost to society. It has been estimated that head injuries occur in up to 1.9 million patients per year at a cost of over $25 billion in the United States alone. However, these figures do not take into account the number of patients with mild injuries who do not seek medical care.

The cost of care of the head-injured patient is not limited to the acute hospitalization. These figures must take into account the expense of rehabilitative therapy, lost workdays and, in many cases, permanent impairment. Furthermore, even patients with mild head injuries can suffer from cognitive difficulties, such as impairments of memory, abstract thinking, and information processing, as well as emotional and behavioral abnormalities.

Young males between the ages of 15 and 24 are at the highest risk for head injury, with a second peak for individuals of either sex over 65 years of age. Risk factors also associated with head trauma include low socioeconomic status and elevated blood alcohol levels. Interestingly, race and ethnicity are of unclear significance in head injuries.

▼

Key Clinical Questions

- ▶ In a patient with traumatic brain injury (TBI), was there a report of seizure activity? Administration of antiepileptic medications for seizure prophylaxis should be considered.
- ▶ In a patient with TBI, what does the pupillary examination demonstrate? Uncal herniation should be considered if one or both pupils appear fixed and dilated. Narcotic use should be considered in the case of pinpoint pupils. Direct injury to the eye and/or orbit (i.e., periorbital ecchymoses, orbital rim fractures) may produce traumatic mydriasis.
- ▶ Does the patient have a reproducible examination that can be followed in lieu of an intracranial pressure monitor?
- ▶ Does the patient demonstrate evidence of a spinal cord injury (SCI; upper motor neuron versus lower motor neuron lesion)?
- ▶ What is the time interval since an acute SCI? Patients presenting within 8 hours of a suspected injury to the spinal cord should be started on high-dose steroid therapy.

The Classification of Head Injury

The grading of head injury has been revised many times over the years. Currently, the most commonly used classification system is the Glasgow Coma Scale (GCS), which has provided a common language with which to assess patients. The GCS has proven useful in guiding the initial and subsequent assessment, management, and determination of prognosis in TBI.

The scoring system relies on the evaluation of three basic categories: eye opening, verbal response, and motor response (Table 16.1). Each category is scored from 1 to 4 or 6, based on the patient's best response, and then summed to determine the patient's total GCS score. Using this system, head injury is then classified as mild, moderate, and severe, based on the initial evaluation of the patient (Table 16.2). Roughly 80% of head-injured patients fall into the mild classification, while the moderate and severe categories each comprise approximately 10%.

Mild head injuries are defined as having a GCS score of 13–15. Mild head injuries can be further stratified into low-, moderate-, or high-risk on the basis of radiographic findings. Low-risk, mild head injuries are defined by a GCS score of 15 without acute radiographic abnormalities. High-risk, mild head injuries are defined by a GCS score of 13–14 or a GCS 15 with acute radiographic abnormalities. Patients with mild TBI may suffer from a documented transient loss of consciousness; loss of memory for the interval before, during, or after

Table 16.2 Classification of head injury	
Category of head injury	**Glasgow Coma Scale (GCS)**
Mild	13–15 (low-, moderate-, or high-risk)
Moderate	9–12
Severe	3–8

the event; and/or an alteration in mental status. The term "mild," however, should not be construed to indicate an insignificant trauma. These patients can suffer from prolonged or delayed cognitive difficulties following the event and are at risk for further complications.

The patient with moderate head injury is defined as having a GCS score from 9–12. These individuals are not comatose, which is defined on the GCS as the inability to open eyes, communicate verbally, or follow commands. However, they do require careful observation and monitoring in an intensive care setting. Although their overall prognosis is generally good, these individuals are at greater risk for cognitive sequelae and posttraumatic epilepsy.

Severe head injury is defined as a score of 3–8 on the GCS. These patients are considered to be comatose, as previously defined. However, there is a wide range of head-injured patients within this single designation. The motor component of the GCS provides a better prognostic instrument within this category. Patients who exhibit flaccidity or extensor posturing have a much worse prognosis than those who localize or flex to noxious stimuli.

Table 16.1 Glasgow Coma Score	
Eye opening (E)	
Spontaneous	4
To voice	3
To pain	2
None	1
Verbal response (V)	
Oriented conversation	5
Disoriented conversation	4
Inappropriate words	3
Incomprehensible sounds	2
None	1
Motor response (M)	
Obeys commands	6
Localizes pain	5
Withdraws pain	4
Flexor posturing	3
Extensor posturing	2
None	1

GCS score = best eye opening + best verbal response + best motor response

The Evaluation of the Head-Injured Patient

Initial Evaluation

Head injuries are classified as "closed" or "penetrating" depending on the mechanism of trauma. As in all initial evaluations, the history surrounding the trauma is of paramount importance. The initial status of the patient immediately following the injury is critical to establish a baseline examination for immediate and longitudinal assessments.

A review of the paramedic's records is central to the reconstruction of the trauma and identifies the use of any paralytic or psychoactive medications in the field. The presence of any seizure activity following the event is potentially important. Patients in the postictal phase following a generalized seizure may show rapid deterioration in neurologic status, followed by a gradual improvement. A focal paralysis may reflect a postictal Todd paralysis. Posttraumatic seizure activity may result from the trauma itself or as a manifestation of a new hemorrhagic mass lesion in the brain, requiring immediate neurosurgical attention.

Physical Examination

Upon arrival of the patient to the trauma unit, multiple concurrent assessments are made in an expeditious manner and a complete battery of laboratory studies are sent. As in all emergency evaluations, the "A, B, C's" of emergency care take precedence. Once, the patient has been stabilized, the neurologic examination is performed along with the examination of all other body systems. The speed and detail of this evaluation takes into account the general medical status of the patient. In a hemodynamically stable patient with a minor head injury, this examination is more thorough and time intensive, as compared to the severe head injury with evidence of significant blood loss. This is left to the discretion of the physician.

In severe TBIs, more than 50% of patients suffer from additional major systemic injuries requiring care from other specialists. In hemodynamically unstable patients, there may be a need for emergent exploratory laparotomy or thoracotomy. This makes the speed of the neurologic assessment an important factor. Intubation for airway protection, pharmacologic sedation or paralysis, hypotension, hypoxia, or intoxication will obscure the neurologic evaluation.

The initial neurologic assessment involves a screening and then a more formal comprehensive examination, as permitted by the patient's medical status. The major objective is to diagnose the presence of any neurologic injury, classify its severity, institute appropriate diagnostic testing, and initiate proper therapeutic interventions. During the neurologic examination, if a patient demonstrates a variable response to stimuli, the best response is more predictive of prognosis than the worst one. Patients in the comatose state have either widespread dysfunction of the bilateral telencephalon or dysfunction of midline structures, such as the diencephalon and brainstem reticular activating system.

The size of the pupils and their response to light is an important aspect of the initial neurologic exam. Pupillary dilation with loss or slowing of the response to light is a well-characterized early sign of temporal lobe herniation. Compression or distortion of the third cranial nerve by the uncus during herniation can impair the function of the parasympathetic axons that travel on its periphery. These fibers transmit the efferent signals for pupillary constriction, thus external compression results in pupillary dilation.

Ocular movements are an important index of the status of the brainstem reticular system. In the cooperative patient, a full range of eye movements confirms the integrity of the ocular motor system within the brainstem.

In the comatose state, when brain death is suspected, the oculocephalic response can be tested. If the cervical spine is considered unstable, testing of the oculovestibular response is necessary. Functional suppression of the brainstem reticular activating system leads to the absence of the fast-phase nystagmus, usually demonstrated in a normal cold caloric evaluation. In TBI with brainstem involvement, this results in tonic deviation of the eyes away from the stimulus.

Diagnostic Imaging

The need and timing for radiologic testing is dictated by the patient's initial presentation, severity of injury, and/or possible neurologic deterioration. In the intact patient with a low-risk, mild head injury (GCS 15), a normal neurologic exam, and only a transient loss of consciousness, no further workup may be necessary. If, however, the patient has more serious injuries or symptoms, further workup is warranted.

A noncontrast computed tomography (CT) scan of the head is the procedure of choice in the evaluation of acute head injury. The conditions to rule out that require emergent neurosurgical attention include any extra-axial collection of blood, intracerebral hemorrhages, contusions, and/or intraventricular hemorrhages. Over 70–90% of patients presenting with severe head injury have abnormalities on the initial CT scan.

All patients with abnormal CT scans warrant a follow-up examination within 24 hours of admission and possibly more frequently, as governed by any deterioration in neurologic status. In certain instances, there may be a role for magnetic resonance imaging, contrast enhanced CT scans, or cerebral angiography.

The Pathophysiology of Head Injury

To competently manage TBI, a thorough understanding of the pathophysiology behind primary and secondary injury is required. Primary injury is defined as the damage sustained by the scalp, skull, and intracranial contents as a result of the initial trauma, and can only be ameliorated by prevention. These injuries can result in physiologic and metabolic derangements, such as ischemia, brain swelling, and electrolyte abnormalities, which characterize secondary brain injury.

Damage to the scalp, skull, or brain occurs when contact or inertial forces strain the structural tolerance of the tissues. Contact forces generally cause contusions or lacerations of the scalp, fractures of the skull, and/or cerebral contusions. Inertial forces are translational, rotational, or angular, and cause injury by acceleration and deceleration. The magnitude and duration of the forces sustained during the injury determine the location and severity of the brain injury. High-velocity acceleration injuries of short duration often cause cerebral contusions and subdural hematomas (SDHs). High-velocity acceleration of longer durations result in diffuse axonal injury and damage to the deeper structures of the brain.

Penetrating injuries vary dramatically depending on the nature of the missile. The danger from low-velocity penetrating injuries arises from potential injury to a major cerebral artery or vein. High-velocity penetrating injuries generally arise from gunshot wounds. The damage of the bullet is related to the velocity at which it strikes the head. Higher-caliber firearms, such as hunting rifles, impart a greater kinetic energy to the brain and surrounding structures. The generated pressure waves can cause injury to structures well away from the missile tract.

Skull Fractures

Head injuries of sufficient force may result in fractures of the skull (Figure 16.1). These are categorized by pattern of injury, anatomic location, and by the condition of the overlying skin.

The pattern of skull fracture is determined by: (a) the force of impact and (b) the ratio of that force to the surface area of impact. Injuries resulting in linear skull fractures arise when the imparted energy is not sufficient to produce elastic deformation of the cranial vault. If the force of the injury is spread over a wide area, there may be little or no skull injury, despite severe intracranial trauma.

If the energy is focused, it can result in multiple fractures radiating from the site of impact. These commin-

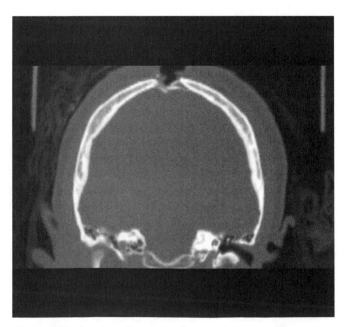

Figure 16.1 Computed tomography scan demonstrating an open, depressed skull fracture over sagittal sinus.

▼

Pearls and Perils

Evaluation of traumatic injuries to the central nervous system

▶ The Glasgow Coma Scale (GCS) is a useful guide to the initial and subsequent assessment, management, and determination of prognosis in traumatic brain injury (TBI). The motor component of the GCS is the best prognostic instrument for the severely head-injured patient. During the neurologic examination, if a patient demonstrates a variable response to stimuli, the best response is more predictive of prognosis than the worst one.

▶ If the multiply injured patient cannot cooperate with the neurologic assessment, they should be presumed to have an injury until it is ruled out.

▶ A noncontrast computed tomography (CT) scan of the head is the procedure of choice in the evaluation of acute head injury.

▶ High-velocity acceleration injuries of short duration often cause cerebral contusions and subdural hematomas, whereas high-velocity acceleration injuries of longer duration often result in diffuse axonal injury and damage to the deeper structures of the brain.

▶ Patients with epidural hematomas may initially present with an intact neurologic examination ("lucid interval"). However, they require vigilant monitoring, as expansion of the hematoma may result in rapid deterioration.

▶ Patients with tenderness along the spinal axis following trauma require further radiographic imaging to assess for fractures. Plain radiographs and CT are excellent for examining the vertebrae; a magnetic resonance image (MRI) is required to evaluate the spinal cord and neighboring soft tissue structures.

▶ Individuals demonstrating a complete loss of motor and sensory function at a dermatomal level are described as having sustained a *complete injury*. Complete spinal cord injuries (SCIs) are described by the last functional and nonfunctional levels (i.e., C6 complete SCI with functional C5 level).

uted fractures result from a greater force, which causes the bone under the impact zone to break into multiple pieces. These fragments can be driven into the underlying parenchyma. Depressed skull fractures are treated conservatively or surgically, depending on the extent of depression, location, and/or other characteristics of the fracture. Generally, depression of the cranial vault greater than the width of the skull is considered for surgical elevation and repair.

The location of the skull fracture is divided into two general areas, skull base and convexity. Skull base fractures, or basilar fractures, run in a longitudinal or transverse fashion in relation to the long axis of the petrous pyramid of the temporal bone. Longitudinal fractures are more common and can involve the tympanic membrane and/or external auditory canal, resulting in otorrhea. Otorrhea following head injury is initially managed conservatively, as most will resolve spontaneously within 5 days. Prophylactic antibiotics are avoided in most patients, unless there is evidence of meningitis. If an initial trial of conservative management fails, then diversion of the cerebrospinal fluid (CSF) by lumbar drainage can be instituted. Failing this, surgical correction is warranted.

Transverse fractures are the result of higher-impact trauma and can cause damage to the ossicles of the middle ear or the facial nerve. Acute surgical decompression of the facial nerve should be considered with progressive deterioration of seventh nerve function.

A compound skull fracture associated with violation of the overlying skin is classified as an "open" fracture, as opposed to "closed." Open skull fractures warrant removal of foreign material and debridement of skin, bone, or brain in an operative setting. This should be performed within 6 hours of the event to limit the opportunity for infection. Closed fractures may be treated conservatively, depending on other factors associated with the injury.

Epidural Hematomas

An acute epidural hematoma (EDH), which occurs in 6% of severe TBI, is an extra-axial blood collection that is located between the skull and dura. Epidural hematomas appear as a biconvex or lenticular-shaped hyperdensity on CT scans (Figure 16.2). Classically, 85% of EDHs are associated with skull fractures that tear the meningeal arteries or, less frequently, one of the major venous sinuses.

Twenty percent of EDHs present with the well-characterized, brief, posttraumatic loss of consciousness, followed by a "lucid interval" for several hours prior to rapid neurologic deterioration. These patients can become rapidly obtunded, display contralateral hemiparesis, and ipsilateral pupillary dilatation. If untreated, they can proceed to decerebrate posturing, respiratory distress, and ultimately death.

Historically, the mortality associated with EDH ranged from 20–55%. However, a prospective study of 107 consecutive cases of EDH demonstrated an overall mortality of 5% with early, aggressive treatment. Any symptomatic EDH or asymptomatic EDH greater than 1 cm is a candidate for surgical treatment. A comparison of hematomas and hemorrhages can be seen in Table 16.3.

Acute Subdural Hematomas

Subdural hematomas, which occur in 24% of severe closed head injuries, require a much higher magnitude of force than for EDH and are uncommon in the pediatric population. They are associated with severe contact injuries or inertial injuries and are often associated with underlying brain injury. Subdural hematomas originate from parenchymal lacerations or from a tear in a surface or bridging vessel during acceleration–deceleration injuries (Figure 16.3).

Subdural hematomas can be associated with contusions and swelling of the ipsilateral cerebral hemisphere (Figure 16.4). This combination, when severe, frequently

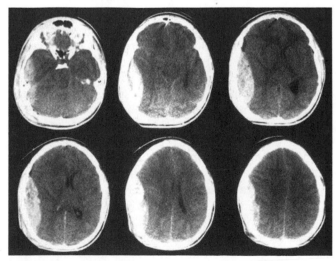

Figure 16.2 Computed tomography scan demonstrating right temporo-parietal epidural hematoma with significant mass effect and midline shift.

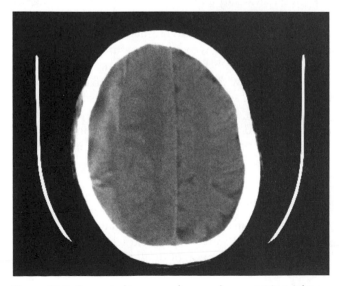

Figure 16.3 Computed tomography scan demonstrating right convexity acute and chronic subdural hematoma with mass effect.

Table 16.3 Hematomas and hemorrhages

Discriminating features	Consistent features	Variable features
Subdural hematomas		
• Crescentic mass of increased attenuation along the inner table of the skull on CT scan	• Classically result from tearing of bridging vessels	• Symptoms may result from compression of the underlying cerebral cortex or from significant midline shift
		• Surgical intervention is considered for SDHs greater than 1cm at the thickest point
Epidural hematomas		
• Biconvex (lenticular) mass of increased attenuation along the inner table of the skull on CT scan	• Classically result from tearing of the middle meningeal artery along the inner table of the skull from an overlying skull fracture	• Surgical intervention is considered for EDHs which are symptomatic and/or >1 cm at its thickest point
	• Classic presentation is a brief post-traumatic loss of consciousness, followed by a lucid interval, and then rapid neurological deterioration from an expanding EDH.	
Intracerebral hemorrhages/contusions		
• Mass of increased attenuation within the cerebral substance on CT scan	• Commonly found adjacent to the skull from sudden acceleration–deceleration of the brain along bony prominences in coup-contrecoup fashion	• Can sometimes enlarge and coalesce over serial CT scans
		• Surgical intervention is considered for large intracerebral hemorrhages or if herniation threatens

CT, computed tomography; EDH, epidural hematoma; SDH, subdural hematoma.

leads to a shift of the intracranial contents and midline structures. The mesial aspect of the temporal lobe can herniate over the tentorial notch, leading to "uncal herniation," with compression of the brainstem.

Rapid identification and surgical evacuation is warranted for any SDH greater than 1 cm at the thickest point, or for any midline shift greater than 5. After hematoma evacuation, the source of the hemorrhage is coagulated, although the source of bleeding may be more difficult to find than in EDH. Smaller SDHs can be observed with serial scans to ensure no further progression.

Mortality with SDH ranges from 30–90%. Variables associated with a worse prognosis include the mechanism of injury, age greater than 65, GCS score less than 8 on admission, and postoperative intracranial pressures greater than 20 mm Hg. Of note, patients on anticoagulation therapy suffer from a much higher incidence of acute SDH following TBI.

Subarachnoid Hemorrhage

Trauma is the most common cause of subarachnoid hemorrhages (SAH) (Figure 16.5). Subarachnoid hemorrhage results from the disruption of small pia-arachnoid vessels. A series of 750 patients with severe TBI reported an initial CT scan positive for SAH in 41%; 10–20% of posttraumatic SAHs lead to clinically symptomatic cerebral vasospasm, which can be corroborated by angiography or transcranial Doppler studies.

Intracerebral Hemorrhages and Contusions

Intracerebral hematomas occur in 10% of patients with severe TBI and result from the injury to parenchymal veins or arteries (Figure 16.6). They are often found in the frontal and temporal lobes.

Posttraumatic cerebral contusions are observed in 20–30% of patients following severe TBI. Contusions directly underlying the focus of impact are known as *coup injuries*. If the head is in motion before an abrupt deceleration, such as in an impact with a stationary object, the brain can be contused at a point remote from the point of contact (*contrecoup*). The areas of the brain most susceptible to this type of injury are found adjacent to bony prominences in the intracranial vault. The base of the skull has many irregularities that can be the point of impact during an acceleration– deceleration injury.

The distinction between an intracerebral hemorrhage and a cerebral contusion has been arbitrarily defined in some sources by the amount of hemorrhage within the lesion. If at least two-thirds of the lesion is comprised of blood, it is defined as an intracerebral hemorrhage.

Contusions are known to expand or "blossom" in 20–30% of patients on serial CT imaging within 24

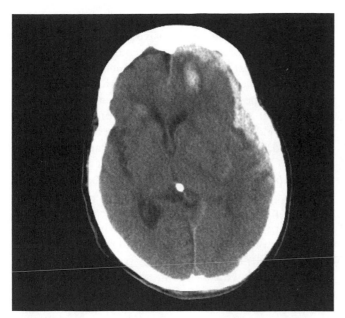

Figure 16.4 Computed tomography scan demonstrating left convexity acute subdural hematoma with cerebral contusions demonstrating mass effect and midline shift.

hours. This is believed to be due to delayed hemorrhage within the original zone of injury. Edema surrounding the contusion peaks 4–6 days following the trauma. This likely represents the effects of increased levels of thromboplastin, hemolytic metabolites, and other neurotoxic elements in the adjacent parenchyma.

The decision to evacuate a cerebral contusion or intracerebral hemorrhage is complex. Lobar hemorrhages

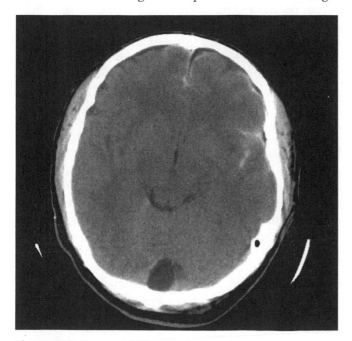

Figure 16.5 Computed tomography scan demonstrating traumatic subarachnoid hemorrhage predominantly in left sylvian fissure and possible incidental posterior arachnoid cyst.

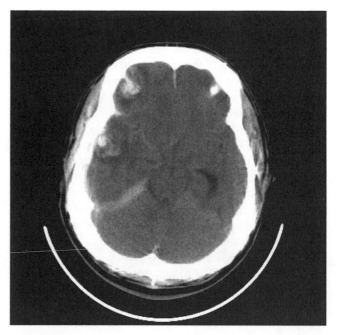

Figure 16.6 Computed tomography scan demonstrating right frontal and temporal cerebral contusions and right temporal and tentorial subdural hematoma with mass effect and midline shift.

less than 25 cm^3 can be managed conservatively if no herniation threatens. However, certain locations, such as the posterior/inferior frontal lobes and medial temporal lobes, are less tolerant to mass lesions and are associated with herniation despite much less mass effect. In these patients, evidence of brainstem distortion should lead one to consider emergent surgical decompression for lesions greater than 15 cm^3. Hemorrhages located in the deep brain structures, such as in the brainstem, basal ganglia, or thalamus, are generally managed conservatively.

Diffuse Axonal Injury

Diffuse axonal injury (DAI) is often cited as the cause of coma that occurs immediately following a head injury. In less severe injuries, DAI may be responsible for the prolonged symptoms experienced by patients with postconcussive syndromes. Mechanisms of injury that cause severe rotational or angular accelerations can lead to shearing of white matter, with microscopic axonal injury that may or may not be evident on CT or MRI scans. In its most severe form, hemorrhagic foci may be seen in the corpus callosum or in the dorsolateral rostral brainstem. Microscopic evidence of axonal damage was seen on autopsy studies in 122 of 434 fatal TBIs.

Secondary Brain Injury

Further damage to an already compromised brain occurs through physiologic or metabolic derangements following TBI. Posttraumatic cerebral blood flow (CBF) is reduced in the region surrounding contusions or underlying SDHs. This reduction of CBF can be immediate, leading to ischemia of the adjacent parenchyma. Pressure and metabolic autoregulatory mechanisms are hampered in injured brain tissue, leading to further damage.

The normal ionic and homeostatic environment is often lost in patients with severe TBI. Several neurotransmitters, which at low levels are crucial for synaptic transmission, appear at elevated levels in the extracellular space following severe TBI. Within minutes of an injury, supranormal levels of glutamate and aspartate, excitatory amino acids, are found in the extracellular space and in the CSF. Research has also found that injured brain parenchyma contains higher levels of oxygen free radicals, which can lyse cell membranes and lead to cytotoxic and vasogenic edema. These mediators of secondary brain injury are the current focus of intense investigations into the molecular and cellular biology following TBI and may lead to more therapeutic interventions to preserve neurologic function.

The Management of Head Injury

Acute Management

Repeat CT scans of head-injured patients are dictated by their initial presentation and diagnostic imaging, generally within 24 hours of their admission. Any evidence of raised ICP in mild, moderate, or severe head injuries warrants serial CT scanning (Box 16.1). The dynamics of ICP have been well characterized by the Monro-Kellie doctrine. The cranial vault in adults has a fixed volume containing three elements: brain parenchyma, blood, and CSF. Any change in volume of one or more elements will lead to elevations in ICP when the compliance of the other elements reaches a maximal point. Thus, if an expanding hematoma surpasses the compliance of the parenchyma and CSF, the pressure within the fixed cranial vault will increase.

The need for ICP monitoring is also dictated by patient presentation. The first, and most essential, tool in monitoring mild to moderate TBI is the neurologic examination. If the patient is able to reproducibly follow simple commands, then this is followed every hour or at

more frequent intervals to assess patient status. However, in severe TBI, continuous, invasive ICP monitoring is required. This is done with the placement of either an intraventricular catheter or intraparenchymal bolt. The ventricular catheter, the gold standard for ICP monitoring, involves the placement of a silastic catheter, attached to an electronic transducer, into the frontal horn of the lateral ventricle. This allows for the direct measurement of ICP and, if needed, treatment of elevated ICP by removal of CSF. The intraparenchymal bolt is an electronically coupled, fiberoptic catheter system that is placed on the surface of the brain parenchyma and is a less invasive monitoring device, without the advantage of treatment.

Emerging noninvasive technology involves the electronic monitoring of pupillary size and reaction to light to determine ICP. The pupillary constriction velocity may slow in patients with a midline shift greater than 3 mm and prolonged elevations of ICP greater than 20 mm Hg following TBI. Clinical trials with a hand-held, point-and-shoot pupillometer to quantitatively assess pupillary function are currently ongoing.

In patients who are unable to follow commands and have an abnormal CT, ICP monitoring is generally warranted, since the incidence of intracranial hypertension is over 50%. In addition to ICP, cerebral perfusion pressure (CPP), which is the mean arterial pressure (MAP) minus the ICP, is also monitored. Therapy is directed at maintaining ICP below 20 mm Hg and CPP above 60 mm Hg. Cerebral perfusion pressure is an indirect measure of the CBF and serves to better address secondary brain injury by ensuring adequate oxygenation and nutritional support of normal and traumatized neuronal elements. However, a greatly elevated CPP (generally greater than 80 mm Hg) can lead to cerebral hyperemia (from loss of vasomotor autoregulatory mechanisms) and a resultant elevation of ICP to a level considered dangerous.

Sustained ICP greater than 20 mm Hg is always abnormal and requires further monitoring and treatment (Table 16.4). Successful treatment requires the identification of the inciting cause and the prevention of secondary brain injury due to limited CBF and ischemia. Basic elements of this care involve elevation of the head of bed to 30 degrees, maintenance of normocarbia or mild hypocarbia for a short period of time ($Pco_2 = 35$ mm Hg), and/or avoidance of jugular venous compression. Patients with extra-axial hematomas or intra-axial hematomas greater than 25 cm^2 should be considered for emergent evacuation.

Osmotic diuretics, such as mannitol, draw excess interstitial fluid from the brain parenchyma into the intravascular space for clearance by the renal system. Mannitol also decreases the viscosity and improves the rheologic properties of blood, allowing for better cerebral perfusion and thus, oxygenation. It is commonly used in intravascular boluses of 0.5–1 g/kg. The patient's electrolytes and serum osmolality are monitored serially, as

---

Box 16.1 Clinical signs of intracranial hypertension

▶ Unilateral or bilateral pupillary dilatation
▶ Asymmetric pupillary response to light
▶ Flexor posturing
▶ Extensor posturing
▶ Unexplained progressive deterioration of the neurologic examination

Table 16.4 Intracranial pressure management guidelines

First-tier treatments

▶ Elevation of head of bed to 30 degrees

▶ Avoid jugular venous compression

▶ Maintain normocarbia or mild hypocarbia (PCO$_2$ >35)

▶ Avoid hypotension (SBP <90 mm Hg)

▶ Avoid hypertension (aim for patient's baseline SBP)

Second-tier treatments

▶ Drain CSF if ventriculostomy in place

▶ Mannitol bolus 0.25–1gm/kg as needed

▶ pofol drip for sedation

▶ Acute hyperventilation for short periods (PCO2 30–35)

▶ High-dose barbiturate therapy

▶ Decompressive craniectomy

SBP, systolic blood pressure; CSF, cerebrospinal fluid

levels greater than 320 mOsm/L have been associated with systemic acidosis and renal failure. Over time, and with repeated boluses, however, mannitol can infiltrate into the interstitial space with loss of the osmotic gradient and worsening cerebral edema.

Hypertonic saline has been increasingly used either as a substitute for mannitol or as adjunctive therapy. Usually, a 3% or 7.5% solution is used, although higher concentrations have been employed. Either small intermittent boluses or a continuous infusion is utilized with the goal of reducing ICP while preventing the serum sodium from climbing above 160. Proposed advantages of hypertonic saline include class two evidence that it is efficacious as a volume expander; thus, avoiding the diuresis associated with mannitol. In a recent editorial in *Critical Medicine*, Hartl and Froelich (2008) provide a succinct summary of the issues with regard to the use of hypertonic saline. Jusson and colleagues (2008) offer a well referenced discussion of the potential advantages of hypertonic saline, although their observations are limited to animal models. Further information is clearly required on the appropriate concentration, dosing schedule, length of treatment, and use of hypertonic saline either alone or in combination with mannitol.

Hyperventilation causes a fall in ICP by reducing the intracranial blood flow and volume through constriction of the cerebral vasculature. This can be instituted in acute management of elevated ICP. However, sustained hyperventilation is not beneficial in treatment of prolonged elevations of ICP, owing to the compensatory mechanisms that offset its effect. Areas of damaged parenchyma have lost the ability to autoregulate blood flow. By decreasing Pco$_2$, it is possible that only the normal areas of parenchyma will respond. Subsequent hypoperfusion may result in ischemia or stroke. Generally,

hyperventilation is safely tolerated from a Pco$_2$ of 30–35 mm Hg. Again, it is important to stress that this should be used in acute settings only for short periods of time, before more definitive treatments are instituted.

Use of other pharmacologic therapies involves sedative medications, such as propofol, opiates, and barbiturates. These are only instituted in patients with ICP monitoring devices, since the ability to follow the neurologic examination is compromised. Induction of high-dose barbiturate therapy is an aggressive and, generally, last-line treatment. Barbiturates limit neuronal destruction by scavenging free radicals from fatty acid peroxidative pathways in mitochondrial metabolism. They limit cerebral metabolism and reduce CBF, thus protecting the brain from damage during the hypermetabolic state following TBI. Barbiturates are administered to maintain ICP less than 20 or until burst suppression is seen on electroencephalography (EEG). The complications following barbiturate therapy limit its use in the clinical setting. Myocardial depression and hypotension may further exacerbate cerebral ischemia, and pulmonary complications from weakened respiratory ciliary function often worsen the overall medical condition of the patient.

Monitoring of electrolytes and fluid balance is integral to the successful care of the head-injured patient. Serum sodium should be monitored closely, as patients with severe head injury can quickly lapse into the syndrome of inappropriate secretion of antidiuretic hormone (SIADH) or cerebral salt wasting (CSW). Furthermore, coagulation profiles should be monitored and corrected to prevent further expansion of intracranial hematomas.

Early posttraumatic seizures occur in 3–9% of all head injuries, with a higher incidence in severe TBI. Patients with intracerebral hemorrhages, traumatic SDHs, depressed skull fractures, EDHs, and prolonged loss of consciousness have a higher risk of seizures. The occurrence of an early posttraumatic seizure can be a harbinger of the development of posttraumatic epilepsy. A large, randomized, double-blind study demonstrated a beneficial effect of phenytoin use in the reduction of seizures during the first week after TBI, but no benefit in the prevention of posttraumatic epilepsy.

Steroids have not been found to improve clinical outcome in multiple studies and have no role in the treatment of elevated ICP in TBI. Hypothermia (cooling) after TBI may reduce mortality and improve neurologic outcome in specific circumstances, but may increase the risk of pneumonia.

Postconcussive Syndromes and Cognitive Sequelae of Head Injury

Following TBI, patients often complain of vague symptoms including headaches, nausea and vomiting, dizziness, anxiety and irritability, and insomnia. They can have difficulties with concentration, memory, cognitive processing, and attention. Of these complaints, posttraumatic headaches are usually the most persistent. These headaches are often variable in nature and can be exacerbated by changes in position, movement, anxiety, or stress. The persistence and severity of these symptoms can be directly related to the severity of the head trauma.

Some patients with mild or moderate head injuries have an identifiable impairment of cognitive processing, inattention, and memory disturbances. These symptoms will generally resolve in 3 months, although in a small minority they may persist. Patients with more severe TBI suffer from greater cognitive deficits for much longer periods of time, possibly permanently.

Posttraumatic complications are treated supportively. Patients are reassured that the symptoms are transient and should resolve with time. Non-narcotic medications are recommended for headaches and low-dose benzodiazepines can be prescribed for vertigo. Posttraumatic depression is best treated with selective serotonin reuptake inhibitors (SSRI). A referral should be made for neuropsychological evaluation for any patient with persistent cognitive difficulties.

Cognitive and behavioral sequelae of blast injury

The war in Iraq has resulted in a much greater incidence of blast-associated injuries, with an increasing recognition that mild TBI is inextricably linked with posttraumatic stress disorder (PTSD). Hoge and colleagues (2008) have recently reported on this association and found that, in returning troops who suffered a brief loss of consciousness following injury, 43.9% developed PTSD. A 27.3% incidence of PTSD occurred in those with an altered state of consciousness, and only a 9.1% incidence in those with no injuries. Of concern is the observation that many troops suffer multiple exposures, making it likely that the typical cognitive and behavioral sequelae of mild TBI, coupled with PTSD, will result in an overwhelming need for long-term care that current facilities will be unable to meet. The interaction of TBI and PTSD must be much better understood in order to develop effective treatment strategies for this increasingly common course of long-term disability in our military forces.

Physical Medicine and Rehabilitation

Comatose patients warrant evaluation by specialists in physical medicine for placement of orthotic splints to limit contractures and for range-of-motion exercises. More mobile patients will benefit from the early initiation of physical and occupational therapy. Speech therapists can assist in the resumption of oral intake. Many TBI patients benefit from further inpatient rehabilitation following discharge from the hospital, whereas patients suffering from mild TBI will benefit from outpatient physical therapy.

Spinal Injury

Injury to the spine and spinal cord occur in an estimated 100,000 individuals each year in the United States. Approximately 8–10% of these patients also suffer from severe neurologic dysfunction. At an estimated cost of $5.6 billion per year, treatment of new and existing patients with SCI takes a significant toll on medical resources.

Spinal column injuries involve the vertebrae and/or its ligamentous attachments, resulting in stable or unstable injuries. The early detection of spinal column injury is necessary to ensure the maximal preservation of neurologic function. Trauma to the spinal cord results in either complete or incomplete injury. Certain characteristics of SCI should be readily identifiable, thus allowing for immediate initiation of treatment.

The Evaluation of the Spine-Injured Patient

Initial Assessment

Early initiation of spine precautions and immobilization is mandatory in any significant trauma to prevent further SCI. Once the patient has been immobilized with a cervical collar and a rigid spine board, she is safe for transportation to a trauma facility.

As in head injury, a detailed history provides insights into the possible spine trauma sustained. For instance, diving injuries result from hyperflexion and compression injuries of the mid cervical region with a characteristic pattern of neurologic loss (Figure 16.7). In these injuries, the vertebral bodies, pedicles, lamina, and ligamentous structures are damaged, resulting in instability. Patients who fall or have other axial compression loading injuries can sustain trauma to the thoraco-lumbar region (T12 and/or L1) with compression or burst fractures of the spinal column (Figure 16.8).

The presence of focal or radicular pain and a detailed motor and sensory examination is critical to localize any potential damage to the spinal cord. Testing of muscle stretch reflexes, the bulbocavernosus reflex, Beevor sign, and anal sphincter tone and wink are essential to rule out cord injury. While maintaining spine immobilization, the patient is examined for any deformity, contusions, or abrasions that might indicate spine injury.

Individuals demonstrating a complete loss of motor and sensory function at a dermatomal level are described as having sustained a *complete injury*. There is bilateral loss of motor function, bilateral loss of all sensory modalities, and incompetent sphincters. Patients presenting with

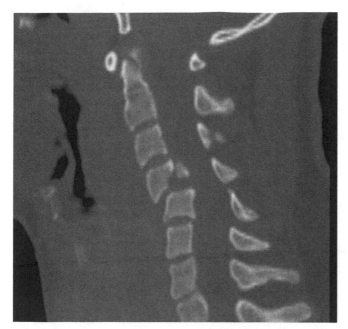

Figure 16.7 Computed tomography scans of cervical spine demonstrating odontoid fracture of C2 and vertebral body fracture and malalignment of C4 following a motor vehicle accident and incomplete C4 spinal cord injury.

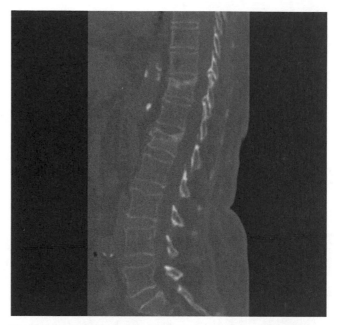

Figure 16.8 Computed tomography scan demonstrating compression fractures following axial loading injury without spinal cord injury.

complete spinal cord injuries are likely to be left with severe and irreversible symptoms, although 2–4% of patients may recover sufficient function for ambulation. Complete SCIs are described by the last functional and nonfunctional levels (i.e., C6 complete SCI with functional C5 level).

Sparing of sensory or motor function is described as an *incomplete injury*. The level is identified as the last completely functional dermatomal level. The focus of care in incomplete SCI is the preservation of the existing function, prevention of further injury, and decompression of any neural elements.

Imaging Modalities

After a detailed assessment, diagnostic imaging is instituted to localize any area of trauma. Plain radiographs of the entire spinal axis are required, with particular attention to levels documented during the examination. Two views, anterior–posterior and lateral, are required for the initial assessment to delineate osseous injury.

Areas of suspicion are further imaged with thin-cut CT scans with sagittal reconstruction of the spine. This modality provides excellent detail of the bone and possible fractures. Axial images can demonstrate compromise of the spinal canal and possible injury to the cord, whereas sagittal images illustrate any loss of height or abnormal angulation of the spine.

Magnetic resonance imaging provides superior resolution of the neural elements and ligamentous structures.

Patients with an identifiable spinal cord injury on physical examination require an MRI, so that they can be evaluated for traumatic disc herniations, hematomas, ligamentous ruptures, and/or high signal cord changes (Figure 16.9).

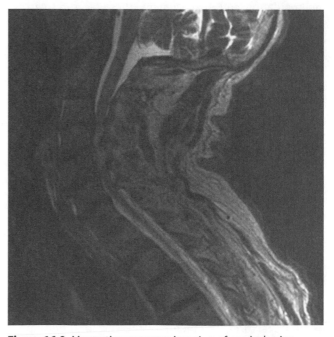

Figure 16.9 Magnetic resonance imaging of cervical spine demonstrating spinal cord contusions over C4–C5 in preexisting degenerative disc disease following hyperflexion injury and C4 incomplete spinal cord injury.

The Mechanisms of Spinal Column Injury

Significant mechanisms of trauma leading to disruption of the bony or ligamentous structures may result in instability of the spine. Depending on the location and degree of injury, treatment may range from bracing and analgesia to surgical fusion of multiple vertebral levels. If there is any question of spinal column instability, the patient is kept under strict spinal precautions and a referral is made to an appropriately trained spine surgeon.

Fractures involving the C1 ring occur in 3–13% of all cervical spine fractures. The classic C1 fracture, known as the *Jefferson fracture*, is described as a "blow-out" fracture involving fractures of bilateral anterior and posterior arches from axial compression. It is an unstable fracture, but usually not associated with neurologic deficits.

The odontoid process of the C2 vertebrae can be fractured through the tip, base, or base and vertebral body, known respectively as types I, II, or III odontoid fractures. Flexion injuries are the most common cause of these fractures. Odontoid fractures are usually unstable and require either immobilization or surgical management, depending on type. However, a high rate of nonunion occurs in certain type II fractures that can require surgical intervention following failure of conservative management.

Fractures through the pars interarticularis of the C2 body are known as "hangman's" fractures. Depending on the angulation and displacement, these fractures can be stable or unstable. Greater than 90% of individuals with hangman's fractures are neurologically intact and these fractures generally heal well with immobilization.

Axial loading injuries of the spine result in compression or burst fractures at the thoraco-lumbar junction. These fractures are well characterized by the three-column model of thoraco-lumbar fractures. The anterior column is composed of the anterior longitudinal ligament (ALL) and anterior half of the vertebral body. The middle column consists of the posterior half of the vertebral body and the posterior longitudinal ligament (PLL). The posterior column is made up of the pedicles, facets, spinous processes, and interspinous ligaments.

Anterior wedge compression fractures are caused by disruption of the anterior column by an axial loading force utilizing the middle column as a fulcrum. Compression fractures involve both the anterior and middle columns, while sparing the posterior column. Generally, no neurologic deficit is associated with this type of injury. In burst fractures, fragments of the vertebral body protrude into the spinal canal and can lead to neurologic injury. These fractures are unstable and require external orthoses or surgical intervention.

Patterns of Spinal Cord Injury

Central Cord Syndrome

The central cord syndrome is the most common incomplete SCI and results from a hyperflexion injury in the setting of cervical degenerative disease. This pattern of injury is associated with weakness of the upper extremities greater than the lower extremities. Sensory changes tend to be variable below the level of injury and myelopathic findings are frequently present. Indications for surgical intervention include continued compression of the spinal cord and/or instability of the spine. However, the timing of the decompression continues to be a matter of some debate. Patients will generally recover some function, with approximately half of patients with cord contusions able to ambulate independently following the injury. Upper extremity weakness with difficulty with fine motor control is often persistent. Bowel and bladder function often recovers with time.

Anterior Cord Syndrome

Injury to the anterior half of the spinal cord is generally a vascular phenomenon involving cord infarction in the distribution of the anterior spinal artery. In the setting of trauma, this occurs from anterior compression of the cord and artery by a dislocated bone fragment or herniated disc. Patients exhibit loss of motor function below the level of the lesion, with a dissociated sensory loss. Involvement of the anteriorly positioned spinothalamic tracts leads to loss of pain and temperature sensation, whereas sparing of the posterior dorsal columns results in preservation of position sense and two-point discrimination. To plan any surgical intervention, radiographic imaging is vital to differentiate surgical lesions due to compressive etiology from vascular lesions. Unfortunately, only 10–20% of patients with injury to the anterior cord recover functional motor control.

Brown-Séquard Syndrome

Penetrating trauma to the spinal cord can result in a cord hemisection with a Brown-Séquard syndrome. Patients exhibit contralateral loss of pain and temperature sensation with ipsilateral loss of proprioception, vibratory sense, and motor control. Penetrating hemisections of the cord are not treated surgically. However, Brown-Séquard syndromes due to traumatic ruptured discs are amenable to surgical intervention.

The Management of Spinal Injury

Acute Management

Following cervical or thoracic SCI, patients may lose sympathetic tone of their vasculature, resulting in hypotension from spinal shock. It is important to maintain adequate systemic pressures via fluid resuscitation and, if necessary, pharmacologic pressors. Antishock trousers can be placed to assist with venous return and increase arterial pressure.

Based on results of the North American Spinal Cord Injury Study II (NASCIS II), steroids have become the mainstay of treatment for all SCI. It was initially believed that steroids could ameliorate the effects of spinal cord edema and inflammation to allow for recovery of neurologic function. However, recent evidence points to their role in limiting secondary injury and cellular damage secondary to lipid peroxidation of cellular membranes. Results from NASCIS II suggest that patients should receive high-dose steroid therapy with clinically detected SCI without waiting for confirmatory radiographic studies. In NASCIS II, methylprednisolone was administered as an initial bolus of 30 mg/kg and a maintenance dose of 5.4 mg/kg/hr for 23 hours to patients presenting within 8 hours of their injury. Patients presenting outside of the 8-hour window, on the other hand, had increased risk of complications from high-dose steroid therapy but no clinical benefit. The NASCIS III trial further refined the use of methylprednisolone, recommending 23 hours of high-dose steroids for patients presenting within 3 hours of SCI and 48 hours of treatment for those presenting from 3–8 hours postinjury.

Prognosis

The likelihood of recovery following complete or incomplete SCI is inextricably linked to age, with younger patients exhibiting a greater potential for recovery. Patients presenting with complete cervical injuries without improvement in the first 24 hours of hospitalization rarely regain significant ambulatory function. Also, the level and degree of an incomplete injury has some prognostic value. Cervical injuries recover more function than thoracic or thoraco-lumbar injuries and, not surprisingly, less severe injuries have a better functional outcome. As patients with incomplete injuries age, they can suffer from progressive loss of neurologic function, which may be related to age-related neuronal loss in the brain and spinal cord.

Summary

Injuries of the central nervous system present difficult management issues for trained medical personnel. Early

---

Pearls and Perils

Management of traumatic injuries to the central nervous system

▶ Skull fractures resulting in depression of the cranial vault greater than the width of the skull should be considered for surgical elevation and repair. Open skull fractures warranting removal of foreign material and debridement should be performed within 6 hours of the event to limit the opportunity for infection.

▶ Surgical evacuation is warranted for any subdural hematoma (SDH) greater than 1 cm at the thickest point or for any midline shift greater than 5.

▶ Any evidence of raised intracranial pressures (ICP) in mild, moderate, or severe head injuries warrants serial CT scanning. In severe traumatic brain injury (TBI), continuous, invasive ICP monitoring is required.

▶ Steroids have not been found to improve clinical outcome and have no role in the treatment of elevated ICP in TBI.

▶ Early initiation of spine precautions and immobilization is mandatory in any significant spinal cord injury (SCI).

▶ Following cervical or thoracic SCI, patients may lose sympathetic tone of their vasculature, resulting in hypotension from spinal shock. It is important to maintain adequate systemic pressures via fluid resuscitation and, if necessary, pharmacologic pressors.

▶ High-dose steroid therapy is the mainstay of treatment for all SCIs presenting within 8 hours of injury.

▶ Patients presenting with complete cervical injuries, without improvement in the first 24 hours of hospitalization, rarely regain significant ambulatory function.

▶ The term "mild head injury" should not be construed to indicate an insignificant trauma, since these patients can suffer from prolonged or delayed cognitive and other difficulties.

▶ Diffuse axonal injury may be responsible for the prolonged symptoms experienced by patients with postconcussive syndromes.

Consider Consultation When...

▶ Patients have head injuries and abnormalities on computed tomography scan.

▶ Patients deteriorate following the initial Glasgow Coma Scale survey.

▶ Patients have fractures of the spinal column.

▶ Patients have suspected or documented injuries of the spinal cord.

identification of the pathophysiology, coupled with quick intervention, is required to optimize patient outcomes in the setting of trauma. The improved care of these patients relies heavily on ongoing clinical and basic science research in the neurosciences.

Annotated Bibliography

Brain Trauma Foundation. *Guidelines for the management and prognosis of severe head injury.* Park Ridge IL: American Association of Neurological Surgeons, Joint Section on Neurotrauma and Critical Care, 2000.
Based upon a comprehensive critical review of the literature, these guidelines make official therapeutic recommendations for the management of severe traumatic brain injury in the United States.

Cooper PR. *Head injury*, 3rd ed. Baltimore: Williams & Wilkins, 1993.
This multiauthored book incorporates the latest information on the advances in the management of patients with head injuries. Epidemiology, acute management, neurodiagnostics, and sequelae are extensively presented.

Cooper PR. *Management of posttraumatic spinal instability.* Park Ridge IL: American Association of Neurological Surgeons, 1990.
Provides a basic working knowledge of a range of spinal injuries. Diagnosis based upon biomechanics and radiography is presented. Treatment strategies are current, including both surgical and conservative management options.

Marshall SB, et al. *Neuroscience critical care*. Philadelphia: WB Saunders, 1990.
This book, by an interdisciplinary care group, delineates the basic principles for the disorders of the nervous system with an emphasis on clinical science as it is applied to the critical care environment. The format converts an intellectually challenging subject to one that is easily readable.

CHAPTER 17

Movement Disorders

Sith Sathornsumetee and Mark A. Stacy

Outline

▶ Evaluation of movement disorders
▶ Characteristics of movement disorders
▶ Anatomy and biochemistry of the basal ganglia
▶ Hypokinetic movement disorders
▶ Hyperkinetic movement disorders
▶ Drug-induced movement disorders

Evaluation of Movement Disorders

Recognition of abnormal clinical phenomenology is the key to the diagnosis and treatment of movement disorders. Hypokinetic movement disorders are associated with slow movement, and are also commonly termed the parkinsonian disorders. Hyperkinetic movement disorders are associated with involuntary movements including tremor, chorea, athetosis, ballism, dystonia, myoclonus, and tics.

Historical information from patients with movement disorders should be comprehensive, with specific information pertaining to age of onset, temporal progression of symptoms, the type of involuntary movements, aggravating factors, and relieving factors (for instance anxiety, stress, sleep, alcohol, food, and medications). Almost all involuntary movements except for segmental myoclonus, tics, and hemifacial spasm disappear during sleep. It is important to obtain past medical history, recent travel history, family history, trauma, toxins/chemical exposure, and information regarding medications used in the past and at present. Dopamine receptor blocking agents (such as neuroleptics and antiemetics) are the most common medications causing drug-induced movement disorders. Although these agents are associated with parkinsonism

and tardive dyskinesia (TD), other agents, such as corticosteroids, are known to produce tremor (Box 17.1). One should always inquire about the history of acute dystonic reaction to any medications.

Neurologic examination should include assessment of language, memory, and other higher cortical functions. Frontal release signs, such as the Myerson sign, are seen commonly in Parkinson disease (PD). Cranial nerve examination with special attention to extraocular movements (vertical saccade) is important, especially when differentiating Parkinson disease from progressive supranuclear palsy, or when evaluating for early signs of Huntington disease. Facial expression and speech pattern should be noted. Motor examination, including muscle tone and power, sensory testing, and assessment of deep tendon and plantar reflexes are also important. Testing for rapid alternating movement, posture, and gait are necessary. In addition, emphasis on postures or movements that increase patient symptoms is helpful in defining particular syndromes.

Special attention should be directed to:

1. the body, neck, and limb posture;
2. ophthalmoscopic examination for Kayser-Fleischer ring;
3. muscle tone (hypotonia versus hypertonia; spasticity, rigidity with or without cogwheeling, or paratonia);
4. maintenance of posture when arms are outstretched anteriorly or in a "wing-beating position" and during a sustained voluntary contraction (for example, firmly holding examiner's fingers);
5. performance of rapid successive and alternating movements;
6. handwriting (not only signature) and drawing an Archimedes spiral (Figure 17.1);

▼

Box 17.1 Drugs that may induce tremor

▶ Caffeine
▶ Cyclosporine
▶ Corticosteroids
▶ Valproic acid
▶ Traditional antipsychotics
▶ Metoclopramide
▶ Reserpine
▶ Metronidazole
▶ Methylxanthines
▶ Lithium
▶ Bronchodilators (-adrenergic agonists)
▶ Serotonin reuptake inhibitors
▶ Tricyclic antidepressants
▶ Verapamil
▶ Atorvastatin
▶ Amiodarone
▶ Thyroxin
▶ Alcohol withdrawal
▶ Tocainamide

7. postural stability (propulsion versus retropulsion);
8. gait (ignition, stride width and length, rate and pattern of walking, arm swing, adventitious limb movement, and steps required for 180-degree turning);
9. facial expression with regards to rate of blinking, blepharospasm, other orofacial spasms or hypomimia ("mask facies");
10. spontaneous speech; and
11. involuntary vocalizations.

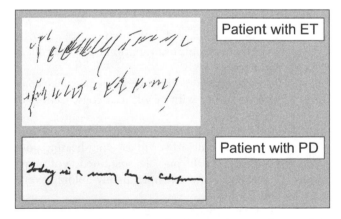

Figure 17.1 Handwriting samples from patients with essential tremor (ET) and Parkinson disease (PD). Courtesy of Dr. Gregory S. Conner, Tulsa, OK.

Abnormal involuntary movements should be described according to distribution (face, neck, trunk, and extremities), frequency and duration, symmetry, characteristic features (rhythmic versus nonrhythmic, synchronous versus asynchronous, stereotyped versus unpredictable or random, simple versus complex, purposeful versus nonpurposeful, suppressible versus nonsuppressible), and occurrence (at rest, during sustention, during voluntary movement or isometric contraction).

Characteristics of Movement Disorders

Hypokinesia refers to a reduced amount of movement, whereas *bradykinesia* refers to slowness of movement or impaired initiation of movement. *Rigidity* is a clinical sign of increased tone of the muscles in a manner velocity-independent of passive movement. It is associated with extrapyramidal tract dysfunction. *Spasticity* refers to increased tone of the muscles in a velocity-dependent manner, and it is a sign of pyramidal or corticospinal tract dysfunction. A rigid limb demonstrates passive resistance throughout a range of motion, whereas a spastic limb has greater initial resistance to movement that diminishes with movement through a range of motion.

Tremor is the most common of the involuntary movement disorders, and it is characterized by rhythmic, oscillatory movement produced by alternating or synchronous contractions of reciprocally innervated muscles. The movement is repetitive and regular in amplitude and frequency. Careful attention must be paid to differentiate a tremor at rest (usually seen in PD) from a tremor with action or posture holding (usually associated with essential tremor) (Table 17.1).

Chorea is characterized by rapid, nonsustained, "dance-like," irregular, nonpatterned, usually asymmetric movements that are purposeless but may be partially incorporated into a purposeful act, such as scratching a nose, pulling on an ear, combing hair, or fixing a dress. The movements are continuous and randomly distributed in space and time. When they are proximal, the movements may result in irregular frontalis contraction, lip pouting, shoulder shrug, or truncal tilt. Distal chorea is manifested by irregular "piano-playing" movements. Certain forms of chorea, for example, Sydenham chorea, are associated with involuntary contractions alternating with relaxations of grip when squeezing the examiner's fingers (milkmaid's grip). Choreatic patients often have difficulty maintaining tongue protrusion and at times develop involuntary rhythmic "in-and-out" movement of the tongue ("darting or serpentine tongue"). The muscle tone in chorea is usually diminished, and reflexes are often pendular or "hung-up."

Athetosis is characterized by a combination of flexion, extension, supination, pronation, abduction, and ad-

Table 17.1 Clinical features of Parkinson disease and essential tremor

Characteristics	Parkinson disease	Essential tremor
Tremor location	Hands, legs, perioral	Hands, head, voice
Bradykinesia	Present	Absent
Rigidity	Present	Absent
Family history	Usually negative	Positive in more than 50%
Alcohol	Minimal reduction	Marked reduction
Age at onset	62.4 years (mean)	42.5 years (mean)
Tremor type	Resting with rarely postural or kinetic	Postural, kinetic, and rarely resting
	Unilateral at onset	Bilateral at onset

duction occurring in a series of coarse, slow, writhing movements. Distal, more so than axial, muscle groups are usually involved, and the muscle tone, in contrast to chorea, is increased. The term *choreoathetosis* is used to describe the combination of choreatic and athetotic movements.

Ballism is an abrupt, forceful, violent, flailing contraction of proximal limb muscles and is usually unilateral (hemiballism). Hemiballism may be an extreme form of hemichorea, which is often the residual motor disturbance in patients who recover from hemiballism. The etiology of hemiballism includes structural lesions such as stroke, tumor, infections (such as acquired immune deficiency syndrome [AIDS] and toxoplasmosis), demyelinating disease, and metabolic disorders such as hyperosmolar hyperglycemic nonketotic state, hypoglycemia, and hypocalcemia. Traditionally, hemiballism is thought to be almost pathognomonic of lesions involving the subthalamic nucleus. However, more recent reports reveal only a minority of cases that have direct involvement of the subthalamic nucleus. Altered firing pattern in basal ganglia structures is in fact more important in the pathogenesis of hemiballism. Because of the rarity of ballism, no large pharmacologic placebo-controlled studies are available. Information on treatment for hemiballism, based on case series or single case reports, includes dopamine receptor blocking drugs such as haloperidol, dopamine depleting agents, such as tetrabenazine, γ-aminobutyric acid (GABA)-ergic drugs such as benzodiazepines, local injection of botulinum toxin, and stereotactic thalamotomy and pallidotomy.

Dystonia is a sustained, patterned, twisting, pulling movement produced by involuntary contraction or relaxation of agonists and antagonists occurring at rest, when maintaining or changing posture, or when performing a specific motor activity. It is usually slow, but in some patients the dystonic movements may be rapid, repetitive, jerky (dystonic spasm) and may progress to fixed contractions (dystonic postures).

Myoclonus is an uncontrollable, sudden, abrupt, brief, jerk-like contraction of one or more muscles. Myoclonus may arise spontaneously in the central nervous system (CNS), or may be provoked by sensory stimuli (cortical reflex myoclonus) or by voluntary movement (action or intention myoclonus). Myoclonus may be focal (jerk restricted to one part of the body), multifocal (asynchronous jerks in different muscle groups), or generalized (massive synchronous jerks involving trunk and limbs). *Asterixis* is viewed as a form of negative myoclonus. Instead of positive muscle contractions, the movements of asterixis are produced by sudden brief lapses in muscle contractions. *Segmental myoclonus* is repetitive, rhythmic, and independent of sensory afferent input, and may even persist during sleep (for example, palatal or brachial myoclonus). Physiologically, segmental myoclonus is characterized by rhythmic co-contraction of agonist muscles. In contrast, tremor is produced by alternating contractions of agonists and antagonists.

Tics are characteristically complex, rapid, sudden, unpredictable, repetitive, stereotypic, purposeless movements of variable intensity and occurring at irregular intervals. They increase with stress and decrease with rest, distraction, and concentration. Tics may be motor or vocal and, in contrast to myoclonus, can be temporarily suppressed by an effort of will. Patients often have a build-up of tension and a rebound exacerbation after voluntary suppression of tics. In some patients with the Tourette syndrome (TS), tics are associated with a premonitory urge to move and a relief with tic performance.

Another neurologic condition which subjects feel the urge to move is *restless leg syndrome*. It is characterized by unpleasant "crawling" sensation in the legs, particularly in the evening when patients are attempting to fall asleep. This sensation usually disappears with voluntary movement of legs or walking. The disorder is not well understood, but it usually responds to dopamine agonists, levodopa, opioids, and gabapentin. Some patients with restless leg syndrome have low serum ferritin, and their symptoms may improve with iron replacement therapy.

Continued muscle stiffness due to continuous muscle firing can result from neuromyotonia, encephalomyelitis with myoclonus and rigidity, and the stiff-limb/stiff-person syndrome. The last tends to involve axial and proximal muscles and has been associated with an antibody to glutamic acid decarboxylase (GAD).

Akathisia refers to "inner" restlessness manifested as voluntary motor activity to relieve unpleasant sensation. It usually takes the form of pacing, trunk-rocking while standing or marching on the spot. Akathisia is usually associated with neuroleptic treatment.

Stereotypies are repetitive, purposeless, and seemingly planned involuntary movements that are associated with the use of dopamine receptor blocking agents (neuroleptics). Because of the strong association between development of movement disorders and antipsychotic and antiemetic drugs, this movement disorder is sometimes used synonymously with *tardive dyskinesia*. However, because tardive parkinsonism, dystonia, akathisia, tremor, tics, and myoclonus are recognized as subcategories of TD, this terminology is potentially confusing. Some neurologists suggest using the term *tardive syndromes* for any of the movement disorders list that are caused by prolonged use of neuroleptics.

Anatomy and Biochemistry of the Basal Ganglia

Parkinsonism, chorea, dystonia, akathisia, ballism, stereotypies, and tics usually result from a disturbance of the basal ganglia. Historically, the basal ganglia comprise the *extrapyramidal pathway*, a term coined by S.A.K. Wilson, to designate a motor system that is not pyramidal (corticospinal) or cerebellar. The basal ganglia, located deep in the cerebral hemispheres and rostral brainstem, include the striatum (caudate and putamen), globus pallidus, subthalamic nucleus, and substantia nigra. Also included are striatum-derived limbic structures such as nucleus accumbens, olfactory tubercle, and parts of the amygdala (Figure 17.2).

The striatum receives a number of inputs from various parts of the CNS and, in turn, connects with important motor and sensory centers. The major striatal input arises from cell layer five of the cerebral cortex. These corticostriatal projections release the excitatory neurotransmitter glutamate. The second major striatal input arises from the dopamine-containing neurons in the pars compacta of the substantia nigra (SNpc). This nigrostriatal pathway is impaired in PD. Abnormalities in the striatolimbic system may be responsible for behavioral disturbances in PD. Serotonergic fibers from the raphe nuclei in the brainstem also project to the striatum. The most important receptive nuclei for these afferent pathways are the caudate and putamen. These striatal nuclei are primarily involved with convergence and integration of the various inputs, and may play a role in depression and obsessive-compulsive disorder.

Within the caudate-putamen, large "aspiny" interneurons contain acetylcholine as one of their neurotransmitters. The medium-sized "spiny" output neurons release the inhibitory neurotransmitter GABA, and also excitatory neuropeptides, substance P and enkephalin. Heterogeneities within the striatum have been described. The matrix (80%) of the striatum receives input from layers III and V of the cerebral cortex, and some thalamic nuclei. The striosomes (20%) receive dopaminergic information from the substantia nigra. The striosomes may also receive cortical input from layer V in the cortex. Both of these structures connect with the ventral lateral and ventral anterior nuclei of the thalamus, which, in turn, project to the motor cortex (from the ventral lateral nucleus) and to the premotor cortex (from the ventral anterior nucleus). In addition, an internal loop connects the globus pallidus, the centromedian nucleus of the thalamus, and the putamen. The external pallidum projects to the subthalamic nucleus (STN), which, in turn, connects with both pallidal segments and with the substantia nigra by excitatory glutamatergic transmission. Thus, the STN modulates the output of the globus pallidus. In addition to its connections with the thalamic nuclei, the striatum provides a feedback to the pars reticulate of the substantia nigra (SNpr). Like the striatothalamic pathway, this striatonigral pathway is also mediated by GABA and by the excitatory neurotransmitter, substance P. Through the cortico-striato-pallido-thalamo-cortical feedback loop, the basal ganglia play a critical role in the control of movement, motor tone, and complex motor behaviors.

Hypokinetic Movement Disorders

Parkinson Disease

Parkinson disease is the second most common neurodegenerative disorder, and its annual incidence rates range from 4.9 to 26 per 100 000. Parkinson disease was first recognized in 1817 by James Parkinson in his monograph "Essay on the Shaking Palsy." Parkinson termed the disease "paralysis agitans" and suggested that the CNS is primarily involved. Charcot subsequently used the term "Parkinson's disease" for paralysis agitans, and differentiated the resting tremor of PD from the cerebellar outflow action tremor seen in multiple sclerosis. In 1912, Wilson linked PD to dysfunction of the extrapyramidal system. Subsequent examinations of the brains of patients dying with idiopathic PD demonstrated depigmentation

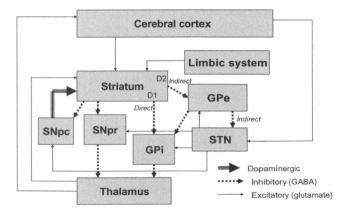

Figure 17.2 Simplified diagram of basal ganglia connections. *SNpc,* substantia nigra pars compacta; *SNpr,* substantia nigra pars reticulate; *GPe,* globus pallidus pars externa; *GPi,* globus pallidus pars interna; *STN,* subthalamic nucleus.

of the substantia nigra in the midbrain associated with a loss of dopamine-producing cells.

Clinical features

Four cardinal signs of parkinsonism include resting tremor, bradykinesia, rigidity, and postural instability. Tremor in PD usually occurs at rest, involving the hand in a pronating–supinating ("pill-rolling") manner at approximately 4- to 6-Hz frequency. Early in the course of the disease, tremor and other parkinsonian signs are usually asymmetric but eventually become bilateral. The tremor in PD may also involve the chin, jaw, tongue, and legs.

Rigidity is an increase of muscle tone in a velocity-independent manner on passive movements in all direction. Steady resistance against passive movements may be interrupted, producing *ratcheting* or *cogwheeling* phenomena. Rigidity may be increased by asking the patient to perform a voluntary act in other parts of body contralateral to the limb being assessed (Froment sign); for example, closing and opening a contralateral fist while passively rotating the patient's wrist. This maneuver enhances the cogwheel phenomenon in the tested wrist.

Bradykinesia (slowness of movement) or *hypokinesia* (poverty of movement) interferes with activities of daily living such as standing, dressing, feeding, brushing teeth, and bathing. On examination, slowness with decreased amplitude in rapid succession movements may be evident. In the advanced disease, early and frequent arrests of movement may be seen with finger tapping, hand clasping, wrist pronation–supination, and heel-tapping.

Postural instability or loss of postural reflexes often occurs in moderate to severe cases of PD and is characterized by propulsion or retropulsion and a tendency to fall. It can be tested by pulling the patient backward while he is standing with his feet together (pull test). The patient often assumes a stooped posture or in cases of unilateral parkinsonism, develops scoliosis away from the affected side.

Most of the other signs in PD are manifestations of these cardinal characteristics either alone or in combination: lack of facial expression (hypomimia), drooling, hypophonia, dysarthria, dysphagia, lack of associated movement such as arm-swing when walking, micrographia, shuffling gait, difficulty standing and turning when walking, difficulty turning in bed, start hesitation, freezing, and festination of gait.

Besides motor symptoms, PD patients often develop depression, passive attitude, and dementia. "Frontal release" signs, such as the Myerson sign, may accompany other mental and motor symptoms of PD, but they are not specific for PD. Sensory symptoms such as pain, burning, coldness, or numbness are reported by about half of PD patients.

Atypical forms of parkinsonism often lead to misdiagnosis. Approximately 12% of patients referred to movement disorder clinics in tertiary care medical centers for PD have parkinsonism-plus syndromes. Some of these disorders are described in Table 17.2. Other conditions that lead to misdiagnosis include drug-induced parkinsonism and other hereditary neurodegenerative conditions. Drugs known to cause or worsen PD are phenothiazines, butyrophenones, metoclopramide, α-methyldopa, reserpine, flunarizine, and tetrabenazine. In addition, environmental toxins such as 1-methyl-4-phenyl-1,2,3,6-tetrahydropyridine (MPTP), carbon monoxide, cyanide, carbon disulfide, manganese, lithium, and even alcohol withdrawal have been associated with parkinsonian features (Table 17.3).

Essential tremor (ET) is often confused with PD when patients present with prominent tremor, although tremor in ET usually does not occur at rest. Bradykinesia, rigidity, postural instability, and other parkinsonian findings are absent in ET. Furthermore, ET often involves the head and responds to alcohol or β-blockers. Family history is not uncommon in ET.

Pathogenesis of Parkinson disease

The pathogenesis of PD remains unclear. It is likely to be a complex interaction between genetic and largely unidentified environmental factors. Most cases of PD are sporadic, but monogenic mutation (at least 10 genes on several chromosomes) can be found in rare, familial cases of PD. Both sporadic and familial cases may have a final common pathway of abnormal protein handling in the ubiquitin-proteasome system (UPS), and/or the impairment of the host defense to inflammation and oxidative stress, which subsequently leads to mitochondrial dysfunction and neuronal cell death in the substantia nigra. Among familial forms of PD, LRRK2 associated with parkinsonism (PARK8) displays phenotype similar to sporadic PD, while Parkin gene mutation (PARK2) is the most common recessive form. The frequency of LRRK2 mutation in all PD cases is approximately 2%. Patients with Parkin mutation usually present at earlier age of onset, more symmetrically with slow progression, and with better response to levodopa. Pathologic studies of the brains from most patients with Parkin mutation reveal the absence of Lewy bodies (pathologic hallmark in sporadic PD). Histologically, Lewy bodies are eosinophilic neuronal inclusions, most often found in the substantia nigra, but also present in the basal ganglia, cerebral cortex, and spinal cord. Lewy bodies consist of α-synuclein and other proteins, such as tau (; microtubule-associated protein seen in neurofibrillary tangles) and synphilin-1. Lewy body formation may represent an epiphenomenon, a direct neuronal toxicity from the protein aggregates, or it may result from impaired cellular segregation of cytotoxic proteins. -Synuclein is a major protein in Lewy bodies and is involved in maintaining the integrity of transmitter-laden vesicles and facilitating vesicular trans-

Table 17.2 Parkinsonism

	Discriminating features	Consistent features	Variable features
Idiopathic Parkinson disease	• Severe neuronal loss and depigmentation in the substantia nigra, corpus striatum, locus ceruleus; Lewy bodies at autopsy	• Asymmetric signs and symptoms at onset • Pronating-supinating 4–7 Hz tremor at rest, bradykinesia, rigidity, postural instability, gait difficulty, handwriting disturbance	• Depression • Dementia • Dysarthria • Drooling • Dysphagia • Hypophonia
Drug-induced parkinsonism	• History of exposure to neuroleptics, metoclopramide, reserpine, or tetrabenazine	• Extrapyramidal signs following drug exposure • Absence of significant resting tremor • Associated akathisia	• With chronic use of neuroleptics, predominance of tardive dyskinesia
Vascular parkinsonism	• History or neuroimaging evidence of multiple strokes	• Gait disturbance, pseudobulbar palsy, spasticity, hyperreflexia, extensor plantar responses	• Dementia • Rarely, tremor
Postencephalitic parkinsonism	• Neurofibrillary tangles and marked gliosis; absence of Lewy bodies at autopsy	• History of encephalitis (1917–1926) with high fever, delirium, or coma • Parkinsonian syndrome • Ophthalmoplegia	• Facial tics • Myoclonus • Oculogyric crises • Bizarre postures and gaits
Multiple system atrophy (Shy-Drager syndrome)	• Neuronal loss in central autonomic neurons, substantia nigra, caudate, locus ceruleus, dorsal motor nucleus of vagus, inferior olives, cerebellum, and lateral horns of spinal cord at autopsy	• Extrapyramidal signs • Orthostatic hypotension and syncope • Cerebellar signs • Pyramidal signs	• Reduced sweating • Iris atrophy • Bladder dysfunction • Amyotrophy
Striatonigral degeneration	• Marked degeneration of the striatum (especially putamen) rather than substantia nigra; absence of Lewy bodies at autopsy	• Similarity to Parkinson disease with greater degree of rigidity • Mild or absent tremor • Rapid course • Poor response to levodopa	• Corticobulbar and corticospinal signs
Progressive supranuclear palsy	• Atypical neurofibrillary tangles and neuronal degeneration in pons, dorsal midbrain, and globus pallidus at autopsy	• Pseudobulbar palsy, gait unsteadiness, and supranuclear ophthalmoplegia (especially vertical gaze) • Extrapyramidal rigidity, particularly in axial musculature	• Dementia, tremor, corticospinal and corticobulbar signs • Modest response to levodopa
Corticobasal ganglionic degeneration	• Enlarged achromatic neurons in cerebral cortex, particularly in frontal and parietal lobes; striatal and nigral neuronal degeneration at autopsy	• Unilateral at the onset with marked rigidity-dystonia on the involved arm • Cortical signs of apraxia, cortical sensory loss and alien limb phenomena	• Hesitant speech, gait disturbance and occasional action tremor
Parkinsonism-dementia-amyotrophic lateral sclerosis complex	• Chamorro population of Guam • Neurofibrillary tangles mainly in the substantia nigra, but also anterior horn cells and corticospinal tract at autopsy	• Parkinsonism with severe progressive dementia and motor neuron disease • Predominantly affects males	• Usually no response to anti-Parkinsonian medications • Motor neuron signs may be upper or lower in nature

Table 17.3 Causes of secondary parkinsonism

▶ Infectious: Infectious and postinfectious encephalitis, Creutzfeldt-Jakob disease, HIV, cryptococcosis

▶ Toxins: manganese, mercury, lead, carbon monoxide, carbon disulfide, cyanide, methanol, lithium, herbicides and ethanol withdrawal

▶ Drugs: phenothiazines, haloperidol, metoclopramide, reserpine, amiodarone, tetrabenazine, alpha-methyldopa, flunarizine

▶ Metabolic: hypoparathyroidism, hyperparathyroidism, chronic hepatocerebral degeneration, folate deficiency

▶ Degenerative: striatonigral degeneration, progressive supranuclear palsy, multiple system atrophy, corticobasal ganglionic degeneration, diffuse Lewy body disease, parkinsonism-dementia-amyotrophic lateral sclerosis complex, neuroacanthocytosis, Alzheimer disease

▶ Hereditary: Parkinsonism associated with monogenic mutations, olivopontocerebellar atrophy, Wilson disease, Huntington disease, Hallervorden-Spatz disease, neuronal ceroid lipofuscinosis, spinocerebellar ataxias

▶ Others: vascular (multi-infarct or lacunar state), brain tumors, trauma, syringobulbia, normal pressure hydrocephalus.

port from cell body to synapse. Dopaminergic neurons are selectively vulnerable to the toxic effects of -synuclein accumulation, providing a plausible link between the accumulation of protein and the topography of the lesions. Dopamine metabolism generates free oxygen radicals leading to cell injury and death. -Synuclein may lead to defective sequestration of dopamine into protective vesicles, leading to unmitigated oxidative injury. In addition, mitochondrial dysfunction, as occurs in the substantia nigra of some PD patients, may contribute to a reduction of protein degradation in the UPS, since it is an energy-dependent pathway. Advances in genomics, proteomics, and molecular cell biology technologies should facilitate the discovery of other genetic and environmental factors, which may subsequently lead to the development of novel neuroprotective therapies for this disorder.

Diagnosis of Parkinson disease

Idiopathic PD accounts for approximately 80% of parkinsonian patients. In this disorder, a detailed neurodiagnostic and metabolic evaluation fails to reveal any specific etiology. Although no laboratory test is available to confirm the diagnosis of PD, the presence of at least two cardinal signs, in combination with some other associated symptoms, is usually sufficient to make the diagnosis. In addition, a response to anti-parkinsonism medications is helpful as a therapeutic diagnosis of PD. The role of neuroimaging in the diagnosis of PD is limited, although it may show basal ganglia infarcts in patients with vascular parkinsonism. Functional imaging

studies such as functional magnetic resonance imaging (fMRI), single photon emission computed tomography (SPECT), and positron emission tomography (PET) are not confirmatory for this diagnosis, but the search for an imaging biologic marker is ongoing.

Treatment of Parkinson disease

Mortality among PD patients before the advent of levodopa in the 1960s was three times than expected. During that era, Hoehn and Yahr reported that 25% of patients after 5 years and 80% of patients after 15 years became severely disabled or died. With the development of levodopa, the overall mortality rate of PD (2.1% per year) is similar to that of an age- and gender-matched control population. At this time, oral levodopa is the single most effective treatment for PD. However, this agent is associated with motor fluctuation and dyskinesia with increased duration of therapy.

Pharmacologic treatment in Parkinson disease. As noted earlier, there is a marked deficiency of dopamine in PD resulting from a loss of dopaminergic neurons in the substantia nigra. These neurons normally synthesize dopamine from the essential amino acid tyrosine. The conversion of tyrosine to levodopa is facilitated by the rate-limiting enzyme tyrosine hydroxylase. Finally, levodopa is converted into dopamine by the nonspecific enzyme dopa decarboxylase.

Five subtypes of dopamine receptors exist; D_1 and D_2 receptors are most prominent in the striatum, whereas D_3, D_4, and D_5 receptors are present mainly in the cerebral hemispheres. The D_2 receptor is activated by dopamine as well as dopamine agonists. The differential role of D_1 and D_2 receptors in regulating striatal function has not been fully defined. D_1 receptors are preferentially distributed in striatum, giving rise to the direct pathway projecting to globus pallidus interna, whereas D_2 receptors are primarily localized in the indirect pathway projecting from the striatum to the globus pallidus externa (Figure 17.2). In the brains of patients with PD, D_1 receptors in the striatum are markedly reduced, whereas D_2 receptors are increased. This upregulation in D_2 receptors may result from striatal denervation supersensitivity in response to the nigrostriatal dopamine deficiency. Because of the supersensitivity, there is an increased responsiveness to dopamine agonists at dosages that would be ineffective in normal subjects.

Pharmacologic therapies in PD can be simply classified into two main categories (Table 17.4). A presynaptic strategy (levodopa/carbidopa, catechol-O-methyl transferase (COMT) inhibitors, monoamine oxidase-B (MAO-B) inhibitors, and amantadine) attempts to maintain physiologic nigrostriatal synaptic concentrations of dopamine. A postsynaptic strategy (pergolide, bromocriptine, pramipexole, ropinirole, cabergoline, and apomor-

Table 17.4 Pharmacologic treatment of parkinsonism

Medication	Mechanism of action	Dosage unit (mg)	Daily dosage
Presynaptic strategy			
Amantadine (Symmetrel)	Release of dopamine; anticholinergic	Capsules (100)	100–300
Carbidopa/levodopa/entacapone (Stalevo)	Dopamine precursor plus dopa decarboxylase and COMT inhibitor	Tablets 50 (12.5/50/200) 100 (25/100/200) 150 (37.5/150/200)	600–800 entacapone
Entacapone (Comtan)	Catechol-O-methyltransferase inhibitor	Tablets (200)	600–1600
Tolcapone (Tasmar)	Catechol-O-methyltransferase inhibitor	Tablets (100, 200)	300–600
Levodopa/carbidopa (Sinemet)	Dopamine precursor plus dopamine decarboxylase	Tablets (10/100, 25/100, 25/250; controlled release 25/100, 50/200)	75/500–200/2000
Selegiline (Eldepryl)	Monoamine oxidase-B inhibitor	Tablets (5)	5–10
Zydis Selegiline (Zelapar)	Monoamine oxidase-B inhibitor	Orally disintegrating tablet (1.25)	1.25-2.5
Rasagiline (Azilect)	Monoamine oxidase-B inhibitor	Tablets (0.5, 1)	1
Postsynaptic strategy			
Apomorphine (Apokyn)	Dopamine agonist	Subcutaneous (10 mg/ml)	2–6
Bromocriptine (Parlodel)	Dopamine agonist	Tablet (2.5)	5–10
Cabergoline (Dostinex)	Dopamine agonist	Tablets (0.5)	0.25–4
Pergolide (Permax)	Dopamine agonist	Tablets (0.05, 0.25, 1)	0.1–3
Pramipexole (Mirapex)	Dopamine agonist	Tablets (0.125, 0.25, 1, 1.5)	1.5–4.5
Ropinirole (Requip)	Dopamine agonist	Tablets (0.25, 0.5, 1, 2, 3, 4, 5)	9–24
Rotigotine (Neupro)	Dopamine agonist	Transdermal (2, 4, 6 mg/d)	2-6
Anticholinergic strategy			
Benztropine (Cogentin)	Anticholinergic	Tablets (0.5, 1, 2)	0.5–8
Trihexyphenidyl (Artane)	Anticholinergic	Tablets (2, 5)	2–20

phine) bypasses degenerating nigrostriatal neurons by stimulating striatal neurons directly. In addition, anticholinergics may play a role in modifying acetylcholine neurotransmission, which counteracts the dopaminergic transmission system.

Levodopa, a dopamine precursor, is converted to dopamine by the enzyme dopa-decarboxylase. This ubiquitous enzyme is present not only in the brain but also in the periphery. As a result of this peripheral action of dopa-decarboxylase, less than 1% of the administered levodopa is actually converted into dopamine in the brain. This peripheral dopamine activates the area postrema, which is not protected by the blood–brain barrier and is largely responsible for some of the side effects of levodopa (nausea, vomiting, and cardiac arrhythmia). *Carbidopa*, a dopa-decarboxylase inhibitor, does not cross the blood–brain barrier, and blocks the conversion of dopa to dopamine only in the periphery. Formulations of the levodopa/carbidopa are available in immediate-release and controlled-release (CR) formulations. Approximately 75–100 mg of carbidopa per day is needed for effective peripheral blockade. This lowers the incidence of gastrointestinal side effects, but psychiatric adverse reactions, such as confusion, delusions, and visual hallucinations may still occur, particularly in patients with

dementia. Dyskinesias, such as chorea, dystonia, or myoclonus, develop in 30% of patients after 3 years of levodopa therapy, and disabling motor fluctuations occur in as many as half of patients after 5 years of treatment. Many of these motor fluctuations may be correlated with plasma levodopa levels. A recent study utilizing an animal model of PD with levodopa-induced dyskinesia revealed an overexpression of D_3 receptors in the brains of MPTP-treated monkeys. Administration of a selective D_3 receptor partial agonist strongly attenuated the dyskinesia induced by levodopa without diminishing its therapeutic effect.

Patients with PD will notice "wearing-off" or end-of-dose deterioration in mobility, thought to result from reduced duration of clinical effectiveness of levodopa. For example, after several years of levodopa therapy, a patient may report only 1–3 hours of benefit, instead of 6 hours of "on-time" seen when this drug was initially begun. A typical patient may also notice dyskinesias or involuntary movements related to peak plasma levodopa levels ("peak-dose dyskinesia"). Treatment of these motor fluctuations is based on "smoothing out" the plasma concentration curves either by more frequent smaller doses of levodopa, conversion to the controlled-release form of levodopa, or adding a COMT or MAO-B inhibitor. Potential problems associated with conversion from immediate- to controlled-release carbidopa/levodopa relate to delayed intestinal absorption of this product and include delayed morning response, prolonged peak-dose dyskinesias, and development of late afternoon–early evening dyskinesias. Both the immediate- and controlled-release carbidopa/levodopa formulations maintained a similar level of control in PD after 5 years compared with baseline. In addition, the incidence of motor complications was not different between the two treatment groups. However, the controlled-release group was superior to the immediate-release group with regard to activities of daily living, a finding possibly explained by higher doses of levodopa in the controlled release group.

With advancing disease and prolonged levodopa and other anti-PD therapies, more complex motor fluctuations occur. These paroxysmal "off" periods and dyskinesias occur at times inconsistent with plasma levodopa levels, and may represent changes in the striatum. In these instances, a consistent levodopa regimen should be found, and other medicines such as dopamine agonists, amantadine, and selegiline should be considered. Levodopa-related dyskinesias and clinical fluctuations are the most serious and therapeutically the most challenging problems associated with chronic use of dopaminergic agents, and many movement disorder neurologists advise withholding levodopa until a patient develops significant physical, occupational, or social disability from the disease. However, data suggesting that levodopa may hasten the progression of the disease is controversial.

Amantadine (Symmetrel) 100–300 mg/day may be useful in the PD patients with dyskinesia and wearing-off phenomenon. It is an antiviral medication with anticholinergic efficacy and may increase dopamine release, block dopamine uptake, and stimulate dopamine receptors. Side effects are similar to those of anticholinergic medications, but it may also cause ankle edema and livedo reticularis at higher doses.

The MAO-B inhibitors *selegiline* was reported in 1987 to delay the need for levodopa use and, perhaps, delay the progression of PD. The large multicenter DATATOP (Deprenyl and Tocopherol Antioxidative Trial of PD) trial used a "time to reach the disease milestone" (i.e., need for levodopa) end-point in untreated PD patients as the primary outcome measure. Statistical analysis suggested that selegiline delayed PD progression. However, because of the long half-life of this drug, its symptomatic effect, and the timing of subject exit evaluations, these data remain difficult to interpret. In a follow-up analysis of DATATOP subjects reaching the primary end-point of requiring levodopa treatment, individuals who had been treated with selegiline demonstrated less progression on the Unified Parkinson Disease Rating Score (UPDRS) and less freezing of gait, but more dyskinesias. Although the "neuroprotective" benefit of selegiline remains controversial, this agent may be clinically useful in PD patients with early gait difficulty, daytime sleepiness, or levodopa addiction. Conventional oral selegiline may be potentially harmful due to its amphetamine metabolites, although metabolite concentrations are significantly lower with a new orally disintegrating tablet (ODT) selegiline formulation. Selegiline ODT (Zydis selegiline, Zelapar) is also absorbed more efficiently and shows less pharmacokinetic variability than conventional oral selegiline. Rasagiline (Azilect) is a novel, second-generation, oral MAO-B inhibitor approved for use as monotherapy and as adjunctive therapy in the treatment of PD. It is well-tolerated and convenient, with once daily dosage. A recent study in early PD subjects using a delayed-start design demonstrated less functional decline in patients whose rasagiline treatment was not delayed. Therefore, rasagiline may have a disease-modifying effect in addition to symptomatic relief. A large-scale, randomized study to confirm this finding is going.

COMT inhibitors are the newest agents in a presynaptic strategy for PD treatment. The use of tolcapone (Tasmar), the first COMT inhibitor marketed in the

---

▼

Pearls and Perils

Hypokinetic movement disorders

▶ Resting tremor is more common in idiopathic Parkinson disease (PD).

▶ Essential tremor (ET) is manifested as an action tremor, but is sometimes misinterpreted as the resting tremor of PD.

▶ Idiopathic PD usually presents with unilateral/asymmetric clinical signs and symptoms.

▶ Brisk levodopa response is more common in idiopathic PD.

▶ Eye movement difficulty is seen in progressive supranuclear palsy.

▶ Apraxia, cortical sensory loss or a patient demonstrating a tendency to hold or rub the more affected limb with the "good hand" suggests corticobasal ganglionic degeneration.

▶ Incontinence, impotence, and orthostatic hypotension are common in multiple system atrophy.

▶ Simultaneous onset of dementia with parkinsonism may suggest Alzheimer disease with parkinsonism, dementia with Lewy bodies, multi-infarct dementia, or frontotemporal dementia.

▶ Lower-body parkinsonism usually suggests normal pressure hydrocephalus (NPH), vascular parkinsonism, or primary gait disorders.

▶ Drugs causing parkinsonian symptoms include anti-emetics, major tranquilizers, α-methyldopa, reserpine, and others.

United States for PD, has been severely restricted by reports of fatal hepatotoxicity. Entacapone (Comtan), however, does not appear to have significant effects on liver functioning and is given in combination with levodopa..It is also now available in a triple combination tablet with levodopa and carbidopa (Stalevo). Entacapone does not cross the blood–brain barrier but acts peripherally to limit metabolism of levodopa. Both of these agents inhibit the COMT enzyme branch of dopamine metabolism, permitting additional levodopa to reach the brain. Several clinical trials have shown consistent benefits of COMT inhibitors in improving motor scores, increasing "on" time, decreasing "off" time, and allowing for an approximately 20% reduction in levodopa dosage. Side effects of entacapone include nausea, vomiting, diarrhea, dyskinesia, urine discoloration, abdominal discomfort, dizziness, somnolence, anxiety, and mood changes.

Dopamine agonists are the most commonly used drugs in a postsynaptic strategy. Dopamine agonists are available in oral, subcutaneous, and transdermal formulations. Recent evidence suggests that the early use of a dopamine agonist is associated with a lower incidence of motor complications than levodopa. However, the long-term impact of delaying dyskinesias in the early years on quality of life is unclear. Bromocriptine, pergolide, pramipexole, ropinirole, subcutaneous apomorphine, and transdermal rotigotine are among the dopamine agonists commonly used in clinical practice as either monotherapy or in combination with levodopa. Studies using functional neuroimaging to monitor dopaminergic neuronal activity in patients given dopamine agonist versus levodopa suggest a reduced loss of uptake in the striatum for dopamine agonist as compared to levodopa. However, differential metabolic changes induced by dopamine on regulation of the dopamine transporter and the concomitant use of supplemental levodopa and other agents, such as selegiline, in some trials, are cited as confounding issues by some, making these data difficult to interpret with regard to the possible neuroprotective benefits of dopamine agonists. Side effects of dopamine agonists include excessive daytime somnolence, peripheral edema, weight gain, impulse dyscontrol behaviors, such as compulsive eating or gambling, and, rarely, sleep attacks. In addition, ergot-derived dopamine agonists such as pergolide and cabergoline (available in Europe) are associated with an increased risk of developing cardiac valvulopathy. Apomorphine, a dopamine agonist in the form of subcutaneous injection, may be used as a "rescue" therapy for off-episodes that occur despite optimized oral therapy. Patients typically benefit within 10–20 minutes after administration, and the effect may last as long as 90 minutes.

Other symptomatic treatments for PD patients include modafinil and amantadine for fatigue, clonazepam for REM-sleep behavior disorder, midodrine and fludrocortisone for orthostatic hypotension, and botulinum toxin injection for excessive salivation. Atypical antipsychotics, such as clozapine (12.5–50 mg/day) and quetiapine (12.5–400 mg/day), with less extrapyramidal side effects, treat symptoms of psychosis, insomnia, and hallucination without worsening PD symptoms. Finally, tricyclics or selective serotonin reuptake inhibitors are important in treating depression.

Surgical treatment of Parkinson disease. When pharmacologic treatments fail to control the motor symptoms of PD, surgical treatment may be an alternative option. Surgical treatments for PD consist of ablative procedures (thalamotomy, pallidotomy, and subthalamotomy) and deep brain stimulation (DBS) in the thalamus, globus pallidus interna (GPi), and subthalamic nucleus (STN). Thalamotomy, lesioning of the ventralis intermedius (VIM) nucleus, is an effective treatment for parkinsonian tremor, but does not influence bradykinesia, freezing, postural instability, or gait disturbances associated with PD. Bilateral thalamotomy is associated with significant speech dysfunction including aphasia, dysarthria, and dysphonia, and is not recommended as the first-line surgical treatment unless alternative approaches such as DBS are contraindicated. Bilateral pallidotomy provides improvement of all cardinal symptoms of PD, but the benefits are variable among clinical studies, being largely dependent on patient selection and the exact location of globus pallidus lesions. The procedure may be associated with speech complications and is effective for only a limited time, usually less than 5 years. Therefore, it is usually not recommended for medically refractory PD patients if DBS is available. Unilateral subthalamotomy was recently reported to be effective for patients with asymmetrical tremor-dominant advanced PD. Deep brain stimulation in the GPi or the STN are relatively safe and effective in controlling motor and gait disturbances in PD, particularly when placed bilaterally. Although there have been no large comparative studies, DBS in the STN is preferable to sites in the GPi. In addition, bilateral DBS in STN has been shown to decrease the required dose of antiparkinsonian medications and improve quality of life at 6 months after operation. A variety of neuropsychiatric symptoms may develop following the STN DBS, thus addressing the importance of preoperative and postoperative neuropsychiatric assessment and intervention. Because of the relatively minor complications from DBS, it is generally considered the first-line surgical therapy for advanced PD with disabling motor fluctuations and dyskinesias in most movement disorder centers in the United States. Other potential targets for DBS may include pedunculopontine nucleus (PPN) in PD patients with ambulatory difficulty.

Novel therapies in Parkinson disease. Although treatment with levodopa results in marked symptomatic improvement, mortality rates of PD have remained relatively unchanged. Recent findings of abnormal protein handling, coupled with mitochondrial dysfunction and oxidative stress, provide a scientific rationale for novel therapeutic strategies to slow disease progression. To be effective, these disease-modifying and neuroprotective therapies must be instituted early in the course of the disease. Early diagnosis and carefully designed clinical trials are therefore critically important. Among antioxidants, creatine and minocycline have been shown to be effective in several animal models of neurodegenerative diseases and are currently being evaluated in clinical trials in PD patients. Similarly, coenzyme Q10 is also effective in animal models and has shown promising effects in human clinical trials of PD as well as Huntington disease. An NIH-sponsored large clinical trial of coenzyme Q10 in PD patients is ongoing. A glial-derived neurotrophic factor (GDNF) administered by intracerebroventricular infusion did not improve parkinsonism in a recent clinical trial, possibly because the GDNF did not reach the target tissues in putamen and substantia nigra. A multicentered clinical trial of intraputaminal GDNF infusion in PD patients has also failed to show clinical benefits. CEP-1347, a novel mixed-lineage kinase (MLK) inhibitor, has recently failed to demonstrated benefit in PD patients. Riluzole, a glutamate release inhibitor, has failed to demonstrate evidence of neuroprotection in a large PD clinical trial. Novel NMDA antagonists such as CP101,606; adenosine 2A antagonists, such as istradefylline (KW-6002); and stem cell transplantation are among other candidates for novel treatments in PD.

Hyperkinetic Movement Disorders

Essential Tremor

Essential tremor is the most common movement disorder, but many affected patients do not seek medical attention. Although central mechanisms are suspected, no specific abnormality is noted in the brains of patients with ET. A recent pathologic study revealed heterogeneous abnormalities with pathology in cerebellum (76%) and Lewy bodies in brainstem (24%). Patients with Lewy bodies in brainstem seem to have a distinct clinical phenotype; however, further larger studies are required. Essential tremor may occur as an autosomal dominant disorder with variable penetrance, sporadically, or in association with various neurologic disorders, including idiopathic torsion dystonia and certain inherited peripheral neuropathies (for example, Charcot-Marie-Tooth disease). Essential tremor has prominent postural (present during maintenance of a position) tremor and action/kinetic tremor. The tremor in ET is typically a flexion–extension movement, whereas pronation–supination oscillation is more characteristic of PD. Essential tremor is of faster frequency (6–12 Hz) than PD tremor (4–7 Hz) and, when fully developed, usually involves the head, neck, jaw, and voice. Furthermore, ET patients do not have parkinsonian features such as hypomimia, shuffling gait, lack of arm-swing, or rigidity, although mild cogwheeling may be present. This action and postural tremor often interferes with handwriting, holding a spoon, using a drinking cup, and manipulating utensils and tools. It is exacerbated during voluntary movement, emotional and physical stress, and diminishes with rest or ethyl alcohol. Essential tremor should be differentiated from other action tremors such as accentuated physiologic tremor seen in anxiety, thyrotoxicosis, alcohol withdrawal, and as a result of taking certain drugs including bronchodilators (β_2-agonists), various CNS stimulants, lithium, and sodium valproate (Box 17.1). Cerebellar kinetic (intention) tremor is most apparent during a goal-directed limb movement such as finger-to-nose and heel-to-shin test. It is usually caused by a lesion in the cerebellar outflow tracts. However, approximately 25% of patients with ET also have intention tremor, which may implicate cerebellar dysfunction in this condition.

The mainstay of treatment for ET is -blockers and primidone (Mysoline), but only about half of patients respond, and the average benefit is only about 50%. Some patients have shown benefit with benzodiazepines, acetazolamide, gabapentin, pregabalin, quetiapine, and levetiracetam. Two randomized controlled studies have confirmed a significant benefit in tremor reduction and functional improvement of topiramate in patients with ET. Injection of botulinum toxin directly into the muscles results in improvement of postural but not kinetic tremor. It also causes significant dose-dependent weakness of the injected muscles. In medically intractable cases, surgical procedures such as DBS in the VIM of thalamus or thalamotomy may produce remarkably gratifying and sustained (>5 years) benefit. One mechanism of DBS-mediated attenuation of tremor may be through activation of adenosine A_1 receptor. Transcranial magnetic stimulation over the cerebellum may provide benefit in some patients with ET.

Huntington Disease

Gradual onset of chorea, dementia, and behavioral abnormalities in a young adult should suggest the possibility of Huntington disease (HD). George Huntington first described this hereditary chorea in 1872. Huntington disease is the most common inherited form of chorea and is transmitted in an autosomal dominant pattern caused by an expansion of unstable trinucleotide (CAG)/polyglutamine (polyQ) of the gene on chromosome 4 encoding the Huntingtin protein. It has the highest prevalence rates in the region of Lake Maracaibo in Venezuela and the Moray Firth region of Scotland, and is relatively rare in

Asia and among African blacks. Initially, the patient may develop facial twitching and grimacing, shrugging of the shoulders, twitching of the fingers ("piano-playing movements"), slight twisting of the trunk, or an extra step or kick when walking. These involuntary movements may be confused with simple restlessness, but with time, the movements become typically choreatic involving the trunk, as well as proximal and distal limbs. The average age of onset is in late 30s or early 40s. In the juvenile form of HD, rigidity, bradykinesia, dystonic postures, ataxia, seizures, pyramidal tract dysfunction, and mental retardation may be the presenting features instead of chorea. This akinetic-rigid form (Westphal variant) is seen most often during the first or second decade of life. This is usually caused by inheritance of the pathogenic gene through the father, as a result of a phenomenon called *anticipation*. In these instances, the triplet repeats become amplified during spermatogenesis via an unknown mechanism. These juvenile HD patients usually have more than 55 CAG repeats. In approximately 85% of patients, regardless of age, chorea is the predominant movement disorder, and in the remaining 10–15% of patients, the motor disorder is characterized by bradykinesia, rigidity, and resting tremor. These parkinsonian features are typically found in the juvenile variant and in the advance stages of HD. In the terminal stage of HD, dysarthria, dysphagia, and respiratory difficulties become the most disabling and life-threatening problems.

Widespread disruption of cognitive functioning results in memory disorder, inability to concentrate, confusion, and forgetfulness. Unlike Alzheimer dementia, the HD patients retain language function and some insight into their illness. This awareness of progressive mental and physical deterioration may contribute to various emotional disturbances, usually in the form of depression. Suicide is a frequent cause of death in HD. Besides depression, other psychiatric disturbances include paranoia, hallucinations, and other delusional and psychotic symptoms.

Pathogenesis

Pathologic changes in the brains of HD patients include generalized atrophy with neuronal degeneration in the cortex and severe loss of small interneurons in the corpus striatum. Marked atrophy of caudate is the pathologic hallmark of HD and can be detected in coronal sections of affected brain on MRI or CT scans. In 1997, Huntingtin (polyQ) aggregates were first found in the brains of HD patients in the form of nuclear inclusions and dystrophic neurites. Since their discovery, the proposed role of polyQ aggregates has remained unclear—ranging from being central to the pathogenesis (toxic gain), a benign epiphenomenon, or even possibly neuroprotective. Wild-type (normal) Huntingtin is necessary for developing and sustaining normal brain function. However, mutant Huntingtin, along with a favorable cellular environment, is associated with

formation of aggregates and neuronal dysfunction and death (particularly in the striatum), via transcriptional dysregulation, proteosome impairment, mitochondrial dysfunction, oxidative damage, disrupted axonal transport, and excitotoxicity. Inhibition of polyQ aggregation has demonstrated benefit in a mouse model of HD. High-throughput screens using in vitro and cell culture assays have been employed to identify compounds that will interfere with the aggregation process. As more of the molecular events in early stages of HD are uncovered, they too will likely serve as potential new therapeutic targets.

Genetic aspects

The development of typical HD features in the setting of a positive family history warrants genetic testing to confirm the diagnosis. Less than 35 CAG repeats is considered normal, whereas 35–39 repeats is associated with an increased risk of developing disease with variable penetrance, and repeats of 40 or more are always associated with disease. The age of onset is inversely correlated with the number of CAG repeats, whereas the relationship between the repeat length and the rate of progression remains unclear. Presymptomatic testing allows at-risk individuals to make informed choices, but requires skilled genetic counseling and supportive care from physicians. In addition, physicians and genetic counselors should always review the potential for a person undergoing genetic testing to experience genetic discrimination, particularly with regard to employment or insurance (Table 17.5).

Differential diagnosis

Besides HD, other less common hereditary choreas include benign familial chorea, paroxysmal choreoathetosis, and neuroacanthocytosis. *Paroxysmal choreoathetosis* is a form of paroxysmal dyskinesia that is manifested by sudden onset of transient choreoathetosis, dystonia, or both (paroxysmal dystonic choreoathetosis). Paroxysmal dyskinesias are subdivided into kinesigenic and nonkinesigenic, depending on whether or not they are induced by sudden movements. In familial (autosomal dominant) kinesigenic paroxysmal choreoathetosis, the episodes are brief (<3 minutes) and occur many times per day (up to 100 times per day), the age of onset is 5–15 years, and the disorder is four times more common in men. This form of paroxysmal dyskinesia may occur as a sporadic or acquired disorder (lesions of premotor cortex or basal ganglia, multiple sclerosis, hypocalcemia). Both familial and sporadic kinesigenic dyskinesias respond well to anticonvulsant medications such as phenytoin, carbamazepine, and phenobarbital. When the attacks are more prolonged (2 minutes to 4 hours), less frequent (three per day), and more dystonic, the disorder is classified as paroxysmal (nonkinesigenic) dystonic choreoathetosis. This is an autosomal dominant disorder with the age of onset as early as infancy. The nonkinesigenic disorder is

Table 17.5 Other movement disorders

	Discriminating features	Consistent features	Variable features
Essential tremor	• Family history (autosomal dominant)	• Action tremor (sustention) relieved by alcohol and propranolol • Onset in second to fourth decade • Resistance to levodopa • Absence of bradykinesia, postural instability, rigidity	• Head and voice involvement
Creutzfeldt-Jakob disease	• Spongiform degeneration of cortex and basal ganglia • Transmissibility	• Subacute progressive course • Dementia, behavioral abnormalities, stimulus-sensitive myoclonus, extrapyramidal signs, and cerebellar dysfunction • Presence of protein 14-3-3 in cerebrospinal fluid	• Amyotrophy, cortical blindness, seizures • 1 Hz periodic discharges on EEG
Huntington disease	• Marked caudate and cortical atrophy • Depletion of small neurons and glia in striatum • Family history (autosomal dominant) • Positive genetic testing	• Chorea, dementia, and psychiatric disturbances (especially depression) • Dysarthria and dysphagia in terminal phase	• Rigid-akinetic form (Westphal variant) in children and young adults
Hallervorden-Spatz disease	• Brown discoloration of the globus pallidus and zona reticulata of substantia nigra	• Juvenile onset, rigidity, stiffness of gait with toe walking, risus sardonicus, anarthria	• Dementia, dystonic posturing, optic atrophy • "Eye of the tiger" sign on brain MRI
Wilson disease	• Hepatic dysfunction, high hepatic content of copper, low serum ceruloplasmin • Kayser-Fleischer ring	• Abnormal movements including rigidity, facial and generalized dystonia, "wing-beating" tremor	• Dementia, behavioral changes, seizures
Olivopontocerebellar atrophy	• Neuronal degeneration in the inferior olives, pons, and cerebellum • Involvement of spinocerebellar and corticospinal tracts, posterior columns, substantia nigra, and basal ganglia	• Progressive cerebellar ataxia, gait impairment, nystagmus, dysarthria, dysphagia, extrapyramidal signs, sphincter dysfunction	• Loss of deep tendon reflexes, extensor plantar responses, mild dementia • Familial inheritance

not precipitated by sudden movement, but by alcohol, coffee, fatigue, stress, or excitement. The treatment of choice is clonazepam or oxazepam rather than other anticonvulsants.

Neuroacanthocytosis is another rare choreiform disorder and is often accompanied by motor and vocal tics, mood disorders, and self-mutilating behavior. Dystonia and chorea involving orofaciolingual structures are the striking features. In addition, sensorimotor neuropathy is also common. The hallmark of the disorder is the presence of acanthocytes on peripheral blood smear. This disorder has been reported in several families, suggesting autosomal dominant or recessive inheritances.

Other neurodegenerative diseases that share the same pathogenesis of polyQ aggregate diseases and may be confused with HD include dentatorubropallidoluysian atrophy and spinocerebellar ataxia type 1, 2, 3, 6, 7, and 17. If family history for the choreatic or psychiatric disorder is lacking, then the following disorders should be considered: senile chorea, TD, CNS vasculitis, subdural hematoma, Wilson disease (WD), neurodegeneration with brain iron accumulation (Hallervorden–Spatz disease; pantothenate kinase associated-neurodegeneration), Sydenham chorea, antiphospholipid antibody syndrome, Creutzfeldt-Jakob disease, paraneo-plastic syndrome, and various toxic and metabolic disorders. The specific toxins causing chorea include oral contraceptives, levodopa, CNS stimulants, neuroleptics, phenytoin, carbamazepine, ethosuximide, and other drugs. Metabolic-endocrine disorders associated with chorea include chorea gravidarum, thyrotoxicosis, hypoparathyroidism, hypernatremia, Addison disease, chronic hepatocerebral degeneration, and others.

Treatment

Pharmacologic manipulation of the cholinergic, dopaminergic, and GABA-ergic systems can alter some symptoms of HD. Dopamine receptor blocking agents (e.g., haloperidol, risperidone, olanzapine, etc.) and dopamine depleting agents (e.g., tetrabenazine) reduce the choreatic movements, but usually do not improve other HD symptoms. Because of potentially serious side effects, including TD and depression, the dopamine blocking drugs should be reserved only for patients with disabling chorea. Amantadine has been shown to be ineffective in HD. Bilateral GPi DBS can improve chorea.

In many patients with HD, depression is more disabling than the chorea. The tricyclic antidepressants and selective serotonin reuptake inhibitors (SSRI) are often helpful in ameliorating the affective disorders. HD results in progressive functional decline and eventual death, usually within 12–15 years of onset. The importance of psychological support, genetic counseling, and long-term planning cannot be overemphasized.

Several clinical trials of putative neuroprotective agents for HD have been carried out recently. A 3-year, randomized controlled study of riluzole in HD patients, revealed no neuroprotective or symptomatic benefits. Vitamin E, a free radical scavenger, and idebenone, a booster of energy metabolism, were not effective. A two-by-two factorial study of coenzyme Q10 and remacemide had no significant effect on disease progression. Apoptosis-modulating agents such as minocycline and creatine were ineffective. Future therapies may involve targeting mutant Huntingtin with small-molecule inhibitors or small-interfering RNA (siRNA). Fetal cell transplantation to the striatum of HD patients was feasible; however, the effects on symptoms and disease progression are not certain.

Dystonia

Dystonia is defined as a sustained, involuntary contraction of muscles, producing an abnormal posture. Because of the characteristic twisting nature of dystonia, the term torsion dystonia has recently been suggested to replace the traditional designation "dystonia musculorum deformans" originally coined by Oppenheim in 1911. The term idiopathic torsion dystonia (ITD) is preferred, since the disorder is not due to muscle abnormality as implied by the word "musculorum," and not all patients with this disorder progress to deformities, as suggested by the word "deformans." At onset, generalized dystonia patients may manifest only transient inversion of the foot, writer's cramp, flexion at the wrist, or dystonic spasms during certain activities. In a recent epidemiologic study in Iceland, the prevalence of all types of dystonia was 37 per 100,000 persons, with cervical dystonia being the most frequent form, followed by limb dystonia, laryngeal dystonia, blepharospasm, and oromandibular dystonia.

Dystonia may be generalized (legs plus other parts of the body), segmental (multifocal), focal, or unilateral. Adult-onset torsion dystonia is usually sporadic and proximal in distribution (for example, torticollis). Distal dystonia, on the other hand, is often seen in children and adolescents, commonly inherited, and usually generalized in distribution. Cranial dystonia (for example, Meige syndrome: blepharospasm and oromandibular dystonia), cervical dystonia (torticollis, anterocollis, or retrocollis), and focal action dystonias (writer's cramp) represent useful terms in categorizing the location of these abnormal involuntary movements. Patients often learn that certain postures or "sensory tricks," such as a counter pressure by a hand against the chin in torticollis, lessen the dystonia. Unilateral dystonia (hemidystonia) is usually associated with a structural lesion in the contralateral striatum, such as an infarction, porencephalic cyst, arteriovenous malformation, or posttraumatic encephalomalacia. In contrast to hemidystonia, the other forms of dystonia are usually idiopathic. When fixed dystonic postures, rather than the more typical mobile dystonia are present, posttraumatic or psychogenic dystonia should be suspected.

Diagnosis of dystonia

The diagnosis of primary dystonia can be made only if there is no other neurologic dysfunction (for example, cognitive, pyramidal, sensory, or cerebellar deficits) and after eliminating secondary causes of dystonia. At the initial evaluation, data pertaining to age of onset; initial and subsequent areas of involvement; course and progression; family history of dystonia, tremor, or other movement disorders; possible birth injury, achievement of developmental milestones; exposure to neuroleptic medications; consanguinity; or Jewish ancestry should be obtained (Table 17.6). The clinical expression of primary dystonia is highly variable even within families, with some patients demonstrating severe problems and requiring extensive assistance in activities of daily living, whereas others exhibit only mild symptoms (for example, foot dystonia or writer's cramp).

Although no consistent structural or biochemical abnormality associated with primary dystonia has been found, the importance of genetic etiology has long been recognized. DYT1 is the most common type of genetically determined dystonia, with a single GAG deletion on the DYT1 (TOR1A) gene encoding torsinA protein. It is inherited in an autosomal dominant pattern with 30–40% penetrance and accounts for approximately 90% of primary dystonia in Ashkenazi Jews. Several other important primary dystonia loci have been mapped to date, associated with gene mutations on chromosomes 8, 18, and 1.

One type of inherited dystonia that deserves special emphasis is dopa-responsive dystonia (DRD), designated as DYT5. It is an autosomal dominant, childhood-onset dystonia that is linked to a locus on chromosome 14. One review of 66 patients found that 76% had diurnal fluctuation, with gait disturbance or abnormal lower extremity posturing occurring particularly in the late afternoon. This disorder is more common in girls (2.5:1), and is frequently associated with parkinsonian features. Therefore, it may be difficult to differentiate this condition from juvenile PD. Most patients report a dramatic improvement with levodopa. Maximum benefit occurs within several days of levodopa therapy and, when combined with a dopa-decarboxylase inhibitor (carbidopa), patients may be maintained on as little as 50 mg/day. Familial myoclonus-dystonia is an autosomal dominant disorder that has genetic heterogeneity and has been associated with mutations of genes on chromosomes 7, 9, 11, and 18. It is characterized by the early onset of dystonia or startle-insensitive myoclonus, normal lifespan; no evidence of seizures, cognitive disability, ataxia, or other neurological deficits; and a dramatic response to alcohol. Most patients report benefit from benzodiazepine therapy. Some of these patients developed associated psychiatric symptoms such as depression, obsessive-compulsive disorder, and alcohol dependence.

When there are other abnormal neurologic findings in addition to dystonia, "secondary dystonias" caused by specific or structural abnormalities should be considered. Of all secondary dystonias, WD is the most common cause, hence underscoring the importance of investigations to rule out this disease. Other secondary dystonias may include drug-induced dystonia (acute dystonic reaction and tardive dystonia), peripherally induced dystonia, reflex sympathetic dystrophy, and neurodegenerative disorders such as neurodegeneration with brain iron accumulation; spinocerebellar ataxias type 3, 6, 16, 17; DRPLA; and recessive ataxias such as Friedreich ataxia, ataxia telangiectasia.

Pathogenesis

The pathophysiology of dystonia is not well understood. Excessive co-contraction of antagonist muscles is one of the pathophysiologic hallmarks of dystonia. Spinal and brainstem reflex abnormalities, including reduced reciprocal inhibition and prolonged stretch reflexes, are also present. Several recent data suggest that dystonia is caused by a functional disturbance of the basal ganglia, particularly in the striatal control of the globus pallidus, coupled with abnormalities of sensorimotor integration at cerebral cortex. These findings suggest that dystonic muscle contraction is associated with changes in the rate and pattern of neuronal firing, somatosensory responsiveness and, perhaps, hypersynchronization of neuronal

---

Table 17.6 Evaluation of dystonia

History:
- Birth injury
- Hypoxic injury
- Head/neck trauma
- Encephalitis
- Prior exposure to dopamine receptor blocking drugs (neuroleptics) and toxins
- Family history of dystonia, tremor or degenerative disorders

Blood studies:
- Ceruloplasmin
- Copper
- Complete blood count
- Erythrocyte sedimentation rate
- Antinuclear antibody
- Protein electrophoresis
- Biochemistry profile
- Arterial blood gas
- Metabolic screen, lactate, pyruvate

Urine for organic acids, oligosaccharides, amino acids
Serum for acanthocytes, amino acids
Magnetic resonance imaging
Electroencephalogram
Muscle biopsy
Psychometric testing

activity. As a result, there is altered thalamic control of cortical motor planning and executive areas, in addition to abnormal regulation of brainstem and spinal cord inhibitory interneuronal mechanisms.

Treatment

Anticholinergic therapy has been found to be effective in ameliorating dystonia, particularly in younger patients. Anticholinergic agents, such as trihexyphenidyl, when slowly increased over a period of weeks or months up to 25 mg/day, may be effective and safe. However, many patients are unable to tolerate such high dosages because of memory difficulties, hallucinations, blurring of vision, and other anticholinergic side effects. Other agents such as benzodiazepines, carbamazepine, tizanidine, and cyclobenzaprine have demonstrated benefit in some dystonic patients. Baclofen may be particularly useful for patients with oromandibular dystonia, whereas tetrabenazine is often beneficial in patients with tardive dystonia. In addition, all childhood-onset dystonia patients deserve a trial of levodopa. Intrathecal baclofen provides symptomatic benefit only in some patients who fail oral therapy.

Intramuscular injection of botulinum toxin A (Botox or Dysport) or botulinum toxin B (Myobloc) is the most effective treatment for focal dystonia, and may be used in a limited setting in patients with generalized dystonia. Acting at the presynaptic membrane, these potent neurotoxins prevent release of acetylcholine at the nerve terminal, thereby causing muscle weakness. Injection into dystonic muscles requires knowledge of muscle anatomy and the site of muscle innervation. Delivery of botulinum toxin through intramuscular injection may be enhanced with electromyographic guidance, but results are dependent on the experience of the injector. To maintain responsiveness to the toxin over repeated injections, use of the lowest dose at the longest dosing interval has been suggested. Treatments are necessary every 3–4 months in most patients, and this therapy has been used safely in some patients for more than 20 years. Resistance to toxins by neutralizing antibodies has been reported. If patients develop clinical resistance to one type of botulinum toxin, the other type may be still effective.

Deep brain stimulation at the internal segment of globus pallidus is effective in primary dystonia (particularly in DYT1 dystonia), myoclonus-dystonia syndrome, and complex cervical dystonia. The outcome of DBS in secondary dystonia is variable. The benefit from DBS in primary dystonia has been reported for at least 3 years. Long-term studies are in progress to assess both motor and neuropsychological sequelae of DBS in dystonia.

Wilson Disease

Wilson disease is one potentially curable form of dystonia. Westphal and Strümpell first described cases of progressive neurologic disease with liver cirrhosis in the 1880s. However, it was S.A.K. Wilson who reported a series of 12 cases of progressive hepatolenticular degeneration in 1912. Approximately 40% of patients with WD initially present with neurologic manifestations. Wilson disease is an autosomal recessive disorder of copper metabolism with onset in children and young adolescents, although symptoms may not become clinically evident until the fourth or fifth decade of life. In children, the characteristic features are facial and generalized dystonia, rigidity, postural instability, dysarthria, drooling, sardonic facial grin, seizures, cerebellar incoordination, tremor, behavioral changes, deterioration in school performance, and evidence of hepatic dysfunction. An adult patient may present with akinetic rigid parkinsonian features, dystonic choreoathetosis, and violent postural tremor, which is characteristically seen when the arms are abducted at the shoulder and flexed at the elbow ("wing-beating" position). The combination of tremor (postural, intention, or resting) and dystonia is present in almost all patients with WD. In contrast to the juvenile form, neurologic symptoms predominate over hepatic dysfunction in the adult variety, and the disorder appears to be less rapidly progressive.

The clinical hallmark of the disorder is the presence of a brownish yellow ring at the corneal rim (Kayser-Fleischer ring), which is due to deposition of copper in the cornea. A slit lamp examination is often necessary to identify this subtle finding. Although almost a pathognomonic sign of WD, the Kayser-Fleischer ring can also be seen with silver intoxication, primary biliary cirrhosis, Addison disease, carotinemia, and chalcosis as a result of unilateral trauma to the eye with copper-containing foreign bodies. Other ocular abnormalities seen in WD include "sunflower" subcapsular cataracts, retinitis pigmentosa, optic nerve atrophy, and impairment of smooth pursuit eye movements.

The diagnosis of WD still depends primarily on the evaluation of clinical and laboratory indices of copper metabolism. Laboratory studies reveal decreased serum ceruloplasmin (less than 20/dL) and increased 24-hour urinary copper excretion (more than 100 µg/24 hours). In WD patients with signs and symptoms only of hepatic dysfunction, liver biopsy may reveal hepatic copper concentrations of more than 100 µg/gm of dry liver. Brain MRI may show signal abnormalities on proton density and T2-weighted images in bilateral putamina and the mesencephalon ("face of giant panda" sign).

Pathogenesis

Wilson disease is due to an inherited defect in copper excretion into the bile by the liver. Several mutations of the ATP7B copper-transporting ATPase gene on chromosome 13q14.3 have been discovered, indicating genetic heterogeneity of WD. It is postulated that most of the symptoms result from failure of copper excretion into bile, which leads to excess deposition of copper in tissues, particularly in the liver and the brain. Brain SPECT study in WD patients showed severe loss of the dopamine transporter (DAT) in the striatum, suggesting significant damage to presynaptic nigrostriatal dopaminergic nerve terminals. Therefore, a presynaptic lesion may contribute to neurological manifestations in WD. One recent study suggests that mitochondrial defects may be important in WD pathogenesis. Interestingly, an individual's apolipoprotein E status may be an important factor in delaying the onset of neurologic and hepatic symptoms.

Treatment

Early treatment usually results in a good recovery of hepatic and neurologic function. The goal of therapy is to reduce copper intake through a low-copper diet and increased copper excretion. D-penicillamine is the agent most often used for acute chelating therapy in WD, however, side effects are potentially serious, including nephrotic syndrome, fever, thrombocytopenia, lymphadenopathy, dermatitis, vitamin B6 deficiency, seizures, and zinc deficiency, causing impairment of taste and smell. Trientine (triethylene tetramine dihydrochloride), an avid copper chelating agent, may be considered in patients who cannot tolerate D-penicillamine. Recent data suggest using tetrathiomolybdate for initial chelation followed by maintenance therapy with zinc sulfate in WD patients with only neurologic manifestations. Only 4% of patients treated with tetrathiomolybdate showed initial neurologic deterioration, compared with an estimated 50% of penicillamine-treated patients. Furthermore, a recent randomized controlled study of zinc in combination with either tetrathiomolybdate or trientine, demonstrated similar efficacy but more side effects with trientine. Zinc is now the recommended therapy for the long-term management of WD. It acts directly on metallothionein, which avidly binds copper in enterocytes, thereby preventing systemic copper accumulation. Elemental zinc of at least 75 mg daily is sufficient. Side effects are usually mild, including gastric irritation and transient elevations of amylase, lipase, and alkaline phosphatase. Orthotopic liver transplantation has been reported to be effective to ameliorate neurologic progression and improve the quality of life in medically intractable WD.

Dietary education regarding high copper-containing foods should be undertaken with specific restrictions on the ingestion of liver and shellfish. Because the disorder is autosomal recessive, it is important to screen other members of the family with neurologic examination, serum ceruloplasmin, 24-hour urine for copper excretion determinations, and slit lamp examination of the corneas. If disease is suspected in a clinically unaffected individual, liver biopsy should be performed to determine hepatic copper content. The clinical manifestations of the disorder may be prevented by early institution of zinc therapy in presymptomatic individuals.

Myoclonus

Myoclonus is a brief jerk-like contraction of a single muscle or muscle group that occurs as an isolated event or may occur in a repetitive regular or irregular manner. Myoclonus may be associated with dementia (Creutzfeldt-Jakob disease, Alzheimer disease, subacute sclerosing panencephalitis, corticobasal ganglionic degeneration), lipidosis (Tay-Sachs and Niemann-Pick diseases), leukodystrophy (Krabbe and Pelizaeus-Merzbacher diseases), cerebellar degeneration (Friedreich ataxia, progressive myoclonic ataxias, olivopontocerebellar atrophy), epilepsy syndromes (juvenile myoclonic epilepsy, Unverricht-Lundborg disease, Lafora disease, myoclonic epilepsy with ragged-red fibers, neuronal ceroid lipofuscinosis, etc.), hypoxia (Lance-Adams syndrome), immune-mediated (Hashimoto encephalopathy) and metabolic encephalopathies (uremic, hepatic), as a remote effect of cancer (infantile myoclonus associated with neuroblastoma), from exposure to drugs or toxins (levodopa, clozapine, bismuth subsalicylate, methylphenidate, amphetamines, lead, mercury, and strychnine), and in a variety of other disorders.

A unique form of myoclonus is the so-called *negative myoclonus* manifested by sudden loss of postural tone. Asterixis, an example of negative myoclonus, has been described in various metabolic or toxic encephalopathies and in certain diencephalic lesions. Unilateral asterixis is most often associated with focal ischemic/hemorrhagic lesion, particularly in the thalamus.

Segmental or spinal myoclonus is characterized by a rhythmic contraction of a group of muscles in a particular segment, such as an arm or leg, or abdominal muscles. Other examples of segmental myoclonus include palatal myoclonus, ocular myoclonus, and hiccups. Palatal myoclonus has been described in patients with infarction, demyelination, and other lesions involving the dentato-rubro-olivary pathway (Mollaret triangle).

Generalized polymyoclonus is repetitive myoclonus of all limbs that often leads to gait disturbance. The clinical feature of whole-body tremulousness may mislead to diagnosis of tremor, however, the surface electromyography may confirm myoclonus with nonperiodic muscle burst durations of less than 50 milliseconds. Etiology may include drugs (opioids, selective serotonin reuptake inhibitors, and serotonin-norepinephrine reuptake inhibitors), or paraneoplastic or autoimmune syndromes associated with putative neuronal autoantibodies.

Startle syndrome is characterized by exaggerated startle responses to sudden unexpected acoustic or tactile stimuli. The precise site of dysfunction in the CNS remains unknown. Familial startle syndrome or hyperekplexia is an autosomal dominant disorder with mutation of the gene encoding the α1 subunit of the inhibitory glycine receptor (*GLRA1*).

Pathogenesis

Neurophysiologic studies have suggested that some forms of generalized myoclonus originate from the cortex (cortical myoclonus), and the electromyographic (EMG) response is time-locked to a cortical electroencephalographic (EEG) discharge. A subtype of cortical myoclonus is cortical reflex myoclonus, which is a brief muscle jerk provoked by sensory stimuli such as a sudden loud noise or a visual threat. Several electrophysiologic studies suggest abnormal hyperexcitability of the somatosensory or motor cortex, or both, underlying the cortical myoclonus. After a cortical potential, the activation proceeds in a rostrocaudal direction, so that contraction of facial muscles is followed by firing in the muscles of the neck, arms, trunk, and legs in descending order. Other forms of myoclonus originate from the caudal brainstem (reticular or subcortical myoclonus). There is no consistent EEG–EMG correlation, although the EEG may reveal generalized spike discharges not necessarily associated with the myoclonic activity. In reticular myoclonus, the neck muscles are activated first, and the excitatory volley propagates in an ascending order up the brainstem and down the spinal cord. A third form of myoclonus, ballistic movement overflow myoclonus, also has no EEG abnormalities associated with the movement, but the duration of contraction is 50–100 msec, as opposed to 10–30 msec in the other two forms of myoclonus. In contrast to most forms of myoclonus (characterized by simultaneous co-contraction of agonist and antagonist muscles), ballistic overflow myoclonus is produced by an alternating agonist and antagonist contraction triggered by a fast ballistic movement of a limb.

Treatment

Several studies have demonstrated decreased levels of 5-hydroxyindoleacetic acid (5-HIAA), the metabolic product of serotonin, in the CSF of patients with posthypoxic action myoclonus. In fact, serotonin precursors (5-hydroxytryptophan), clonazepam, sodium valproate, and piracetam have produced clinical improvement of myoclonus in some patients. However, direct examination of the serotonergic median raphe nuclei fails to reveal any specific abnormalities. Therefore, further studies are needed to elucidate the biochemical, neurophysiologic, and pharmacologic mechanisms of myoclonus. In segmental myoclonus, presynaptic depleting agents such as tetrabenazine and drugs used for treatment of generalized myoclonus may be of benefit. Several new antiepileptic drugs such as levetiracetam (Keppra) and zonisamide (Zonegran) may also be useful in some cases of generalized and segmental myoclonus.

Tics and Tourette Syndrome

Tourette syndrome is characterized by chronic waxing and waning motor and vocal tics ,usually beginning between the ages of 2 and 15 years and affecting boys more frequently than girls. Prevalence of this disorder is estimated to be 31–157 cases per 1,000 in children aged 13–14 years. About half of the patients start with simple motor tics such as frequent eye blinking, facial grimacing, head jerking, shoulder shrugging, or with simple vocal tics such as throat clearing, sniffing, grunting, snorting, hissing, barking, and other noises. Most of the patients then develop more complex tics and mannerisms such as squatting; hopping; skipping; hand shaking; compulsive touching of things, people, or self; and other stereotyped movements. The tics may change from one form to another. Although described as a lifelong condition, up to one-third of the patients eventually achieve spontaneous remission during adulthood. The tics can be voluntarily suppressed for seconds to hours, but this may be followed by a rebound burst of exaggerated abnormal involuntary movements. The temporary voluntary suppression of tics and the subjective urge experienced by most patients before each tic helps to differentiate tics from myoclonus.

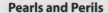

Pearls and Perils

Hyperkinetic movement disorders

- ▶ The presence of stereotypies in an adult almost always suggests the diagnosis of tardive dyskinesia (TD).
- ▶ The presence of more than one movement disorder in one patient (unless tremor and dystonia) suggests the diagnosis of TD.
- ▶ Wilson disease should be ruled out in all young patients presented with tremor and dystonia.
- ▶ Tic disorders and myoclonus do not abate with sleep.
- ▶ Tics are voluntarily suppressible, at least temporarily.
- ▶ Chorea and family history for Huntington disease in the elderly may be subtle and should not preclude genetic testing.
- ▶ Essential tremor is associated with idiopathic torsion dystonia, restless legs syndrome, bruxism, and writer's cramp.
- ▶ The ingestion of neuroleptic drugs can rarely produce acute dystonia.
- ▶ Acute dystonia is treated with anticholinergic drugs (e.g., diphenhydramine).
- ▶ Features of psychogenic movement disorders may include abrupt onset with rapid progression, inconsistent movements, presence of false weakness or sensory loss, and suppression of movements with distraction.

In the original description of the disorder by Gilles de la Tourette in 1885, five out of the nine original patients had coprolalia (involuntary shouting of obscenities) and echolalia (involuntary repetition of words or phrases). Two of the patients had echopraxia (imitation of certain motor acts). Coprolalia, echolalia, and echopraxia are the most dramatic symptoms of TS, but are present in a minority of patients.

Recent studies have emphasized the familial nature of this disorder, suggesting that approximately one-third of the probands have a positive family history of simple tics and another one-third have a positive family history of the full TS. This suggests that TS represents one extreme of a spectrum, of which the mildest manifestation is a simple or transient tic of childhood. This clinical heterogeneity makes specific definition of TS problematic. In addition to the motor and vocal tics described earlier, many patients have behavioral disorders including obsessive-compulsive disorder, attention deficit-hyperactivity disorder, self-destructive behavior, depression, and sexual disturbances.

Pathogenesis

The etiopathogenesis of TS is poorly understood. It is likely a complex interaction between genetic and environmental factors. Several candidate genes have been assessed in patients with TS. Perinatal injuries, drug abuse, and recurrent streptococcal infections with postinfectious autoimmune response are among possible risk factors for the development of TS. Favorable response to dopamine-blocking and dopamine-depleting agents gives some support to involvement of the dopaminergic axis, and the obsessive-compulsive symptoms suggests the involvement of serotonergic pathways. Sensorimotor integration is abnormally processed in TS. A motor evoked potential study in patients with TS showed evidence of abnormal premovement motor cortex excitability. Magnetic stimulation studies demonstrate a shortened cortical silent period and reduced intracortical inhibition. Functional MRI, SPECT, and PET studies show abnormal activation of various cortical and subcortical areas. Dysfunction of basal ganglia-thalamo-cortical projections affects sensorimotor, language, and limbic cortical circuits, and may explain why patients with TS have difficulty in inhibiting unwanted behaviors and impulses.

Treatment

Because of the fluctuating nature of this illness, treatment of TS should be initiated with a clear goal for improvement. Tics most often respond to neuroleptics but sometimes will benefit from α_2-adrenergic agonists such as guanfacine and clonidine. Since they have fewer short-term and long-term side effects compared to neuroleptics, guanfacine and clonidine may be reasonable first-line agents in some TS patients with previously untreated mild to moderate tics. When tics become severe or unresponsive to α_2-adrenergic agonists, neuroleptics are usually considered. Fluphenazine, pimozide, and haloperidol are effective, but may have serious long-term side effects. Of these three agents, fluphenazine seems to cause the least difficulties with sedation. All neuroleptics carry a risk of TD and require regular follow-up to prevent its development. Other new atypical antipsychotics such as risperidone, olanzapine, quetiapine, and aripiprazole may be of benefit, with fewer side effects. Tetrabenazine seems effective; however, it is not widely available. Botulinum toxin injection has been shown to decrease premonitory sensory urges in patients with simple motor tics. Deep brain stimulation to infrathalamic and thalamic targets may be useful in some intractable TS patients. The Tourette Syndrome Association has recently released a guideline to select patients with TS for DBS treatment. The obsessive-compulsive symptoms often respond to SSRIs such as sertraline (Zoloft), fluoxetine (Prozac), or paroxetine (Paxil), however, they may occasionally exacerbate tics at higher dosages. Patients who have difficulty with obsessive-compulsive symptoms and also report problems with falling asleep or bedwetting may be good candidates for the tricyclic antidepressant clomipramine (Anafranil). Specific cognitive behavioral techniques might be useful in selected patients with obsessive-compulsive symptoms associated with Tourette's syndrome.

In addition to pharmacologic therapy, psychotherapeutic attention to difficulties of self-esteem, social coping, family issues, and school adjustment is important.

Consider Consultation When...

▶ A patient with otherwise typical parkinsonism features lacks tremor, has unusual neurologic findings such as vertical ophthalmoparesis, apraxia, weakness, early dementia, hallucinations, dysautonomia, or is unresponsive to levodopa.

▶ A patient complains of writer's cramp, involuntary eye closure, or twisting of the neck, suggesting focal dystonias that are amenable to botulinum toxin injection.

▶ There is strong family history of movement disorder.

▶ The patient or his family report frequent blinking, jerk-like movements, involuntary vocalizations, and other noises such as sniffing, throat clearing, coughing, and other phonic tics.

▶ A patient presents with complex involuntary movement that is difficult to characterize.

▶ A patient is willing to participate in clinical trials at the movement disorder center.

The Tourette Syndrome Association and its local chapters are excellent resources for patients and their families.

Drug-Induced Movement Disorders

Since the introduction of chlorpromazine in 1952, the beneficial effects of antipsychotic medications have been clearly established. However, a variety of movement disorders may be observed in patients treated with the traditional major tranquilizers and some antiemetic drugs (neuroleptics). All movement disorders described in the phenomenology section of this chapter have been associated with dopamine receptor blocking drugs (DRBDs).

The most dramatic early side effect of neuroleptic therapy is an acute dystonic reaction, usually in the form of torticollis, oromandibular dystonia, or dystonic posturing of the limbs or trunk. Up to 10% of patients who take neuroleptic drugs develop these highly distressing symptoms, usually after only one or two doses, but this reaction is reported after as long as 2 weeks of therapy. This acute dystonic reaction is most often seen in young male patients and is dramatically reversed by intravenous or oral administration of diphenhydramine (Benadryl) or other antihistamines, benztropine mesylate (Cogentin) or other anticholinergic agents, or muscle relaxants (diazepam). On rare occasions, the dystonia can become permanent.

Parkinsonism is seen in 20–40% of patients treated with DRBDs and usually occurs within the first 3 months of drug exposure. This condition is dose-dependent and usually improves with dosage reduction or discontinuation, although it can take up to 12 months to resolve.

Akathisia (an urge to move) and motor restlessness of the legs, manifested by continual shifting, tapping, crossing and uncrossing of the legs, and marching in place is seen in approximately 10% of patients during the early phase of neuroleptic administration. The mechanism of this paradoxical hyperactivity is unknown, but may be related to selective blockade of the mesocortical dopamine system rather than the nigrostriatal system.

The neuroleptic malignant syndrome (NMS), manifested by a severe form of rigidity, fever, and unresponsiveness, is a potentially fatal idiosyncratic reaction to neuroleptics. These symptoms begin in 90% of affected patients within the first 2 weeks of therapy and may last up to 8 weeks after drug discontinuation. Patients almost always require supportive care to monitor cardiac and autonomic status and follow sometimes significantly elevated creatine kinase (CK) levels. Dantrolene, levodopa, and dopamine agonists have been used to treat the muscle rigidity.

Tardive dyskinesia (TD) is a drug-induced movement disorder that persists beyond 2–6 months after discontinuation of an offending DRBD. The most common movement disorder seen in this condition is stereotypy. These movements are usually patterned and repetitive, such as chewing, lip smacking, rocking or thrusting movements of the trunk and pelvis, and shoulder shrugging. Respiratory dyskinesia can produce grunting vocalizations, hyperventilation, and shortness of breath. Other tardive movement disorders include dystonia, akathisia, parkinsonism, tremor, myoclonus, chorea, and tics. Tardive dystonia tends to occur in younger men and may present with severe retrocollis and hyperextension of trunk. Identification of stereotypic movements and one other movement disorder in an adult almost always suggests the diagnosis of TD and the need to identify the offending medication.

A number of possible explanations of TD have been offered. The emergence of striatal dopamine D_2 receptor supersensitivity due to chronic dopamine blockade by neuroleptics appears to be the most likely pathophysiological mechanism. GABA-ergic hypofunction and oxidative damage in the basal ganglia due to free radicals generated by neuroleptics is another possible mechanism. In addition, several genetic studies have suggested that the D_3 receptor genotype may play an important role in the development of TD.

Early detection of abnormal involuntary movements should alert the clinician to reduce the dosage and, if possible, discontinue the use of an offending drug. Up to one-third of patients, particularly children, with TD achieve spontaneous and permanent remission within 1 year of discontinuation of the offending drug, but most patients continue to have abnormal involuntary movements indefinitely. Other therapeutic approaches have included the use of dopamine-depleting agents, such as tetrabenazine, for stereotypies and tremor, and botulinum toxin for (focal) dystonias. Sodium valproate, ondansetron, branch-chain amino acids, piracetam, levetiracetam, and vitamin B_6 have been effective in reducing the symptoms of TD in few clinical studies. However, well-designed, large, prospective, trials are needed to address the long-term outcome and side effects. The use of levodopa and other dopaminergic medications for parkinsonism may not be feasible because of the high risk of aggravating psychiatric symptoms in patients already requiring DRBDs. In TD patients who require neuroleptics for controlling their psychiatric symptoms, atypical antipsychotics with modest (clozapine) or mild (quetiapine) antagonistic effect on D_2 receptors should be considered.

Annotated Bibliography

Brewer GJ, Fink JK, Hedera P. Diagnosis and treatment of Wilson's disease. *Semin Neurol* 1999;19:261–270.
  A review of the pathophysiology, clinical presentation, and treatment of Wilson disease.
Jankovic J. Tourette's syndrome. *N Engl J Med* 2001;345:1184–1192.

A review of the diagnosis, pathogenesis, and treatment of Tourette syndrome.

Louis ED. Essential tremor. *Lancet Neurol* 2005;4:100–110.
An excellent recent review of essential tremor.

Jankovic J, Stacy M. Medical management of levodopa-associated motor complications in patients with Parkinson's disease. *CNS Drugs* 2007;21(8):677–692.
Strategies for treating common complications in the advanced Parkinson disease patients.

Stacy M, Cardoso F, Jankovic J. Tardive stereotypy and other movement disorders in tardive dyskinesias. *Neurology* 1993;43(5):937–941.

A review of medical records and videotapes of 100 patients with tardive dyskinesia at a movement disorders clinic.

Stacy M, Galbreath A. Optimizing long-term therapy for Parkinson disease: Levodopa, dopamine agonists, and treatment-associated dyskinesia. *Clin Neuropharmacol* 2008;31:51–56.
A recent review on long-term pharmacological therapy in patients with Parkinson disease.

Tarsy D, Simon DK. Dystonia. *N Engl J Med* 2006;355:818–829.
A recent clinical review on dystonia.

CHAPTER 18

Neuromuscular Diseases

Nayan P. Desai and Richard K. Olney

▼

Outline

▶ Selected features of the neuromuscular examination
▶ Tests for neuromuscular diseases
▶ Common clinical problems in neuromuscular disease
▶ Peripheral neuropathy
▶ Generalized symmetrical polyneuropathies
▶ Generalized neuronopathies
▶ Focal or multifocal neuropathies
▶ Radiculopathy
▶ Myopathy
▶ Neuromuscular junction disorders

Selected Features of the Neuromuscular Examination

Cranial Nerve Signs

Cranial nerve signs develop in a minority of neuromuscular diseases. Table 18.1 summarizes the neuromuscular diseases that have cranial nerve findings.

Extraocular muscle weakness that limits eye movement is a consistent feature of most neuromuscular junction disorders, including myasthenia gravis, congenital myasthenic syndromes, and botulism. In myasthenia gravis, this weakness develops insidiously and varies through the course of the day with fatigue. In congenital myasthenic syndromes, extraocular weakness is present in infancy and persists into adulthood, at which time it may be initially noticed rarely. In food-borne botulism, it develops over several hours to 2 days, is constantly present for weeks, and then resolves over several months. Weakness that limits eye movement also occurs acutely over several days to 4 weeks in approximately 10% of patients with the Guillain-Barré syndrome (GBS; all pa-

tients with the Miller-Fisher variant and occasionally in patients with the acute inflammatory demyelinating polyneuropathy variant of the GBS). Constant extraocular muscle weakness that limits eye movement is a consistent feature of certain mitochondrial myopathies that develop insidiously in teens and young adults, and of centronuclear myopathy that persists from childhood into adult life. The extraocular weakness of oculopharyngeal muscular dystrophy is limited to constant severe ptosis that develops insidiously in middle or late adult life.

Among neuromuscular diseases, clinically obvious pupillary involvement is typical only of food-borne botulism. Whereas this is a relatively consistent feature of botulism, pupillary reactivity is normal in a significant minority of patients with botulism and is absent in rare cases of the GBS, so pupillary signs are used with great caution in distinguishing these two diseases, which are treated quite differently.

Facial and bulbar weakness develops acutely over hours in botulism and over days to 4 weeks in the GBS. Facial and bulbar weakness often develop over weeks or months in amyotrophic lateral sclerosis (ALS), polymyositis, and myasthenia gravis, with variation through the course of the day, and with fatigue characterizing the latter. Facial weakness without bulbar weakness is a consistent feature of fascioscapulohumeral dystrophy, but may be subtle unless carefully sought. The insidious onset of bulbar weakness without facial weakness (except for ptosis) is a consistent feature of oculopharyngeal dystrophy.

Motor Examination

The motor examination involves observation of muscle bulk, tone, and strength. Severe muscular atrophy is almost always secondary to loss of most motor axons and may be obvious within 1 to 3 months after acute loss.

Table 18.1 Cranial nerve involvement in neuromuscular diseases

	Extraocular muscle weakness	Pupillary abnormalities	Facial weakness	Bulbar weakness
Myasthenia gravis	+++		++	++
Congenital myasthenic syndromes	+++			
Food-borne botulism	+++	++	++	++
Mitochondrial myopathies	++			
Centronuclear myopathy	++		+	
Oculopharyngeal dystrophy	+++ (ptosis only)			+++
Fascioscapulohumeral dystrophy			+++	
Polymyositis			+	++
Guillain–Barré syndrome	++	+	++	++
Amyotrophic lateral sclerosis			++ early; +++ late	++ early; +++ late

+++ Common; ++ variable; + rare

Mild muscular atrophy may occur from mild loss of motor axons or from chronic myopathy or disuse. In radiculopathy, neuropathy, or anterior horn cell disease, patterns of muscular atrophy may be as important as patterns of weakness in determining the localization. Fasciculations are due to spontaneous discharges of single lower motor neurons. Although common in motor neuron diseases such as ALS, fasciculations occur without weakness in benign fasciculation syndrome or in localized distributions with other forms of lower motor neuron disease or injury. Muscle tone is normal or reduced in most neuromuscular diseases, with the exception of diseases that also involve upper motor neurons and are associated with spasticity (for example, ALS and compressive cervical myelopathy). Muscle strength is reduced distally in most neuropathies and proximally in most myopathies, with occasional exceptions. The methods for assessing and grading strength are discussed in Chapter 1.

Coordination is not usually affected out of proportion to weakness in neuromuscular diseases, except in those that cause spasticity. Because normal walking requires intact sensory function, leg strength, and coordination, clinical analysis of gait is an important aspect of the neuromuscular examination. Myopathies usually cause a waddling gait from proximal weakness. A peroneal neuropathy or a severe unilateral L5 radiculopathy causes a unilateral foot drop, whereas weakness from a polyneuropathy or bilateral lumbosacral polyradiculopathy causes a bilateral foot drop or steppage gait in which the patient lifts the legs higher while walking to compensate for bilateral weakness in ankle dorsiflexion. Loss of large sensory nerve fibers that carry joint position information causes a sensory ataxia in which the gait is unsteady and worsens dramatically with eye closure (Romberg sign). Subtle gait disturbances can be elicited by having the patient walk quickly or having the patient walk heel to toe (tandem gait).

Reflexes

Muscle stretch reflexes are typically reduced or absent in diseases that affect large-diameter sensory axons from the muscle spindles. This mechanism underlies focal reflex loss in radiculopathy and distal or generalized reflex loss in neuropathies. Other than neuropathic disorders, depressed or absent reflexes are typical of only rare syndromes, such as the Lambert-Eaton myasthenic syndrome. Stretch reflexes are normal or reduced in proportion to weakness in diseases without sensory involvement, such as anterior horn cell disease, myopathy, and myasthenia gravis. Plantar responses are flexor, except in diseases that have also affected the upper motor neuron.

Sensory Examination

Sensory loss is caused by neuromuscular diseases that affect peripheral nerves, dorsal root ganglia cells, or nerve roots, or by non-neuromuscular diseases that affect the central sensory pathways. Focal peripheral nerve injuries result in a better-demarcated pattern of sensory loss than radiculopathies or sensory loss from central nervous system (CNS) injury. For example, a patient with an ulnar neuropathy usually has a well-demarcated sensory loss that encompasses the little finger, splits the ring finger, and extends proximally to the wrist, whereas a patient with a C8 radiculopathy has sensory impairment of the little finger with vague boundaries over the other digits and sensory symptoms proximal to the wrist over the medial forearm.

When considering sensory loss as a part of a neuromuscular disease, impairment of pain sensation (ability to differentiate pin-prick from dull touch) and temperature (the ability to accurately identify warm and cold) are considered signs of a disease that is affecting small-diameter sensory nerve fibers, rather than the spinothalamic tract. Vibratory sensation and proprioception (joint position sense) reflect large-fiber function peripherally or posterior column function centrally. Certain neuropathies primarily affect large-fiber sensory nerves (for example, vitamin B12 deficiency), and others characteristically affect small-fiber sensory nerves (for example, amyloidosis). Most polyneuropathies affect both small and large sensory fibers, with one fiber type occasionally affected more than the other.

Tests for Neuromuscular Diseases

Serum Creatine Kinase and Other Muscle Enzymes

Elevated serum creatine kinase (CK) is a useful laboratory test for muscle disease. A CK level over 10 times the upper limit of normal is almost always indicative of a clinically significant muscle disease. A moderate (6–10 times the upper limit) elevation of CK is supportive of muscle disease, but may also be seen in neuropathic diseases with active, widespread denervation, such as ALS and the spinal muscular atrophies (especially X-linked bulbospinal muscular atrophy, which is also known as Kennedy disease). A mild (2–5 times the upper limit of normal) elevation of CK in a patient with weakness is more suggestive of muscle than nerve disease, but may be seen with either. A mild elevation of CK in a patient who is not weak may also represent a variation of normal. In contrast to the relative specificity of CK elevation for muscle involvement, aspartate aminotransferase (AST),

alanine aminotransferase (ALT), and lactate dehydrogenase (LDH) are elevated in muscle or liver disease. γ-Glutamyl transpeptidase (GGT) is found in liver, but not in muscle, so it is useful to differentiate liver from neuromuscular disease.

Electrodiagnostic Studies

Electrodiagnostic studies are an integral part of the evaluation of neuromuscular disease. They are usually arranged at the same time that the initial CK level is drawn, and are obtained before finalizing decisions for invasive tests such as muscle or nerve biopsy and for treatment. Because needle electromyography increases the CK level, CK levels should be tested either before the electrodiagnostic studies or several days later. Electromyography and nerve conduction studies are discussed in Chapter 3.

Muscle Biopsy

A muscle biopsy is performed to confirm the specific findings in a clinically diagnosed myopathy if its pathology is likely to support an inflammatory or genetic mechanism. Muscle biopsy is rarely performed without clear evidence for myopathy from the clinical examination, laboratory testing, and electrodiagnostic studies. The biopsy is usually performed on the biceps in the upper extremity or the quadriceps in the lower extremity. The muscle selected for biopsy is usually moderately affected. Biopsy of a markedly weak or atrophic muscle often reveals the less diagnostic features of end-stage muscle disease. Clinically unaffected muscles may not provide a specific pathologic diagnosis. Clinical examination and electromyography are usually used to select muscles that are moderately affected. Muscle biopsy is performed on the opposite side from electromyographic (EMG) testing to avoid EMG needle-induced inflammatory tracts on the biopsy, unless the biopsy is delayed for more than 1 month after the EMG study.

Muscle biopsy may be performed with a needle or open technique. The needle biopsy is less invasive and leaves less of a scar than an open biopsy. However, the needle biopsy obtains several small pieces of muscle that may be difficult to orient and interpret. The open biopsy requires the involvement of a surgeon in most hospital settings, so is more expensive. Usually, the decision to obtain a needle or open biopsy is based on the experience of the neuromuscular physician and the pathology laboratory at the institution. The care and handling of the muscle tissue after biopsy is crucial. Unlike many other types of surgical pathology specimens, muscle must be processed immediately and cannot be stored in saline or left overnight before processing. Muscle biopsies are often of limited value due to extensive artifacts, if not performed at an institution that has experience with the han-

---

Key Clinical Questions

▶ Is the pattern of motor weakness proximal or distal?

▶ Did the symptoms develop acutely (over days to weeks) or subacutely (over weeks to months)?

▶ Does the patient's symptoms fluctuate?

▶ Is the weakness associated with cranial nerve findings?

▶ Is there muscular atrophy? Fasciculations?

▶ Is sensory loss a feature of the neuromuscular process?

▶ Is there a significant elevation of serum creatine kinase (CK)?

▶ Does the patient have medical conditions (e.g., diabetes, thyroid disease, human immunodeficiency virus, malignancy) that might predispose to neuromuscular disease?

▶ Is there a family history of similar neuromuscular disease?

Pearls and Perils

Electrodiagnostic testing

▶ The sensitivity and specificity of results from electro-diagnostic testing depend on the experience and training of the physician who performs the testing, especially for less common neuromuscular diseases.

▶ The results of nerve conduction testing need to be interpreted with caution during the first 3–12 days after an acute injury, because the size of sensory and motor responses can be deceptively normal before Wallerian degeneration is complete.

▶ Fibrillation potentials develop in acutely denervated or injured muscle over 1–4 weeks, depending on the site of injury.

▶ Although marked slowing indicates demyelination, slowing also occurs from axonal loss and with decreased temperature of the limb; conduction velocity is normally lower below age 3 years and over age 50 years.

▶ Weakness from myopathy, and lower motor neuron and upper motor neuron diseases, produces three distinctive patterns of electromyographic (EMG) abnormality; however, decreased effort and upper motor neuron weakness cannot be differentiated by EMG testing.

▶ Sensory nerve conduction studies test large-diameter sensory fibers; patients with selective sensory loss for small-diameter sensory fiber modalities (pain and temperature) have normal results for sensory nerve conduction studies.

▶ Clinical sensory loss for vibration or proprioception with normal results for sensory nerve conduction studies supports the idea that the lesion is proximal to the dorsal root ganglia (radiculopathy or central nervous system sensory loss).

Table 18.2 Classification of neuromuscular diseases by patterns of presentation

1 Acute generalized weakness
  Guillain-Barré syndrome
  Food-borne botulism
  Acute necrotizing myopathy
  Acute poliomyelitis syndrome
  Periodic paralysis
2 Subacute or chronic generalized weakness
  Motor neuron diseases
  Chronic demyelinating polyneuropathy
  Myopathies
  Neuromuscular junction diseases
3 Subacute or chronic weakness more than distal numbness
  Demyelinating polyneuropathies
4 Subacute or chronic distal numbness more than weakness
  Distal axonal polyneuropathies
5 Numbness, weakness, or pain limited to one limb
  Radiculopathy
  Plexopathy
  Compressive neuropathy
  Initial nerve affected by mononeuritis multiplex

dling and processing of specimens. Special stains may be necessary to arrive at a specific diagnosis.

Genetic Testing

Many of the inherited neuropathies and muscular dystrophies can be detected using serologic genetic tests for known mutations. These are performed in specialized commercial laboratories or at specialized laboratories based at university medical centers.

Common Clinical Problems in Neuromuscular Disease

The clinical approach to neuromuscular disease is facilitated by recognition of five common clinical patterns, as summarized in Table 18.2. The most common patterns are the last two. The presentation of a patient with subacute or chronic distal numbness more than weakness is typically a distal axonal polyneuropathy, which is often due to diabetes mellitus or alcoholism. The presentation of a patient with numbness, weakness, or pain limited to one limb is usually due to a radiculopathy or a compression neuropathy (for example, a carpal tunnel syndrome), but is rarely caused by a plexopathy or the initial nerve to be affected by a mononeuropathy multiplex. Such patients are usually managed by their primary care physicians, so long as pain is controlled or resolved by non-narcotic medications and disability is mild or absent, remaining confined within one limb. Consultation is often advisable for patients with these presentations who are more severely affected, and for patients with the other patterns of presentation, most urgently for patients with acute generalized weakness (Table 18.3). The consultation usually includes both clinical and electrodiagnostic evaluation, so it is most efficiently performed by a consultant who is knowledgeable in each. Neurologists and physiatrists who are familiar with radiculopathy, compression neuropathy, and distal axonal polyneuropathy are usually available in the community. Patients with less common neuromuscular diseases may benefit more from consultation with a neuromuscular disease subspecialist, who may be available in some community settings and in most university medical centers (Table 18.4).

Table 18.3 Acute generalized weakness

Discriminating features

▶ Guillain-Barré syndrome
  1 Generalized areflexia
  2 Distal tingling with little sensory loss
  3 Elevated CSF protein
▶ Food-borne botulism
  1 Symmetric weakness including extraocular muscles
  2 Normal CSF and CK
  3 Other affected family members
▶ Acute necrotizing myopathy
  1 Markedly elevated CK
  2 Normal CSF
▶ Acute poliomyelitis syndrome
  1 CSF pleocytosis
  2 Fever
▶ Periodic paralysis
  1 Symmetric weakness that reverses within 1 day
  2 Normal CSF and CK

Consistent features

▶ Guillain-Barré syndrome
  1 Symmetric weakness
  2 Antecedent infection
▶ Food-borne botulism
  1 Gastrointestinal symptoms
  2 Maximum within 2 days
▶ Acute necrotizing myopathy
  1 Symmetric weakness
  2 No respiratory failure
  3 Normal extraocular eye movements
▶ Acute poliomyelitis syndrome
  1 Asymmetric weakness
  2 Maximum within 3 days
▶ Periodic paralysis
  1 No respiratory failure

Variable features

▶ Guillain-Barré syndrome
  1 Extraocular weakness
  2 Respiratory failure
  3 Normal CSF protein during first week
▶ Food-borne botulism
  1 Fixed pupils
▶ Periodic paralysis
  1 Positive family history

CK, creatine kinase; CSF, cerebrospinal fluid

Table 18.4 Subacute or chronic generalized weakness

Discriminating features

▶ Motor neuron diseases
  1 Weakness with atrophy and fasciculations
  2 EMG signs of lower motor neuron loss and decreased recruitment
▶ Chronic inflammatory demyelinating polyneuropathy
  1 Weakness without atrophy
  2 EMG signs of decreased recruitment
  3 Nerve conduction studies slowing or conduction block
▶ Myopathy
  1 Weakness without atrophy
  2 EMG signs of rapid recruitment
▶ Neuromuscular junction disorder
  1 Weakness without atrophy
  2 Extraocular weakness
  3 EMG signs of rapid recruitment

Consistent features

▶ Motor neuron diseases
  1 Distal > proximal asymmetric weakness
  2 Preservation of reflexes unless severe weakness
▶ Chronic inflammatory demyelinating polyneuropathy
  1 Distal > proximal symmetric weakness
  2 Absent reflexes
▶ Myopathy
  1 Symmetric proximal weakness
  2 Elevated CK level
▶ Neuromuscular junction disorder
  1 Symmetric proximal weakness with fatigue
  2 Normal CK level

Variable features

▶ Motor neuron diseases
  1 Elevated CK level
  2 Upper motor neuron signs
  3 Proximal symmetric weakness
▶ Chronic inflammatory demyelinating polyneuropathy
  1 Fasciculations
  2 Asymmetric weakness
  3 Atrophy

CK, creatine kinase; EMG, electromyograph

Peripheral Neuropathy

Classification

Peripheral neuropathy is a disease that affects motor, sensory, or autonomic axons distal to the nerve roots that leave the spinal canal. By clinical convention, peripheral neuropathy also encompasses diseases that affect the cell bodies of sensory axons (located in the dorsal root ganglia) and the cell bodies of lower motor neuron axons (located in the anterior horn of the spinal cord and motor nuclei of the brainstem). A clinically useful classification of peripheral neuropathies is one that has three divisions by an anatomic distribution (Table 18.5). Generalized symmetrical polyneuropathies have symmetrical involvement of sensory, motor, and autonomic fibers, but clinical signs of one fiber type often predominate. Generalized neu-

Table 18.5 Peripheral neuropathy

Discriminating features

▶ Generalized symmetric polyneuropathies
  1 Symptoms and signs include sensory and motor features
  2 Symmetric
▶ Generalized neuronopathies
  1 Symptoms and signs limited to sensory or motor features
  2 Symmetric or focal
▶ Focal or multifocal neuropathies
  1 Symptoms and signs include sensory and motor features
  2 Focal or multifocal

Consistent features

▶ Generalized symmetric polyneuropathies
  1 Tingling in both feet
  2 Numbness, weakness, or both in feet
  3 Ankle reflexes depressed or absent
▶ Generalized neuronopathies
  1 Numbness or weakness (but not both) in any distribution
▶ Focal or multifocal neuropathies
  1 Numbness, weakness, or both in the distribution of one or
    more nerves

Variable features

▶ Generalized symmetric polyneuropathies
  1 Numbness or weakness to knees and wrists
  2 Pain in feet, hands, or back
  3 Proximal weakness
  4 Generalized areflexia
▶ Generalized neuronopathies
  1 Tingling, pain, or reflex depression with numbness
  2 Cramping or fasciculations with weakness
▶ Focal or multifocal neuropathies
  1 Tingling, pain, reduced reflexes, cramping, or fasciculations in
    affected distributions

Table 18.6 Symmetric neuropathies

Discriminating features

▶ Distal axonal polyneuropathy
  1 Length dependent symptoms and signs
  2 Numbness more severe than weakness
  3 Electrodiagnostic signs or distal axonal loss
▶ Demyelinating polyneuropathy
  1 Weakness and reflex depression more severe than numbness
  2 Electrodiagnostic signs of demyelination
  3 Elevated CSF protein

Consistent features

▶ Distal axonal polyneuropathy
  1 Numbness and weakness in feet more severe than in lower
    legs and hands
  2 Absent ankle reflexes
▶ Demyelinating polyneuropathy
  1 Moderate distal and mild proximal weakness
  2 Mild distal numbness
  3 All tendon reflexes absent

Variable features

▶ Distal axonal polyneuropathy
  1 All reflexes absent
  2 Burning or lancinating pain in feet
  3 Weakness more severe than numbness
▶ Demyelinating polyneuropathy
  1 Tingling in hands and feet, but little numbness
  2 Aching pain in back or limbs

CSF, cerebrospinal fluid

ronopathies affect the cell bodies of only one type of peripheral neuron. Sensory neuronopathies affect the dorsal root ganglia cells and produce numbness that may begin in a focal/asymmetrical distribution or in a distal symmetrical fashion. However, motor function is affected only by loss of proprioceptive feedback. Motor neuronopathies are more commonly referred to as *anterior horn cell diseases*. They produce weakness that may begin in asymmetrical or symmetrical distribution, depending on the specific disease process. Focal or multifocal neuropathies affect sensory and motor fibers in one or more nerves.

Generalized Symmetrical Polyneuropathies

Generalized symmetrical polyneuropathies are further subdivided into distal axonal polyneuropathy and demyelinating polyneuropathy (Table 18.6). Distal axonal polyneuropathy predominantly affects the peripheral axons and is the common type of generalized peripheral neuropathy. The clinical features of distal axonal polyneuropathy form a distinctive pattern that is important for primary care physicians to recognize. A patient with a generalized peripheral neuropathy that does not fit this pattern is appropriate to refer for neurologic consultation and evaluation. Demyelinating polyneuropathy is the uncommon type that predominantly affects the myelin or Schwann cells around the axons.

Distal Axonal Polyneuropathy

The clinical features of a distal axonal polyneuropathy are length-dependent impairment of sensory function that is more severe than motor involvement. Length dependency refers to a pattern of deficits in which increasing severity of symptoms is directly proportional to increasing distance from the spinal cord. Thus, a distal axonal polyneuropathy typically presents with symptoms and signs of sensory impairment in the toes and feet, which are innervated by the axons that extend the farthest from the spinal cord. It may be manifest initially as pain, tingling, or numbness in the feet. If the only symptom is pain, a burning or lancinating quality for the pain is sufficiently specific to strongly suggest peripheral neuropathy as the explanation for the pain. Aching pain as the only symptom may be caused by ligamentous or skeletal disease or injury more commonly than peripheral neuropathy. However, the association of tingling or numbness with aching pain is sufficient to infer a peripheral neuropathy. On examination, the threshold for perception of pin-prick, warmth, or vibration is reduced in the feet, and the ankle reflex is depressed (relative to the knee reflex) or absent. Muscle bulk and strength are usually normal, even in the feet.

Over time, the upper margin of sensory symptoms gradually spread proximally. By the time the upper margin of tingling or numbness is at the mid-calf level, tingling or numbness typically begins in the fingertips. Patients often additionally complain of imbalance or of stubbing their toes with this severity of a distal axonal polyneuropathy. On examination, the threshold for perception of pin-prick, warmth, or vibration is reduced in a graded fashion in the distal leg and fingers. Ankle reflexes are usually absent and other reflexes depressed. Weakness of toe movement and wasting of intrinsic foot muscles are commonly present with such moderate sensory impairment.

Distal axonal polyneuropathy has many causes. The etiology is usually attributed by association to concurrent diseases or toxic exposures that are known to produce neuropathy. The two most common causes in Western societies are diabetes mellitus and alcoholism. An occasional etiology is exposure to neurotoxic prescription drugs. If the symptoms and signs are mild, these neuropathies are typically managed by primary care physicians. If the distal axonal polyneuropathy is not typical for one caused by diabetes mellitus, alcoholism, or prescription medications, or if signs are moderate or severe, referral to a neurologist is strongly considered. In these latter patients, diagnostic evaluation will include a detailed family history for symptoms that suggest neuropathy, a focused history for possible exposure to occupational or environmental toxins, electrodiagnostic studies, and laboratory studies. These latter include complete blood count (CBC), chemistry tests of renal and liver function, vitamin B_{12} level, thyroid stimulating hormone level, and serum protein electrophoresis. For many such patients, subsequent studies will include serum immunofixation (even if the protein electrophoresis is normal) and 24-hour urine for light chain analysis. Heavy metal studies are obtained only if a history for possible exposure, associated gastrointestinal or CNS symptoms, and abnormalities on the CBC suggest the need for further evaluation of this possible etiology.

▼

Pearls and Perils

Distal axonal polyneuropathy

▶ The two most common causes are diabetes mellitus and chronic alcoholism.
▶ Prescription drugs are occasionally the cause.
▶ Consider referral if one of these three causes is not present.
▶ Consider referral if signs or disability is moderate or severe.

Diabetic polyneuropathy

Diabetes mellitus is the most common cause of generalized symmetrical polyneuropathy that is predominantly due to distal loss of axons. It accounts for one-quarter to one-third of distal axonal polyneuropathies. Diabetic polyneuropathy is the most common form of diabetic neuropathy, but the latter term also encompasses proximal motor neuropathy, cranial mononeuropathy, truncal neuropathy, and polyradiculopathy. The development of diabetic polyneuropathy is related to the type of diabetes mellitus, the age of the individual, and the length of diabetes. Individuals under 40 years of age with type I diabetes mellitus for less than 10 years rarely have diabetic polyneuropathy. However, because the onset of diabetes mellitus is at an earlier age, and the average duration of survival is well beyond 10 years, over half of these patients eventually develop subclinical polyneuropathy, and 10–20% will have symptomatic polyneuropathy. Individuals over age 50 years with type II diabetes mellitus may have diabetic polyneuropathy as the presenting symptom of the diabetes mellitus. Because of the later age at onset, the average duration of survival is shorter; however, the incidence of polyneuropathy in type II diabetics is similar to that of type I patients. The major risk factor for diabetic polyneuropathy that can be modified is the control of serum glucose. Poor control increases the risk, and tight control decreases the risk for the development and progression of diabetic polyneuropathy. However, the correlation between control and the polyneuropathy is not direct. Occasionally, diabetics with long-term tight control will have severely disabling polyneuropathy and, conversely, occasional individuals with poor control will remain free of polyneuropathy for many years. Impaired glucose tolerance is increasingly being implicated as a cause for previously labeled idiopathic polyneuropathy, and more rigorous testing of glucose handling with an oral glucose tolerance test is warranted when no other cause for a polyneuropathy is forthcoming. Up to a third of previously idiopathic cases can potentially be reclassified as polyneuropathy associated with impaired glucose tolerance. A current trial at the Mayo Clinic is seeking to clearly define the causal relationship between impaired glucose tolerance and polyneuropathy.

The most common presenting symptoms are those typical for a distal axonal polyneuropathy, with burning pain, tingling, or impairment of sensation in both feet and subsequent distal weakness beginning in the toe extensors and flexors only after the upper margin for sensory impairment is above the ankle level. Autonomic involvement is common and may include postural hypotension, resting tachycardia, painless myocardial infarction, impaired gastric emptying, nocturnal diarrhea, or impotence. The etiology of diabetic polyneuropathy is not fully established. Impaired glucose regulation is an important contributing factor. The final step in the pathogenesis is the accumulation of multiple microinfarctions of nerve due to capillary closure. The relative role of impaired regulation of glucose, polyol pathway activity, nonenzymatic glycosylation of proteins, or other undefined mechanisms in producing capillary basement membrane thickening is uncertain.

The conventional treatment of diabetic polyneuropathy consists of optimal glucose control, preventive foot care, and symptomatic treatment of pain. The Diabetes Control and Complication Trial provided convincing evidence that tight control reduces the incidence of new cases of diabetic polyneuropathy. No treatment other than tight control has been demonstrated to alter the rate of progression. Therapeutic trials with several generations of aldose reductase inhibitors have failed to provide significant benefit with safety. Current research is evaluating the role of vascular endothelial growth factor (VEGF) in arresting further progression and perhaps reversing the course of diabetic polyneuropathy. Other important measures include good nutrition and avoidance of alcohol or other agents that are neurotoxic. Adequate foot care is essential to avoid Charcot joints or other foot injuries resulting from decreased sensation. Neuropathic pain can be treated with older agents like tricyclic antidepressants or gabapentin or newer agents like pregabalin or duloxetine.

Distal axonal polyneuropathy caused by alcoholism or nutritional deficiency

Polyneuropathy is a common neurologic complication of chronic alcoholism and accounts for 20–30% of distal axonal polyneuropathies in some populations. The symptoms are those typical of distal axonal polyneuropathy. The incidence of polyneuropathy among men and women is similar, although there is a much higher incidence of alcoholism among men, suggesting that women may be more susceptible than the numbers suggest. Most cases occur in alcoholics over the age of 30, with a history of heavy alcohol consumption (at least 100 g of ethanol per day or the equivalent of more than six standard alcohol-containing drinks per day) over 3 years or more in a dose-related fashion. A direct toxic effect of alcohol on peripheral nerves is usually considered to be the predominant mechanism. If this is true, humans must be significantly more sensitive to this toxic effect than Macaque monkeys, because monkeys fed diets with 50% of the calories replaced with alcohol for 5 years were not found to have electrophysiological or histological evidence for neuropathy. Nutritional deficiency may act synergistically with the toxic effect of alcohol to produce polyneuropathy.

Symptoms of alcohol-related neuropathy are typical to those of a distal symmetric axonal polyneuropathy discussed previously. Tingling, numbness, or pain begin gradually in the feet and spread above the ankles before weakness of toe movements develops. Symptoms and signs improve and may even fully resolve with the cessation of alcohol consumption. Improvement is usually apparent only after 3–6 months of abstinence, and pain may increase initially as axonal regeneration begins after cessation of alcohol, so symptomatic treatment for pain is usually necessary.

Distal axonal polyneuropathy caused by prescription medications

Distal axonal polyneuropathy may be produced by a large number of prescription medications. Table 18.7 presents a list of some of the more common offending drugs, although this is not an exhaustive list. If a patient who is treated with any prescription drug presents with symptoms and signs of distal axonal polyneuropathy, a literature search is performed on every medication that the

---

Table 18.7 Prescription medications that cause distal axonal polyneuropathy

Medication	Frequency	Associated features
Sensory		
Cisplatin	Common	Also ototoxic
Metronidazole	Occasional	
Misonidazole	Occasional	
Pyridoxine (vitamin B$_6$)	Rare	Common if >200 per day
Sensory > motor		
Amiodarone	Occasional	
Colchicine	Common	Also myopathy with fibrillation potentials
Disulfiram	Common	
Gold	Rare	Also rash and renal failure
Isoniazid	Occasional	Common without pyroxamine
Nitrofurantoin	Occasional	
Taxol	Common	
Thalidomide	Common	
Vincristine	Common	Rarely, motor more than sensory
Motor > sensory		
Dapsone	Occasional	

person takes for possible reports of polyneuropathy. Furthermore, even if such reports are not found, consider withdrawing any medication that was initiated within several months of the first neuropathic symptoms.

Monoclonal protein-associated distal axonal polyneuropathy

After diabetes mellitus and alcoholism, hematologic disorders that produce monoclonal proteins are the third most common identifiable systemic disease associated with distal axonal polyneuropathy. These polyneuropathies account for 5% of distal axonal polyneuropathies. Some patients will have multiple myeloma or other well-defined hematologic disease, but the majority of patients with polyneuropathy have a monoclonal gammopathy of undetermined significance. These patients have normal CBCs, often have normal results for serum protein electrophoresis, and rarely have plasma cell dyscrasia with bone marrow aspiration. The main clinical significance of the monoclonal protein is its probable role in causing the polyneuropathy. The age of the patient is an important factor in estimating the probability that the monoclonal protein is causally related to the polyneuropathy. Causation is highly probable if the patient is under age 50 years, but becomes dubious over age 70 years. By the age of 70 years, more than 5% of asymptomatic men will have a monoclonal protein.

Even if causation is considered highly probable, the benefits of aggressive treatment are uncertain for patients with mild distal axonal polyneuropathy. Response to intensive immunosuppression may occur, but is uncertain. Treatment is usually symptomatic unless disability is moderate or severe, or unless clinically significant hematologic disease becomes manifest over time.

HIV-associated distal axonal polyneuropathy

This polyneuropathy becomes increasingly common with increasing duration of human immunodeficiency virus (HIV) infection and increasing severity of immunosuppression. In patients with acquired immune deficiency syndrome (AIDS) who complain of this neuropathy, their presenting complaint is burning pain in the feet. More commonly, mild sensory impairment in the feet is a sufficiently minor symptom that the neuropathy is recognized by a physician only when the patient presents for unrelated reasons. The specific mechanisms may involve increased macrophage activity with release of toxic cytokines, such as tumor necrosis factor- , increased viral replication with release of toxic proteins, such as gp120, or less likely, increased nutritional deficiency. No treatments are yet known that alter the rate of progression. Both lamotrigine and recombinant nerve growth factor have been shown to reduce pain significantly. Other agents are the standard treatments for neuropathic pain, such as gabapentin and antidepressants.

Hereditary distal axonal polyneuropathy

Many hereditary disorders are associated with distal axonal polyneuropathy. Many produce disease in the central and peripheral nervous systems, and some cause only peripheral neuropathy. The most common of these that produces only polyneuropathy is hereditary motor sensory neuropathy (HMSN) type 2, which is also known as the neuronal form of Charcot-Marie-Tooth disease. This is an autosomal dominant disease with variable penetrance that causes skeletal deformities in childhood and usually presents during adulthood with distal weakness. The skeletal deformities most often consist of high arches and hammer toes, but less often include scoliosis. On examination, the main clinical features are distal wasting and weakness of foot and lower leg muscles with absent ankle jerks. Although sensory impairment is often not clear clinically, electrodiagnostic studies confirm distal loss of sensory and motor axons, with absent sensory responses at the ankle level and small motor responses that have normal or nearly normal latencies and velocities. The common absence of clinically observable sensory impairment may be explained by the insidious loss of sensory fibers over decades that is associated with CNS amplification of the minimal sensory input. Gene mutations have been found in fewer than 2% of cases with HMSN-2, so genetic testing is not recommended at this time. Diagnostic evaluation involves examination of other family members, ideally both parents. Establishment of an autosomal dominant inheritance is the best confirmatory test. The treatment is symptomatic and rehabilitative. Bilateral plastic ankle-foot orthoses are often important to maintain function through the remainder of a normal lifespan.

The autosomal dominant form of hereditary sensory and autonomic neuropathy (HSAN) presents in adulthood with small-fiber sensory symptoms and signs. Although occasionally presenting with foot pain, loss of pain perception often causes significant foot injuries.

Among those associated with CNS diseases, distal axonal polyneuropathy is most common with a number of spinocerebellar syndromes, in which it is a common or essential feature of certain autosomal dominant and autosomal recessive types.

Idiopathic distal axonal polyneuropathy

In one-quarter to one-half of patients who have distal axonal polyneuropathy but do not have diabetes mellitus or alcoholism, no causative factors are identified despite thorough evaluation. These patients are said to have an *idiopathic distal axonal polyneuropathy*. Idiopathic polyneuropathy becomes more common with advancing age. Minor disability is often produced by pain in the feet, numbness in the feet, sensory ataxia, or bilateral partial foot drop. Lifespan is not shortened by this disease, and disability is palliated with symptomatic treatment of pain, use of bilateral plastic ankle-foot orthoses for partial foot drop, and a cane for sensory ataxia. Because no associated disease is present, no conventional treatment is available to alter the insidiously progressive course of the disease. However, ongoing research is assessing the potential benefit of weight loss and exercise in patients with impaired glucose tolerance.

Symptomatic treatment of distal axonal polyneuropathy

When a precise etiology is not found, or the disease does not have a definitive treatment, symptomatic treatment of neuropathic pain becomes an especially important therapeutic strategy. Neuropathic pain is commonly described using adjectives such as burning, tingling, shooting, electric-like, or lancinating. This spontaneous pain is often accompanied by painful perception of normal sensory stimuli (this is referred to as *allodynia*), especially light touch. Neuropathic pain is usually worse late in the day or during the night and often interferes with sleep. Symptomatic treatment usually includes low doses of tricyclic antidepressants (amitriptyline, nortriptyline, or desipramine) or gabapentin. Amitriptyline tends to produce benefit more rapidly, in part, because it is most sedating and improves sleep within days. However, it produces the most anticholinergic side effects (dry mouth, dry eyes, constipation), so may be less well tolerated. Desipramine has a much lower incidence of anticholinergic side effects and is usually better tolerated. However, the dosage may need to be increased gradually to higher levels before it benefits the pain. Both drugs are usually given at bedtime, starting with 10 mg tablets. The dosage is increased by 10 mg every 2–5 days, if no side effects have developed. The dosage is not increased after benefit is achieved or side effects develop. Tricyclic antidepressants are usually effective for pain at doses lower than those used to treat depression. Benefit is often achieved around 50 mg/day for amitriptyline or 80 mg/day for desipramine, but the effective dosage varies widely among different patients. Gabapentin is usually effective at a dose of 900–1,800 mg/day, in divided doses, although doses as high as 3,600 mg/day have also been used.

Severe shooting, electric-like, or lancinating pain is often improved with a membrane-stabilizing drug. Carbamazepine or lamotrigine is usually more effective than phenytoin. Treatment is started with very low dosages that are gradually increased. Newer agents like pregabalin and duloxetine have been shown to be effective in clinical trials of diabetic polyneuropathy, but are more expensive. Narcotics and nonsteroidal anti-inflammatory drugs (NSAIDs) are much less effective at treating neuropathic pain, but are sometimes useful adjuncts.

Demyelinating Polyneuropathy

Demyelinating polyneuropathies are far less common than distal axonal polyneuropathies. Furthermore, the number of diagnostic possibilities is far more limited. Demyelinating polyneuropathies usually present with weakness as the chief complaint. On examination, weakness is more severe than sensory impairment, and reflexes are usually absent in the arms and the legs. For the inflammatory demyelinating polyneuropathies, weakness is usually more severe distally than proximally, but includes more proximal weakness than occurs in a length-dependent, distal axonal polyneuropathy. Once this pattern that differs from a length-dependent, distal axonal polyneuropathy is recognized, consider referral to a neurologist with subspecialty expertise in neuromuscular diseases for further evaluation. The consultation usually includes clinical and electrodiagnostic evaluation. With all types of demyelinating polyneuropathy, motor nerve conduction velocities are slowed considerably relative to age-matched control subjects. The three most common diagnostic possibilities for this neuropathy are inflammatory demyelinating polyneuropathy, monoclonal protein-associated demyelinating polyneuropathy, and hereditary demyelinating polyneuropathy. The inflammatory demyelinating polyneuropathies are further subdivided into those with acute and chronic onset, which have important differences in treatment.

Acute inflammatory demyelinating polyneuropathy

Acute inflammatory demyelinating polyneuropathy (AIDP) is the most common form of the GBS in developed countries. It causes acute symmetrical non–length-dependent weakness more than sensory symptoms, as well as reduced or absent reflexes. Symptoms develop rapidly over 1–2 weeks in most patients and reach a maximum within 4 weeks in all patients. Generalized weakness is so severe as to cause respiratory failure in about 30% of patients. For those with this severity of weakness, ventilatory support is often required for 1–2 months, but rarely for 6 months or longer. For those without respiratory failure, weakness remains at a plateau for 1–2 weeks, before improvement begins. A vast majority of patients without respiratory failure recover fully over several months, and a majority of patients with respiratory failure make a good recovery. Cranial nerve involvement occurs in 10–20% of cases, with weakness of extraocular, facial, or palatal muscles being far more common than impairment of pupillary function. Approximately 5% of cases of GBS have the Miller-Fisher variant, in which ataxia, areflexia, and ophthalmoplegia are the predominant symptoms and signs. Less than 5% of cases of the GBS have severe loss of sensory and motor axons. These are the small minority of patients who often remain ventilator-dependent for 6 or more months. Autonomic involvement with labile vital signs is common and may be life-threatening in a minority who develop an arrhythmia or refractory hypotension. The cerebrospinal fluid (CSF) protein is almost always elevated, without elevation of white blood cells after the first week. The presence of elevated white cell count in the spinal fluid raises the possibility of infection, such as recent HIV seroconversion or Lyme disease. Electrodiagnostic testing confirms signs of an acute polyneuropathy, often with subclinically multifocal demyelination. If subclinical multifocal demyelination with conduction block and multifocal slowing is documented, AIDP is well established. If signs are those of an acute polyneuropathy without definite demyelination, the differential diagnosis includes acute intoxication with heavy metals or hexacarbons, as well as one of the porphyrias. Treatment involves close cardiovascular and respiratory monitoring for signs of potentially life-threatening bulbar, respiratory, or autonomic involvement and administration of either plasmapheresis or intravenous (IV) immunoglobulins. Each of these latter treatments has been proven to improve the speed of recovery, with the average length of time to regain independent walking and, if necessary, to breathe independently of a respirator reduced by half. Administration of one of these two treatments is now standard therapy for all patients with acute inflammatory demyelinating polyneuropathy who are unable to walk independently.

Chronic inflammatory demyelinating polyneuropathy

Chronic inflammatory demyelinating polyneuropathy (CIDP) presents with similar clinical features to AIDP, but has a slower course of onset. Symmetrical weakness evolves over 2–6 months or longer. On examination, non–length-dependent weakness is more severe than sensory impairment. Reflexes are usually absent in the arms and legs. Electrodiagnostic studies reveal marked slowing of motor conduction that is often subclinically multifocal and associated with conduction block. Cerebrospinal fluid shows elevated protein usually without white blood cells, unless the patient is HIV-positive. If subclinical multifocal slowing and conduction block are found electrodiagnostically, the differential diagnosis is between idiopathic CIDP and CIDP associated with monoclonal protein or other systemic disease (such as HIV). Evaluation for associated monoclonal protein disorder consists of obtaining serum protein electrophoresis, serum immunofixation, 24-hour urine for light chain analysis, and skeletal survey. If slowing is uniform and conduction block is not found, the differential diagnosis also includes hereditary demyelinating polyneuropathies. Treatment of idiopathic CIDP may be curative and may include prednisone, plasmapheresis, or IV immunoglobulins acutely, or prednisone or azathioprine chronically. Rare patients require cyclophosphamide or other cytolytic immunosuppressive treatment. In CIDP associated with HIV infection, treatment is similar but does not include azathioprine or cyclophosphamide.

Chronic demyelinating polyneuropathy associated with monoclonal protein disorders

Patients with this neuropathy present in the same manner neurologically as those with CIDP. Some patients will have Waldenstrom macroglobulinemia or other well-defined hematologic disease, but the majority of patients who present with polyneuropathy have a monoclonal gammopathy of undetermined significance that was first identified by the serum protein electrophoresis, serum immunofixation, or 24-hour urine for light chain analysis. A skeletal survey is obtained to determine if an osteosclerotic myeloma is present. This myeloma is often a single sclerotic lesion and remediable with surgical or radiation therapy. In contrast to the relationship between distal axonal polyneuropathy and monoclonal proteins, the presence of a monoclonal protein is almost always relevant to the cause for a demyelinating polyneuropathy. Furthermore, treatment is often initiated for the neuropathy, because these patients are more disabled by weakness and are more likely to improve with therapy.

Hereditary demyelinating polyneuropathy

Several hereditary disorders are associated with demyelinating polyneuropathy. In some, the peripheral neuropathy is only one aspect of disease that also affects the CNS or eyes (for example, Refsum disease, metachromatic leukodystrophy, and adrenomyeloneuropathy). In others, the peripheral neuropathy is the only primary manifestation of the disease, although secondary manifestations may still include skeletal deformities (for example, hammer toe formation and high foot arches). The most common disease among the latter group is hereditary motor sensory neuropathy (HMSN) type 1, which is also known as the hypertrophic form of Charcot-Marie-Tooth disease. HMSN 1 is usually inherited as an autosomal dominant trait, but it can be X-linked. HMSN type 1 is usually manifest in the first or second decade of life, with subtle intrinsic foot weakness and foot deformities (high arches and hammer toes). However, patients may not present with bilateral partial foot drop until their teens or adulthood. In addition to the signs of distal weakness and muscular atrophy, tendon reflexes are absent at the ankles and reduced or absent at the knees and often in the arms at the time of presentation. Sensory loss is often not apparent clinically. Electrodiagnostic studies reveal uniform and marked slowing of motor nerve conduction velocity by the age of 5 years. With increasing severity of the disease, the size of motor responses becomes smaller. Although clinical sensory loss is usually mild or absent, sensory nerve responses are usually absent at the ankles and small and slow in the hands. Cerebrospinal fluid protein is often elevated. The most common genetic abnormality that produces HMSN 1 is a duplication on chromosome 17 that encodes for peripheral myelin protein-22 (PMP-22). This is available as a routine commercial test. If the duplication is found, this is diagnostic of HMSN type 1A. A deletion of this gene produces a different syndrome, hereditary liability to pressure palsies. These patients usually have an underlying polyneuropathy with palpably enlarged nerves, and there is a history of multiple compressive neuropathies. Other forms of HMSN are due to mutations of the myelin P0 protein gene on chromosome 1 and mutations of the connexin gene on the X chromosome. Genetic testing is often diagnostically useful in cases of HMSN 1, since a specific gene defect is found in two-thirds to three-quarters of cases.

Generalized Neuronopathies

Motor Neuronopathy

Motor neuronopathy is produced by degeneration of anterior horn cells in the spinal cord or motor neurons in brainstem motor nuclei with secondary Wallerian degeneration of motor axons. The primary clinical manifestations of motor neuronopathy are weakness and atrophy of muscles without sensory involvement. It is usually associated with fasciculations and cramping of muscles. Most motor neuronopathies affect the anterior horn cells first and most severely, so the term of *anterior horn cell disease* is used more commonly than motor neuronopathy by many clinicians. Anterior horn cell disease may present in isolation or in combination with degeneration of other neurologic systems (Table 18.8).

Amyotrophic lateral sclerosis

The most common disease that includes anterior horn cell involvement is ALS (or Lou Gehrig disease). Nearly half of patients who are eventually found to have ALS present with weakness or incoordination of one hand due to either anterior horn cell disease or upper motor neuron disease that is asymmetrically affecting the cervical segment. Other patients present with dysarthria from bulbar onset of disease or leg weakness or incoordination from lumbosacral involvement. Amyotrophic lateral

sclerosis is usually rapidly progressive and leads to respiratory weakness and death in an average of about 4 years. In 5–10% of patients, ALS is an autosomal dominant disorder that follows autosomal dominant inheritance, with one of the parents having been known to have died from the disease. Differential diagnosis depends on the presenting symptoms. After thorough evaluation, a presumptive diagnosis of possible or probable ALS is usually made, with the diagnosis of definite ALS delayed until progression produces signs of generalized upper and lower motor neuron involvement. With the presentation of lower motor neuron weakness in the upper limbs and spasticity in the lower limbs, cervical spondylosis with central canal stenosis producing myelopathy and foraminal stenosis causing polyradiculopathy is a common disease that must be distinguished. Other rare diseases of the cervical spinal cord (for example, syringomyelia or tumor) may present in a similar manner. Magnetic resonance imaging (MRI) of the cervical spine is an important diagnostic test for these patients. The differential for upper motor neuron onset of ALS includes compressive myelopathy, multiple sclerosis, hereditary spastic paraparesis, and primary lateral sclerosis. With this presentation, an MRI at the highest level of upper motor neuron signs (usually either head or cervical spine) is usually necessary. The differential for lower motor neuron onset of ALS includes multifocal motor neuropathy, polyradiculopathy, and spinal muscular atrophy. Electrodiagnostic studies performed by a physician who has experience in distinguishing these disorders is the most important diagnostic step, as the electrophysiologic signs of demyelination to identify multifocal motor neuropathy are often present over a short nerve segment that may not be included in a routine nerve conduction test.

Although there was no treatment known to alter the course of ALS until recently, treatments are starting to become available that modestly slow progression. Riluzole is the first drug to receive approval from the U.S. Food and Drug Administration (FDA) to delay the progression of ALS. Celecoxib and minocycline demonstrated promising results in the mouse model for ALS, but large, phase III clinical trials have failed to demonstrate efficacy. Current research is evaluating the efficacy of ceftriaxone, arimoclomol, and lithium in ALS. Other empirical treatments include antioxidant vitamins and coenzyme Q10. Symptomatic treatments include antispasticity medications (such as baclofen or tizanidine), physical therapy programs (to maintain strength of good muscles and to reduce spasms and stiffness with stretching), bracing (for example, plastic ankle-foot orthoses for foot drop), speech therapy (to instruct in modification of swallowing, to help advise in the timing of gastrostomies, and to assist with alternative communication methods), and respiratory therapy (to help prevent atelectasis and aspira-

---

Table 18.8 Classification of anterior horn cell diseases

Isolated
- ▶ Infectious: poliovirus or other enterovirus
- ▶ Hereditary: autosomal recessive or X-linked spinal muscular atrophies
- ▶ Fazio-Londe disease

Occurring in association with degeneration of other neurologic systems
- ▶ Amyotrophic lateral sclerosis (pyramidal)
- ▶ Multiple systems atrophy (parkinsonism, cerebellar, autonomic, cognitive, and pyramidal disease)
- ▶ Hexosaminidase A deficiency (cognitive, pyramidal, cerebellar, tremor)

tion pneumonia). An emerging practice pattern is the long-term management of patients with ALS by multidisciplinary groups in specialized centers.

Hereditary motor neuronopathies

The next most common type of anterior horn cell diseases are autosomal recessive or X-linked. These diseases affect only anterior horn cells and are called *spinal muscular atrophies*. Autosomal recessive proximal spinal muscular atrophy type III starts in late childhood. Patients may not present for medical attention until young adulthood. Autosomal recessive proximal spinal muscular atrophy type IV presents with very slowly progressive proximal weakness in adulthood that is usually indistinguishable clinically from a chronic myopathy. Electrodiagnostic studies reveal EMG evidence for acute and chronic partial denervation with reinnervation and nerve conduction study evidence for normal sensory nerve action potentials. Kennedy disease is an X-linked recessive disease that is classified as a hereditary motor neuronopathy. It presents with slowly progressive weakness, cramping, twitching, or tremor. The examination reveals perioral facial twitching when the lips are pursed and gynecomastia. Although sensation is normal clinically, sensory nerve conduction studies reveal small responses as a subclinical feature of the more severe anterior horn cell involvement.

No treatment has yet been proven to alter the course of these diseases. Diagnosis is important to provide prognostic information to the affected patients and genetic counseling for the patient and their family.

Viral paralytic poliomyelitis

Poliovirus or certain other enteroviruses that cause acute infectious anterior horn cell disease usually begin with fever, malaise, headache, and gastrointestinal symptoms. Currently in North America, West Nile virus is the most common cause for acute viral paralytic poliomyelitis. Lower motor neuron weakness usually begins within the first 2 weeks of the systemic infection. Progression of weakness is rapid, with the nadir of weakness following within 5 days of the first sign of weakness. The CSF has inflammatory results, with elevated white blood cells (usually 100–200 with predominantly mononuclear cells during the first week or two), elevated protein, but normal glucose. Recovery is usually slow and often incomplete.

Other anterior horn cell diseases

Rare forms of anterior horn cell disease include Fazio-Londe disease and hexosaminidase deficiency. Fazio-Londe disease is an anterior horn cell disease confined to bulbar musculature in patients in their late teens or twenties. Hexosaminidase deficiency typically presents as Tay-Sachs disease. In rare cases, it has presented with slowly progressive generalized anterior horn cell disease affecting proximal muscles in childhood or adulthood. This may be associated with pyramidal signs and mimic ALS. Later cognitive changes such as dementia, psychosis, or personality change and a tremor may become evident. There is no cherry red spot on the macula as in Tay-Sachs, but leukocyte or cultured fibroblasts show severe deficiency or absence of hexosaminidase A.

Sensory Neuronopathy

Sensory neuronopathy presents with numbness or sensory ataxia of a single limb or of both lower limbs distally. On examination, sensation is reduced and tendon reflexes are reduced or absent in affected limbs. Strength is usually normal, although severe sensory ataxia may produce such severe incoordination that strength is impaired late in its course. Sensory neuronopathy can be classified into to one of four groups.

Paraneoplastic sensory neuronopathy

Paraneoplastic sensory neuronopathy is the most serious and life-threatening form of the disease, with death from the underlying neoplasm occurring within 1 year in most cases. Sensory impairment may be asymmetrical or symmetrical. A small-cell carcinoma of the lung is by far the most common neoplasm. The neoplasm is usually unknown at the time of neurologic presentation and may not become manifest for many months. Chest computed tomography (CT) is an important part of the evaluation. The presence of an anti-Hu antibody in the serum is specific for the paraneoplastic etiology, but this antibody is not always present.

Sjögren syndrome

Sensory neuronopathy is rare presentation for Sjögren syndrome. Sensory impairment may be asymmetrical or symmetrical. Symptoms and signs of the sicca syndrome (dry eyes and dry mouth) are usually obvious at the time of neurologic presentation. Intensive immunosuppression is often tried to arrest progression if diagnosis precedes severe disability. Such treatment has not been proven effective, but several anecdotes suggest benefit.

Toxic sensory neuronopathy

Several toxins are known to produce sensory neuronopathy, including pyridoxine (vitamin B_6 in doses above 200 mg/day) and cisplatin. Sensory symptoms are always distal and symmetrical with these. Progression is arrested within weeks of discontinuation of the toxic exposure, and subsequent improvement is expected, although often incomplete.

Idiopathic sensory neuronopathy

Cases without identifiable cause are not unusual. Sensory impairment may be asymmetrical or symmetrical. Progression is usually slow and self-limited after several months or years. Disability is usually less severe than with paraneoplastic cases and those associated with Sjögren syndrome. After spontaneous stabilization, improvement is expected, although often incomplete.

Focal or Multifocal Neuropathies

Common Compressive Neuropathies

Median nerve

The most common compressive neuropathy is the carpal tunnel syndrome, which is secondary to compression of the median nerve as it passes under the transverse carpal ligament at the wrist. It usually presents with intermittent tingling, numbness, and pain of a hand, usually the dominant one. About half of patients have milder symptoms or signs in the other hand. Worsening of symptoms at night that causes nocturnal awakening several hours into sleep is a characteristic symptom. Symptoms typically occur during daytime activity, such as driving or repetitive use of the hands. However, activity-related symptoms are also typical of arthritis and tendonitis. The pain is typically aching and felt in the hand and forearm, but sometimes also in the arm and shoulder. The numbness often causes clumsiness that interferes with opening jars and may be confused with weakness.

A mild carpal tunnel syndrome may produce no signs on examination. The most common abnormality is a positive Tinel sign (tingling in the fingers with gentle tapping over the nerve where it passes through the carpal tunnel for this syndrome) or a positive Phalen maneuver (tingling and pain with wrist flexion for 60 seconds). Persistently altered sensation over the thumb, first two fingers, and the lateral half of the ring finger is a sign of a moderate carpal tunnel syndrome. Weakness and wasting of the abductor pollicis brevis and other median innervated thenar muscles are the signs of a severe carpal tunnel syndrome.

The carpal tunnel syndrome is more common during middle and late adulthood in women than in men, probably because women tend to have narrower carpal tunnels congenitally and their median nerves become compressed with lesser amounts of arthritis or tenosynovitis. Carpal tunnel syndrome seems to be caused in some individuals by repetitive wrist or finger movement and thus is common in workers who spend much of their day typing on a computer keyboard. However, the relationship between repetitive, low-force activity and carpal tunnel syndrome remains controversial. Pregnancy, rheumatoid arthritis, and hypothyroidism are also common causes. Uncommon causes include chronic hemodialysis, multiple myeloma, and type II familial amyloidosis. Diabetic polyneuropathy and perhaps other neuropathies increase the risk of developing carpal tunnel syndrome.

Differential diagnosis includes sensory symptoms from a C6 or C7 radiculopathy, weakness from a C8 or T1 radiculopathy, a proximal median neuropathy, and a brachial plexus lesion. Electrodiagnostic studies are important to document the presence and severity of the carpal tunnel syndrome, or to make one of these other diagnoses before proceeding with treatment.

Treatment is either conservative or surgical, in part depending on the severity of nerve injury. The cornerstone of conservative treatment is the use of a neutral-position wrist splint (especially while sleeping at night). Steroid injection at the proximal edge of the carpal tunnel, a short course of oral steroids, or oral NSAIDs are often administered, as an adjunct. If conservative treatment fails, if repetitive hand activity cannot be avoided, or if the nerve deficits are moderate or severe, surgical treatment is indicated. This consists of sectioning the transverse carpal ligament.

Other median nerve compression or entrapment syndromes include the anterior interosseus neuropathy and the pronator teres syndrome. The anterior interosseus nerve is a pure motor branch of the median nerve at the elbow. Thus, an anterior interosseus neuropathy causes weakness of the flexor pollicis longus, the flexor digitorum profundus of the index and long fingers, and the pronator quadratus muscles, the first two of which allow pinching of the thumb and index and long fingers together. The pronator teres syndrome is not clearly a neuropathy because, often, electrophysiologic evidence of median nerve injury is not present. It involves aching and pain in the anterior forearm with focal muscle tenderness. Symptoms are worsened by repetitive pronation of the arm. Some presume that the syndrome is caused by median nerve entrapment at the point at which it passes between the two heads of the pronator teres. Signs and symptoms of median nerve or anterior interosseus nerve motor or sensory loss are usually absent. Treatment involves avoidance of repetitive pronation of the arm. Corticosteroid injections into the pronator muscle can improve symptoms. Surgical exploration is considered occasionally as a last resort.

Ulnar nerve

The second most common compressive neuropathy is an ulnar neuropathy at the elbow. Ulnar neuropathies usually present with sensory loss or tingling in the little finger. Aching pain of the elbow, forearm, or hand is an occasional complaint. Motor symptoms vary from none to severe weakness and atrophy of ulnar intrinsic hand muscles. On examination, sensory impairment involves the little finger, the medial half of the ring finger, and the palmar and dorsal aspect of the medial hand, with normal sensation over the medial forearm. Weakness and wasting of the interosseus and hypothenar muscles are common. Mild weakness for flexion of the tips of the ring and little fingers and of the wrist is common if hand weakness is severe. Reflexes are normal and symmetric. A positive Tinel sign at the elbow is occasionally observed.

With ulnar neuropathy at the elbow, the ulnar nerve is usually compressed in the condylar groove of the humerus or in the cubital tunnel. Compression at the condylar groove is usually external, from a single severe traumatic injury (such as motor vehicle accident or fall) or from repetitive minor injury (such as habitually leaning on the elbow). The cubital tunnel syndrome is a commonly bilateral form of ulnar neuropathy at the elbow. It is often produced by repetitive flexion and extension of the wrist or by repetitive hammering movements. During these activities, the nerve is compressed between the two heads of the flexor carpi ulnaris. Other causes for ulnar neuropathy at the elbow include stretch of the nerve over an elbow deformity that has resulted from an old supracondylar or medial condylar fracture (this is referred to as a *tardy ulnar neuropathy*), or from recurrent subluxation of the nerve out of the condylar groove.

The differential diagnosis includes C8 radiculopathy, lower trunk or medial cord brachial plexus lesions, and ulnar neuropathy at the wrist. Electrodiagnostic localization of an ulnar neuropathy at the elbow relies on identification of loss of ulnar motor or sensory axons in an appropriate distribution and slowing or conduction block of ulnar motor conduction across the elbow.

Initial treatment of an ulnar neuropathy at the elbow involves the use of elbow pads or avoidance of external pressure from leaning on the elbow. If symptoms worsen or do not significantly improve despite conservative treatment, or if there is evidence of a structural process compressing the nerve, then surgical treatment is considered. Surgery involves decompression of the ulnar nerve in the cubital tunnel, transposition of the nerve to the front of the elbow, or medial epicondylectomy. A majority of patients stabilize or improve with surgery.

Ulnar neuropathy at the wrist usually presents with weakness of ulnar intrinsic hand muscles that more severely affects the interosseus than the hypothenar muscles. Sensory loss occurs in a minority of cases. If present, it affects the little and medial ring fingers and the palmar (but not the dorsal) medial hand. Electrodiagnostic studies are important to distinguish ulnar neuropathies at the wrist from those at the elbow and from C8 radiculopathy.

Ulnar neuropathies at the wrist or hand often occur because of repeated pressure on the nerve at the wrist or hand from using tools or bicycling, in which case they are commonly bilateral. Ganglia may also compress the nerve in this location. If external compression has not obviously occurred, surgical exploration is considered.

Peroneal nerve

Peroneal neuropathy is the most common focal neuropathy of the lower limbs. Patients with it usually present with a foot drop. If weakness is limited to foot and toe dorsiflexion, a deep peroneal neuropathy is present. In this situation, a patch of numbness is often present between the great and second toes over the dorsum of the foot. If weakness includes eversion of the ankle, then a common peroneal neuropathy is present. It usually causes numbness over the anterolateral leg and dorsal foot. Pain is either absent or a minor complaint in most patients.

Because of its superficial course, the common peroneal nerve is commonly compressed during prolonged squatting or leg crossing (especially in thin persons who lack the subcutaneous adipose tissue to protect the nerve) or during surgery in the lithotomy position. The peroneal neuropathy less often results from compression by synovial cysts, the peroneus longus muscle at the fibular tunnel or other structures, or traumas at the fibular head. The peroneal nerve is also the most common nerve to be affected first in vasculitic mononeuropathy multiplex.

The differential diagnosis includes sciatic neuropathy and L5 radiculopathy. Electrodiagnostic studies are important to localize the lesion and assess its severity.

If due to compression, treatment of peroneal neuropathy is conservative, with instruction to avoid leg crossing during close clinical follow-up. If the pathophysiology is predominantly conduction block from compression, improvement is common over 1–3 months. If compression is not likely, or if systemic symptoms are present, evaluation includes blood tests for vasculitis.

Sciatic nerve

Sciatic neuropathy is the second most common lower limb focal neuropathy. Pain is common in association with weakness and numbness. The peroneal division of the sciatic nerve is usually more severely affected than the tibial division, so distinction of it from common peroneal neuropathy may be difficult. The ankle reflex is an important sign in such cases. Even when tibial division involvement is minor, the ankle reflex is usually depressed or absent in sciatic neuropathy, whereas it is normal in common peroneal neuropathy. The most common causes for sciatic neuropathy are total hip arthroplasty and trauma (for example, vehicular accidents and gunshot wounds). Electrodiagnostic studies are important to localize the lesion and provide prognostic information. The pathophysiology is usually axonal loss. Treatment is usually conservative, with medication to control pain and the prescription of a plastic ankle-foot orthotic to improve walking. The majority of patients make a good but incomplete recovery over 2–3 years.

Plexopathy (Multifocal Neuropathies within a Limb)

Brachial or lumbosacral plexopathies occur secondary to trauma, infiltration by neoplasm, radiation injury, idiopathic inflammation, or, for the lumbosacral plexus, microvascular disease from diabetes mellitus. Idiopathic brachial neuritis (idiopathic brachial plexopathy, idiopathic brachial plexus neuropathy, or the Parsonage-Turner syndrome) is a relatively common cause for a plexopathy. It presents with excruciating unilateral shoulder pain that interferes with sleep. A preceding history of an immunization or viral infection is common. Weakness follows pain by several days to 2 weeks. The shoulder pain dissipates in 1–2 months, leaving the patient with severe weakness and atrophy of shoulder girdle muscles. The three most commonly affected nerves are the long thoracic (which causes winging of the scapula from serratus anterior weakness), the suprascapular (which causes weakness with external rotation of the shoulder from infraspinatus involvement), and the axillary (which causes weakness of shoulder abduction from deltoid involvement). Thus, idiopathic brachial neuritis may be confused with a C5 radiculopathy. Numbness is inconspicuous. Less commonly, other arm muscles are affected. Improvement in strength begins about 2–3 months after onset. Recovery is slow over 1–2 years, but is usually complete. Except in rare familial cases, symptoms rarely recur. No known treatment is known to alter the course of disease, but high-dose daily prednisone is often tried and may lessen the severity of the attack. Pain control is important. The initial use of narcotics is reasonable, whereas a sedative antidepressant, such as amitriptyline, is begun for longer-term pain management.

A metastatic brachial plexopathy in a cancer patient is a relatively common acute syndrome. If the primary lung or breast cancer was treated with radiation near the brachial plexus, the differential is between radiation-induced versus malignant infiltration of the brachial plexus.

Radiation plexopathies may be secondary to radiation-induced changes in the endothelium of the vasa nervorum causing ischemic injury to the plexus. Treatment

with heparin has suggested stabilization in a few cases of radiation plexopathy, but no controlled data has been provided yet.

Idiopathic lumbosacral plexopathy is a rare syndrome that is similar to idiopathic brachial neuritis, but affects the lumbosacral region. Occasionally, the erythrocyte sedimentation rate is elevated and prednisone is beneficial. Several other cases have been chronic but responsive to IV immunoglobulins. Patients with diabetes mellitus over the age of 50 years occasionally develop a syndrome in which weakness develops in the distribution of the femoral and obturator nerves in association with pain, weight loss, and often more diffuse weakness. This syndrome was termed *diabetic amyotrophy* in the 1950s and has since been referred to with many different names. Electromyographic studies often reveal acute denervation of the paraspinal muscles, so *diabetic radiculoplexopathy* is one name for it. Treatment includes control of glucose and pain management.

Multifocal Axonal Neuropathy (Mononeuritis Multiplex)

Mononeuritis multiplex is a neuropathy that affects multiple single nerves and is usually caused by vasculitis. The vasculitis is limited to peripheral nerve in a majority, but in a significant minority is associated with systemic vasculitis. The initial symptom is often a deep aching proximal limb pain that is followed in days by painful numbness in the distribution of one nerve within this limb. Over days to weeks, multifocal or asymmetric sensory loss and pain develop. Weakness, especially foot drop, is common, because the peroneal nerve is the most common to be affected by vasculitis. Symptoms initially present as acute loss of sensation and weakness in individual nerve territories, but this can become confluent and resemble an axonal symmetric polyneuropathy. Because of its association with vasculitis, mononeuritis multiplex is a neurologic emergency that must be evaluated and treated promptly.

The most common causes of vasculitic mononeuritis multiplex are the polyarteritis nodosa group of systemic vasculitides and rheumatoid arteritis. Essential mixed cryoglobulinemia, which is often associated with viral hepatitis, may present as a mononeuritis multiplex. Causes of mononeuritis multiplex other than vasculitis include Lyme disease, herpes zoster, leprosy, tumor infiltration of nerve, and cytomegalovirus infection in late stage AIDS.

Electrodiagnostic testing is useful to confirm the asymmetric loss of sensory and motor axons and quantitate the degree of nerve injury. The workup for mononeuritis multiplex includes a serologic workup with CBC, erythrocyte sedimentation rate, liver and renal function tests, HIV antibody, rheumatoid factor, antinuclear anti-

---

▼

Pearls and Perils

Radiation-induced versus Malignant Infiltration of the Brachial Plexus

▶ Radiation plexopathies are often associated with myokymic discharges on needle EMG of affected arm muscles.

▶ Malignant infiltration of the brachial plexus is usually painful, whereas radiation-induced plexopathies are usually painless.

▶ Malignant invasion of the brachial plexus usually affects the lower brachial plexus and may be associated with an ipsilateral Horner syndrome (miosis in dark illumination, ptosis, and/or anhidrosis of the face).

body, ANCA, and urinalysis. In contrast to demyelinating inflammatory neuropathies, CSF protein is usually normal because there is rarely involvement of nerve roots. Other tests may be indicated in specific patients. Sural nerve biopsy is often used to diagnose vasculitis pathologically. The yield of sural nerve biopsy is improved by selecting a sural nerve that is abnormal electrophysiologically. Treatment usually includes prednisone and often azathioprine or cyclophosphamide. If an underlying systemic vasculitis is present, treatment focuses more on the underlying vasculitis than the mononeuritis multiplex and usually includes cyclophosphamide. The neuropathy makes a good recovery in most patients who survive the systemic vasculitis.

Radiculopathy

Radiculopathy refers to pain, numbness, or weakness that results from injury of sensory or motor nerve roots as they leave the spinal canal. Injury usually occurs from bony changes of the neural foramen (spondylosis) or from an intervertebral disc herniation that is compressing the nerve root. Radiculopathies are rarely caused by metastasis to vertebral pedicles, by inflammation of nerve roots from herpes zoster or sarcoid, or by infiltration from carcinomatous meningitis. Painful thoracic radiculopathies are usually associated with diabetes mellitus or herpes zoster. The characteristic features of a radiculopathy are pain in the area of nerve root compression, numbness or tingling in the appropriate dermatome, a depressed tendon reflex, and often weakness in a myotomal pattern. Localization of the symptomatic root is primarily clinical. If clinically indicated, laboratory assessment often includes electrodiagnostic testing and imaging studies. Electromyographic studies identify functional significant injury to motor roots and often aid the clinical decision regarding the symptomatic root. Imaging studies have a high false-positive rate and are used to assess the anatomy of the symptomatic root. If an inflammatory or malignant radiculopathy is suspected, then CSF analysis is performed. Table 18.9 lists the clinical features of common nerve root compressions.

Myopathy

Myopathy is disease of muscle tissue. The fundamental symptom of myopathy is weakness. Patients with weakness from myopathy occasionally have pain from muscle (myalgia). However, the vast majority of patients who have myalgia without weakness do not have a form of myopathy that can be objectively documented by currently available diagnostic tests, including biochemical analysis of biopsied muscle tissue.

Patients with myopathy usually present with subacute or chronic proximal weakness associated with an elevated CK level in the serum. Occasionally, patients with myopathy present with acute, generalized, or distal weakness. For further evaluation and treatment, patients with myopathy need to be distinguished from patients with weakness caused by diseases of the lower motor neuron and the neuromuscular junction. Although clinical features alone are not sufficiently accurate to distinguish these, the pattern of motor unit recruitment as recorded during an EMG study of a moderately weak muscle reliably separates lower motor neuron and myopathic weakness, and the results of additional electrophysiological testing (such as repetitive nerve stimulation) distinguish myopathy from neuromuscular junction disease.

Myopathy results from several different disease processes. The primary care physician is most likely to be involved in the initial diagnosis of inflammatory myopathy and of myopathy that results from systemic disease or toxic exposure. These myopathies often present acutely or subacutely. Many other myopathies present with chronic or recurrent symptoms, and outpatient referral to a neuromuscular specialist is arranged more routinely. These latter myopathies include the muscular dystrophies, congenital myopathies, metabolic myopathies, mitochondrial myopathies, and those diseases with defects of muscle membrane channels (periodic paralysis and my-

Table 18.9 Clinical features of common nerve root compressions

Root	Distribution of sensory symptoms	Muscle weakness	Decreased tendon reflexes
C6	Lateral forearm and thumb	Elbow flexion, pronation, and wrist extension	Biceps
C7	Index and middle fingers	Elbow and wrist extension, pronation, supination	Triceps
C8	Little finger and medial forearm	Finger flexion and extension, intrinsic hand movements	Finger flexor
L4	Medial shin	Knee extension, ankle dorsiflexion	Knee
L5	Lateral shin, dorsal and medial foot	Dorsiflexion, inversion and eversion of ankle; toe dorsiflexion	
S1	Posterior leg, plantar and lateral foot	Ankle and toe flexors	Ankle

otonia). Many of these myopathies are hereditary and may have remained undiagnosed in other family members because of subtle presentations.

Inflammatory Myopathies

Inflammatory myopathies include myopathies for which treatment may be curative (Table 18.10). Although their incidence is about one per 100 000, their potential for reversibility make them important for recognition by primary care physicians. The vast majority are included in the three types of primary inflammatory myopathies: polymyositis, dermatomyositis, and inclusion body myositis. Less commonly, systemic inflammatory diseases, such as connective tissue diseases or HIV infection, may secondarily involve muscle.

The primary inflammatory myopathies in adulthood present with symmetric weakness that is usually painless. Occasionally, muscles are painful and tender in dermatomyositis more often than polymyositis, usually when onset is more acute (over several days to a few weeks), and the CK level is exceptionally high. If pain is prominent, and the CK is normal or mildly elevated, polymyalgia rheumatica (in a person over 60 years with an elevated erythrocyte sedimentation rate), joint disease, or fasciitis is far more likely than an inflammatory myopathy.

Polymyositis

Polymyositis is a primary inflammatory myopathy that develops in patients over the age of 20 years without associated inflammation of the skin. Symmetric, painless proximal weakness usually develops over several weeks to several months. Less commonly, it develops acutely or insidiously. The proximal weakness usually includes the shoulder girdle, the pelvic girdle, and the neck flexor muscles. Dysphagia occasionally accompanies the proximal weakness and rarely occurs without it. Respiratory weakness is rare, except in advanced cases. Myocarditis is rarely manifest clinically as congestive heart failure or arrhythmia. Interstitial lung disease occurs in 5–10% of patients, who often have an autoantibody test directed against the Jo-1 nuclear protein. An increased incidence of malignancy may be present in patients with polymyositis, but this is controversial.

The CK is consistently elevated, often severely (>10 normal). Electromyographic studies reveal small-amplitude, short-duration motor unit action potentials that recruit early and are associated with fibrillation potentials. Nerve conduction studies have normal results. The muscle biopsy shows scattered muscle fiber necrosis and regeneration with inflammatory infiltrate within endomysium, including invasion of non-necrotic muscle fibers. There is no evidence of perifascicular atrophy or complement deposition in capillaries. The diagnostic sen-

---

Table 18.10 Inflammatory myopathies

General features
► Symmetric weakness
► Elevated CK
► EMG: myopathy with fibrillation potentials
► Muscle biopsy: inflammatory infiltration

Discriminating features
► Polymyositis
  – Muscle biopsy:
    • scattered muscle fiber degeneration
    • mononuclear cell invasion of non-necrotic fibers
    • absence of inclusion bodies and perifascicular atrophy
► Dermatomyositis
  – Muscle biopsy:
    • perifascicular atrophy
    • perimysial and perivascular infiltrate
  – Rash
► Inclusion body myositis
  – Muscle biopsy:
    • inclusion bodies
  – Prominent weakness of finger flexors or extensors and quadriceps
  – No improvement with steroids

Consistent features
► Polymyositis
  – Weeks or months of proximal weakness
  – No rash
  – Improvement with steroids
► Dermatomyositis
  – Weeks or months of proximal weakness
  – Improvement with steroids
► Inclusion body myositis
  – Insidiously progressive weakness over years
  – No rash
  – Age over 50 years

Variable features
► Polymyositis
  – Dysphagia
  – Interstitial lung disease
  – Malignancy?
► Dermatomyositis
  – Dysphagia
  – Interstitial lung disease
  – Malignancy
► Inclusion body myositis
  – Previous muscle biopsy interpreted as polymyositis

CK, creatine kinase; EMG, electromyograph

---

sitivity of EMG is higher than muscle biopsy, probably due to its ability to sample more muscle tissue. The diagnostic specificity is higher for muscle biopsy, but two or more biopsies may be necessary to obtain the most specific findings.

Treatment is usually initiated with high-dose, daily prednisone (1.0–1.5 mg/kg/day; usually at least 60 mg to no more than 100 mg/day in adults). This usually results in improvement in muscle strength. As strength improves, a gradual, slow taper of prednisone with alternate day dosing over a period of 8–24 months is usually effective. Patients may require treatment for years. The second-line drug of choice is either azathioprine or methotrexate. One is often begun after 1 or 2 months of prednisone treatment to avoid the long-term corticosteroid side effects. Objective improvement in muscle strength is the most important guide to treatment success. Improvement is strength is accompanied by a rapid reduction in the CK level. However, even a moderate decrease in the CK level without improvement in strength may occur in patients who become refractory to high-dose, daily prednisone. An increase in proximal weakness after the first month of prednisone treatment without an interval increase in CK should alert the clinician to the possibility of a superimposed steroid myopathy, which requires a decrease in steroid dosage. If patients start to develop significant side effects from prednisone, a cytotoxic agent such as azathioprine or methotrexate is begun to decrease the effective long-term dosage of prednisone. These steroid-sparing agents take 3–6 months to reach their maximum effect. Other therapeutic options for unresponsive cases may include mycophenolate, IV immunoglobulins, cyclophosphamide, chlorambucil, and total lymphoid irradiation.

Adult dermatomyositis

Dermatomyositis in adulthood differs clinically from polymyositis by the presence of skin changes. The eyelids develop a violaceous appearance (the heliotrope rash), especially the lower margin of the upper eyelid. The cheeks have an erythematous and telangiectatic malar rash. The knuckles often have erythematous, scaling papules (Groton papules). The muscle symptoms of adult dermatomyositis are quite similar to those of polymyositis. In contrast to polymyositis, in which the association is still debated, a significantly increased risk of malignancy (especially adenocarcinoma) is well established in patients over 40 years of age with dermatomyositis.

The results of CK and EMG are the same as for polymyositis. Muscle biopsy in dermatomyositis shows characteristic atrophy of muscle fibrils at the edges of the fascicle (perifascicular atrophy), which is secondary to vascular injury caused by pericapillary inflammation. The mononuclear infiltrate is predominantly perimysial and perivascular. Immune deposits of IgM>IgG antibodies and components of the complement membrane attack complex are found on the microvascular walls, supporting the concept of dermatomyositis as a vascular disease.

The treatment of dermatomyositis is the same as for polymyositis, with initial usage of daily prednisone 1.0–1.5 mg/kg/day (usually at least 60 mg or up to 100 mg/day in adults).

Inclusion body myositis

Inclusion body myositis is an inflammatory myopathy in persons over 50 years of age that has several distinctive features. Unlike the other primary inflammatory myopathies, muscle weakness in inclusion body myositis is more insidiously progressive over many months or years (rather than weeks or months). The pattern of weakness is also characteristic: severe weakness occurs, with atrophy of the quadriceps and forearm flexor muscles; ankle dorsiflexors and proximal upper limb muscles may also be affected, but less severely. Dysphagia is not unusual. A rash or an association with malignancy is not expected. Inclusion body myositis accounts for about 25% of cases of inflammatory myopathy.

The CK is usually normal or only mildly elevated; EMG studies reveal either small-amplitude, short-duration motor unit action potentials or a mixture of these with long-duration polyphasic motor unit action potentials. Fibrillation potentials are usually present if carefully sought, but are not prominent. The muscle biopsy shows features of a low-grade inflammation, in which mononuclear cells invade non-necrotic muscle fibers, rare degenerating and regenerating fibers, and fibers with multiple rimmed vacuoles lined with granular material (inclusion bodies). The rimmed vacuoles are seen within the cytoplasm of muscle fibers on routine light microscopic hematoxylin and eosin or modified trichrome stains. The specific inclusion bodies are seen with congo red stain on light microscopy or under electron microscopy.

Unfortunately, other than supportive care, no treatment has been effective for inclusion body myositis. Rare cases have been reported to respond to prednisone, azathioprine, methotrexate, or IV immunoglobulins, but the vast majority do not.

Inflammatory myopathies associated with connective tissue disease

Inflammatory myopathies do not commonly occur as a part of well-defined connective tissue disorders, such as systemic lupus erythematous or rheumatoid arthritis, but can be a part of overlap syndromes, such as mixed connective tissue disease. Alternatively, blood vessels in muscles can be involved as a part of a systemic vasculitis. The treatment for these inflammatory myopathies is similar to that for polymyositis and dermatomyositis.

Human immunodeficiency virus–associated myopathy

Two main types of myopathy are associated with HIV: an inflammatory myopathy that is similar to polymyositis, and a mitochondrial myopathy that is secondary to chronic use of zidovudine. Often, the differentiation of these two types of myopathy is unclear, and both can co-exist.

HIV-associated inflammatory myopathy typically occurs in the early stages of HIV infection and can be the presenting symptom of HIV. The clinical symptoms are similar to polymyositis: painless proximal weakness that most commonly affects the shoulder girdle and spares bulbar muscles. The muscle biopsy is similar to polymyositis, with the rare addition of subsarcolemmal inclusions, nemaline bodies, which are seen in a few biopsies. Treatment of HIV-associated polymyositis is with prednisone, plasmapheresis, or IV immunoglobulins. Azathioprine, methotrexate, or other cytotoxic drugs are not used in these patients.

Zidovudine causes a myopathy with myalgias more than weakness, commonly when it has been used over an extended period of time (usually with cumulative doses >250 g). This occurs because zidovudine is a mitochondrial toxin and produces an iatrogenic mitochondrial myopathy. Typically, patients with zidovudine-associated myopathy are in the later stages of HIV. If present, weakness is similar to that of HIV-associated inflammatory myopathy. Muscle biopsy often reveals changes typical of a mitochondrial myopathy: subsarcolemmal accumulations of abnormal mitochondria, which on trichrome stain are called *ragged red fibers*. However, similar changes may be seen in asymptomatic patients who take zidovudine.

Because it is difficult to differentiate HIV-inflammatory myopathy from zidovudine-associated mitochondrial myopathy, HIV patients who have features of myopathy on examination and EMG testing, and who have been taking significant doses of zidovudine, are treated with an empiric trial of discontinuation of zidovudine for 4–12 weeks. If weakness does not improve, then a muscle biopsy is performed and, if inflammatory myopathy is found, the patient is treated with prednisone.

Inflammatory myopathies associated with trichinosis

Trichinosis, caused by the nematode *Trichinella spiralis* found in uncooked meat (especially pork), presents as myalgias and weakness that begins within a week after the organism is ingested. These symptoms are usually preceded by a diarrheal illness 1–7 days after infection. Systemic features include fever, periorbital edema, pulmonary involvement, congestive heart failure, and a focal or generalized encephalitis with normal CSF. Eosinophilia is almost always present, and CK is elevated. The EMG shows features typical of a myopathy with fibrillation potentials. The muscle biopsy usually reveals inflammation and often the trichinosis larvae. However, the larvae are not always seen. Therefore, any patient with an acute inflammatory myopathy and eosinophilia on blood smear should be suspected of having trichinosis and

treated empirically awaiting definitive diagnosis. Treatment involves prednisone with antitrichinella therapy.

Myopathy with Systemic Diseases or Toxic Exposures

Endocrine myopathies

Corticosteroid-associated myopathy is the most common endocrinologic myopathy and is more frequently caused by iatrogenic treatment with corticosteroids than by Cushing disease. Daily doses of 30 mg or more of prednisone are part of the usual clinical context for steroid myopathy, but daily doses as low as 15 mg may sufficient to cause it. Alternate day dosing of steroids lessens, but does not remove, the risk of steroid myopathy. Clinically, patients present with painless, proximal weakness without CK elevation. The EMG is often normal but occasionally reveals mild signs of myopathy (small motor unit action potentials that recruit early) without fibrillation potentials in patients with severe weakness. Muscle biopsy features are nonspecific, showing type 2 fiber atrophy. Steroid withdrawal is usually performed empirically, if possible. Muscle biopsy is usually obtained only if strength does not improve after discontinuation of steroids.

Hypothyroidism commonly causes neuromuscular symptoms, including myalgia, muscle stiffness, muscle fatigue, and, in about one-quarter of patients, overt muscular weakness. The CK is usually markedly elevated in the range of 10–100 times normal, even in patients who do not have definite weakness. A low thyroxine level establishes the diagnosis. The muscle symptoms rapidly reverse with thyroid supplementation. Other neurologic features of hypothyroidism include a mild sensorimotor polyneuropathy with an increased incidence of entrapment neuropathies like carpal tunnel syndrome. Hyperthyroidism is usually without neuromuscular complications, but it rarely causes proximal muscle atrophy and weakness, often in association with fasciculations. Other distributions are affected less often. Myasthenia gravis and periodic paralysis are less frequent associations of hyperthyroidism. Hyperparathyroidism rarely presents with proximal weakness and atrophy, often with hyperreflexia and fasciculations. Weakness usually improves when calcium homeostasis is restored. Acromegaly causes proximal muscle weakness after years of the disease. The serum CK is normal or mildly elevated, and the EMG reveals findings of myopathy without fibrillation potentials.

Electrolyte disturbances

Hypokalemia often causes proximal or generalized weakness that is usually painless. With acute hypokalemic paralysis, serum potassium is well below 3.0 mEq/L. Weakness improves within 1–2 hours and resolves over several hours or days with potassium replacement. However, if hypokalemia has been severe or associated with alcoholism, an acute necrotizing myopathy with rhabdomyolysis and renal failure may result, which improves partially or completely over days to weeks. Hyperkalemia has severe and acute effects on both skeletal and cardiac muscle, causing rapidly ascending quadriparesis, frequent respiratory failure, and cardiac arrest. Serum potassium is usually over 7.5 mEq/L. The CK and muscle biopsy are usually normal. Skeletal muscle weakness usually resolves within hours, even if serum potassium has not changed. The common presence of paresthesias and a Chvostek sign suggests that hyperkalemia causes weakness more through its effects on nerve than muscle. Hypocalcemia causes paresthesias and motor dysfunction from tetany more than weakness with presence of Chvostek and Trousseau signs. Thus, its symptoms and signs are better explained by spontaneous peripheral nerve activity than by myopathy. Hypercalcemia causes weakness with hyperreflexia, so this may relate more to CNS effects than those on muscle. Severe hypophosphatemia (serum phosphate <0.4 mM/L) causes acute and severe areflexic weakness with rhabdomyolysis. Because mild hypophosphatemia can be caused by hyperventilation, only serum phosphorus levels <1.0 mM/L should be considered as severe enough to cause weakness or rhabdomyolysis. Hypomagnesemia is often associated with hypocalcemia and may contribute to signs of tetany with weakness. Hypermagnesemia is rarely encountered and usually due to exogenous administration of it. If serum magnesium levels exceed 9.0 mEq/L, severe generalized weakness with respiratory failure usually develops.

Myopathies associated with drugs and toxins

Alcohol can cause acute rhabdomyolysis through pressure from obtundation or from toxic effects of alcohol on muscle, usually in the setting of malnutrition and hypokalemia. Alcohol can also cause weakness secondary to associated hypokalemia or hypophosphatemia. It is unclear whether alcohol itself directly damages muscle, and the existence of an alcohol related chronic myopathy is disputed. Cocaine or impurities in the street drug formulation can cause rhabdomyolysis from a direct myotoxic effect, which is presumably from the cocaine-induced vasoconstriction that causes muscle infarction.

A variety of prescription drugs cause myopathies that are usually reversible with discontinuation of the drugs. A few produce the clinical picture of an acute necrotizing myopathy, but most develop subacutely or chronically. The most common category of drugs that produce acute necrotizing myopathies are diuretics that cause hypokalemia. Less commonly, ε-aminocaproic acid or the combination of vecuronium and steroids in the intensive care unit may cause a severe acute myopathy. The list of drugs that causes subacute or chronic myopathy is much

longer. As described previously in the section on inflammatory myopathies, zidovudine causes a mitochondrial myopathy when a cumulative dose of greater than 250 g is given. Colchicine may cause neuropathy and myopathy when large doses are given or in the presence of renal disease. Chloroquine may cause a vacuolar myopathy, a neuropathy, and a defect in neuromuscular transmission that is similar to myasthenia gravis. Cholesterol-lowering agents that are HMG-CoA reductase inhibitors, such as lovastatin or simvastatin, cause a myopathy with elevation of CK. Niacin can potentiate the effects of HMG-CoA reductase inhibitors on muscle and, in high doses (>1 g/day), can cause weakness and muscle pain by itself. Other drugs that are potentially myotoxic include emetine and rarely adrenergic blockers (such as labetalol and sotalol). Penicillamine can cause an inflammatory myopathy or a myasthenia-like disorder with elevated antibodies to acetylcholine receptor antibodies. Injection of heroin, pentazocine, and meperidine can cause severe local muscle damage when injected repeatedly (usually through self-administration).

Muscular Dystrophies

Muscular dystrophies are hereditary diseases that cause progressive muscle weakness and characteristic "dystrophic" changes on muscle biopsy. These dystrophic pathologic signs are degeneration of muscle fibers; variability of muscle fiber size, including hypertrophic fibers; an increase proportion of muscle fibers with central nuclei; and replacement of muscle tissue with fat and connective tissue (Table 18.11).

Duchenne and Becker muscular dystrophies are the most common and occur in one out of 3,300 live male births. However, the milder Becker phenotype is present in only 5–10% of cases. Both are caused by X-linked recessive mutations in the dystrophin gene, so the term *dystrophinopathy* is sometimes used to refer to them. Boys with Duchenne muscular dystrophy rarely live past the age of 20 years, so this is not a diagnostic consideration in adults who present with progressive weakness. Becker muscular dystrophy is a milder phenotype than Duchenne, and often presents in young adults. Symptoms of muscle weakness usually develop in the early teens to young adulthood in Becker muscular dystrophy. Cardiac, respiratory, and skeletal (scoliosis and contractures) involvement are present in Becker dystrophy but are less severe than in Duchenne. Life expectancy is reduced in Becker muscular dystrophy, but most patients survive into their 40s or 50s. Therapeutic interventions for dystrophinopathies involve supportive measures like bracing, scoliosis surgery, preventing pressure sores, and maintaining an effective pulmonary toilet. This is best achieved through the multidisciplinary efforts of a muscular dystrophy clinic.

Table 18.11 Muscular dystrophies

General features
- ▶ Hereditary weakness
- ▶ Elevated CK
- ▶ EMG: myopathy usually with fibrillation potentials
- ▶ Muscle biopsy: degeneration and regeneration of muscle cells with increased connective tissue

Discriminating features
- ▶ Becker or Duchenne dystrophy
  - Muscle biopsy:
    - absent or decreased staining for dystrophin membrane protein
  - X-linked recessive inheritance
- ▶ Emery-Dreifuss dystrophy
  - Contractures limiting neck flexion, elbow extension
  - Cardiac involvement
- ▶ Fascioscapulohumeral and scapuloperoneal dystrophy
  - Fascioscapulohumeral:
    - scapular winging, arm and facial weakness
  - Scapuloperoneal:
    - scapular winging and peroneal weakness
- ▶ Oculopharyngeal dystrophy
  - Muscle biopsy:
    - 8.5 nm intranuclear inclusions on EMG
  - Late onset (>40 years) ptosis and dysphagia
  - Autosomal dominant

Consistent features
- ▶ Becker or Duchenne dystrophy
  - Scoliosis
  - Normal brain MRI
  - Respiratory and cardiac involvement
  - Moderate-severe proximal muscle weakness
- ▶ Emery-Dreifuss dystrophy
  - X-linked recessive inheritance
- ▶ Fascioscapulohumeral and scapuloperoneal dystrophy
  - Other family members unaware of weakness
  - Autosomal dominant with variable penetrance
  - Nonprogressive or slowly progressive
- ▶ Oculopharyngeal dystrophy
  - Muscle biopsy:
    - inclusion bodies
  - No fluctuations in symptoms with fatigue
  - No cardiac or respiratory involvement

Variable features
- ▶ Becker or Duchenne dystrophy
  - Low IQ
  - Mild improvement with steroids
- ▶ Emery-Dreifuss dystrophy
  - Early pacemaker placement
  - Female carriers of gene have cardiac involvement
- ▶ Fascioscapulohumeral and scapuloperoneal dystrophy
  - Fascioscapulohumeral:
    - hearing loss and/or retinal disease (Coats disease)
- ▶ Oculopharyngeal dystrophy
  - Mild neck or proximal extremity weakness

CK, creatine kinase; EMG, electromyograph; MRI, magnetic resonance imaging

---

Emery-Dreifuss muscular dystrophy is an X-linked recessive disorder that is much less common than dystrophinopathies. Emery-Dreifuss muscular dystrophy presents in males in their early childhood or teenage years as prominent contractures, especially at the elbows, neck, and Achilles tendons, giving the typical appearance of fixed flexed elbows. Symmetric weakness occurs in the proximal arm muscles and the peroneal muscles of the legs, sparing scapular muscles, after the development of contractures. Patients usually survive well into their adult life. Symptom severity is variable, so that some patients lose the ability to walk during the third decade and others are relatively asymptomatic throughout life. Cardiac involvement, including atrial arrhythmias and heart block, can be severe even in the absence of severe muscular weakness. Patients often need pacemaker placement at an early age, and all patients and female carriers must be monitored closely for signs of cardiac involvement.

Fascioscapulohumeral and scapuloperoneal dystrophies and limb girdle dystrophies are disorders with specific patterns of weakness that follow predictable patterns of progression. Fascioscapulohumeral and scapuloperoneal dystrophies are autosomal dominant disorders that involve prominent serratus anterior weakness with scapular winging. Fascioscapulohumeral dystrophy causes scapular winging, facial weakness, and arm weakness with variable peroneal weakness and affects about one of 100,000 adults. Scapuloperoneal dystrophy causes scapular winging with peroneal weakness but little facial or arm weakness. There is variable penetrance; some family members are severely affected and other family members are only mildly affected. Fascioscapulohumeral dystrophy is usually caused by deletions of 3.3 kB D4Z4 repeats on chromosome 4q35, which can be tested in individual patients.

Limb girdle dystrophies cause proximal or diffuse limb muscle weakness, usually without discrete patterns of involvement as in fascioscapulohumeral or scapuloperoneal dystrophies. Approximately 90% of cases are autosomal recessive. These tend to be more severe and present in young adulthood. The less common, autosomal dominant cases tend to be less severe and present in midlife. At least 15 different genetic mutations are now recognized. The specific genetic mechanism can be determined in a majority of affected individuals. Such knowledge is predictive of the likelihood of life-threatening cardiac involvement. For forms with cardiac involvement, pacemaker placement may be indicated. Treatment is supportive and involves genetic counseling and the use of splints and appliances to improve functional capabilities.

Oculopharyngeal muscular dystrophy is an autosomal dominant disease that presents late in life, between the fourth and sixth decades. The initial symptom is usually ptosis (which can be asymmetric), but presentation is often delayed until the usually later onset of dysphagia. There is no evidence of the fatigability (i.e., dramatic improvement in symptoms after rest) that is seen in myasthenia. Late in the course of the illness, mild neck and proximal extremity weakness occur. Dysphagia progresses, so that severe malnutrition or aspiration can occur. Diagnosis is based on family history and muscle biopsy features of a chronic myopathy with rimmed vacuoles on standard stains and a pathognomonic 8.5-nm diameter tubular intranuclear filament on electron microscopic examination of muscle. Treatment is supportive and includes genetic counseling, eyelid surgery to relieve ptosis, and cricopharyngeal myotomy to improve dysphagia.

Congenital Myopathies

Congenital myopathies are inherited diseases of muscle that have less evidence of fulminant destruction of muscle (dystrophic features) than the muscular dystrophies and are usually nonprogressive or slowly progressive. The three most common types of congenital myopathies are central core disease, nemaline myopathy, and centronuclear myopathy. Clinical features of congenital myopathies overlap, and muscle biopsy is usually necessary to differentiate these disorders. Of great importance to the primary care physician, a high incidence of malignant hyperthermia occurs during anesthesia in central core disease.

Metabolic Myopathies

Metabolic myopathies include a variety of rare muscle diseases that are caused by abnormalities in muscle glycogen or lipid metabolism.

McArdle disease or myophosphorylase deficiency

This is a rare muscle disorder in which the conversion of glycogen to glucose is impaired (glucose is metabolized to lactate through glycolysis). It usually presents in the teenage or adult years with exercise-related muscle pain, cramps, easy fatigability, and muscle stiffness or contractures. Myoglobinuria is common with significant exertion. Muscle weakness at rest is present in about a third of patients. Patients commonly report a "second-wind: phenomenon, in which improved exercise tolerance occurs after initial fatigue. The disease is usually autosomal recessive, but at least 50% of patients have a positive family history. Serum CK is elevated in about 90% of patients with McArdle disease. Decreased lactate production during forearm ischemia is a good screen for abnormal glycolysis, but must be performed cautiously to avoid severe muscle injury or false-positive tests. Referral to a neuromuscular specialist should be considered if this disorder is suspected.

Carnitine palmitoyl transferase

Carnitine palmitoyl transferase (CPT) deficiency causes recurrent rhabdomyolysis with pain, stiffness, and weakness of muscles associated with fasting and/or prolonged exercise, as a result of impaired metabolism of long chain fatty acids. Unlike McArdle disease, there are no contractures of muscles with exertion and no second-wind phenomenon. Attacks usually begin in adolescence, but may appear later. Most patients are normal between attacks, with normal serum CK, normal EMG, normal forearm ischemia test, and usually normal muscle biopsy (except for reduced CPT activity using specialized assays). Treatment involves frequent meals with high-carbohydrate low-fat foods and avoidance of prolonged exercise and fasting.

Acid maltase deficiency

Acid maltase deficiency is an autosomal recessive disease that is secondary to a deficient lysosomal enzyme in muscle, liver, and heart (glucosidase). Adult acid maltase deficiency causes a slowly progressive myopathy after age 20, which may present with respiratory failure or pulmonary hypertension. Lifespan can be normal or reduced secondary to respiratory muscle involvement. Serum CK is usually normal or slightly elevated; EMG shows evidence of a myopathy with fibrillation potentials. Complex repetitive discharges and myotonic discharges are seen, most prominently in paraspinal muscles. Muscle biopsy shows intralysosomal glycogen deposits. There is no known treatment other than supportive care, although a high-protein diet has been advocated.

Malignant hyperthermia

Malignant hyperthermia is a rare but potentially lethal rhabdomyolysis associated with general anesthesia (especially halothane and succinylcholine). Patients with certain neuromuscular disorders such as central core disease, carnitine palmitoyl transferase deficiency, the myotonic disorders, and dystrophinopathies (Duchenne and Becker muscular dystrophies) are at increased risk. Early manifestations of malignant hyperthermia include increased end-tidal carbon dioxide with both metabolic and respiratory acidosis, rhabdomyolysis, and rigidity. Temperature elevation may be delayed and is seen in only in one-third of patients. Life-threatening arrhythmias and hypertension are common. Some patients have prior exposure to anesthetic agents without symptoms of malignant hyperthermia. Treatment with dantrolene (an agent that inhibits calcium release from the sarcoplasmic reticulum) should be initiated immediately if malignant hyperthermia is suspected. Patients should be well hydrated, and renal function should be followed closely to avoid damage from rhabdomyolysis-induced acute tubular necrosis. Cardiovascular function should also be monitored closely. Prophylactic treatment prior to anesthesia with dantrolene and avoidance of halothane-like anesthetics and depolarizing muscle relaxants are important in susceptible patients.

Mitochondrial Myopathies

Mitochondrial myopathies often manifest with multisystemic features. Common, neuromuscular features include muscle fatigue, weakness, or ophthalmoplegia. Nonmuscular manifestations of mitochondrial disease include deafness, intermittent ataxia, neuropathy, seizures, strokes, short stature, diabetes, cardiomyopathy, cardiac conduction abnormalities, cataracts, retinitis pigmentosa, and multiple lipomas. The most common mitochondrial myopathy syndromes are Kearns-Sayre syndrome, familial progressive external ophthalmoplegia (PEO), myoclonic epilepsy and ragged red fibers (MERRF), and mitochondrial myopathy, encephalopathy, lactic acidosis, and stroke-like episodes (MELAS). Features of these syndromes often overlap. A single mitochondrial DNA defect usually presents with several different phenotypes. Patients with mitochondrial myopathies often have depressed ventilatory drive and are at increased risk for respiratory arrest with sedation.

The primary feature of both Kearns-Sayre syndrome and familial PEO syndrome is a gradually progressive ptosis and ophthalmoplegia (usually without diplopia), which can vary in severity from mild unilateral ptosis to complete ophthalmoplegia and severe bilateral ptosis. Ragged red fibers are present on skeletal muscle biopsy. MERRF is characterized by proximal limb weakness (with little or no ophthalmoplegia or ptosis), myoclonus, generalized seizures, intellectual deterioration, ataxia, and hearing loss. MELAS is a multisystemic mitochondrial disorder that begins in childhood or early adulthood with stunted growth and recurrent stroke-like episodes that have a predilection for the posterior fossa and often cause visual field defects or cortical blindness. Other features include a mitochondrial myopathy with proximal weakness, as well as episodic vomiting, hearing loss, elevated serum and CSF lactate, and myoclonic epilepsy. Some patients have ataxia from a cerebellar syndrome and ophthalmoplegia or ptosis. Marked overlap often occurs between mitochondrial syndromes. Diagnosis is important for proper genetic counseling. Effective treatments for inherited mitochondrial myopathies have not been established.

Periodic Paralysis and Myotonia

These disorders are due to defects in ion channels in muscle membrane. Whereas many forms of these channelopathies exist in isolation, some forms of periodic paralysis coexist with paramyotonia.

Periodic paralysis

Many patients complain of episodic fatigue from temporal exacerbations of neurologic, medical, or psychiatric diseases. True episodic paralysis is very rare, and it is important to consider more common diagnoses before making a diagnosis of a potassium-related periodic paralysis. There are two major forms of periodic paralysis: hypokalemic periodic paralysis and hyperkalemic periodic paralysis. Both involve episodes of transient limb weakness, usually without significant bulbar or respiratory involvement. Both are autosomal dominant with variable penetrance. In between episodes, in the initial decades of symptoms, strength is normal. The EMG testing may reveal signs of myotonia in hyperkalemic periodic paralysis. In both hypokalemic and hyperkalemic periodic paralysis, a characteristic increase in the amplitude and area of the compound muscle action potential (CMAP) occurs after 3–5 minutes of exercise, which is followed 20–35 minutes later by a significant decrease in CMAP amplitude and area. If a diagnosis of periodic paralysis is suspected, referral to a neuromuscular specialist is advised.

Myotonia

Myotonia is demonstrated on clinical examination by abnormal relaxation of muscles: the inability to rapidly release a grip, delays in relaxation of joint reflexes, or delayed opening of the eyelid after forceful closure. Abnormal relaxation of muscle can also be demonstrated by a persistent indentation of muscle after percussion by a reflex hammer. On needle EMG testing, myotonic discharges are characterized by spontaneously waxing and waning discharges of muscle fibers, which sound like a dive bomber on the speaker.

Myotonic dystrophy is the most common myotonic disorder and the most common adult muscular dystrophy. It is an autosomal dominant multisystem disease caused by a protein kinase gene defect that affects about 1 in 8,000 adults. The myotonia is usually clinically asymptomatic and is seen only in some muscles during clinical examination or needle EMG testing. Patients present in any decade. Presentation is usually earlier in each successive generation (anticipation). Because myotonic dystrophy affects multiple organ systems, the presenting features vary. Neurologically, patients complain more often of weakness than of stiffness or myotonia. Slowly progressive muscle wasting is especially noticeable in the masseters and temporalis muscles, giving patients a hatchet-faced appearance. Ptosis is mild. Pharyngeal weakness with dysphagia and aspiration is common in middle and late life. Limb weakness occurs in a peculiar pattern, affecting distal arm and leg muscles but sparing intrinsic foot and intrinsic hand muscles. First- and second-degree heart block are common, and elective pacemaker placement is often indicated. Various personality traits such as apathy or paranoia have been ascribed to myotonic dystrophy patients, and intelligence is often below average. Ophthalmologic features include cataracts and retinal and macular pigmentary degeneration. Genetic counseling is important, as 25% of offspring of myotonic dystrophy mothers will have congenital myotonic dystrophy, a severe disorder with mental retardation, respiratory distress, and poor suck and swallowing ability.

Myotonia congenita is a rarer disease with myotonia. The autosomal dominant form is called Thomsen disease, and the autosomal recessive form is called Becker disease. Thomsen disease can present as asymptomatic myotonia on needle EMG testing in one family member, and as severe myotonia with generalized stiffness and increased muscle bulk beginning in infancy in another family member. In Becker myotonia congenita, symptoms appear later in childhood and present as unusual stiffness in cold or transient stiffening of muscles that can sometimes cause falls. In both types of myotonia congenita, succinylcholine, anticholinesterase drugs, and potassium administration can exacerbate myotonia and should be avoided. Treatment with mexiletine, Dilantin, or quinine can dramatically improve symptoms of myotonia.

Paramyotonia is the rarest disorder with myotonia. These patients rarely present for medical attention because of stiffness. Symptoms are so tightly associated with cold or exercise that patients learn to alter their activities to avoid symptoms and often do not seek treatment. If these patients seek medical attention, it is usually for weakness caused by periodic paralysis.

Neuromuscular Junction Disorders

Myasthenia Gravis

Myasthenia gravis is the most common neuromuscular junction disease. It is an autoimmune disorder that is associated with antibodies to acetylcholine receptors on skeletal muscle. Myasthenia gravis usually presents with fluctuating, fatigable diplopia or ptosis that may be associated with dysarthria, dysphagia, dyspnea, or fatigable proximal limb weakness. Ocular myasthenia gravis refers to patients in whom symptoms and signs are limited to extraocular muscles. Generalized myasthenia gravis develops in most patients over time, with involvement of proximal limb, pharyngeal, or respiratory muscles. Thus, it may imitate a variety of neurologic diseases. Because there are many effective treatments for myasthenia gravis, accurate diagnosis is important. In both ocular and generalized myasthenia, the key clinical feature that differentiates myasthenia from other neurologic disorders is muscle fatigue with dramatic fluctuations in symptoms over time.

Ocular myasthenia gravis usually presents subacutely, with fluctuating diplopia and ptosis. The neurologic examination reveals fatigable ophthalmoparesis and ptosis without abnormalities in pupillary function. The differential diagnosis includes acute brainstem lesions (stroke, malignancy, or multiple sclerosis) and botulism as well as chronic diseases such as Graves disease (thyroid ophthalmopathy), chronic progressive external oph-

thalmoplegia (CPEO), and oculopharyngeal muscular dystrophy. The dramatic worsening of symptoms with fatigue and improvement with rest helps to differentiate ocular myasthenia from these other disorders. Lack of pupillary involvement helps to exclude brainstem lesions. Improvement in ptosis and eye movement with administration of an anticholinesterase medication (for example, IV edrophonium) is a useful diagnostic test for myasthenia gravis.

Generalized myasthenia gravis usually presents with fluctuating dysarthria, dysphagia, and shortness of breath or proximal limb fatigue after several weeks or months of fluctuating diplopia and ptosis. These nonocular symptoms may have been precipitated by intercurrent infection or illness. The neurologic examination reveals fluctuating ptosis, ophthalmoparesis, dysarthria, dysphagia, or proximal limb weakness. Reflexes and sensation are normal. The differential includes inflammatory myopathy (which is usually associated with an elevated CK) and ALS (which has signs of spasticity and normal extraocular movement). Improvement in the presenting nonocular complaint with administration of anticholinesterase inhibitors (for example, IV edrophonium) is a useful diagnostic test.

The diagnosis of myasthenia gravis is based on the preceding clinical features together with one or more of the following: a positive acetylcholine receptor antibody (AChRAb), objective improvement in response to pharmacologic testing with edrophonium, a decremental response with repetitive nerve stimulation testing, or increased jitter with single-fiber EMG studies. The most specific test of myasthenia gravis is an elevated AChRAb titer. This has an extremely low rate of false positives. Unfortunately, the AChRAb test is positive in only 85–90% of patients with generalized myasthenia gravis and 50–70% of patients with myasthenia restricted to ocular muscles. The 10–30% of patients without an elevated AChRAb titer represent a difficult diagnostic dilemma. Muscle-specific kinase (MuSK) antibodies may be found in 40–50% of patients with no antibodies to the acetylcholine receptors. These patients tend to have more oculobulbar involvement, with neck extensor weakness and respiratory symptoms. Pharmacologic test results are neither highly sensitive nor specific. The improvement is often subjective, and a placebo response provides a false-positive result. Patients, especially older ones with ocular symptoms, often do not respond to acetylcholine esterase inhibitors, and this produces false-negative results. Electrophysiologic testing becomes especially useful in antibody-negative patients. The results of repetitive nerve stimulation are influenced by a number of technical problems, so are most meaningful if performed by an electrodiagnostic medical consultant who is experienced in assessment of neuromuscular junction disorders. With repetitive stimulation testing of several nerves (including proximal ones), these results have a high sensitivity and specificity. Single-fiber EMG is the most sensitive electrophysiologic test for myasthenia gravis. If this study is performed on a muscle with fatigue, normal results virtually exclude myasthenia gravis. However, single-fiber EMG is not specific for myasthenia gravis and is abnormal with several other neuromuscular diseases.

Once a diagnosis of myasthenia gravis is made, a chest CT and thyroid function tests are obtained. Myasthenia is associated with thymic hyperplasia in most patients under age 50 years and with thymoma in about 15%. The chest CT is quite sensitive in detecting thymoma. Approximately 10% of myasthenics have associated thyroid disease, roughly equally split between hyperthyroidism and hypothyroidism. Hyperthyroidism, if present, usually precedes myasthenia. The presence of thyroid disease is usually due to autoimmune disease that requires separate treatment.

Several effective treatments are available for myasthenia gravis. A major initial decision regards thymectomy. If a thymoma is present, a thymectomy should be performed. Controversy exists as to which patients without thymoma should be treated with thymectomy. Although definitive randomized, placebo-controlled study is lacking, thymectomy is usually recommended for adults with generalized myasthenia gravis who are under age 50 years. Thymectomy is usually avoided in patients with generalized myasthenia gravis over age 65 years, unless thymoma is suspected. If weakness is purely ocular, thymectomy is not recommended. For patients between age 50 and 65 years, individual patient circumstances and the local surgical experience has a strong influence on the decision to recommend thymectomy. Patients with MuSK myasthenia do not seem to respond to thymectomy.

Standard treatment of generalized myasthenia gravis includes symptomatic treatment with pyridostigmine and immunosuppressive treatment. If weakness is moderate or severe, immunomodulatory treatment is often initiated with plasmapheresis or IV immunoglobulins to rapidly restore strength before use of prednisone. Outpatient prednisone therapy is initiated cautiously in myasthenia gravis, because weakness often increases during the initial 10–14 days of therapy before improvement begins. Long-term medical therapy often includes mycophenolate or azathioprine as steroid-sparing agents. Less often, cyclophosphamide is necessary for myasthenia patients who are more refractory. Because of the side effects of prednisone and the cost and transient improvement with plasmapheresis and IV immunoglobulins, ocular myasthenia is often treated only with symptomatic measures like pyridostigmine or eye patching to eliminate diplopia. Myasthenia may also transiently worsen with infections and with the use of several drugs, especially aminoglycosides, procainamide, quinine, quinidine, and β-adrenergic blocking agents.

Lambert-Eaton Myasthenic Syndrome

This is an autoimmune disorder associated with antibodies to calcium channels on the presynaptic nerve terminals of skeletal muscle and autonomic ganglia. In approximately one-half to two-thirds of cases, the syndrome is paraneoplastic. The neoplasm is usually a small-cell lung carcinoma, but the Lambert-Eaton myasthenic syndrome is occasionally seen with other malignancies. Neuromuscular symptoms usually antedate the diagnosis of the malignancy by months or years. In up to one-half of cases, and in most cases that present at younger than 30 years, the syndrome is not associated with malignancy.

Symptoms usually involve proximal leg weakness with difficulty arising from a chair or climbing stairs, or shoulder girdle weakness. Dysarthria and dysphagia are common only when limb weakness is severe. However, in contrast to myasthenia gravis, ptosis and diplopia are rare. Also in contrast to myasthenia gravis, reflexes are usually reduced or absent in the Lambert-Eaton myasthenic syndrome. Furthermore, parasympathetic symptoms are common and include dry mouth, dry eyes, constipation, urinary retention, and impotence.

The diagnosis is usually made through electrodiagnostic testing. Nerve conduction testing identifies small compound muscle action potentials with normal sensory nerve action potentials. Electromyographic studies reveal findings typical for a myopathy with small-amplitude, short-duration motor unit action potentials recruited rapidly. In this context, the diagnosis is established by recording a compound muscle action potential before and after 10–20 seconds of exercise. A post-exercise facilitation of more than 200% is diagnostic of the Lambert-Eaton myasthenic syndrome.

Treatment of Lambert-Eaton involves a thorough search for malignancy (especially small-cell lung cancer with chest CT) and repeated surveillance if no malignancy is found. Treatment of the underlying tumor may be associated with improvement in symptoms of Lambert-Eaton syndrome. Pyridostigmine treatment modestly improves symptoms in some patients. The addition of 3-4-diaminopyridine to pyridostigmine is more dramatically beneficial. Immunosuppression with prednisone, plasmapheresis, or IV immunoglobulin may result in improvement, but does not produce the dramatic improvement that is seen in myasthenia gravis.

Botulism

Botulism is a rare disorder in which a biologic toxin irreversibly blocks the release of acetylcholine from autonomic and skeletal motor nerve terminals. The toxin is released by the bacterium *Clostridium botulinum*. In adults, the disease is most commonly caused by eating poorly cooked food contaminated with the bacterium

▼

Consider Consultation When...

▶ Chronic distal numbness more than weakness is not explained by diabetes or alcohol abuse, or if distal numbness or weakness is progressive or severe.

▶ Patient has acute generalized weakness.

▶ Patient has subacute or chronic weakness or distal weakness more than numbness.

▶ Pain in one limb does not resolve with symptomatic treatment for radiculopathy or compressive neuropathy, or if significant numbness or weakness accompanies pain.

▶ Recommendations are needed for specific diagnostic tests or interpretation of tests.

during canning, but cases of contamination of wounds (especially in IV drug abusers who "skin-pop" black tar heroin) have been reported. Botulism usually presents within 12–36 hours after exposure to the toxin. Initial symptoms are nausea, vomiting, and anorexia or severe constipation, followed by blurred vision and diplopia. This is followed by dysarthria, dysphagia, dyspnea, and limb weakness, often associated with autonomic dysfunction. Botulism may be confused with GBS. In contrast to GBS, onset is more fulminant, extraocular muscles and pupils are more commonly affected, and the CSF protein is normal.

Early in the course of the disease, there may be an increase in the area and amplitude of the compound muscle action potential with exercise or 50-Hz repetitive stimulation. Later, motor nerves can become unexcitable.

Needle EMG shows a myopathic pattern, and fibrillation potentials can develop in muscles after a few weeks to a month. Definitive diagnosis is based on identification of botulinum toxin in serum. Treatment involves IV trivalent antiserum within 2–3 days of onset and supportive care. For patients with wound infection, the wound must be found and drained. Recovery occurs over weeks to months.

Annotated Bibliography

Dyck PJ, Thomas PK, Griffin JW, Low PA, Poduslo JF. *Peripheral neuropathy*, 4th ed. Philadelphia: W. B. Saunders, 2005. *This two-volume book is the most comprehensive single source for description of the clinical features, differential diagnosis, pathophysiology, pathology, and treatment of the various forms of peripheral neuropathy.*

Engel AG. *Myology*, 3rd ed. New York: McGraw-Hill, 2004. *This two-volume book is the most comprehensive single source for description of the clinical features, differential diagnosis, pathology, and treatment of the various forms of myopathy and neuromuscular junction disorders.*

Griggs RC, Mendell JR, Miller RG. *Evaluation and treatment of myopathies*. Philadelphia: F.A. Davis, 1995. *An excellent initial reference to look up a specific myopathy and review its clinical features, genetics, course, and management.*

Layzer RB. *Neuromuscular manifestations of systemic disease*. Philadelphia: F.A. Davis, 1985. *An excellent reference to look up a known systemic disease for its potential neuromuscular complications.*

Stewart JD. *Focal peripheral neuropathies*, 3rd ed. Philadelphia: Lippincott Williams & Wilkins, 2000. *An excellent reference to look up a known focal neuropathy or radiculopathy and review its clinical features, distinguishing features, and treatment.*

CHAPTER 19

Infections of the Nervous System

Anita A. Koshy and Cheryl A. Jay

Patients with nervous system infections challenge primary care physicians and specialists alike. Although any given nervous system infection may be uncommon, as a group, neurologic infections occur frequently and appear in the differential diagnosis of many neurologic syndromes. The limited ability of the brain and spinal cord to recover from injury makes rapid, accurate diagnosis and early, definitive treatment essential. The urgency clinicians typically feel when a nervous system infection is suspected is warranted, since the earlier therapy is instituted, the better the outcome.

The ever-expanding array of pathogens, diagnostic tests, and antimicrobial agents makes a rational clinical approach to neurologic infections especially important. Indeed, the diagnostic and therapeutic complexity inherent in these disorders frequently requires expertise from many specialties, including neurology, infectious disease, neurosurgery, neuroradiology, critical care, otolaryngology, ophthalmology, and oral surgery. By understanding the basic principles of how the nervous system becomes susceptible to and recovers from infection, and by being familiar with the more common clinical syndromes, clinicians can effectively evaluate, manage, and coordinate care for patients with these serious, but treatable, disorders.

Pathogenesis and Clinical Approach

All infections, neurologic and otherwise, occur when an organism capable of causing disease encounters a suitable host and successfully eludes its defense mechanisms. Host defenses include anatomic barriers and the immune system. The blood–brain barrier (BBB), formed by tight junctions unique to central nervous system (CNS) capillaries, supplements the substantial protection afforded by the skin, skull, spine, and meninges. Infections of the nervous system are frequent and feared complications in patients with defective cellular or humoral immunity, highlighting the critical role the immune system plays in neurologic, as well as systemic, infections. Even in the normal host, however, pathogenic organisms have evolved diverse and ingenious strategies to evade host defenses. Once established, neurologic infections produce disease by several mechanisms: (a) direct neuronal or glial infection; (b) mass lesion formation; (c) inflammation with subsequent edema, interruption of cerebrospinal fluid (CSF) pathways, neuronal damage, or vasculopathy; and (d) secretion of neurotoxins. In addition, the systemic consequences of infection and sepsis, such as shock, disseminated intravascular coagulation, and multiorgan failure, may also cause neurologic dysfunction.

The diagnostic approach, then, for the patient with the cardinal signs of nervous system infection—fever, head or spine pain, and generalized or focal neurologic dysfunction—combines rapid assessment of the host–pathogen interaction with classic neuroanatomic localization. Because the host must first encounter a pathogen, history regarding travel, occupation, recreational activities, or pets may be critical to identifying the responsible pathogen. Factors known to increase or otherwise influence vulnerability to neurologic infections must be sought systematically, including prior trauma, neurosurgical procedures, recent or ongoing bacteremia or other infection (particularly involving eye, ear, sinus, or teeth), immune status, and antibiotic use. In immunocompromised patients, the same immune suppression that confers vulnerability to CNS infections may make some of the classic manifestations, such as fever and meningismus, subtle or even absent. As with all neurologic disorders, the time course of symptoms yields important diagnostic clues. For example, a severe, rapidly evolving meningitis brings to mind suppurative bacterial pathogens, in contrast to a more subacute clinical picture that might suggest *Mycobacteria*. Initial neurologic examination not only helps define the clinical syndrome—meningitis versus encephalitis, for example—but also establishes a baseline from which response to therapy may be inferred.

Diagnostic evaluation includes blood and CSF studies as well as neuroimaging, supplemented at times by cultures from other sites, and occasionally skin testing and biopsy. In addition to culture, blood may be tested for specific antigens, bacterial toxins, and acute and convalescent antibody responses. Cerebrospinal fluid protein, glucose, and cell count determination forms the cornerstone for diagnosing many CNS infections. In addition, CSF may be examined directly for bacteria, fungi, and some parasites, as well as cultured and tested for antigens of selected organisms. Polymerase chain reaction (PCR) testing for nucleic acids of selected pathogens, particu-

▼

Key Clinical Questions

Neurologic infections

▶ Where have you lived or traveled outside the area? (For returning travelers: In what kinds of activities did you participate while away?)

▶ What is your living situation?

▶ What kind of work do you do?

▶ Do you consume unpasteurized dairy products?

▶ Do you have any pets?

▶ Have you had any problems with your eyes, ears, sinuses, or teeth?

▶ Have you ever had brain or spine surgery or trauma?

▶ Have you ever used injection drugs or have any other reason to think you might have been exposed to human immunodeficiency virus (HIV)?

▶ Have you ever been exposed to tuberculosis or taken medications for it? (If yes: which medications and for how long?)

▶ Do you take chronic steroids?

▶ Have you ever had chemotherapy or taken other medications that suppress the immune system?

▶ Have you taken any antibiotics recently?

larly viruses, has assumed a more prominent role in diagnostic evaluation in recent years. For all microbiologic testing, specimens must be handled properly to ensure the highest possible yield and most accurate results. Biopsy of sites such as skin, lymph nodes, or bone marrow may yield evidence of disseminated infection, suggesting the neurologic infection may share the same cause. Biopsy of neural tissue is sometimes solely diagnostic, as in nerve biopsy for leprosy or brain biopsy for some mass lesions in human immunodeficiency virus (HIV)-infected patients. In other situations, such as brain or spine abscess, definitive therapy with surgery also affords an opportunity to obtain culture material.

Neuroimaging with computed tomography (CT) and magnetic resonance imaging (MRI) has greatly improved diagnosis of CNS infections, particularly cerebral mass lesions, herpes simplex virus (HSV) encephalitis, and spinal epidural abscesses. In these situations, pre- and postcontrast images should be obtained whenever possible. Neuroimaging has also greatly improved the ability to detect neurologic complications of meningitis such as hydrocephalus and stroke. In these situations, noncontrast images may provide sufficient information to guide management.

Antimicrobial agents are a mainstay of therapy, supplemented occasionally by surgery, antitoxins, or hyperimmune globulin, and accompanied always by meticulous supportive care and close surveillance for systemic and secondary neurologic complications (Box 19.1). As for all infections, antibiotic selection depends on the susceptibility of the suspected or proven pathogen and local antibiotic resistance patterns. Additional important considerations for CNS infections include the ability of antibiotics to cross the BBB and the selection of "cidal" agents that kill organisms, rather than "static" drugs, which simply inhibit their growth.

Some nervous system infections require surgical management in addition to medical therapy. Neurosurgical intervention plays a central role in definitive management of many cerebral infectious mass lesions and spinal infections, and may be indicated when hydrocephalus or intracerebral hemorrhage develops as a complication of meningitis. Cerebral infections complicating eye, ear, sinus, or dental infections may require surgical management of the primary infection concurrent with therapy for its secondary neurologic complications. In tetanus and wound botulism, mediated by clostridial neurotoxins, surgical treatment is also important, in the form of aggressive debridement of infected tissue. Antitoxin is typically administered as well.

Close neurologic monitoring and meticulous supportive care are critical. In situations in which initial treatment is empiric, neurologic improvement is an important sign that therapy, particularly antimicrobial selection, is appropriate. Neurologic deterioration suggests that an-

> **Box 19.1** Treatment of nervous system infections
>
> **Medical management of infection**
> ▶ Antimicrobial agents
>   – Choose cidal, not static, drugs that reach infected site at adequate levels
>   – Empiric coverage (pending cultures) depends on likely pathogens, given clinical situation
>   – Specific coverage depends on culture and sensitivity
> ▶ Adjuncts: steroids, antitoxins, hyperimmune globulin
>
> **Surgical management of infection**
> ▶ Neurosurgery for infectious cerebral mass lesions, spinal epidural abscess
> ▶ Surgery for adjacent infected sites: eye, ear, sinus, teeth, mediastinum, retroperitoneum
> ▶ Debridement of infected tissue: clostridial neurotoxins (botulism, tetanus)
>
> **Anticipate and manage neurologic complications**
> ▶ Seizures: anticonvulsants
> ▶ Cerebral infarction
> ▶ Hydrocephalus: ventriculostomy
> ▶ Increased intracranial pressure: head elevation, osmotic agents, steroids, hyperventilation
>
> **Anticipate and manage medical complications**
> ▶ Immobilization: thromboembolism, decubiti
> ▶ Cerebral dysfunction: aspiration pneumonia, diabetes insipidus, syndrome of inappropriate secretion of antidiuretic hormone, cerebral salt wasting
> ▶ Acute illness: malnutrition, gastrointestinal hemorrhage
> ▶ Infection: sepsis, disseminated intravascular coagulation
>
> **Assess need for public health intervention**
> ▶ Notification for reportable conditions
> ▶ Prophylaxis for contacts

tibiotic therapy is inadequate, that secondary neurologic complications have occurred, or that sepsis, hypotension, or metabolic derangements have developed. Seizures, increased intracranial pressure (ICP), hydrocephalus, and strokes frequently complicate cerebral infections and must be promptly recognized and treated. Electrolyte disturbances, particularly the syndrome of inappropriate secretion of antidiuretic hormone, diabetes insipidus, and cerebral salt wasting, must be anticipated and managed. Prophylactic therapy for gastrointestinal hemorrhage, decubitus ulcers, deep venous thrombosis, and contractures can reduce both morbidity and mortality.

Finally, it is important to remember that treatment for neurologic infections may extend beyond the patient. Some nervous system infections, such as meningococcal meningitis, obligate prophylactic therapy for close con-

tacts, which may include medical professionals as well as family members. Others, such as viral encephalitis and botulism, require reporting to public health authorities for surveillance or to obtain specialized diagnostic testing and treatment.

Classic Neuroinfectious Syndromes

Acute Bacterial Meningitis

Bacterial meningitis typically presents as an acute febrile illness with prominent headache, neck stiffness, photophobia, and often abnormal mental status. Infants and the elderly, the patients most at risk for bacterial meningitis, are important exceptions and may demonstrate only mild behavioral changes with low-grade fever and little clinical evidence of meningeal inflammation. Bacterial meningitis may develop as a consequence of parameningeal infection (ear, sinus, dental, or paraspinal sites), impairment in the brain's anatomic barriers (trauma or following neurosurgery), or, rarely, when a brain abscess ruptures into the ventricular system or subarachnoid space. More commonly, however, bacterial meningitis develops when pathogenic bacteria colonizing the nasopharynx cause bacteremia and manage to breach the BBB.

In adults with intact structural and immune defenses, *Streptococcus pneumoniae* and *Neisseria meningitidis* are the most common meningeal pathogens, due to their ability to colonize the nasopharynx and cross the BBB. Meningococcal meningitis may occur as an outbreak in institutional settings, such as college dormitories and military barracks. *Haemophilus influenza*, type b, previously a classic childhood meningeal pathogen, has become a less common cause of bacterial meningitis in the United States, due to routine childhood vaccination against this pathogen. Similarly, in developed countries, invasive pneumococcal disease is on the decline given the recent widespread vaccination against this agent. Staphylococcal species, particularly *S. epidermidis* and *S. aureus*, often cause meningitis in patients with ventricular shunts. Gram-negative bacilli may also cause meningitis, particularly in hospitalized (including post neurosurgery) and neutropenic patients. Patients most at risk for meningitis from *Listeria monocytogenes* include neonates, patients older than 50 years of age, and immunocompromised hosts, including those with alcoholism.

In general, CSF examination reveals elevated pressure and protein (100–500/dL, normal 15–45), decreased glucose (<40% serum glucose,) and marked pleocytosis (100–10 000/mm^3, normal 5) with polymorphonuclear predominance. The sensitivity for any single parameter in the CSF is poor. The CSF Gram's stain is positive in at least 60% of cases, and CSF culture positive in about 75%. Blood cultures reveal the causative organism in

50% of cases. Peripheral leukocytosis and left shift are common. Neuroimaging studies may be negative or reveal complications of bacterial meningitis, such as cerebral edema, communicating or obstructive hydrocephalus, cerebral infarction, or venous sinus thrombosis.

For the acutely ill, febrile patient with meningeal signs, altered mental status, and inflammatory CSF with polymorphonuclear pleocytosis, the differential diagnosis also includes chronic meningitis and meningitis due to parasites. In the aseptic meningitis syndrome, discussed in the next section, symptoms and signs of meningeal irritation are prominent, but mental status is normal. When meningeal signs are less prominent, other diagnostic considerations include brain abscess, subdural empyema, cranial epidural abscess, and viral encephalitis. It should be emphasized that elderly, immunosuppressed or otherwise chronically ill patients may not manifest the full clinical syndrome, and a high index of suspicion is necessary to make the diagnosis.

Therapy for all types of acute bacterial meningitis includes prompt antibiotic administration and aggressive management of systemic and neurologic complications. For community-acquired bacterial meningitis, dexamethasone administered before or with the first dose of antibiotics and continued for 4 days decreases morbidity and mortality. Antibiotic selection depends on clinical setting, local resistance patterns, allergy history, and CSF results. The emergence of resistant pneumococcus, with approximately a quarter of isolates resistant to penicillin and nearly 10% resistant to third-generation cephalosporins (such as ceftriaxone or cefotaxime), has significantly influenced empiric therapy for community-acquired bacterial meningitis. Penicillin and ampicillin reliably cover *Listeria* spp., meningococcus, and many (but not all) pneumococcus, but not *Staphylococcus* spp. or gram-negative bacilli. Third-generation cephalosporins are effective against most standard meningitis pathogens, including intermediate-grade resistant pneumococcus, but not *Listeria* or *Staphylococcus* spp. Vancomycin covers highly resistant pneumococcus and Staphylococcal spp. (but not *Listeria*), and has become part of typical empiric regimens for community- or hospital-acquired bacterial meningitis in adults. Ceftazidime, unlike other third-generation cephalosporins, and cefepime, a fourth-generation cephalosporin, cover *Pseudomonas* spp. and are reserved for situations in which meningitis with this organism is suspected or proven. Doses for many antibiotics used to treat bacterial meningitis are higher than those recommended for systemic infections.

Although infectious disease consultation is prudent for most patients with bacterial meningitis, guidelines for empiric antibiotic coverage allow therapy to be started quickly. For the healthy young or middle-aged adult, a third-generation cephalosporin and vancomycin comprise a typical regimen. Because of the rising incidence of resistant pneumococcus, most authorities advise against initial empiric therapy with penicillin or ampicillin alone. However, in patients older than 50 or otherwise at risk for *L. monocytogenes*, such as patients with alcoholism, chronic renal failure, or immunosuppression, penicillin or ampicillin should be added to the regimen, because vancomycin and cephalosporins do not cover *Listeria*. In hospital-acquired meningitis, including postoperative neurosurgery patients or neutropenic patients, consideration should be given to anti-*Pseudomonas* coverage agents, such as ceftazidime. Antibiotic coverage can be narrowed once culture and sensitivity results are known. Infectious disease consultation is mandatory when meningitis develops in a patient who is already hospitalized, chronically ill, or elderly, or has a history of neurosurgery, recent head trauma, or antibiotic allergies. When meningococcal meningitis is proven or strongly suspected, the patient should be in contact isolation, and chemoprophylaxis must be provided for close contacts, which may include medical personnel.

Two other practical points regarding antibiotic therapy deserve mention. First is the situation in which a delay in lumbar puncture (LP) occurs. An example would be the patient with suspected meningitis whose focal findings or clinical evidence of increased ICP warrants a head CT before LP. Antibiotics, and dexamethasone, as appropriate, should be given after blood cultures are drawn, prior to LP. Since antibiotic therapy takes several hours to sterilize CSF, cultures may still be helpful even when obtained after antibiotics are begun, and antibiotics generally will not affect the cell count, glucose, or protein for days or longer. Second, the CSF Gram's stain provides useful information when experienced personnel examine a well-prepared smear. Outside these circumstances, the test may provide inaccurate information. Even under ideal conditions, recent antibiotic therapy may alter bacterial morphology enough to cause errors. Hence very narrow antibiotic coverage based on a CSF Gram's stain in a very sick patient may be ill advised.

As for the role of dexamethasone, benefit was shown for adults with community-acquired bacterial meningitis, most of whom had *S. pneumoniae* meningitis, when administered prior to or with the first dose of antibiotics. The current recommendation is that patients with suspected community-acquired bacterial meningitis who are not septic receive dexamethasone intravenously with or before the first dose of antibiotics. Patients whose culture results document *S. pneumoniae* meningitis should continue dexamethasone every 6 hours for 4 days. There is no clear consensus about whether steroids should be stopped if the pathogen is not *S. pneumoniae*. It should be emphasized that the benefit of dexamethasone or other steroid therapy has not been shown for patients with acute bacterial meningitis complicating neurosurgical pro-

▼

Pearls and Perils

Bacterial meningitis

▶ Classic, acute presentation of fever and altered mentation with meningeal symptoms and signs may not be fully expressed in individuals evaluated early in the infection or who are immunosuppressed, elderly, or taking antibiotics.

▶ If cerebrospinal fluid (CSF) examination is delayed for any reason in suspected community-acquired bacterial meningitis, obtain blood cultures and administer dexamethasone and antibiotics prior to lumbar puncture. Dexamethasone should be started prior to or with the first dose of antibiotics.

▶ Due to the increasing incidence of resistant pneumococcus, initial empiric therapy with ampicillin or penicillin alone is not recommended.

▶ Avoid narrow antibiotic coverage on CSF Gram's stain alone in severely ill patients.

▶ Failure to improve within several days should prompt consideration of alternative etiologies, in particular tuberculosis (TB), spirochetes, parasites, fungi, or drugs.

▶ Deteriorating mental status or focal cerebral dysfunction may suggest associated electrolyte disturbance, seizure, cerebral infarction, or hydrocephalus, alone or in combination.

▶ Meningitis occasionally complicates brain abscess, but the reverse is far less common in adults. Coexisting meningitis and abscess may suggest a shared risk factor, such as bacteremia or contiguous craniofacial infection.

cedures or open head trauma or in patients who are severely immunocompromised or with less likely diagnoses of acute bacterial meningitis, particularly in the developing world.

Neurologic consultation should be sought in patients with persistently altered mental status despite treatment, focal neurologic findings, or seizures at any time. Appropriate specialty consultation (otolaryngology, ophthalmology, oral surgery) should be obtained when meningitis complicates ear, sinus, orbital, or dental infection. A neurosurgeon should evaluate any patient with meningitis who has a ventricular shunt or history of other neurosurgical procedure, recent head trauma, or if hydrocephalus or cerebral edema requires ventricular drainage or ICP monitoring.

Before antibiotics, bacterial meningitis was nearly uniformly fatal. Currently, the case fatality rate for pneumococcal meningitis is 21%, higher for gram-negative bacilli and lower for *Meningococcus*. Neurologic sequelae, ranging from mild cognitive deficits, deafness, and other cranial neuropathies to hemiparesis, epilepsy, or persistent vegetative state, are common in survivors.

Aseptic Meningitis Syndrome

The aseptic meningitis syndrome applies to the patient who develops over hours to days, the signs, symptoms, and CSF profile suggestive of meningeal inflammation, in which evidence of typical bacterial or fungal pathogens or parameningeal infection cannot be found. Implied is the absence of parenchymal brain dysfunction, such as depressed level of consciousness, seizures, or focal cerebral deficit. Clinical or radiologic evidence of cerebral or cord involvement suggests encephalitis, meningoencephalitis, myelitis, or brain or spinal abscess. Also implied is a benign and self-limited course. Perhaps because CSF inflammatory cells are usually lymphocytic and monocytic, "aseptic meningitis" has, over the years, evolved into a more generic diagnosis applied to any patient with a lymphocytic pleocytosis in CSF. Defining aseptic meningitis by CSF profile alone can be dangerous. Not all causes of lymphocytic pleocytosis are benign, and distinguishing aseptic meningitis from early meningoencephalitis or chronic meningitis can be difficult. Early in the course, then, aseptic meningitis must remain a provisional diagnosis; any neurologic deterioration or persistent symptoms beyond 3–4 weeks warrants reconsideration of the diagnosis.

Viruses cause most cases of aseptic meningitis. Nonpolio enteroviruses, such as echovirus and Coxsackie virus, are the common viral agents, either sporadically or as the classic summer outbreak. Enterovirus 71 has recently emerged as a neurotropic nonpolio enterovirus that causes aseptic meningitis, as well as rhombencephalitis and a motor neuron infection resembling polio. The paramyxovirus that causes mumps also causes viral meningitis, favoring winter and spring; this pathogen had declined by 99% in the United States by 2003. Unfortunately, it has had a resurgence in developed countries including the United Kingdom, Canada, and the United States. Thus, in epidemic aseptic meningitis, mumps virus should be on the differential and can be found by PCR in the nasopharynx, saliva, blood, urine, and CSF. Lymphocytic choriomeningitis (LCM) virus also strikes more commonly in autumn/winter, and may cause encephalitis as well as meningitis. Arboviruses more frequently cause encephalitis, but can cause meningitis, with summer and fall the more characteristic times of the year. The herpes viruses (HSV-1, HSV-2, varicella zoster virus [VZV], Epstein-Barr virus [EBV], and cytomegalovirus [CMV]) can cause meningitis, encephalitis, or both, year-round. HIV also causes aseptic meningitis, particularly at seroconversion and early in its course (Table 19.1).

Aseptic meningitis may also result from nonviral and noninfectious causes (Box 19.2). Nonviral infectious

---

Table 19.1 Aseptic meningitis

Discriminating features
- ▶ Signs, symptoms, and CSF profile consistent with meningeal inflammation
- ▶ Absence of parenchymal CNS involvement
- ▶ Benign, self-limited course

Consistent features
- ▶ Viral prodrome
- ▶ Mildly elevated CSF protein
- ▶ Normal CSF glucose
- ▶ Lymphocytic pleocytosis

Variable features
- ▶ Viral etiology
- ▶ May occur as late summer outbreak

▼

Box 19.2 Causes of aseptic meningitis

Infectious
- ▶ Viruses: enteroviruses (echovirus, Coxsackie virus, enterovirus 71), mumps, lymphocytic choriomeningitis (LCM), herpes viruses ([HSV-1, HSV-2], Epstein-Barr virus [EBV], varicella zoster virus [VZV], cytomegalovirus [CMV]), arboviruses, human immunodeficiency virus
- ▶ Spirochetes: syphilis, Lyme disease, *Leptospira*
- ▶ Other: *Chlamydia, Rickettsia, Ehrlichia, Mycoplasma, Brucella, Bartonella,* Whipple disease

Parainfectious
- ▶ Partially treated bacterial meningitis, parameningeal infection, endocarditis/bacteremia, postvaccination

Noninfectious
- ▶ Medications: nonsteroidal anti-inflammatory drugs, trimethoprim, sulfamethoxazole, azathioprine, γ-globulin, OKT3, among others; intrathecal administration of chemotherapy or dye
- ▶ Tumors: craniopharyngioma, epidermoid cyst
- ▶ Collagen-vascular diseases: including primary CNS vasculitis
- ▶ Other: sarcoidosis, Vogt-Koyanagi-Harada syndrome, Behçet disease, migraine, seizures

Note: causes refer to aseptic meningitis, as defined by a self-limited course. See text and Box 19.3 for causes of chronic meningitis.

---

causes include spirochetes (syphilis, Lyme disease, and *Leptospira*), discussed later in this chapter, as well as rickettsiae, mycoplasma, and cat-scratch disease. Partially treated bacterial meningitis should be considered in the patient recently or currently taking antibiotics. Parainfectious causes include endocarditis or other bacteremic states in addition to parameningeal infections, such as sinusitis, mastoiditis, otitis, subdural empyema, cranial or spinal epidural abscess, and cranial osteomyelitis. Among noninfectious causes, meningitis caused by drugs may be easily overlooked. Commonly implicated agents include nonsteroidal anti-inflammatory drugs (NSAIDs), trimethoprim-sulfamethoxazole, other antibiotics, γ-globulin, and other antibody preparations. Additional noninfectious causes include intracranial tumors and cysts, sarcoidosis, collagen-vascular disorders, spinal anesthesia, intrathecal diagnostic procedures or chemotherapy, and occasionally following migraine or seizures. Meningitis due to carcinoma, mycobacteria, fungal pathogens, or malignancy more typically follows a progressive, rather than self-limited, course and is discussed in the next section.

Special mention should be made of recurrent meningitis, characterized by discrete, repeated episodes of meningitis. Recurrent bacterial meningitis suggests an anatomic defect (such as basilar skull fracture with CSF leak or spinal dermal sinus), parameningeal infection involving craniofacial structures or spine, or impaired immunity (as in hypogammaglobulinemia, complement deficiency, or postsplenectomy states). For recurrent aseptic meningitis, infectious causes include HIV, Whipple disease, some parasitic infections, and treatment failures of atypical bacterial or fungal pathogens. Mollaret meningitis, a benign variant of recurrent aseptic meningitis, has recently been linked to HSV-2, and occasionally HSV-1, infection. Noninfectious causes include drug-related meningitis, repeated rupture of cerebral cysts and cystic

tumors into the subarachnoid space, neurosarcoidosis, uveomeningitic syndromes such as Behçet disease and Vogt-Koyanagi-Harada syndrome, familial Mediterranean fever, and migraine with pleocytosis.

As a syndrome that can be confidently diagnosed only after a period of observation and with many causes ranging from the ominous and treatable to the benign and self-limited, aseptic meningitis can pose challenges to the clinician. Several points merit particular attention. A prior history of meningitis should raise concern that the current episode warrants detailed evaluation, as should aseptic meningitis in the elderly, immunosuppressed, chronically ill, or person at risk for HIV infection. Medication history, with particular attention to antibiotics and including over-the-counter drugs, should be reviewed to exclude partially treated bacterial or drug-related meningitis. Although patients with aseptic meningitis may appear uncomfortable, a toxic clinical picture, significantly impaired mentation, or focal neurologic dysfunction suggests another diagnosis, such as acute bacterial meningitis, chronic meningitis, meningoencephalitis, subdural empyema, epidural abscess, or viral encephalitis. For most patients with aseptic meningitis, CSF shows normal glucose, mild protein elevation (50–80/dL) and mild to moderate pleocytosis (10–1,000 white blood cells [wbc]/mm^3), predominantly consisting of lymphocytes. Low CSF glucose should raise suspicion for alternative diagnoses, although mumps and LCM have been associated with mildly decreased CSF glucose. Polymorphonuclear pleocytosis may be seen early in viral meningitis, changing to mononuclear cells within 1–2 days, as well as in meningitis due to drugs, parasites and, of course, bacteria. West Nile virus and CMV are viral pathogens that can cause persistent polymorphonuclear pleocytosis.

The clinical approach thus varies depending on the clinical setting. For many patients, sending CSF for VDRL, cryptococcal antigen, and fungal, AFB, and viral cultures, in addition to routine studies (bacterial culture and Gram's stain) is reasonable, as is freezing acute-phase serum, in case it should be needed later. Obtaining history concerning acuity of symptoms, travel, and HIV risks and serum syphilis serologies are also part of a reasonable initial evaluation. Close outpatient monitoring may be appropriate for the otherwise healthy patient with typical aseptic meningitis during a recognized community outbreak. In the patient whose initial CSF examination reveals polymorphonuclear pleocytosis, some clinicians would empirically cover for bacterial meningitis pending cultures. Others would watch closely without antibiotics, repeating the CSF examination in 6–12 hours to confirm the expected shift to a mononuclear profile. The approach should be individualized, depending on the specifics of the clinical situation. In patients at high risk for HIV infection, an initially negative HIV test should be followed by a repeat test in 3–6 months, since aseptic meningitis may accompany seroconversion Patients who are elderly, immunosuppressed, systemically ill, or experiencing recurrent meningitis require more extensive evaluation, which should probably begin with infectious disease and neurology consultations.

Prognosis for aseptic meningitis, by definition, is good. In general, in the immunocompetent patient, the treatment for viral meningitis is supportive, including hydration and management of pain and nausea. The challenge, as has been emphasized, is to distinguish aseptic meningitis from the early stages of more ominous conditions such as acute bacterial or chronic meningitis, meningoencephalitis, or viral encephalitis.

Chronic Meningitis

The patient with a 4-week or greater course of headache, fever, neck stiffness, and photophobia, in addition to a CSF profile demonstrating elevated protein, low or normal glucose, and a mono-nuclear pleocytosis, fulfills the definition of chronic meningitis. Practically speaking, most patients come to medical attention, and often empiric therapy, before 4 weeks, particularly when altered mentation, cranial neuropathies, or other neurologic symptoms de-

velop. The progressive (rather than self-limited or relapsing) course distinguishes chronic meningitis from aseptic or recurrent meningitis. The relatively stereotyped clinical presentation of chronic meningitis frequently provides few clues to its numerous etiologies, which may be infectious, neoplastic, or vasculitic, among others.

In generally healthy patients, common infectious causes of chronic meningitis include TB, cryptococcosis and syphilis. Lyme disease, histoplasmosis, coccidiomycosis, and cysticercosis should also be considered in patients who have spent time in endemic areas. Less commonly, anaerobic bacteria and other atypical bacteria, fungi, and parasites may cause chronic meningitis. Parameningeal infections may also cause chronic, as well as aseptic, meningitis. Important noninfectious causes include drugs, meningeal spread of carcinoma or lymphoma, recent subarachnoid hemorrhage, neurosarcoidosis, systemic or primary CNS vasculitis, and uveomeningitic syndromes. The overlap with entities that cause aseptic meningitis is substantial (Box 19.3).

Recognizing the clinical syndrome is not usually difficult, in contrast to identifying the specific cause among so many possibilities. History should focus on constitu-

---

Box 19.3 Causes of chronic meningitis

Infectious
▸ *Mycobacteria tuberculosis*
▸ Spirochetes: syphilis, Lyme disease, *Leptospira*
▸ Other bacteria: *Brucella, Nocardia, Actinomyces,* anaerobes
▸ Fungi: *Cryptococcus,* Coccidiomycosis, Histoplasmosis, Blastomycosis, among others
▸ Parasites: Neurocysticercosis, among others
▸ Viral: human immunodeficiency virus, enteroviruses in agammaglobulinemia; rarely mumps, LCMV, herpes viruses

Parainfectious
▸ Partially treated bacterial meningitis, parameningeal infection, endocarditis/bacteremia

Noninfectious
▸ Medications: see Box 19.2
▸ Neoplasms
  – Primary: glioma, medulloblastoma, craniopharyngioma, ependymoma, epidermoid cyst
  – Metastatic: lymphoma, leukemia, carcinoma
▸ Collagen-vascular disorders: including primary CNS vasculitis
▸ Other: neurosarcoidosis, unrecognized subarachnoid hemorrhage, Vogt-Koyanagi-Harada syndrome, Behçet disease, Fabry disease, idiopathic

tional and systemic symptoms as well as travel, work, or possible infectious contacts. Weight loss and suspected postobstructive pneumonias in a patient with a long smoking history might suggest carcinomatous meningitis, whereas chronic meningitis in a livestock worker should raise concern for brucellosis. Examination may provide clues, such as uveitis in sarcoidosis, Behçet disease, and Vogt-Koyanagi-Harada syndrome, or palmar rash in secondary syphilis.

Laboratory studies obtained will vary widely, depending on the specifics of the clinical setting, but reasonable initial studies to obtain include: blood count with differential, electrolytes, liver panel, sedimentation rate, antinuclear antibody, syphilis serology, serum cryptococcal antigen, blood cultures, urinalysis, and chest film. Consideration should be given to serologic testing for HIV, *Histoplasma*, *Coccidioides*, *Brucella*, and Lyme disease in appropriate patients. A CSF examination will often need to be performed repeatedly and sent for cytology, as well as cultures. The likelihood of detecting many causes of chronic meningitis, in particular TB, fungi, and neoplastic cells, is highest from high-volume CSF collections. In addition, serial CSF examinations allow therapeutic response to be monitored, which is particularly important when empiric treatment is necessary. The CT or MRI may be entirely negative or show meningeal enhancement, an abnormal, but nonspecific, finding. Neuroimaging studies may be quite helpful, for example, in revealing a clinically inapparent brain tumor or parameningeal infection. Angiography may be necessary if vasculitis is suspected. If the clinical situation suggests paraspinous infection as a cause, chest or abdominal CT, or spine MRI may be indicated to demonstrate or exclude these considerations.

Skin testing for TB, if positive, may increase suspicion for TB meningitis, although a negative test does not exclude the diagnosis. As chronic meningitis not infrequently develops as a manifestation of disseminated infectious or systemic disease, careful eye examination, biopsy of skin lesions, enlarged lymph nodes, or bone marrow may provide useful information. Given the broad differential, infectious disease and neurology consultation are indicated in most cases of chronic meningitis, to help prioritize what can be an extensive workup and assist with decisions about empiric therapy. Meningeal biopsy, and thus neurosurgical consultation, may be necessary in selected cases.

Obviously, both treatment and prognosis depend on specific etiology. Many clinicians institute empiric anti-TB therapy in patients with chronic meningitis, even without evidence of systemic TB. Empiric antifungal therapy is less common, and a therapeutic trial of steroids should be undertaken only if the potential risks of worsening some infectious causes and obscuring the ability to diagnose some noninfectious causes can be justified. Until diagnostic methods improve, chronic meningitis will continue to prove a major diagnostic and therapeutic challenge.

Suppurative Cerebral Mass Lesions

Patients with brain abscess present with signs and symptoms of an expanding mass lesion, namely progressively worsening headache accompanied by altered mentation or focal deficit. Nausea and vomiting or fever occurs in about half of cases, hence the absence of these should not be used to exclude the diagnosis on clinical grounds. Brain abscesses develop most frequently by spread from a contiguous infected cranial site, such as ear (causing cerebellar or temporal lobe abscess), sinus (causing frontal lobe abscess), or teeth (especially molars). Open head trauma, previous neurosurgery or craniofacial osteomyelitis are other sites from which brain abscess may develop. Hematogenous spread from remote infection may also cause brain abscess, particularly in the setting of congenital heart disease with right-to-left shunt, or pulmonary sources such as lung abscess, bronchiectasis, or arteriovenous fistula. Although up to 20% of brain abscesses occur without these predisposing craniofacial, cardiac, or pulmonary conditions, early diagnosis of brain abscess frequently depends on considering the diagnosis in the at-risk patient with cerebral dysfunction and headache, even without fever.

Pearls and Perils

Chronic meningitis

▶ Although defined as meningitis, usually with lymphocytic pleocytosis lasting longer than 30 days, patients frequently come to medical attention sooner.
▶ Consider the diagnosis in patients with a working diagnosis of the aseptic meningitis syndrome who develop cranial neuropathies, parenchymal cerebral involvement, hydrocephalus, myelopathy, or polyradiculopathy.
▶ Also consider the diagnosis, particularly tuberculous meningitis, in patients with suspected bacterial meningitis and negative blood and cerebrospinal fluid cultures, and who do not improve with antibacterial agents.
▶ Pay particular attention to human immunodeficiency virus (HIV) risks, travel, occupational exposures, medications, and systemic symptoms and signs (particularly uveitis, skin lesions, adenopathy, joints, visceral involvement).
▶ Infectious disease and neurologic consultations are appropriate in most cases of chronic meningitis to assist in evaluation and guide and monitor empiric therapy, if needed.

Frequently composed of mixed infections, brain abscess pathogens vary depending on the clinical setting. Aerobic and microaerophilic streptococci may be isolated from most bacterial brain abscesses. Other important pathogens include anaerobes, gram-negative bacilli, and *S. aureus*. Important associations include: pneumococcus with sinus source, *Bacteroides* and *Enterobacter* with ear source, anaerobic streptococci with pulmonary infections, and *S. aureus* in the patient with head trauma, recent neurosurgery, or cranial osteomyelitis. In immunocompromised patients, fungi and atypical pathogens frequently cause brain abscess, as discussed later in this chapter.

Cranial CT and MRI have dramatically improved the ability to diagnose and manage brain abscess, which typically appears as a ring-enhancing lesion, surrounded by edema. Enhancement pattern plays an important role in neuroradiologic diagnosis of cerebral mass lesions and, hence, precontrast and postcontrast images must be obtained when brain abscess is a diagnostic consideration. Multiple lesions frequently, but not invariably, suggest a hematogenous source. Cranial imaging may also identify associated sinus or ear infection, although dedicated sinus or temporal bone CT may be necessary as well. Peripheral leukocytosis may be mild or absent, and should not be relied upon for considering the diagnosis. Because of the risk of herniation, LP is contraindicated in suspected or proven brain abscess. The CSF typically reveals nonspecific findings (elevated protein and lymphocytic pleocytosis with normal glucose) and rarely yields positive cultures unless the abscess has ruptured into the subarachnoid space.

The diverse clinical presentations of brain abscess lead to a broad differential diagnosis, depending on which clinical features are prominent. In the febrile patient with headache, altered mentation, and lateralizing findings, other infectious etiologies, such as subdural empyema, epidural abscess, viral encephalitis, acute bacterial meningitis, and endocarditis (with septic embolism or mycotic aneurysm rupture) should be considered. When fever is low-grade or absent, primary or metastatic brain tumor enters the differential. Pre- and postcontrast CT or MRI reliably distinguishes among many of these diagnostic possibilities, although deciding whether a ring-enhancing lesion represents an abscess or tumor can be difficult, even for an experienced neuroradiologist.

Successful treatment of brain abscess requires antibiotics in all patients and surgery in many, and hence infectious disease and neurosurgical consultations should be obtained in all cases, in addition to neurologic consultation typically obtained during diagnostic evaluation. Because brain abscesses are frequently polymicrobial, combination antibiotic therapy is the rule. Antibiotic selection, timing, and steroid therapy should be determined in consultation with infectious disease, neurology, and neurosurgery. The same considerations regarding resist-

ant pneumococcus discussed for bacterial meningitis apply to brain abscess, and vancomycin has largely supplanted penicillin as part of an empiric regimen. Metronidazole provides excellent anaerobic coverage and penetrates well into brain abscesses, although it does not cover *Actinomyces*, which are oral flora that can rarely cause brain abscesses. Third-generation cephalosporins (typically cefotaxime or ceftriaxone, or ceftazidime if *Pseudomonas* is a concern) provide gram-negative coverage, an important consideration in an abcess that is hospital-acquired or from an otic source. Hence, current empiric antibiotic therapy for brain abscess often includes vancomycin, metronidazole, and a third-generation cephalosporin (typically cefotaxime, ceftriaxone, or ceftazidime). Adjunctive medical therapy includes management of cerebral edema and increased ICP with dexamethasone, mannitol, fluid restriction, and other maneuvers, and prophylactic or symptomatic anticonvulsant therapy in appropriate situations.

Medical therapy alone has led to cure in patients with abscesses in inaccessible locations, such as the brainstem, but surgical intervention should be considered. Controversy persists as to whether aspiration or total excision produces better results. Computed tomography-guided stereotactic neurosurgical techniques have made serial aspirations more feasible. Operative specimens should be handled carefully, with specimens sent for atypical pathogens such as mycobacterial and fungal smears and cultures when appropriate. The frequency with which anaerobes cause brain abscess means that even "routine" cultures must be handled carefully, to ensure highest diagnostic yield. When brain abscess occurs in association with suspected or proven sinus, ear, or dental infection, otolaryngologic or oral surgical consultation should be obtained.

Prognosis has improved significantly over the past 15 years, probably related to improved neuroimaging and neurosurgical techniques. Mortality has decreased from over 50% to 5–10%. Of survivors, half are neurologically normal and about 10% severely impaired.

Although less common than brain abscess, subdural empyema and epidural abscess are extra-axial suppurative cranial infections that share many clinical features with brain abscess (Table 19.2). Subdural empyema, a collection of pus between dura and arachnoid, develops most commonly in adults as a consequence of ear or sinus infection, and occasionally in association with trauma or neurosurgery. Patients often present acutely, with prominent headache, fever, stiff neck, seizures, and focal cerebral symptoms and signs. There is significant overlap between brain abscess and subdural empyema with regard to pathogenesis and clinical presentation, and the disorders share many features of diagnosis and management. Pathogens for both disorders are similar and neuroimaging, generally MRI if feasible, not CSF

Table 19.2 Suppurative cerebral mass lesions: clinical features

	Infected site	Predisposing conditions	Acute onset	Fever/ leukocytosis	Organisms
Brain abscess	Brain parenchyma	Contiguous site (ear, sinus, teeth, skull) Hematogenous source (lung, congenital heart disease)	Varies	Varies	Often mixed: streptococci, anaerobes, gram-negative, *S. aureus*
Subdural empyema	Between dura and arachnoid	Ear or sinus infection; trauma or neurosurgery (rare)	Common	Common	Similar to brain abscess except less often mixed
Epidural abscess	Between dura and skull	Ear, sinus, orbital infection; cranial osteomyelitis	Varies	Varies	Streptococci, *S. aureus*

examination, is the diagnostic test of choice. Subdural empyema is a neurosurgical emergency because of the rapidity with which acute neurologic decompensation can occur. In fact, untreated, subdural empyema is uniformly fatal. With aggressive neurosurgical, and sometimes otolaryngologic, intervention and antibiotic therapy, over half of patients do well. Cranial epidural abscess, an infection in the space between dura and skull, begins as cranial osteomyelitis complicating ear, sinus, or orbital infection. Diagnosis, management, and prognosis are similar to subdural empyema. Important differences are the more indolent course characteristic of cranial epidural abscess and the particular importance of covering for staphylococcus, in addition to typical abscess or empyema pathogens. Because they share many of the same risk factors, brain abscess, subdural empyema, epidural abscess, and bacterial meningitis may occur in varying combinations in the same patient.

Septic Venous Sinus Thrombosis

Antibiotics have rendered this grim complication of facial, sinus, ear, or dental infection relatively uncommon. Depending on the site of primary infection, thrombosis may develop in the cavernous, superior sagittal, or lateral sinuses. Specific presenting features vary with the site involved, although headache, altered mentation, cranial neuropathies, seizures, and increased ICP occur frequently. When these symptoms develop in association with craniofacial infection, septic venous thrombosis should be considered, along with bacterial meningitis and the suppurative cerebral mass lesions just discussed. The CT or MRI may demonstrate the primary infection or venous infarction and sometimes reveal thrombosis, although conventional angiography with venous phase studies may be necessary to confirm the diagnosis. In general, treatment consists of empiric antibiotics and surgical debridement of the primary source. The role of anticoagulation

remains controversial, due to the risk of hemorrhage, although it may be beneficial in selected patients with a heavy clot burden or who progress despite aggressive antibiotic therapy and surgical intervention. The decision to anticoagulate a patient with septic venous sinus thrombosis should be made in consultation with neurology and neurosurgery. Thrombolytics for this entity are still considered experimental, and should be reserved for those cases that are severe and continue to progress despite maximal medical and surgical therapy. Even with aggressive antibiotic therapy and surgical management of the craniofacial infection, morbidity and mortality remain high.

Acute Viral Encephalitis and Related Disorders

Viral encephalitis presents acutely with fever, headache, altered mentation, and evidence of parenchymal brain involvement, such as seizure or focal cerebral dysfunction. Viruses enter the CNS by hematogenous or neuronal routes. Blood-borne spread is the more common mechanism, with CNS seeding during viremia. A few viruses, such as HSV and rabies, use neuronal routes to invade the CNS. Given the paucity of highly specific antiviral agents, the difficult task of identifying particular viral pathogens may seem to be of little practical importance, but prognostic information and public health concerns often justify the effort. In any case, even in its currently limited state, available antiviral therapy makes rapid recognition of viral encephalitis important.

Arthropod-borne viruses, or arboviruses, cause viral encephalitis in the United States and worldwide. Important American arboviruses include Western equine, Eastern equine, Venezuelan equine, St. Louis, LaCross, and, most recently, West Nile virus. West Nile encephalitis first appeared in the United States in a classic summer outbreak in and around New York City in 1999. Since then, the epidemic has spread west, and, as of January 2008, every state in the continental United States, except for

▼

Pearls and Perils

Suppurative cerebral mass lesions

▶ Consider the diagnosis in the patient with headache, impaired mentation, and seizure or focal cerebral dysfunction, particularly if there is coexisting craniofacial infection. Fever may not be prominent in brain abscess.

▶ Contiguous craniofacial infection (orbit, sinus, ear, teeth, skull) predisposes to brain abscess, subdural empyema, and epidural abscess, which may exist in varying combinations in an individual patient.

▶ Magnetic resonance imaging is the diagnostic test of choice, although computed tomography with and without contrast can be adequate. Lumbar puncture is often contraindicated, and rarely yields helpful information.

▶ Consider fungi and parasites, as well as bacteria, in immunocompromised patients with brain abscess.

▶ Consultation with a neurosurgeon is indicated in all instances. If orbital, sinus, ear, or dental infection is the source of infection, consultation with an ophthalmologist, otolaryngologist, or oral surgeon should be obtained.

▶ Complications include increased intracranial pressure, seizures, venous sinus thrombosis, and meningitis.

Maine, has reported human cases. Most arboviruses, including West Nile, typically cause nonspecific febrile illnesses. Older and immunosuppressed patients appear to be at increased risk for CNS involvement. In addition to altered mentation, ataxia, or extrapyramidal syndromes, West Nile may cause a paralytic syndrome resembling polio. In China and Southeast Asia, Japanese B encephalitis, a significant public health problem in these regions, is caused by a mosquito-borne arbovirus. Encephalitis due to polio, an enterovirus, and mumps and measles, both paramyxoviruses, has significantly decreased in the United States secondary to vaccination programs, although recent outbreaks of mumps have occurred (see aseptic meningitis.) Enterovirus 71, as previously mentioned, has a neurotropism similar to polio viruses, and has become an important cause of epidemic encephalitis and myelitis in Asia, and it may be an underrecognized cause of similar syndromes in the United States. Other enteroviruses, such as echovirus and Coxsackie virus, more typically cause viral meningitis, but occasionally cause encephalitis.

Herpes simplex virus is the most common cause of focal nonepidemic encephalitis in the United States. HSV-1 accounts for essentially all adult cases. HSV encephalitis (HSVE) develops as a consequence of either primary infection spreading along the olfactory tract or reactivated infection in trigeminal ganglia, accounting for its predilection for orbitofrontal and temporal cortex. The efficacy of high-dose IV acyclovir in reducing mortality from HSVE has made empiric therapy the standard in suspected viral encephalitis.

Rabies, another important endemic cause of encephalitis worldwide, illustrates another approach to therapy. Although not all individuals bitten by a rabid animal will develop encephalitis, the absolute fatality of the disease, once symptomatic, justifies vaccination of those at particular risk, antitoxin administration to anyone bitten by a proven or suspected rabid animal, and aggressive capture and quarantine efforts in all cases.

Time of the year may assist in diagnosis. Arbovirus infections occur more frequently in summer and fall, paramyxovirus infections more commonly in winter, and HSVE year-round. Neuroimaging studies, particularly MRI, may show temporal lobe or orbitofrontal enhancement and edema in HSVE, particularly several days or more into the course. In most cases of acute viral encephalitis, however, neuroimaging findings are nonspecific, with the study serving to exclude brain abscess or extracranial suppurative infection. Computed tomography or MRI can also help determine whether it is safe to proceed with LP, which usually shows normal or elevated pressure, elevated protein (usually <200/dL), normal glucose, and up to several hundred white cells, which are usually mononuclear. When CSF is examined very early, polymorphonuclear cells may predominate, raising concern for bacterial meningitis. Very rarely, CSF may be relatively normal very early in the course. In such patients, CSF should be re-examined in 12–36 hours, depending on clinical course. Xanthochromia and red cells are a classic, but not particularly common, CSF finding in HSVE. In rabies, CSF and other body secretions are highly infectious, and appropriate precautions should be taken.

Viral CSF cultures and acute and convalescent serum titers rarely yield diagnostic information rapidly enough to influence management, but may be helpful in determining prognosis and are important for epidemiologic surveillance during outbreaks. Infectious disease consultation should be obtained for guidance as to which titers to order and when. Acute-phase serum may be frozen, with the decision on specific testing made later, depending on the clinical course. Electroencephalogram (EEG) may be helpful in HSVE, demonstrating periodic lateralized epileptiform discharges, although these may be seen in other viral encephalitides and acute cerebral disorders. Given the high sensitivity and specificity of CSF HSV-1, PCR for diagnosing HSVE has largely replaced brain biopsy in establishing the diagnosis. Because acyclovir is the only antiviral agent clearly shown to be effective against any form of viral encephalitis, empiric therapy with this usually well-tolerated drug has been used in favor of biopsy in most cases. Whether biopsy will again become important as antiviral agents for other causes of encephalitis are developed will depend on whether noninvasive techniques such as CSF PCR for specific viral nucleic acids eventually provide accurate, timely identification of encephalitis pathogens.

In the acutely ill, febrile patient in whom evidence of parenchymal cerebral involvement (seizure, altered mentation, and focal cerebral signs) is more prominent than signs of meningeal irritation, the differential diagnosis includes brain abscess, subdural empyema or epidural abscess, nonviral causes of meningoencephalitis (atypical bacteria, fungi, parasites), postinfectious encephalomyelitis, endocarditis, Reye syndrome, and collagen vascular diseases. Recognizing parenchymal CNS involvement is critical to avoid mistaking viral encephalitis (with its guarded prognosis and need for early treatment) for viral meningitis (which has a benign course). Neurologic consultation can assist with defining the clinical syndrome as well as managing seizures and other complications of viral encephalitis.

Because it is well tolerated and has been shown to improve outcome in HSVE, high-dose IV acyclovir is customarily given to all patients with viral encephalitis, even though HSV causes only about 10% of viral encephalitis in the United States. Renal insufficiency is the major serious, although usually reversible, side effect of acyclovir, and often can be avoided with adequate hydration of pa-

tients during their course of acyclovir. Seizures and increased ICP should be anticipated and managed if they develop.

Prognosis depends on the causative agent, with overall mortality of about 10%. California encephalitis is rarely fatal, in contrast to rabies, which is uniformly fatal once symptoms develop. For HSVE, mortality with acyclovir therapy is 20%, compared with 70% in historical controls. Neurologic sequelae likewise vary by pathogen, affecting the majority of patients who survive eastern equine or Japanese B encephalitis and relatively few patients with Venezuelan equine encephalitis. For patients with HSVE treated with acyclovir, just over a third recovered to mild or no neurologic impairment. For all types of viral encephalitis, neurologic sequelae include mild cognitive impairment, behavioral and personality changes, epilepsy, hemiparesis, or persistent vegetative state.

Postinfectious encephalomyelitis, an autoimmune demyelinating syndrome, most commonly follows influenza infection in the United States and measles infection worldwide. The disorder may also develop after vaccination. Days to weeks after recovery from a viral syndrome, patients acutely develop fever, decreased level of consciousness, seizures, and focal signs referable to brain, cord, or both. Differential diagnosis on clinical grounds includes bacterial meningitis, viral encephalitis, or Reye syndrome. The CSF may be normal or show nonspecific changes. A CT typically is also unrevealing, but MRI may show demyelinating lesions in brain and cord. Severe symptoms usually create no diagnostic confusion with multiple sclerosis, but the rarer less dramatic presentation may raise the issue of whether the patient is experiencing a first attack of multiple sclerosis. Although vaccines themselves have been associated with postinfectious encephalomyelitis, their widespread use for exanthematous conditions has been credited with decreasing the frequency of this severe condition. Steroids are usually administered (although their efficacy has never been proven in a controlled study), along with supportive care, often in an intensive care unit (ICU) setting. Both intravenous immunoglobulin (IVIg) and plasmapheresis have been used as adjunct therapy.

Prion Diseases and Related Disorders

Clinically distinct from acute viral encephalitis and postinfectious encephalomyelitis, prion diseases are devastating disorders that may be infectious or genetic. Prions, novel proteinaceous agents highly resistant to common disinfectants, can cause disease after incubation periods of years or even decades. Creutzfeldt-Jakob disease (CJD), a condition of middle age and later life, presents most commonly in its sporadic form (sCJD) as a rapidly progressive dementia with prominent ataxia and

---

Pearls and Perils

Viral encephalitis

▶ Consider the diagnosis in the patient with acute onset of fever, headache, and altered mentation, with concomitant seizure or other evidence of focal cerebral dysfunction.

▶ Pre- and postcontrast computed tomography or magnetic resonance imaging (MRI) and cerebrospinal fluid (CSF) examination can help exclude suppurative cerebral mass lesions and postinfectious encephalomyelitis.

▶ Xanthochromic CSF, characteristic electroencephalographic (EEG) patterns and temporal lobe changes on MRI support a diagnosis of herpes simplex virus (HSV) encephalitis, although the absence of some of these features does not exclude the diagnosis. CSF HSV-1 polymerase chain reaction (PCR) is highly sensitive and specific for the diagnosis.

▶ Even though HSV accounts for about 10% of American encephalitis cases, acyclovir should be given in all cases of suspected viral encephalitis, since it is usually well tolerated and improves outcome.

▶ Prognosis depends on the viral pathogen. This and public health concerns frequently justify viral cultures and serologic studies to identify the specific agent.

myoclonus. Iatrogenic cases are occasionally seen in recipients of cadaver tissues or extracts. A cluster of cases related to cadaver-derived growth hormone (GH) therapy prompted development of recombinant GH, which does not transmit this relentlessly fatal disease. Neuroimaging studies and CSF, obtained in the search for treatable causes, are unrevealing. Diagnosis depends on recognizing the clinical syndrome and the characteristic periodic complexes on EEG. Brain biopsy may be performed to confirm the diagnosis, posing uncertain risks to the surgical team and pathologist. There is no known treatment. Neurologic deterioration progresses rapidly, with death occurring within months in most cases.

Variant CJD (vCJD) has attracted significant media attention as "mad cow disease." It followed the appearance, in 1986, of the prion disease bovine spongiform encephalopathy (BSE) in cows in the United Kingdom. Cattle feed containing contaminated cow products contributed to the outbreak. The human disease vCJD has been linked to consumption of BSE-contaminated cattle products. Compared with sCJD, vCJD affects younger patients and presents with psychiatric or behavioral symptoms first, followed by frank cognitive impairment, movement disorders, and ataxia. The characteristic EEG findings of sCJD are uncommon in vCJD. Until very recently, import restrictions and elimination of the practice of using rendered cow products as cattle feed appeared to limit the epidemic to Europe, with cases in the United Kingdom thought to have peaked in 1993. The discovery of BSE in a cow in Canada and in the United States in 2003 has raised concern that locally acquired vCJD cases will be seen in North America.

Although not a prion disorder, subacute sclerosing panencephalitis (SSPE) is a clinically similar syndrome that follows a very small fraction of measles infections. Consequently, it develops most frequently in children, although it may manifest in early adulthood. Subacute sclerosing panencephalitis commences with the insidious onset of personality change, visual disturbance, and intellectual dysfunction, beginning months to years after typical measles, progressing to frank dementia with prominent myoclonus over months. The etiology of SSPE—defective virus versus an abnormal immune response—remains controversial. In the typical clinical picture, elevated measles titers in the CSF and characteristic periodic discharges on EEG confirm the diagnosis. Typically fatal in months to years, widespread vaccination has made this disorder rare in the United States, although it remains a problem in parts of the world where measles vaccination is not routine.

Spinal Epidural Abscess

The combination of fever, back pain with local spine tenderness, and radiculopathy or myelopathy obligates emergent evaluation for spinal epidural abscess. Infection develops in the epidural space either by hematogenous spread (particularly from skin infections or related to intravenous [IV] drug use) or by direct extension of vertebral osteomyelitis or soft tissue infections, such as retropharyngeal, mediastinal, perinephric, or psoas abscesses. Radicular pain is a common early symptom, frequently overshadowed by rapidly progressive paraparesis or quadriparesis, depending on the spinal level involved. Local tenderness over the infected site is a useful diagnostic sign. S. aureus causes most spinal epidural abscesses. Other important pathogens include gram-negative bacilli and aerobic streptococci.

Peripheral white count and erythrocyte sedimentation rate are usually elevated. Plain films are abnormal in about half of cases, and should not be used to exclude the diagnosis if normal. The diagnosis depends on MRI, or CT myelography if MRI cannot be performed. Blood cultures are often positive, usually correlating well with abscess cultures. A CSF examination may be risky both because of risk of spinal herniation and of spreading infection to the subarachnoid space, should the needle pass through the abscess. Computed tomography-guided aspiration of the abscess has become more common and increases the yield of identifying causative agent.

Differential diagnosis includes other spinal infections, such as M. tuberculosis, Histoplasma, Coccidioides, and occasionally other fungi such as Aspergillus or Candida. Other diagnostic considerations include epidural metastases, primary spinal tumors, or transverse myelitis. Most case series emphasize the delay in diagnosis, which can have adverse consequences for neurologic recovery.

Once MRI or myelography establishes the diagnosis and blood cultures have been drawn, antibiotics to

---

Pearls and Perils

Spinal epidural abscess

▶ The patient with fever, back pain with local spine tenderness, and radiculopathy or myelopathy, particularly with proven or suspected recent bacteremia, has a spinal epidural abscess until proven otherwise.

▶ Diagnosis depends on spine magnetic resonance imaging or computed tomography myelography. Urgent neurosurgical consultation should be obtained.

▶ Common bacterial pathogens include skin flora and gram-negative bacilli. Consider also TB and, particularly in immunocompromised patients, fungi.

▶ Prognosis depends on duration and severity of neurologic deficit prior to surgery, highlighting the importance of rapid diagnosis.

cover *S. aureus* and gram-negative bacilli should be administered. Emergent neurosurgical consultation should be obtained, as surgical drainage may be indicated to relieve spinal cord compression and obtain cultures to identify the pathogen. Steroids are frequently administered preoperatively and postoperatively. Prognostic factors for recovery in spinal epidural abscess underscore the need for early diagnosis. Prognosis for neurologic recovery depends on the severity and duration of cord dysfunction prior to surgery. When motor involvement is severe or neurologic signs are present for more than 24 hours, significant neurologic recovery is unlikely.

Specific Pathogens of Neurologic Importance

The previous section focused on clinical neurologic infectious syndromes. Some pathogens, however, figure in the differential diagnosis of so many infections or are of sufficient epidemiologic or historical importance to warrant separate discussion.

Mycobacteria

Obligate aerobes, mycobacteria can cause CNS and peripheral nerve disease. *Mycobacterium tuberculosis* is spread by infected droplets, first causing pulmonary infection, followed by tuberculemia. Neurologic complications develop in up to 10% of TB infections, either as tuberculous involvement of the spine with myelopathy (Pott disease) or as meningitis or tuberculoma (Figure 19.1). Meningeal seeding during tuberculemia results in Rich foci (small subpial or subependymal foci of caseous lesions), which, upon rupture, result in meningitis. Because neurologic TB may develop during primary infection or reactivate during immunosuppression, TB is a consideration in the differential diagnosis of meningitis, focal brain lesions, and compressive myelopathy in normal and immunocompromised patients. Suspected or proven systemic TB usually prompts consideration of the diagnosis, but neurologic involvement may develop without positive skin tests or chest film indicating active disease. Hence, ensuring that surgical specimens from cerebral or spinal infectious mass lesions are sent for AFB smears and culture is prudent in most circumstances, especially in recent immigrants from countries with a high incidence of TB. Tuberculosis should also be considered when meningitis fails to respond to antibacterial therapy. The CSF demonstrates elevated protein, normal or decreased glucose, and moderate pleocytosis, usually lymphocytic, with all indices usually less strikingly abnormal than for acute bacterial meningitis. Because a negative AFB smear does not rule out TB meningitis, and cultures may not yield organisms for weeks, antituberculous ther-

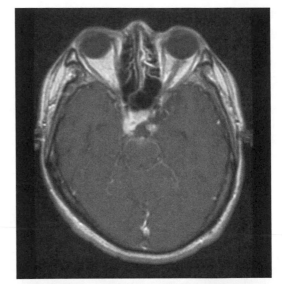

A

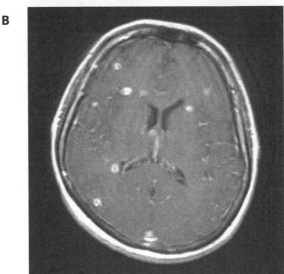

B

Figure 19.1 Neurotuberculosis: Gadolinium-enhanced T1 brain magnetic resonance imaging from a patient with new-onset focal motor seizures and disseminated tuberculosis demonstrate basilar enhancement (A), consistent with tuberculous meningitis and multiple, small enhancing lesions (B), consistent with tuberculomas. Aspirated material from the patient's thyroid mass was positive of AFB and ultimately grew *M. tuberculosis* in culture. Courtesy of Anita Koshy, Stanford University.

apy with at least four drugs frequently is started before microbiologic confirmation is available. The yield of CSF AFB smears and mycobacterial cultures improves with repeated, high-volume LPs. The difficulty in confirming the diagnosis has prompted interest in PCR techniques, although these are not yet in wide clinical use. The exuberant basilar exudates accompanying TB meningitis can interfere with CSF flow, causing obstructive or communicating hydrocephalus, or injure cranial nerves or cerebral vessels with subsequent cranial neuropathy or

---

▼

Pearls and Perils

Tuberculosis (TB) and the nervous system

▶ Consider the diagnosis in all cases of meningitis, spinal epidural infection, and brain mass of obscure cause.

▶ Pulmonary or non-neurologic extrapulmonary disease may not be evident, and hence negative skin tests and chest film should not be used to exclude the diagnosis.

▶ For TB meningitis, highest diagnostic sensitivity of AFB smears and culture requires high-volume cerebrospinal fluid examinations, performed serially.

▶ Empiric therapy often with steroids may be necessary, since cultures may take up to 6 weeks to turn positive.

▶ Meningeal exudate and arachnoiditis can cause vasculitis with subsequent cerebral infarction, cranial neuropathy, and hydrocephalus. Adjunctive steroids, serial lumbar punctures or shunting procedures may be necessary.

---

cerebral infarction. In immunocompetent adults, adjunctive steroid therapy lowers mortality, although not morbidity, and is typically administered in conjunction with a four-drug antituberculous regimen.

Mycobacterium leprae causes leprosy, or Hansen disease, one of the most common causes of peripheral neuropathy in the world. The spectrum of disease depends on the patient's cell-mediated immune response. At one end is the lepromatous form of diffuse, cutaneous disease with a poor prognosis, seen in immunocompromised hosts. At the other is tuberculoid leprosy, the more localized, neural form with a better prognosis. Patients demonstrate hypopigmented, anesthetic skin lesions and thickened nerves. The predilection for superficially located nerves such as cranial nerves V and VII and greater auricular, ulnar, and common peroneal nerves has been attributed to the organism's preference for cooler temperatures. Trophic changes, such as skin ulcers and arthropathy, develop commonly. Demonstration of AFB in skin scrapings or nerve biopsy establishes the diagnosis. Treatment consists of dapsone, clofazimine, and rifampin in varying combinations.

Spirochetes

Treponema pallidum, Borrelia burgdorferi, and *Leptospira interrogans* cause syphilis, Lyme disease, and leptospirosis, respectively. These infections cause a variety of acute and chronic neurologic disorders. Syphilis and Lyme disease share several important features: early manifestations that may be dramatic but self-limited, multifocal neurologic involvement causing CNS and peripheral

nerve disease, suboptimal diagnostic methods, and the potential to relapse despite therapy.

Neurologic disease is not a feature of primary syphilis, although asymptomatic spread to the CNS has been documented in 30% of early syphilis cases. Disseminated disease characterizes secondary syphilis, manifesting systemically with flu-like illness and rash and neurologically as syphilitic meningitis or cranial neuropathies, including hearing loss. In meningovascular syphilis, cerebral or spinal cord infarction with positive serum serologies and abnormal CSF develops, typically within about 5 years of primary infection. Latent syphilis is asymptomatic, with disease apparent only by serology or CSF abnormalities. In tertiary syphilis, cardiac and neurologic disease develops years and sometimes decades after primary infection. Parenchymal forms include the dementia known as *general paresis* and a myeloneuropathy, *tabes dorsalis*. Syphilitic gummas (granulomas that manifest as space-occupying lesions in brain or cord) can occur throughout the course of syphilis, but have become rare in the penicillin era.

Neurosyphilis is thus a consideration in the diagnostic evaluation of dementia, cranial neuropathy, aseptic or chronic meningitis, stroke in the young patient, unusual CNS mass lesions, or myelopathy. In addition, the diagnosis of asymptomatic neurosyphilis is not always easy. Confusion persists in the literature and in practice for several reasons. The technical difficulty and high false-positive and false-negative rates of direct examination and culture techniques, combined with the limitations of nonspecific and treponemal tests in both serum and CSF, can make it difficult to decide who does and does not have asymptomatic neurosyphilis. A positive CSF-VDRL, in an atraumatic tap, is very specific, but not highly sensitive, for the diagnosis of neurosyphilis. The CSF may show only elevated protein with or without pleocytosis in documented neurosyphilis, and serum nontreponemal tests may revert to negative in late syphilis. Hence, a negative CSF-VDRL does not rule out the diagnosis of neurosyphilis. Cerebrospinal fluid treponemal specific tests are sensitive, but not specific, for neurosyphilis, and thus may be helpful in excluding the diagnosis. Regardless, when neurosyphilis is suspected, at minimum, both screening and treponemal specific serum tests should be obtained.

The U.S. Centers for Disease Control and Prevention (CDC) recommends lumbar puncture in patients with positive serum syphilis serologies and associated neurologic or ocular disease, evidence of active tertiary disease such as aortitis or gumma, treatment failure, or coexisting HIV infection with late latent syphilis or syphilis of unknown duration. Patients with positive serum syphilis serologies should be offered HIV testing (and vice versa), since the disorders potentiate each other's transmission and share risk factors.

For all forms of neurosyphilis, the CDC recommends high dose IV penicillin (3–4 million units every 4 hours) for 10–14 days or, intramuscular (IM) benzathine penicillin with oral probenecid. For the IM regimen, it is important to ensure that patients will adhere to the four times daily dosing of probenecid and that IM therapy is with benzathine penicillin, not the combined benzathine and procaine penicillin preparations intended for other infections. Finally, defining which serum and CSF parameters indicate treatment failure, and how often and for how long these should be monitored, remain unsolved problems. The CDC recommends repeat CSF examinations every 6 months until CSF normalizes. Neurologic, ophthalmologic, or dermatologic consultation to document the presence of nervous system, eye, or skin disease consistent with syphilis may be helpful. In all but the most straightforward situations, particularly patients with penicillin allergies or concurrent HIV infection, infectious disease consultation can guide evaluation, therapy, and follow-up.

Many of the same uncertainties in diagnosis and optimal antibiotic therapy that make neurosyphilis challenging apply to Lyme disease and its neurologic consequences. In contrast to syphilis, and complicating the situation further, is continuing debate over the spectrum of Lyme-related neurologic disease (neuroborreliosis). Best agreement exists for the early neurologic syndromes, which include cranial neuropathy (including unilateral or bilateral Bell palsy), meningitis, and painful radiculoneuritis. Late neurologic disorders continue to be defined, ranging from encephalomyelitis and neuropathy to post-Lyme syndromes resembling fibromyalgia. Current guidelines recommend a 2-week course of parenteral ceftriaxone or cefotaxime for early neuroborreliosis (meningitis, cranial neuritis, or radiculopathy). Oral doxycycline is likely to be equivalent, but less commonly used or recommended in the United States. There is no consensus as to whether or not patients with an isolated facial nerve palsy secondary to Lyme must have an LP to rule out concurrent meningitis. If an LP is done and is negative, then oral treatment for 14 days with doxycycline, amoxicillin, or cefuroxime can be used. If the CSF has evidence of active inflammation, then the previously mentioned parenteral antibiotics are recommended. Patients with late neurologic complications of partially treated or previously untreated Lyme disease usually have abnormal CSF, neuropsychiatric studies, or neuroimaging. In these patients, treatment with parenteral ceftriaxone for 2–4 weeks is recommended. Adjunctive steroids have no evidence for benefit or harm in patients with neuroborreliosis. In patients with post-Lyme syndrome, characterized by continued musculoskeletal pain, fatigue, and neuropsychiatric complaints despite appropriate antibiotic courses for Lyme disease, and without objective measures of ongoing CNS inflammation, recurrent or prolonged antibiotic courses do not improve outcomes and are not recommended. Despite these recently published guidelines, ambiguity still exists regarding diagnosis and management of neuroborreliosis and thus justifies neurologic and infectious disease consultation in these patients.

Many domestic and wild animals carry *L. interrogans*. Rather than full-blown leptospirosis, exposed individuals most commonly develop mild or subclinical infection. Leptospirosis is usually a biphasic illness, although it can be difficult to distinguish the initial phase from the second phase, especially in severe infections. The initial bacteremic phase is characterized by fevers, conjunctival suffusion, myalgia, and headache. A brief period of apparent recovery will often be followed by recurrent symptoms and hepatic and renal involvement. During this phase, the organism is found in most organs, but is less readily cultured from the blood. In Weil disease, the fulminant form of the second or immunologic phase, hepatic and renal failure with impaired consciousness and high mortality rates are seen. It is also in this second stage that asymptomatic and occasionally symptomatic meningitis, typically with lymphocytic pleocytosis, occurs. More severe CNS complications, such as meningoencephalitis or myelitis, may occur during this phase, but are rare. Postinfectious Guillain-Barré syndrome (GBS) after leptospirosis has been reported. Diagnosis depends on culturing the organism or demonstrating increasing antibody titers in acute and convalescent serum. Meningitis will often resolve without therapy, although tetracyclines or β-lactam antibiotics are usually given. Late neurologic complications, as occur in syphilis and Lyme disease, do not appear to be an important feature of leptospirosis.

Other Atypical Bacteria

Rickettsiae, obligate intracellular parasites whose transmission often depends on arthropods, cause febrile illnesses with ulcerative skin lesions, rash, and meningoencephalitis. In the United States, epidemiologically important rickettsial illnesses include Rocky Mountain spotted fever (RMSF), Q fever, ehrlichiosis, and scrub typhus. The CSF usually demonstrates an aseptic meningitis profile and skin biopsy, and serologic tests confirm the diagnosis. Tetracycline, doxycycline, and chloramphenicol are among the effective antibiotics. Special mention should be made of RMSF, which is caused by *R. rickettsii*, and is seen most often in the South Atlantic region of the United States, although an outbreak of RMSF occurred in Arizona during 2002–2004. If not recognized and promptly treated, the mortality rate can be as high as 23%. Rocky Mountain spotted fever presents as an acute meningitis and is usually seen in the late spring to early fall and in those under the age of 16. A petechial rash that begins on the extremities, and can involve the palms and soles, and moves centrally may begin several days after the onset of fever. The treatment of choice is doxycycline.

Whipple disease, caused by the recently characterized gram positive bacillus *Tropheryma whippelii*, is a multisystem disorder characterized by gastrointestinal disease, arthritis, lymphadenopathy, and protean neurologic manifestations including dementia, supranuclear ophthalmoplegia, meningitis, neuropathy, and myopathy. Classically, the disease manifests as coexisting neurologic and gastrointestinal disease, although rarely it can primarily involve the CNS alone. If the disease is suspected, periodic acid–Schiff (PAS)-positive bacilli identified on duodenal biopsy, PAS-positive cells on CSF cytospin, or positive PCR from CSF, blood, or tissue are considered diagnostic. In its numerous other presentations, sarcoidosis and collagen vascular disease may be other diagnostic considerations. Trimethoprim-sulfamethoxazole is the treatment of choice.

Bacterial Toxins

Rather than causing neural injury by direct invasion or inflammation, a few bacteria cause neurologic disease by secreting specific neurotoxins. In developed countries, vaccination has decreased, but not eliminated, diphtheria and tetanus, whose clinical presentations can rapidly evolve from subtle and puzzling to dramatic and life-threatening. Both continue to cause serious morbidity and mortality where immunization is not offered or encouraged, and highlight the importance of vaccination as an effective public health strategy.

An exotoxin secreted by *Clostridium botulinum* causes botulism, a presynaptic disorder of neuromuscular transmission. The toxin, ingested in contaminated food or synthesized in situ in an infected wound or gut, blocks acetylcholine release at the neuromuscular junction. Beginning typically with diplopia and dysarthria, the initial weakness of extraocular and bulbar muscles rapidly descends to include limb and respiratory muscles. Paralytic ileus occurs frequently. Pupils may be large and sluggishly reactive, distinguishing the disorder from myasthenic crisis, another cause of diplopia and rapidly progressive weakness. The CSF is normal in botulism, in contrast to the elevated CSF protein often seen in GBS. Electromyographic (EMG)/nerve conduction studies with repetitive stimulation distinguishes the presynaptic defect of neuromuscular transmission seen in botulism from the postsynaptic disorder of myasthenia and from the peripheral nerve demyelination of GBS. Poliomyelitis, tick paralysis, and vascular or demyelinating brainstem events usually can also be excluded by examination, CSF, and electrophysiologic studies. Rapid determination of the toxin source is critical, to allow expeditious wound debridement in wound botulism and identification of at-risk individuals in food-borne cases. Blood, stool, and potential food sources should be assayed for toxin and cultured for *C. botulinum*. Antitoxin is usually recommended. Because of its equine source, hypersensitivity must be excluded prior to administration. Whether antibiotics active against *C. botulinum*, such as penicillin or metronidazole, should be administered remains controversial, since the resulting bacterial lysis might lead to increased toxin release. Respiratory function should be monitored with serial bedside pulmonary function tests, which are more sensitive than blood gas determinations in diagnosing ventilatory failure. Long-term ventilatory support and tracheostomy may be necessary, and full recovery may take years.

In tetanus, a toxin elaborated by *Clostridium tetani* in an infected wound inhibits release of brainstem spinal cord inhibitory neurotransmitters such as glycine and γ-aminobutyric acid (GABA). The resulting net excitation of motor circuits leads to uncontrolled muscle contractions, which may remain localized to the wound-bearing limb, but are more commonly generalized. Jaw and facial muscle involvement cause trismus and risus sardonicus. Axial muscle involvement causes opisthotonus which, combined with limb contractions, may be severe enough to compromise respiration. Frequently stimulus-sensitive and painful spasms may be complicated further by autonomic instability. As with botulism, a critical goal of therapy is to decrease toxin production and binding to neural targets by administration of hyperimmune globulin and wound debridement. Penicillin is customarily given to eliminate the organism, but does not substitute for wound debridement. Patients frequently require ventilatory support and symptomatic therapy for spasms by minimizing stimuli and administering high-dose benzodiazepines, or sedative-anesthetics such as propofol. In addition, continuous or intermittent intrathecal baclofen has been used safely in severe tetanus, and may cause less sedation and lead to earlier weaning from the ventilator. The high potency of tetanus toxin means that clinical tetanus may not result in functional immunity, and hence vaccine or booster should be administered.

Diphtheritic polyneuropathy has become rare in the United States, owing largely to routine vaccination. *Corynebacterium diphtheriae* elaborates a toxin that is especially active against heart, kidney, and peripheral nerve. Cardiac and neurologic manifestations develop in a minority of cases, typically several weeks to months after the pharyngitis, and are proportional to the severity of the initial disease. Ciliary and palatal weakness are prominent early, and manifest as blurred vision, dysarthria, and dysphagia, followed by a more generalized sensorimotor polyneuropathy, which may be severe enough to cause quadriparesis and respiratory failure. Treatment for acute diphtheriae involves antitoxin and appropriate antibiotics, but for neurologic complications is largely supportive. Neurologic recovery is the rule, although arrhythmias from cardiac involvement may be fatal. In addition, like tetanus, clinical disease may not result in functional immunity, and vaccination or booster should be given.

Fungi

Fungal infections cause brain abscess, meningitis, meningoencephalitis, and occasionally spinal cord lesions. In most cases, these complications develop in the context of disseminated infection, which may not always be recognized when neurologic manifestations appear. Cryptococcosis (discussed later in the chapter, in the section on acquired immune deficiency syndrome [AIDS]) is a notable exception, as this fungus appears to possess specific tropism for the nervous system. Diagnosing fungal CNS infections depends on maintaining a high index of suspicion and recognizing high-risk clinical settings.

Pathogenic fungi can cause disease in immunocompetent hosts. In blastomycosis, *Blastomyces dermatitidis*, endemic to the Midwest United States, establishes infection through the respiratory tract. In about 15% of patients with disseminated infection, meningeal, cerebral or cord involvement occurs. Another infection endemic to the Midwest as well as Appalachia is histoplasmosis. *Histoplasma capsulatum* may cause meningitis, brain mass, or cord lesion, and should be considered when these neurologic syndromes evolve in a systemically ill patient from an endemic area. Coccidiomycosis, endemic to the southwestern United States, usually causes a nonspecific febrile illness conferring lifelong immunity. Occasionally, *Coccidioides immitis* infection disseminates, especially in patients of Filipino, African American, or Latino descent, causing brain or cord mass or meningitis. Serum and CSF complement fixation studies can help establish the diagnosis.

Opportunistic fungal pathogens infect immunologically impaired hosts. Aspergillosis can cause meningitis, brain abscess, and spinal cord lesion, in association with fungemia and sinus infection. *Aspergillus* tends to invade blood vessels, leading to ischemic, and occasionally hemorrhagic, cerebrovascular complications. Candidiasis causes brain abscess, and occasionally meningitis or cord lesions, typically in association with IV drug use, hyperalimentation, central venous lines, and broad-spectrum antibiotic therapy. Patients with ventricular shunts are predisposed to candidal meningitis without concomitant candidemia. Mucormycosis causes sinusitis and orbital cellulitis, and then rapidly invades the meninges, the cerebral vessels, and the brain. Diabetics are at particular risk, accounting for 70% of cases of this devastating infection. Even with extensive debridement and antifungal therapy, mortality exceeds 20%.

The grave nature of CNS fungal infections warrants IV amphotericin B in most cases, although the newer azole and echinocandin antifungals, such as voriconazole and caspofungin have their role as well. Additionally, intrathecal amphotericin may be required, and fungal brain or cord abscesses require surgical therapy. Unfortunately, the severely debilitated patients who most often acquire opportunistic fungal infections are the highest-risk surgical candidates. When meningitis, cerebral mass lesion, or cord compression develop in an immunosuppressed host, or have a seemingly obscure cause in an individual from an endemic area, fungal infection should be considered.

Parasites

Although few parasites that cause neurologic infection are endemic in the United States, immigration and the ease of international travel mean that these infections are not mere curiosities. Indeed, travel history may be the key to considering the diagnosis. Both helminths and protozoa may infect the nervous system, typically causing meningitis or cerebral mass, and occasionally myopathy or myelopathy.

Neurocysticercosis (NCC) results from ingestion of larva of the pork tapeworm *Taenia solium*. Endemic to Central and South American, as well as southeast Asia, the high frequency with which autopsies demonstrate cysticercosis in these areas may make this the most common neurologic infection in the world. Central nervous system involvement includes parenchymal, meningeal, and intraventricular forms, which may coexist in a particular patient. The diagnosis should be considered in the patient from an endemic area with seizures, hydrocephalus, cerebral mass lesion(s), or meningitis. Ocular infection may coexist, but a search for extraneural infection (with eosinophilia, stool ova and parasites, or soft tissue calcification on plain film) is rarely helpful. Serum cysticercal titers may support the diagnosis, although high seropositivity rates among individuals living in endemic areas make the test suggestive, but not diagnostic. On neuroimaging studies, inactive cysts appear as scattered small calcifications, and active cysts are cystic structures without enhancement and often without edema. The degenerating cyst is ring-enhancing and usually surrounded by edema. Both old and new lesions may be seen on a given scan, providing an important diagnostic clue. The CSF may show changes consistent with aseptic or eosinophilic meningitis, as well as positive cysticercal titers, which strongly support the diagnosis. The most important treatment for patients with NCC presenting with neurologic symptoms is appropriate interventions for their seizures and increased ICP, if evident. Antiparasitic treatment in these patients is complicated and depends on many factors including the number of cysts, the anatomic location, and the developmental state of the cysts. For active or degenerating parenchymal lesions of 20 or fewer, albendazole should be administered, in conjunction with steroids to attenuate the intense inflammatory reaction evoked by dying cysts. In patients with heavy infections (100+ cysts), treatment may lead to symptomatic increased ICP, and the optimal treatment for these patients is unclear. A single enhancing lesion usually suggests a degenerating cyst and can be treated with albendazole alone with steroids added if side effects occur. There are no trials to help guide therapeutic decisions about subarachnoid cysts, which can cause chronic meningitis, leading to lacunar infarcts and cranial nerve palsies. The treatment options include albendazole and steroids for 4+ week, and/or surgical removal of the cyst. Intraventricular disease often requires surgical therapy, as the ball-valve effect of the cyst within the ventricular system can cause acute hydrocephalus and death. The role of antiparasitic and anti-inflammatory treatment in these patients is unclear. In both subarachnoid and ventricular NCC, hydrocephalus necessitating placement of a ventricular shunt may occur. Unfortunately, these shunts often become obstructed. There is limited evidence that antiparasitic therapy decreases the risk of shunt complications. Clearly, except for patients with single lesions, the treatment decisions for NCC are complicated and neurologic, infectious disease, and neurosurgical consultations are appropriate.

Trichinosis, acute infection with *Trichinella spiralis*, is acquired by ingestion of undercooked pork, bear, or walrus. A difficult diagnosis in isolated cases, trichinosis presents as a febrile illness with gastrointestinal symptoms beginning 1–2 days after ingestion. Periorbital edema and subconjunctival hemorrhages often accompany muscle invasion. Altered mental status and seizures suggest cerebral involvement, which occurs in about 10% of cases. Treatment consists of steroids and thiabendazole.

Other helminths cause meningoencephalitis, including schistosomiasis, particularly *Schistosoma japonicum* in Asia, and paragonimiasis, the lung fluke found in Central and South America, southeast Asia, and Africa. *Angiostrongylus cantonensis*, the rat lungworm endemic to the tropical Pacific, including Hawaii and southeast Asia, may cause eosinophilic meningitis, the differential diagnosis of which also includes other parasites, coccidiomycosis, tuberculosis, foreign bodies, drug-induced meningitis, and neoplasm. Treatment is supportive, although steroids may shorten the durations of symptoms. Prognosis for spontaneous recovery is excellent.

Several protozoa cause cerebral infection. Most common is cerebral toxoplasmosis, discussed later in the section on HIV/AIDS. Cerebral malaria results from sludging in small vessels in the brain during severe *Plasmodium falciparum* infection. Mortality exceeds 15%. Aggressive antimalarial therapy may be beneficial, but steroids may be harmful. African sleeping sickness is a chronic meningoencephalitis due to *Trypanosoma brucei*. *Entamoeba histolytica* rarely causes cerebral amebiasis or brain abscess, and should be considered in patients with a history of amebiasis and focal findings or isolated brain abscess on neuroimaging. Most commonly, it is associated with other extraintestinal amebic disease (liver or lung abscess.) Primary amebic meningoencephalitis may occur acutely due to *Naegleria fowleri*, and recent freshwater exposure is a key risk factor. The diagnosis can be made by visualization of ameba on a fresh CSF wet prep or by PCR. Granulomatous amebic encephalitis is caused by *Acanthamoeba spp.* (immunocompromised hosts) or *Balamuthia mandrallis* (immunocompetent and immunocompromised hosts) and generally follows a more indolent course. Diagnosis is made by finding organisms on brain biopsy or rarely in CSF wet prep, or, from tissue, culturing the organisms or isolating the DNA by PCR.

Shingles and Postherpetic Neuralgia

Herpes zoster, or shingles, classically presents with paresthesias and pain in a cranial or spinal dermatome, sometimes preceded by a viral prodrome and usually followed by vesicular lesions in the affected dermatome. The incidence increases with age, coincident with declining cell-mediated immunity to varicella zoster virus (VZV). Despite evidence that the VZV vaccine decreased the incidence of zoster and postherpetic neuralgia (PHN) by 50%, few elderly patients receive appropriate zoster vaccination.

Postherpetic neuralgia, persistent neuropathic pain in the affected dermatome, is a feared complication whose frequency and severity also increase with age. Antiviral therapy started within 72 hours of the appearance of the rash decreases acute pain, although it remains unclear whether it, with or without concomitant steroid therapy, decreases risk or severity of PHN. The thrice-daily dosing of famciclovir or valacyclovir is an advantage over oral acyclovir, which must be taken five times per day. Ophthalmologic consultation should be obtained in patients with shingles affecting the trigeminal nerve, to preserve vision. For PHN, tricyclic antidepressants, the antiepileptic drugs gabapentin and pregabalin, topical capsaicin, and lidocaine patches are treatment options. Some patients require chronic opiate therapy.

Other Viruses

Human T-lymphotropic virus type I (HTLV-I), a retrovirus endemic to the Caribbean, South America, and Japan, causes tropical spastic paraparesis (TSP), a progressive myeloneuropathy, and leukemia, although rarely do both disorders coexist in the same patient. Related to HIV, HTLV-I shares a similar transmission pattern, specifically sexual contact, breast milk, IV drug use, and transfusion. Patients develop back and radicular pain with dysesthesias, sphincter dysfunction, and spastic paraparesis, evolving over months to years. HTLV-I antibodies may be detected in blood and CSF. Routine CSF studies typically show elevated protein, normal glucose, and mild lymphocytic pleocytosis. For the patient from an endemic area with a progressive myelopathy or myeloneuropathy, the differential diagnosis should include TSP, along with B_{12} deficiency, neurosyphilis, demyelinating disease, and compressive cauda equina or conus medullaris syndrome. Steroids may yield short-term improvement, although treatment remains largely symptomatic and supportive.

Poliomyelitis presents as an acute febrile illness typically with meningeal symptoms, followed within days by asymmetric flaccid paralysis that may be severe enough to compromise respiration. Although classically an epidemic disease of childhood, poliomyelitis can be sporadic or develop in adults. Poliovirus, an enterovirus, multiplies in gut lymphoid tissue, causing viremia. In 1–2% of patients, the infection spreads to neural tissue, where its predilection for motor neurons causes poliomyelitis. Lumbar puncture reveals elevated CSF pressure and protein in addition to pleocytosis, typically polymorphonuclear early, but shifting to lymphocytic within several days. Recovering virus from throat washings, blood, stool or, occasionally, CSF, confirms the diagnosis. Vaccination programs have nearly eradicated the disease in the United States, but the disease may develop in nonimmunized individuals. With no specific antiviral therapy available, treatment consists of aggressive supportive care with particular attention to respiratory status. The acute febrile presentation and active CSF usually distinguish poliomyelitis from other causes of acute generalized weakness, such as GBS, myasthenic crisis, botulism, diphtheritic polyneuropathy, and tick paralysis. Postpolio syndrome develops in some polio survivors, characterized by subacute muscular weakness and atrophy developing subacutely 15–30 years after the acute illness. Physical therapy helps preserve function. Of note, both West Nile Virus and enterovirus 71 can cause polio-like myelitis syndromes.

Immunocompromised Patients

Nervous system infections in immunocompromised patients differ significantly from those occurring in immunologically normal individuals. Subtle clinical presentations and unusual pathogens cause diagnostic confusion, particularly in a patient whose medical situation is already complex. Understanding specific clinical syndromes and the specific type of immunosuppression allows clinicians to maintain the high index of suspicion required to recognize and successfully manage these potentially disabling or fatal, yet frequently treatable, disorders.

Human Immunodeficiency Virus/Acquired Immune Deficiency Syndrome

HIV infection is a common context in which health care providers encounter immunosuppressed patients. Prior to the widespread use of potent combination antiretroviral therapy (ART), neurologic disease was evident clinically in about half of HIV-infected patients and present neuropathologically in nearly all. ART can suppress HIV replication, assessed clinically by viral load testing, to undetectable levels in plasma, often leading to improved immune function, monitored by CD4 count. ART has led to dramatic declines in AIDS-related opportunistic infections (OIs) and deaths, including those affecting the nervous system, such as cerebral toxoplasmosis, progressive multifocal leukoencephalopathy (PML), and cryptococcal meningitis. The same is true for HIV-related neoplasms, both extraneural (Kaposi sarcoma) and cerebral (primary CNS lymphoma). In the ART era, primary HIV-related neurologic disorders, such as HIV-related dementia, appear to be less common, and also less relentlessly progressive than before effective antiretroviral therapy. Distal symmetric polyneuropathy (DSP) can also be a primary HIV-related condition or a complication of antiretroviral drugs, in particular, the "d-drug" nucleosides didanosine (ddI), dideoxycytidine (ddC), and stavudine (d4T). These toxic neuropathies are a manifestation of nucleoside mitochondrial toxicity, which can also cause acute generalized weakness with lactic acidosis. Zidovudine (ZDV) causes mitochondrial myopathy, and can resemble inflammatory myopathies, which also occasionally complicate HIV infection. Finally, atypical inflammatory reactions in the first several months of ART can lead to the development of autoimmune disorders or unusual manifestation of infections. These so-called *immune reconstitution syndromes* sometimes affect the nervous system.

The approach to the HIV-infected patient with signs or symptoms of nervous system dysfunction requires assessment of immune and virologic status and definition of the neurologic syndrome. Immune function is defined by CD4 count—the lower the value, the greater the risk of serious neurologic disease. At CD4 counts less than 200/mm³, patients are at particular risk for the major cerebral OIs (toxoplasmosis, PML, and cryptococcal meningitis), primary CNS lymphoma, and the primary HIV-related syndromes (dementia, myelopathy, and neuropathy). ART can lead to substantial increases in CD4 count, raising the question of whether the most recent value or the lowest (nadir) CD4 count is more important. Recent CD4 count may be more relevant if viral load is fully suppressed and both parameters have been stable for 6 months or more. In patients with detectable or rising viral loads, it is prudent to use nadir CD4 count in evaluating the patient. The same is true when neurologic symptoms or signs develop in the first few months of ART. In addition, the immune reconstitution inflammatory syndrome should be considered when patients develop new neurologic symptoms in the first weeks to months of ART. Major neurologic syn-

> ## Box 19.4 Neurologic complications of HIV infection: overview
>
> **Central nervous system syndromes**
> ▶ Focal brain disorders: (focal or multifocal cerebral dysfunction prominent)
>   – Cerebral toxoplasmosis
>   – Primary central nervous system lymphoma
>   – Progressive multifocal leukoencephalopathy
>   – Other causes: stroke, brain abscess (bacterial, fungal, parasitic), syphilitic gumma
> ▶ Diffuse cerebral disorders: (focal signs and symptoms occur rarely)
>   – HIV-related: AIDS dementia complex
>   – Other causes: cytomegalovirus (CMV), varicella zoster virus (VZV), metabolic encephalopathy
> ▶ Meningitis: (altered mentation may overshadow meningeal signs)
>   – HIV-related: aseptic meningitis, recurrent meningitis, chronic meningitis
>   – *Cryptococcus neoformans*
>   – Other causes: syphilis, *Coccidioides*, *Histoplasma*, tuberculosis
> ▶ Myelopathy:
>   – HIV-related myelopathy
>   – Other viruses: VZV, herpes simplex virus, CMV, HTLV-I
>   – Compressive lesions: lymphoma, fungi, *Toxoplasma*
>
> **Neuromuscular syndromes**
> ▶ Peripheral neuropathy:
>   – Demyelinating neuropathies: acute or chronic
>   – Nucleoside neuropathy: ddl, ddC, d4T
>   – AIDS neuropathy
>   – CMV polyradiculitis
> ▶ Myopathy:
>   – HIV-associated inflammatory myopathy
>   – Zidovudine (ZDV) myopathy

dromes (Box 19.4) include focal versus diffuse cerebral brain dysfunction, meningitis, myelopathy, peripheral neuropathy, and myopathy.

Therapy may involve specific antibiotic therapy, such as pyrimethamine, sulfadiazine, and folinic acid for toxoplasmosis or antifungal agents for cryptococcal meningitis. Before ART, chronic suppressive therapy was mandatory to prevent relapse. Patients who develop these infections while not on antiretroviral drugs may be candidates for stopping chronic suppressive therapy if they achieve stable CD4 counts over $200/mm^3$ with full viral load suppression for at least 6 months on ART. Suppressive therapy should be resumed if CD4 count falls again. Other interventions include optimizing ART and managing pain, seizures, or increased ICP. Many drugs, including anticonvulsant agents, interact with ART. Interactions that decrease the efficacy of ART can cause regimen failure and viral resistance. Care in prescribing is critical in patients on ART.

Focal brain disorders typically complicate advanced (CD4 $<200/mm^3$) HIV disease, with toxoplasmosis, primary CNS lymphoma, and PML the most common diagnoses. Cerebral toxoplasmosis, caused by the parasite *Toxoplasma gondii*, has become less common because of ART, and because some antibiotics prescribed as prophylaxis for *Pneumocystis jiroveci* pneumonia also provide excellent primary prophylaxis for toxoplasmosis. Fever, headache, altered mentation, and focal cerebral dysfunction, evolving over days to weeks, are typical presenting features. Computed tomography (or MRI) with and without contrast shows ring-enhancing lesions, multiple in over 70% of cases, with a predilection for the basal ganglia and gray–white junctions (Figure 19.2). Serum toxoplasma IgG titers are usually positive. They do not establish the diagnosis, but negative titers should prompt early consideration of alternative etiologies. Most commonly, the diagnosis is made by clinical and radiologic improvement during a therapeutic trial of pyrimethamine and sulfadiazine, with concurrent folinic acid to help prevent bone marrow suppression from pyrimethamine. Clindamycin may be given as a second-line agent in sulfa-allergic patients or if drug toxicity occurs with first-line therapy. Regression of lesions by repeat neuroimaging study after 10–14 days of therapy, when accompanied by clinical improvement, may be taken as empiric evidence of cerebral toxoplasmosis. Response to therapy can be difficult to interpret in the patient treated with other antibiotics and steroids, as occurs when there is concern for increased ICP at presentation. Steroids alone can yield marked clinical and radiologic improvement of many cerebral mass lesions. Secondary prophylaxis should be continued until patients have a greater than 6-month history of a CD4 $>200/mm^3$.

Primary CNS lymphoma presents with headache, altered mentation, and focal cerebral dysfunction evolving over weeks or months. Computed tomography (or MRI) with and without contrast shows one or more homogeneously enhancing mass lesions, often favoring periventricular regions or corpus callosum. Solitary lesions are more common, but multifocal lesions can occur. Toxoplasmosis and primary CNS lymphoma thus share many clinical and radiologic features, with primary CNS lymphoma more likely in patients with negative toxoplasma IgG, on chronic trimethoprim/sulfamethoxazole as PCP prophylaxis, or when both patient and repeat scan progress despite empiric antitoxoplasma therapy. Biopsy tissue reveals high-grade B-cell lymphoma. Tumor cells frequently show evidence of EBV infection. If LP can be safely done, CSF cytology will occasionally establish the diagnosis, obviating the

A

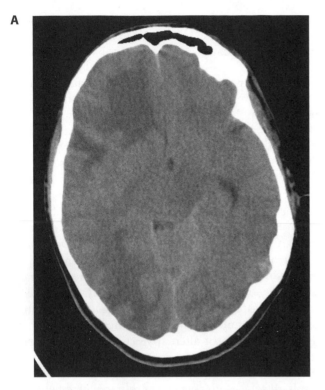

B

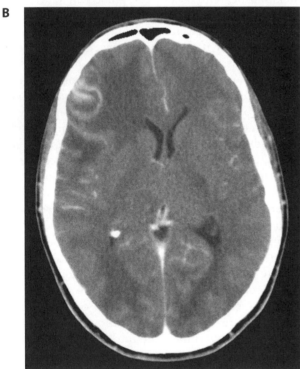

Figure 19.2 Cerebral toxoplasmosis: Noncontrast (A) and contrast (B) head computed tomography images from an AIDS patient with fever, progressive headache, photophobia, nausea, vomiting, and lethargy show edema, mass effect, and multiple ring-enhancing lesions consistent with cerebral toxoplasmosis. Toxoplasma immunoglobulin (IgG) was positive, and the patient improved clinically and radiographically with empiric anti-*Toxoplasma* therapy. Courtesy of Anita Koshy, Stanford University.

need for biopsy. Cerebrospinal fluid EBV PCR appears more specific than sensitive for the diagnosis of primary CNS lymphoma, but is not routinely available. Before ART, prognosis was about a month without therapy and several months with steroids and radiotherapy. Prognosis has improved in the ART era, particularly in patients who develop primary CNS lymphoma while not on antiretroviral therapy. Starting ART (or optimizing it in patients already on treatment) may be a reasonable adjunct to steroids and chemotherapy or radiation in patients with primary CNS lymphoma.

Progressive multifocal leukoencephalopathy typically manifests as focal cerebral dysfunction progressing over weeks to months, without fever or headache. Reactivated JC virus infection of oligodendroglia leads to the characteristic demyelinative lesions of PML. Neuroimaging studies, particularly MRI, show nonenhancing white matter lesions, without mass effect, in contrast to the enhancing lesions, frequently surrounded by edema, characteristic of toxoplasmosis and lymphoma. Before ART, PML was often fatal within several months. In the ART era, about half of patients survive a year or more, and sustained remissions may occur in untreated patients placed on ART.

The question of whether to perform brain biopsy arises when a course of empiric antitoxoplasma therapy has failed, or less frequently, when broad-spectrum antibiotic coverage, steroids, or both were required during initial management. Both hemorrhagic and ischemic strokes may cause focal brain dysfunction in HIV-infected patients. Clinical course and radiologic findings usually allow stroke to be diagnosed securely. Other, less frequent causes of cerebral mass lesion reported in HIV infection include bacterial brain abscess, granulomatous amebic encephalitis, cryptococcoma, tuberculoma, *Nocardia*, *Aspergillus*, *Candida*, *Mucor*, Chagas disease, and syphilitic gumma. The decision to proceed with a brain biopsy to look for these and even rarer brain lesions should be made in consultation with infectious disease, neurology, and neurosurgery departments.

Diffuse cerebral disorders have a broad differential diagnosis, including medication side effects and metabolic disturbances. In patients with mid- to late-stage HIV disease and cognitive impairment, HIV-associated neurocognitive disorders, typically begin with apathy and social withdrawal that resembles depression. In the pre-ART era, the disease often progressed relentlessly over months, with memory impairment and motor slowing, usually accompanied by hyperreflexia and Babinski signs. Occasional patients present with delirium or psychosis. Focal findings, such as aphasia, hemianopsia, or hemiparesis are unusual, and should prompt consideration of an alternative diagnosis. Patients with advanced dementia are mute, spastic, incontinent, and bed-bound. Evaluation is geared toward identifying treatable causes of cognitive impairment, such as thyroid disease, B_{12} deficiency, neurosyphilis, neurologic opportunistic infections (cryptococcal meningitis and as discussed above), or CNS lymphoma. Pre- and postcontrast neuroimaging shows atrophy and sometimes ill-defined, nonenhancing white matter lesions, better demonstrated by MRI than by CT, which correlate with demyelination seen pathologically. The CSF shows nonspecific HIV-related changes of normal or elevated protein and moderate lymphocytic pleocytosis. ZDV at doses higher (1,200–1,500 daily) than currently used has been shown to arrest disease, at least transiently. With widespread use of ART, cognitive impairment is less common, and its course more indolent and with less motor involvement.

Cytomegalovirus encephalitis may cause acute or subacute cerebral dysfunction, typically in the severely immunocompromised patient with a CD4 count of less than 50/mm³. Brainstem symptoms and signs and neuroimaging studies showing periventricular enhancement are clues to the diagnosis. Evidence of systemic CMV infection, such as retinitis or positive urine or blood cultures, may suggest, but does not necessarily establish, the diagnosis. Polymerase chain reaction for CMV nucleic acids in CSF confirms the diagnosis, although the sensitivity is unknown. Ganciclovir and foscarnet, individually or in combination, have been used with some success. Cidofovir is another option, although there is less experience with this agent for CMV encephalitis.

Meningitis, typically aseptic or chronic, may occur throughout the course of HIV infection. Particularly in advanced disease, manifestations of meningeal inflammation such as headache, neck stiffness, and photophobia may be subtle or absent, and hence diffuse cerebral dysfunction may be the predominant clinical picture. Acute aseptic meningitis occasionally accompanies HIV seroconversion, commonly called acute retroviral syndrome, or may occur during early HIV infection, possibly representing viral entry into the CNS. Recurrent aseptic meningitis may also occur. More commonly, mild to moderate lymphocytic pleocytosis and protein elevation in CSF occur without meningeal symptoms or signs. Low CSF glucose, protein exceeding 100/dL, or pleocytosis greater than 50 cells/mm³ should prompt a continued search for a cause other than HIV.

In advanced HIV infection, meningitis may present with cognitive impairment, personality change, or cranial neuropathy, without significant headache, fever, or meningeal signs. *Cryptococcus neoformans* is an important consideration in such patients, particularly when the CD4 count falls below 200/mm³. Although CSF may show the expected profile of elevated protein, low glucose, and lymphocytic pleocytosis, these changes may be mild enough to fall into the range attributable to HIV infection alone. India ink smear will reveal *Cryptococcus* in many cases. Better still is CSF cryptococcal antigen, which is

over 90% sensitive when compared to fungal cultures, which may take weeks to grow. Most patients begin therapy with daily amphotericin B, switching to fluconazole for maintenance. Fluconazole may be used as primary therapy, although many practitioners initiate therapy with amphotericin B, particularly in the acutely ill patient. Depressed level of consciousness and increased ICP are worrisome prognostic markers. Neurologic and neurosurgical consultation should be obtained if the initial CSF examination reveals elevated ICP, since serial LPs and other interventions may be necessary. Relapse risk is high, and chronic suppressive therapy is usually necessary. Patients who develop cryptococcal meningitis in the first months of ART may experience prominent meningismus, as an immune reconstitution event. Longer term, if the CD4 count rises above 100–200/mm³ with fully suppressed viral load for 6 months or more, consideration may be given to stopping secondary prophylaxis with fluconazole.

Meningeal lymphomatosis, due to either known systemic lymphoma or as a presenting manifestation, also causes meningitis in late-stage HIV infection. Cerebrospinal fluid cytology, ideally from high-volume and sometimes repeated LPs, establishes the diagnosis. Other causes of meningitis occurring throughout the course of HIV infection include neurosyphilis, *Coccidioides*, *Histoplasma*, and *M. tuberculosis*. The abnormal CSF profile and immune response caused by HIV itself can make these infections difficult to diagnose.

Subacute spinal cord dysfunction in HIV-infected patients may indicate AIDS myelopathy. Sometimes coexisting with dementia and neuropathy, this disorder of advanced HIV infection manifests as gait difficulty with prominent sphincter dysfunction progressing over weeks to months. Examination demonstrates spastic paraparesis, hyperreflexia especially in the legs, and Babinski signs. Sensation is also usually impaired, although a definite sensory level is uncommon. Arms are usually spared until late in the course. Pathologic findings resemble those of subacute combined system degeneration, although serum B_{12} determination is usually normal. Suspected, but not proven, to be directly related to HIV itself, myelopathy does not appear to improve with antiretroviral therapy. Rehabilitation with attention to range of motion, mobility, and bladder and bowel care can help prevent contractures, decubiti, urosepsis, and fecal impaction. Other, less common and usually more acute causes of myelopathy in HIV infection include herpes virus infections such as CMV, HSV, and VZV; compressive lesions due to bacterial spinal osteomyelitis or epidural abscess in patients with IV drug use; lymphoma; TB; and fungal infection. Concomitant HTLV-I infection can cause chronic progressive myeloneuropathy.

Various peripheral neuropathies complicate HIV infection. The inflammatory demyelinating neuropathies (IDPs) occasionally develop in early HIV disease, possibly from the immune dysregulation that precedes the frank immunosuppression of later HIV infection. Whether acute (known also as AIDP or GBS) or chronic (CIDP), the IDPs that develop during HIV infection resemble in most aspects those seen in seronegative patients. A monophasic illness, GBS presents as cranial and limb numbness and weakness, over days to weeks. Sensory complaints and motor signs, particularly weakness and depressed or absent reflexes, are prominent. Weakness may be severe enough to cause respiratory failure. In contrast, sensory and motor symptoms in CIDP fluctuate, and significant respiratory muscle weakness is rare. Whether acute or chronic, markedly elevated CSF protein without pleocytosis (so-called albuminocytologic dissociation), the classic CSF profile of seronegative IDPs, is less typical in HIV-positive patients, in whom both protein and cell counts may be elevated. Indeed, a diagnosis of an IDP should prompt an inquiry into HIV risk factors, and an IDP with CSF pleocytosis warrants consideration of HIV testing. Management for seronegative and seropositive patients is similar: plasmapheresis or γ-globulin accompanied by close monitoring of respiratory status for GBS and steroids or γ-globulin for CIDP.

Acute generalized weakness, resembling GBS, has been reported in association with lactic acidosis in patients on ART. Recognizing this unusual syndrome is important, because stopping antiretroviral therapy can be life-saving.

Other neuropathic syndromes complicate later HIV infection. Distal symmetric polyneuropathy complicates mid- to late-stage HIV infection. This axonal neuropathy often begins as foot pain, typically most bothersome at night. Hands are often spared. Examination shows depressed or absent ankle jerks, with distal sensory loss. Despite the lack of motor involvement, DSP can be disabling, because of severe pain. The clinical syndrome is usually distinctive enough so that electrophysiologic studies and LP are not required. Other causes of axonal neuropathy, such as diabetes and alcoholism, should be considered. Neurotoxic drugs commonly used to manage HIV infection or its complications include the nucleoside antiretrovirals ddI, ddC, and d4T (discussion follows) as well as isoniazid, dapsone, metronidazole, hydroxyurea, and vincristine. There is no specific therapy for DSP and no U.S. Food and Drug Administration (FDA)-approved drugs for symptomatic management. Neurotoxic exposures should be minimized as much as possible. Careful consideration should be given to drug–drug interactions, in particular with components of ART, in managing neuropathic pain. Symptomatic therapy includes tricyclic antidepressants, gabapentin, pregabalin, NSAIDs, topical capsaicin, or transcutaneous electrical nerve stimulation (TENS) units, often in combination. Chronic narcotic therapy may be necessary, and referral to a multidisciplinary pain management center is appropriate in selected patients.

Nucleoside neuropathy, mediated by mitochondrial dysfunction, is a reversible axonal neuropathy, associated with the "d-drug" antiretroviral, ddI, ddC, and d4T. A major dose-limiting toxicity of these agents, its clinical features closely resemble HIV-related DSP. The pace of symptoms can help distinguish DSP from nucleoside neuropathy, the former typically evolving over months and sometimes years, and the latter occasionally escalating more rapidly, over weeks. A curious phenomenon of the nucleoside neuropathies is "coasting," in which discontinuing the drug leads to transient worsening of symptoms for as long as 1–2 months before more sustained improvement. Since nucleoside neurotoxicity is dose-related, some patients may tolerate reinstitution of therapy at a lower dose. Alternatively, a different antiretroviral nucleoside may be used, but cross-neurotoxicity among these agents has been noted. Another common clinical problem is whether to use neurotoxic antiretrovirals in patients with preexisting DSP. Decisions should be individualized depending on the severity of DSP and HIV treatment history. Patients taking "d-drugs" should be monitored for development of neuropathic signs and symptoms.

A less common, but clinically distinct and fatal if untreated, neuropathic syndrome of very late-stage HIV infection (usually CD4 <50/mm³) is CMV polyradiculitis. Patients present with leg weakness and prominent sphincter dysfunction, usually over several weeks. The disorder thus resembles AIDS myelopathy. However, instead of the spasticity, hyperreflexia, and Babinski signs that accompany weakness in AIDS myelopathy, lower motor neuron signs predominate in CMV polyradiculitis. Hence, tone is normal or decreased, reflexes decreased or absent, and toes silent or downgoing. This cauda equina syndrome frequently prompts MRI imaging of the lumbosacral spine, which may be normal or show nerve root enhancement. The CSF profile is unusual and distinctive: elevated protein, normally or mildly decreased glucose, and polymorphonuclear pleocytosis. Polymerase chain reaction in CSF for CMV nucleic acids can confirm the diagnosis. Untreated, the disorder is fatal within weeks to months. Ganciclovir or foscarnet, alone, or in combination, can be life-saving. If therapy begins early in the course, before nerve root necrosis occurs, neurologic function stabilizes and improves quickly. Neurologic recovery occurs much more slowly once radicular necrosis has developed. Differential diagnosis includes neurosyphilis and lymphomatous radiculitis. In both conditions, CSF pleocytosis tends to be lymphocytic rather than polymorphonuclear. Serum and CSF syphilis serologies and CSF cytology can confirm these diagnoses.

Muscle disease can be difficult to diagnose in HIV infection, particularly in advanced disease when weakness may be attributed to systemic illness. HIV-associated inflammatory myopathy (HIV-IM) resembles polymyositis, both clinically and pathologically. Proximal weakness develops subacutely, manifest as difficulty climbing stairs or rising from chairs. Creatine kinase (CK) is usually elevated, and EMG shows mixed myopathic and neurogenic features. This disorder is unusual among HIV-associated neurologic conditions in that it may occur at any stage of HIV infection, including in asymptomatic individuals. Muscle biopsy reveals myopathic changes, with endomysial inflammation. HIV-IM may be mild and nonprogressive. When weakness is functionally limiting, steroids can improve strength and normalize CK. The potential need for chronic steroid therapy can be problematic in an already immunosuppressed host. γ-Globulin may be used, although its efficacy is better established in seronegative dermatomyositis and polymyositis than in HIV-IM. Whatever therapy is used, it should be titrated to strength and functional status, rather than to CK in isolation.

In patients taking ZDV for more than 6 months, proximal weakness may be due to HIV-IM or ZDV myopathy, a toxic mitochondrial disorder. The CK may be normal or elevated. Although clinically similar, muscle biopsy can distinguish these disorders. Alternatively, clinical response to medication holiday or dose reduction may be monitored.

Although most of the neurologic disorders related to HIV/AIDS have declined with the use of ART, it should be noted that cognitive impairment and most CNS OIs have been noted to occur in treated patients with CD4 of over 500 mm³, suggesting that even in the face of what is generally considered to be an acceptable response by CD4 criteria, immune function may continue to be significantly impaired.

Transplant Recipients

With increasing numbers of solid organ transplants (SOT) and hematopoietic stem cell transplants (HSCT), more patients are at risk for infectious and noninfectious neurologic complications of transplantation. The risk of infectious complications is proportional to the intensity of immunosuppression, hence patients who have required additional therapeutic immunosuppression to manage host-versus-graft disease in SOT or graft-versus-host disease in HSCT are at especially high risk. Although transplant recipients and HIV/AIDS patients are both immunosuppressed, key differences exist between the two groups. Transplant patients generally are under close medical supervision when immunosuppression begins, receive early and timely prophylaxis for fungal and viral infections, and the intensity of immunosuppression, as well as the type of cell types affected, is limited as much as possible. In HIV/AIDS, CD4 count serves as a useful and simple guide to the degree of immune compromise and likely infectious complications. In transplant recipients, the immunosuppressant regimen, cell counts, and time from

---

▼

Pearls and Perils

Neurologic complications of HIV infection

▶ Central and peripheral nervous system disorders develop commonly during HIV infection, due to complications of immunosuppression, neurotropic properties of the virus, and consequences of therapy and systemic illness.

▶ HIV infection may present as neurologic disease, and should be considered in the differential diagnosis of aseptic and chronic meningitis, atypical dementia, focal or multifocal cerebral mass lesions, subacute myelopathy, demyelinating or axonal neuropathies, and polymyositis.

▶ The stage-specific nature of many HIV-related neurologic conditions makes a recent CD4 count a useful diagnostic tool. The risk for serious neurologic disease increases as CD4 count falls.

▶ As in other immunocompromised states, a high index of suspicion facilitates early diagnosis of HIV-related neurologic infections.

▶ Many HIV-related neurologic infections require chronic suppressive therapy to prevent relapse. In patients with sustained virologic and immunologic response to highly active antiretroviral therapy, suppressive therapy can sometimes be discontinued. It should be restarted if CD4 count falls and remains persistently low.

---

transplant influence the differential diagnosis. In both groups, current or recent antibiotic prophylaxis influences the spectrum of likely pathogens. For transplant recipients, discontinuing prophylaxis has made some infectious complications previously characteristic of the early post-transplant period serious diagnostic considerations in later posttransplant periods. In both groups, the clinical approach depends on defining the neurologic syndrome and assessing the degree of immunosuppression.

A common clinical feature of neurologic disease in transplant recipients and HIV-infected patients is subtle signs and symptoms, particularly compared to the immunocompetent host. Headache and minor cognitive or focal cerebral symptoms should be monitored closely, with a low threshold for diagnostic evaluation, even in the afebrile patient. Often, CNS infections occur as part of disseminated disease. Hence, a careful search for an extraneural focus of infection, in particular in lungs, sinuses, and skin, is important. Important meningitis or meningoencephalitis pathogens in both SOT and HSCT patients include *Listeria*, *Cryptococcus*, *M. tuberculosis*, human herpes virus-6, and VZV. In addition, OKT3 monoclonal antibody and γ-globulin therapy can cause aseptic meningitis. When the clinical picture is that of a focal brain lesion, *Aspergillus*, *Nocardia*, *Toxoplasma*, post transplant lymphoproliferative disorder and primary CNS lymphoma should be considered. The ordering of these diagnoses can depend on whether the clinical setting is SOT or HSCT, and as stated previously, how far out the patient is from the transplant. Ideally, rather than the trial of empiric antitoxoplasma therapy often pursued in HIV-infected patients, definitive diagnosis by biopsy of an extraneural site or the CNS should be considered early in the diagnostic evaluation. Unfortunately, especially in HSCT patients who have a number of blood dyscrasias during their transplant, including severe thrombocytopenia, definitive diagnosis is often not possible, and broad empiric coverage and close monitoring of clinical status and neuroimaging findings and CSF results are sometimes required.

For reasons poorly understood, infections with *Listeria*, *Nocardia*, and *Aspergillus* occur more frequently in transplant recipients than in HIV-infected patients. Patients with lymphoma, particularly Hodgkin disease, and individuals on chronic steroids develop neurologic complications similar to those seen in transplant recipients.

Other Immunosuppressed States

Defective granulocyte function develops during chemotherapy or in aplastic anemia, particularly when absolute neutrophil count is less than 500/mm^3. Important meningitis pathogens include gram-negative bacilli, *S. aureus*, and pneumococcus. *Candida*, *Aspergillus*, and *Mucor* are important causes of focal brain lesions in such patients. In addition, immunomodulatory therapy is being used more often for autoimmune diseases such as multiple sclerosis and rheumatoid arthritis, potentially placing these groups at risk for unusual opportunistic infections.

Impaired humoral immunity and B-cell dysfunction occurs with congenital immune deficiencies, as well as in

chronic lymphocytic leukemia, myeloma, and post-splenectomy, including sickle cell anemia. Such patients are at particular risk for infection with encapsulated bacteria such as pneumococcus, *H. influenza* type B, and meningococcus.

Summary

The immune system and multiple anatomic barriers protect the nervous system from infectious agents. When organisms develop strategies to evade host defenses, or when host defenses are impaired, a neurologic infection may develop. Diagnosis begins with classic neuroanatomic localization and rapid assessment of the host–pathogen relationship. Occasionally, a specific causative organism may be identified at presentation. More frequently, however, initial evaluation generates a list of potential pathogens. Because the outcome for most infections of the nervous system depends so heavily on instituting treatment early, initial therapy is frequently empiric and subject to modification as the diagnostic evaluation continues. Elderly or immunocompromised patients pose particular challenges, since presentations may be subtle, without the fever, head or spine pain, or marked neurologic dysfunction that signal nervous system infection in the immunocompetent individual. Moreover, immunologic impairment significantly alters the spectrum of pathogens, which may cause a particular neuroinfectious syndrome. Rapid, accurate diagnosis for all infections of the nervous system depends on intelligent use of neuroimaging studies and of microbiologic and serologic tests, particularly of blood and CSF, supple-

---

▼

Consider Consultation When...

▶ An infectious mass lesion is suspected or proven.

▶ A central nervous system (CNS) infection is thought to result from an orbital, ear, sinus, or dental source.

▶ A CNS infection is suspected or proven in a patient with a ventricular shunt or other neurosurgical procedure or recent head trauma.

▶ A CNS infection is complicated by hydrocephalus, increased intracranial pressure, stroke, or seizure.

▶ Close neurologic monitoring, for example, in an ICU setting, is indicated.

▶ Management of the neurologic infection requires assessment and potential treatment of family members and other close contacts.

▶ The patient presenting with an infectious neurologic illness is elderly, immunosuppressed, otherwise chronically ill, or has antibiotic allergies.

▼

Pearls and Perils

Nervous system infections in the immunocompromised host

▶ Classic symptoms of neurologic infection such as fever, headache, meningismus, and marked focal deficit may not be present in immunologically impaired patients.

▶ Infection should be considered as a potential cause of acute or subacute neurologic symptoms in immunocompromised patients.

▶ Unusual pathogens, particularly fungi, atypical bacteria, and viruses, are common.

▶ The specific type of immunosuppression and time from transplant frequently define the most likely pathogens.

mented by a broad range of other tests including culture from other sites, skin testing, and biopsy of neural or other tissues. Surgical intervention, antitoxins, and hyperimmune globulins supplement aggressive supportive care and antimicrobial agents, which ideally should get into the nervous system at levels adequate to kill, rather than simply inhibit, organisms. Infectious disease, neurology, neurosurgery, neuroradiology, otolaryngology, ophthalmology, and oral surgery are among the consultants who can assist the clinician in managing these serious and complex but, frequently treatable, disorders.

Annotated Bibliography

Cohen BA. Clinical applications of new cerebrospinal fluid analytic techniques for the diagnosis and treatment of central nervous system infections. *Curr Neurol Neurosci Rep* 2001;1:518–25.
Review covering CSF testing beyond protein, glucose, cell counts, and cultures, with an emphasis on polymerase chain reaction testing for bacterial, viral, and parasitic CNS pathogens.

Deisenhammer F, Bartos A, Egg R, et al. Guidelines on routine cerebrospinal fluid analysis: Report from an EFNS task force. *Eur J Neurol* 2006;13:913–922.
Guideline for recommendations for CSF testing in infectious and noninfectious neurologic disorders.

Marra CM, ed. *Neurologic clinics: Central nervous system infections.* Philadelphia: WB Saunders, 1999.
Multi-authored collection of articles covers the diagnosis and management of bacterial, fungal, and viral CNS infections.

Scheld WM, Whitley RJ, Marra CM, eds. *Infections of the central nervous system,* 3rd ed. Philadelphia: Lippincott Williams & Wilkins, 2004.
Comprehensive reference is detailed and thorough, while remaining readable and practical.

Trunkel AR, Hartman BJ, Kaplan SL, et al. Practice guidelines for the management of bacterial meningitis. *Clin Infect Dis* 2004;39:1267–1284.
The guidelines to know and follow for acute bacterial meningitis.

CHAPTER 20

Demyelinating Diseases

Edward Kim, Michele K. Mass, Ruth H. Whitham, and Dennis N. Bourdette

▼

Outline

- ▶ Demyelinating diseases: definition, pathophysiology, and classification
- ▶ Monophasic/focal demyelinating disease
- ▶ Clinically isolated syndromes
- ▶ Monophasic/multifocal demyelinating disease
- ▶ Polyphasic/multifocal demyelinating disease

Demyelinating diseases of the central nervous system (CNS) are a family of related immune-mediated illnesses. Important demyelinating diseases include multiple sclerosis (MS), acute optic neuritis (AON), acute transverse myelitis (ATM), acute disseminated encephalomyelitis and its variants, and neuromyelitis optica.

Demyelinating Diseases: Definition, Pathophysiology, and Classification

Demyelinating diseases share the common feature of inflammation and destruction of CNS myelin with relative sparing of axons, referred to as *primary demyelination*. Although primary demyelination remains an important feature of demyelinating diseases, it is now recognized that axonal destruction also occurs in these disorders. In all demyelinating diseases, the inflammatory response within the CNS mediates the demyelination and axonal injury. The inflammatory response, in which lymphocytes and macrophages typically predominate, appears directed at antigens within the myelinated tissue. The pathogenic immune targets are unknown for all of the demyelinating diseases, but they may be normal myelin proteins, such as myelin basic protein, myelin oligodendrocyte glycoprotein or proteolipid protein, or viral antigens. Since normal neural function depends on the integrity of the myelin sheaths around axons, immune-mediated destruction of myelin can result in significant neurologic dysfunction. However, considerable improvement can follow episodes of primary demyelination once the pathologic immune response abates. Following demyelination, repair processes, including remyelination and axonal ion channel remodeling, can restore neural function. Because of these repair processes, significant, even dramatic, improvement of neurologic function can occur following acute episodes of demyelination. However, when axonal destruction accompanies the lesions, repair is incomplete, as CNS axonal regeneration is largely ineffective. Permanent disability in these disorders is now believed to largely reflect axonal loss.

Despite the underlying pathologic similarity, the disease course and clinical manifestations of the demyelinating diseases vary considerably. Demyelinating diseases include acute monophasic illnesses, such as acute optic neuritis, and chronic recurrent and progressive illnesses, most notably multiple sclerosis (MS). Demyelinating diseases also may affect only one part of the CNS, as in acute transverse myelitis, or involve multiple parts of the CNS, as occurs in acute disseminated encephalomyelitis and MS. Classifications of demyelinating disease are based on the temporal pattern and anatomic localization of the disorders (Box 20.1). Since there are no diagnostic "tests" for any of the demyelinating disorders, accurate diagnosis rests on the knowledge of the physician and the appropriate use of tests to help confirm the diagnosis and exclude the presence of other disorders that can mimic the various demyelinating disorders.

▼

Box 20.1 Classification of demyelinating diseases

Monophasic/focal demyelinating diseases (Clinically isolated syndrome)
▶ Acute optic neuritis
▶ Acute transverse myelitis (complete and incomplete)
▶ Acute brainstem demyelination

Monophasic/multifocal demyelinating diseases
▶ Acute disseminated encephalomyelitis and its variants (postinfectious or parainfectious encephalomyelitis; postvaccination encephalomyelitis; rabies vaccine encephalomyelitis; measles encephalomyelitis; chicken pox encephalomyelitis)

Polyphasic/multifocal demyelinating diseases
▶ Multiple sclerosis
▶ Neuromyelitis optica

▼

Key Clinical Questions

▶ Is the temporal pattern of the demyelinating illness monophasic or polyphasic?
▶ Is the demyelination an isolated event or part of a multifocal demyelinating process?
▶ Is there evidence of neurologic dysfunction separated in time and in space?
▶ Have other disorders that might explain the patient's neurologic symptoms been excluded?

Monophasic/Focal Demyelinating Disease

Acute Optic Neuritis

Acute optic neuritis (AON) results from immune-mediated demyelination of one or both optic nerves. It may occur as an isolated event or as part of a multifocal demyelinating disease, such as MS or acute disseminated encephalomyelitis. Acute optic neuritis affects females more than males and young and middle-aged adults more than children or the elderly. The principal symptom of optic neuritis is visual loss that typically worsens over several days. Most patients complain of periorbital pain, usually with eye movement. Ophthalmologic examination discloses loss of visual acuity, which can vary from minimal to complete loss. A variety of visual field abnormalities can occur, including central or paracentral scotomas, hemianopsias, quadrantanopsias, and altitudinal defects. Color vision, as measured with Ishihara color plates, is also impaired in the majority of patients. Initially, the funduscopic examination is often normal. However, a swollen optic disc, which is often subtle, occurs in about one-third of cases. When dramatic optic disk edema is present, the AON is referred to as *acute papillitis*. Within a few weeks of onset, optic disk pallor appears in most but not all cases. Reaction of pupils to light is often abnormal, with impaired direct responses but intact consensual responses. This can be best demonstrated by performing the "swinging flashlight test," which allows comparison of the extent of direct and consensual pupillary constriction in the symptomatic eye. Magnetic resonance imaging (MRI) can demonstrate increased signal in the involved optic nerve and gadolinium enhancement. Cerebral MRI can be normal or can demonstrate white matter abnormalities, even in patients whose neurologic symptoms are only referable to their AON (Table 20.1).

Acute optic neuritis must be differentiated from other causes of acute or subacute monocular vision loss, including acute ischemic optic neuropathies, retinal artery occlusion, acute narrow angle glaucoma, retinal hemorrhage and detachment, and central serous maculopathy. Definitive diagnosis usually requires consultation with an ophthalmologist. A careful funduscopic examination and measurement of intraocular pressures will exclude most of the intraocular disorders. However, central serous maculopathy, which occurs in a similar age group and causes only subtle changes on routine funduscopic examination, can sometimes be confused with AON. Use of an Amsler grid to demonstrate the characteristic distortion of vision along with fluoroscopy allows differentiation from AON. Acute ischemic optic neuropathies (AION) result in optic disc edema with or without hemorrhages and may have associated retinal ischemia. Acute ischemic optic neuropathies tends to occur in middle-aged and elderly patients with risk factors for arteriosclerosis, and it affects

---

Table 20.1 Acute optic neuritis

Discriminating features
▶ Subacute monocular vision loss
▶ Abnormal color vision
▶ Ocular pain

Consistent features
▶ Age 20–55
▶ Central or paracentral scotoma
▶ Relative afferent pupillary defect
▶ Abnormal magnetic resonance imaging (MRI) of optic nerve

Variable features
▶ Optic disk edema
▶ Retinal venous sheathing
▶ Posterior uveitis
▶ Bilateral vision loss
▶ Abnormal brain MRI

males and females equally. The more dramatic optic nerve and retinal changes and the older population in AION generally assists in its differentiation from AON. However, AION and acute papillitis may be difficult to distinguish.

The prognosis for improvement of vision following AON is generally good. Almost all patients experience some improvement in vision. Over 50% of patients will have their vision return to normal, and less than 10% will have a poor recovery of vision (visual acuity of >20/50).

Acute optic neuritis can be the first symptom of MS. The risk of MS following AON varies widely among published series, depending in part on the length of follow-up and the characteristics of the population studied. Length of follow-up is critical. Within 2 years of developing AON, about 20% of patients with AON will have a definite diagnosis of MS. Within 10–15 years, 50% of patients will have a diagnosis of MS. Gender, MRI findings, and cerebrospinal fluid (CSF) abnormalities influence the risk of developing MS following AON. The presence of asymptomatic white matter lesions on the brain MRI is the most significant predictor of risk of subsequently developing MS. Patients with AON and a normal brain MRI have about a 20% risk of developing MS over the ensuing 5–10 years. Patients with two or more white matter lesions have a risk of 50–60% of developing MS by 10 years. Females with AON appear to be at a higher risk of developing MS than males. Cerebrospinal fluid oligoclonal IgG bands or an elevated IgG index at the time of the AON also increases the risk of MS. Thus, a female patient with CSF oligoclonal bands and an abnormal brain MRI scan may have a risk of developing MS as high as 80–90%. A male with normal CSF and MRI scan at presentation may have a risk as low as 10–20%. Unfortunately, gender, brain MRI, and CSF studies alone or together do not allow one to predict with complete certainty whether or not a given patient with AON will develop MS. Despite limitations in predicting actual MS risk, it is important for patients with AON to undergo a brain MRI to help define the risk of developing MS. Physicians should inform patients with AON about their increased risk of developing MS and advise them to seek appropriate evaluation if they develop new neurologic symptoms.

Traditionally, AON has been treated with corticosteroids. The Optic Neuritis Treatment Trial showed that a combination of methylprednisolone (1 g intravenously per day) for 3 days followed by oral prednisone (1 mg/kg/day) for 11 days resulted in faster recovery of vision but provided no significant long-term improvement of vision. Treatment with *oral* prednisone (1/kg/day) for 14 days was no more effective than placebo, and was associated with a twofold increase in the risk of recurrent attacks of optic neuritis. In addition, an extension study of the Optic Neuritis Treatment Trial suggested that the subset of patients with two or more periventricular or ovoid white matter lesions 3 mm or larger in size on cerebral MRI scan who received intravenous (IV) methylprednisolone had a reduced occurrence of MS within 2 years of the optic neuritis compared with similar patients treated with placebo. This apparent protective effect disappears after 2 years, however. As a consequence of these results, we recommend that patients with AON undergo a cerebral MRI scan. If two or more periventricular or ovoid white matter lesions 3 mm or larger are present on cerebral MRI scan, some physicians will treat acutely with a 3-day course of IV methylprednisolone with or without an oral prednisone taper. If there is no or only one lesion present, we do not always treat, unless the patient has significant eye pain or vision loss, since treatment with corticosteroids will reduce pain as well as time of recovery. We do not use low-dose oral prednisone alone. For optic neuritis patients with two or more lesions, careful consideration should also be given to early initiation of MS disease-modifying therapy because of the high risk for these patients to convert to clinically definite MS (see the section Clinically Isolated Syndrome for a discussion of potential benefits of early therapy).

Acute Transverse Myelitis

Acute transverse myelitis results from immune-mediated demyelination of the spinal cord. Like optic neuritis, ATM may occur as an isolated event or as part of a multifocal demyelinating disease, such as MS or acute disseminated encephalomyelitis. Importantly, there are two distinct clinical syndromes: complete and incomplete ATM. Complete ATM is a dramatic condition that often follows a viral illness after a 1- to 4-week interval, but may occur without an antecedent infection. Patients typically present with paralysis affecting the legs with or without arm weakness, urinary retention, and sensory abnormalities below the affected spinal cord segment. The symptoms typically evolve over hours to days. About 50% of patients will have back pain and tenderness at the level of spinal cord involvement. Fever occurs in many patients and may be secondary to an identifiable infection, such as a urinary tract infection, or may be secondary to the ATM. Some patients will present with "spinal cord shock" similar to acute spinal cord injury with a flaccid paraplegia, areflexia, and urinary retention. Incomplete ATM presents with sensory symptoms and signs referable to the thoracic or cervical spinal cord with little or no weakness. Gait imbalance and Babinski signs are variably present. Patients with cervical involvement may have a "Lhermitte's sign," which is really a symptom consisting of electric shock sensations or paresthesias that extend down the back and into the legs or arms elicited by neck flexion. Systemic signs and symptoms, such as fever, are generally absent. There are important prognostic differences between the two syndromes. Only about 15% of

Table 20.2 Acute transverse myelitis

Discriminating features

▶ Absence of compressive lesion on spinal magnetic resonance imaging (MRI)

▶ Increased signal on T2-weighted images of spinal cord with or without gadolinium enhancement on MRI scan

▶ Cerebrospinal fluid (CSF) pleocytosis

▶ Elevated IgG index and synthesis rate; CSF oligoclonal bands

Consistent features

▶ Subacute onset

▶ Signs and symptoms referable to the thoracic or cervical cord

▶ Paraparesis or quadriparesis

▶ Sensory level

▶ Back pain

Variable features

▶ Enlarged spinal cord on MRI scan

▶ Fever

▶ "Spinal cord shock" with flaccid paralysis, areflexia, and urinary retention

patients with complete ATM will subsequently develop MS, whereas 50–90% of patients with incomplete ATM will eventually develop MS (Table 20.2).

Acute transverse myelitis must be differentiated from acute spinal cord compression resulting from tumor, abscess or herniated disk, and from acute spinal cord in-

farction. Spinal imaging, usually with MRI scan, is generally necessary in cases of suspected ATM to exclude spinal cord compression. In ATM, spinal MRI may be normal or may disclose an area of increased signal on T2-weighted images with or without gadolinium enhancement (Figure 20.1). Complete ATM can present with an abrupt onset similar to that of acute spinal cord infarction. Acute spinal cord infarction should be suspected as an alternative diagnosis to ATM in patients who have the clinical picture of the anterior spinal artery syndrome. With this syndrome, resulting from occlusion of the anterior spinal artery, ischemia to the anterior two-thirds of the spinal cord occurs, resulting in weakness and light touch/pinprick sensation abnormalities below the spinal level of involvement, but with sparing of vibratory and position sense. This clinical picture is unusual in ATM and suggests acute spinal cord infarction. Dural arteriovenous fistulas can also cause ischemia of the spinal cord, which may mimic ATM and involve vibration and position sense. Abnormal blood vessels, particularly posterior to the cord, are usually apparent on the spinal MRI scan but the findings may be subtle.

Cerebrospinal fluid examination in cases of ATM may be normal or show a mild to moderate pleocytosis. In cases of complete ATM, the pleocytosis can be marked with cell counts up to 500 cells/mm^3, and may acutely include granulocytes as well as lymphocytes and monocytes. Cerebrospinal fluid IgG abnormalities, including oligoclonal bands and elevated total IgG, IgG index, and

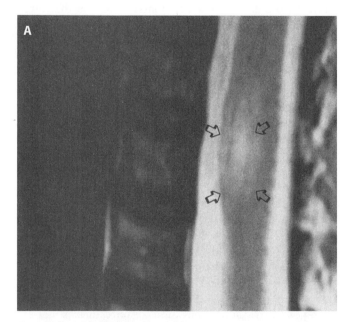
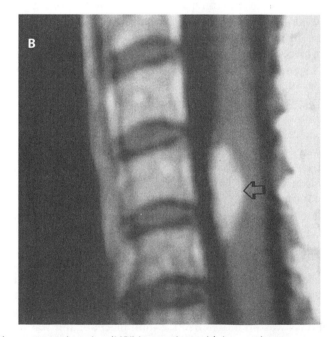

Figure 20.1 Acute transverse myelitis. A: T2-weighted spinal magnetic resonance imaging (MRI) in a patient with incomplete transverse myelitis shows enlargement of the cervical spinal cord and increased signal (*arrows*). B: T1-weighted spinal MRI in the same patient with gadolinium shows increased signal within the spinal cord at the same area as the T2 abnormality, indicating a breakdown in the blood–spinal cord barrier (*arrow*).

IgG synthesis rate, may be present and, in the case of incomplete ATM, increases the likelihood of subsequently developing MS.

Recovery from ATM is quite variable. Patients with complete ATM who present with total, flaccid paralysis often make a poor recovery, whereas those with incomplete paralysis can make significant, even complete, recovery. As mentioned previously, the risk of MS following complete ATM is low, with about 15% of patients developing MS. However, some of these patients may have neuromyelitis optica (Devic syndrome), and this possibility should be considered in patients who have contiguous spinal cord abnormalities extending over three or more vertebral segments. The risk of MS following incomplete ATM is probably similar to, if not somewhat higher than, that of AON. Patients with CSF oligoclonal bands and those with cerebral white matter lesions on MRI scan may have a risk of subsequently developing MS that approaches 90%, whereas those with normal CSF and cerebral MRI scans have a lower risk around 20%. As for optic neuritis, however, one cannot predict with certainty the actual risk of developing MS in individual cases.

Patients with ATM often are treated with corticosteroids, although there is no conclusive evidence that treatment alters the course of the illness. We generally treat patients with significant weakness with methylprednisolone (1 g/day IV for 3–5 days) without a prednisone taper. We do not treat patients with incomplete ATM with corticosteroids unless there is weakness or imbalance that significantly affects daily activities.

Acute Brainstem Syndromes

Acute demyelination of the brainstem may occur in isolation or as part of MS or acute disseminated encephalomyelitis. Although a considerable literature exists on AON and ATM, much less is published about acute demyelinating brainstem syndromes. Patients may present with a variety of symptoms referable to the brainstem, including numbness restricted to one side of the face, facial weakness, diplopia, vertigo, and imbalance. Symptoms may evolve over hours to days. Neurologic examination varies depending on the tracts of the brainstem involved. Findings may include loss of light touch and pin-prick sensation involving all divisions of the trigeminal nerve, unilateral or bilateral internuclear ophthalmoplegia, lateral rectus palsy, nystagmus, peripheral type facial weakness, gait imbalance, cerebellar tremor, and pyramidal tract signs. Usually, focal brainstem ischemia or tumor is initially suspected, and the MRI scan discloses a focal abnormality, suggesting acute demyelination (Figure 20.2). Cerebrospinal fluid examination may disclose a mild pleocytosis, oligoclonal bands, and elevated IgG index and synthesis rate, although the CSF can be normal.

Unless the demyelination is severe and extensive, pa-

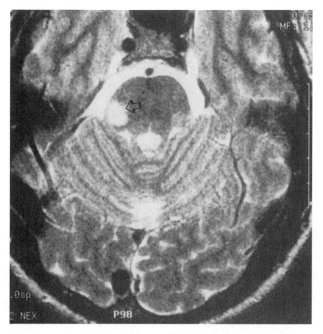

Figure 20.2 Acute brainstem demyelination. T2-weighted brain magnetic resonance imaging (MRI) in a patient presenting with acute right facial numbness and gait imbalance reveals an area of increased signal (*arrow*) in the right lateral pons.

tients generally make a good recovery following acute brainstem demyelination. The risk of MS following an initial episode of acute brainstem demyelination is similar to that of incomplete ATM. Presence of cerebral lesions on MRI and CSF IgG abnormalities increases the risk of developing MS, whereas a normal cerebral MRI scan and CSF decrease the risk.

The authors treat patients with disabling symptoms with corticosteroids as described for ATM.

Clinically Isolated Syndrome

Optic neuritis, transverse myelitis, or a demyelinating brainstem syndrome may represent an acute monophasic disease, or clinically isolated syndrome (Table 20.3). Or, each may represent the initial symptom of MS (a polyphasic demyelinating disease). One of these entities in combination with two or more periventricular or ovoid T2 abnormalities on the brain MRI puts an individual at high risk of developing clinically definite MS. For individuals at high risk for development of MS after a first demyelinating event, the onset of clinically definite disease was delayed in those receiving early initiation of MS disease-modifying therapy compared with those who received placebo. This effect was demonstrated for interferon β-1a by the CHAMPS and ETOMS trials, for interferon β-1b by the BENEFIT trial, and for glatiramer acetate by the PreCISe trial.

Treatment should be considered in patients with a clinically isolated syndrome (CIS) based on the results of the CHAMPS, ETOMS, BENEFIT, and PreCISe trials. Disease-modifying treatment should be initiated by physicians familiar with the agents available. Patients with CIS who choose not to initiate treatment should be closely monitored clinically and by MRI for disease progression. The clinician should consider a repeat MRI in 3–6 months after the first scan. If new brain lesions appear on follow-up MRI scans or the patient has a second clinical event, treatment should be readdressed, as this individual now meets McDonald criteria for definite MS (Table 20.3).

Monophasic/Multifocal Demyelinating Disease

Acute Disseminated Encephalomyelitis

Acute disseminated encephalomyelitis (ADEM) is a monophasic demyelinating disease affecting the CNS in multiple areas (Table 20.4). Acute disseminated encephalomyelitis can follow a variety of viral infections, particularly the viral exanthems of childhood. The most commonly implicated viruses are rubeola, rubella, varicella, and influenza. Acute disseminated encephalomyelitis can also follow immunizations, including those for measles, mumps, rubella, influenza, and rabies. Young children seem to be most susceptible to ADEM, probably because they are the most commonly vaccinated or infected with viruses. Acute disseminated encephalomyelitis, however, can affect any age group, and there may be no identifiable antecedent event.

Acute disseminated encephalomyelitis typically develops about 3–4 days after the onset of rash when associated with a viral exanthem or 1–4 weeks after an immunization or nonspecific viral upper respiratory infection. Acute disseminated encephalomyelitis evolves over a few hours or days and can cause headache, fever, drowsiness or even coma, seizures, and focal neurologic

---

Table 20.3 Clinically isolated syndrome

Discriminating features
▶ Absence of other diseases to explain neurological symptoms

Consistent features
▶ A clinical episode of acute optic neuritis, incomplete transverse myelitis or brainstem syndrome
▶ High risk of development of clinically definite multiple sclerosis if two or more periventricular or ovoid lesions on magnetic resonance imaging (MRI) scan

Variable features
▶ Elevated cerebrospinal fluid (CSF) IgG index and synthesis rate; CSF oligoclonal bands

---

Table 20.4 Acute disseminated encephalomyelitis

Discriminating features
▶ Monophasic illness
▶ Signs and symptoms of multifocal white matter disease of the central nervous system
▶ History of antecedent viral illness or vaccination
▶ Multiple white matter abnormalities on cerebral magnetic resonance imaging (MRI) scan
▶ Absence of other diseases to explain neurologic problems

Consistent features
▶ Optic neuritis
▶ Transverse myelitis
▶ Alteration of level of consciousness
▶ Cerebrospinal fluid (CSF) pleocytosis

Variable features
▶ Elevated CSF IgG index and synthesis rate; CSF oligoclonal bands
▶ Coma
▶ Seizures

---

abnormalities. The focal neurologic abnormalities vary, depending on the parts of the CNS involved. Patients may have signs and symptoms of optic neuritis, brainstem demyelination, and ATM. Severity is variable, with some patients having a mild, transient illness and others having a fulminant course ending in coma and death. Recovery often is complete but patients may be left with permanent neurologic sequelae. Death occurs in 5–10% of cases. Recurrent episodes of ADEM rarely occur, and typical MS generally does not occur after an episode of ADEM. However, acute MS with significant cerebral involvement can be difficult to differentiate clinically from ADEM.

Diagnosis relies on the constellation of signs and symptoms. Acute disseminated encephalomyelitis is readily diagnosed in patients with a typical clinical course following a recent vaccination or exanthematous illness, but may be more difficult to diagnose if there is no apparent antecedent exposure. In severe cases with cerebral involvement without evidence of optic neuritis or transverse myelitis, viral encephalitis and bacterial meningitis will enter into the differential diagnosis. Acute MS often is considered in adults presenting with ADEM. The simultaneous onset of disseminated signs and symptoms reflecting demyelination of the optic nerves, cerebral hemispheres, brainstem, and spinal cord is common in ADEM but rare in MS. Differentiation of acute MS from ADEM often depends either on postmortem neuropathology or on long-term follow-up of patients. Magnetic resonance imaging and CSF studies are useful in evaluating patients with suspected ADEM. Cerebral MRI scan typically reveals relatively symmetric white matter and often gray matter lesions that diffusely

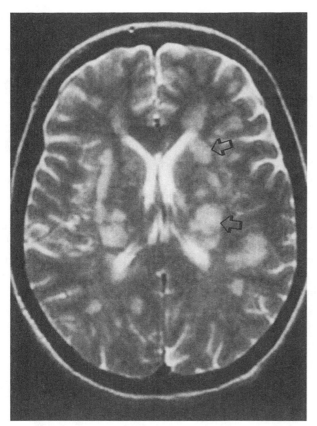

Figure 20.3 Acute disseminated encephalomyelitis. T2-weighted brain magnetic resonance imaging (MRI) in a patient with acute disseminated encephalomyelitis discloses multiple areas of increased signal involving both white and deep gray matter (*arrows*).

enhance with gadolinium (Figure 20.3). Cerebrospinal fluid examination may demonstrate a mild pleocytosis consisting principally of lymphocytes and a normal glucose and total protein. Cerebrospinal fluid IgG abnormalities (oligoclonal bands, elevated IgG index, and synthesis rate) are variably present. However, there are neither absolute MRI nor CSF criteria to definitively distinguish ADEM from an initial demyelinating attack of MS. Patients with ADEM often are treated with corticosteroids, but without good evidence that it is beneficial. We generally will treat ADEM in adults with corticosteroids as described for ATM.

Polyphasic/Multifocal Demyelinating Disease

Multiple Sclerosis

Multiple sclerosis is the most common, progressive neurologic disease of young and middle-aged adults in North America. Although the cause of MS is uncertain, considerable evidence suggests that MS is an immune-mediated disease. T lymphocytes, macrophages, inflammatory cytokines, and perhaps antimyelin antibodies all appear to participate in the multiple episodes of CNS demyelination that characterize MS. Development of the disease appears to be influenced by both genes and the environment. Although only 5% of patients with MS have a family history of the disease, clear evidence suggests that multiple genes influence susceptibility to MS. Caucasians are more susceptible to MS than other racial groups. Having a family history of MS increases the risk of MS five- to 10-fold, and identical twins have a 25% concordance rate for MS compared with a 1–2% concordance rate for nonidentical twins. Until recently, the only clear gene associated with an increased risk of MS was HLA-DR2, but it has long been believed that multiple genes modestly alter the risk of MS. A recent genomewide association study confirmed the association of MS risk with the HLA-DR2 gene. The study also identified two new genes encoding IL-2R and IL-7R-α to be associated with an increased risk of MS. Although variants in each of these genes remain a limited predictor of MS risk, their association provides evidence that multiple genes related to immune response regulation are important factors in MS. These results further reinforce the concept of MS as an autoimmune-based disease with a multifactorial risk, including heterogenous genetic predisposition. Environment also influences the risk of developing MS. In North America and Europe, MS is more prevalent in northern latitudes, suggesting an environmental influence. Epidemiologic studies also suggest that environmental exposure before the age of 15 influences the risk of MS in adulthood. The environmental factors that influence the risk of MS are uncertain but may be one or more viruses or dietary factors, such as vitamin D. Multiple sclerosis thus appears to be an immune-mediated disease induced in genetically susceptible individuals by one or more environmental exposures.

Multiple sclerosis usually begins between the ages of 20 and 55, although it can occur at any age, and it affects women more than men by a ratio of approximately 2:1. In the United States, the prevalence of MS is about 50–100/100,000. The natural history of MS is highly variable. Based upon older natural history data obtained from untreated MS patients, about 10–15% would have a benign course and never develop any permanent disability from the illness. Most patients, however, would eventually develop some permanent disability, and less than 50% of patients would remain employable 10 years after onset. One-third of patients would eventually become nonambulatory from the disease, and 5% or fewer would have a malignant course resulting in severe disability within 5–7 years of onset. The influence of early use of disease-modifying therapies on the natural history of untreated MS is uncertain. It is probable that this natural history is now improved with the introduction of MS disease-modifying therapies.

About 90% of patients with MS have a relapsing-remitting course from onset (Figure 20.4). During a relapse, the disease is active, and acute demyelination occurs. Patients may develop new neurologic signs and symptoms, recurrence of old problems, or worsening of existing problems. Symptoms typically worsen over several days to weeks, then patients begin to improve as the relapse resolves. Patients may recover completely from a relapse or be left with some residual neurologic impairment. The phase following a relapse in which the disease is relatively quiescent is the "remission." Most patients have persistent neurologic symptoms during their remissions, which may last months to years. The frequency of relapses varies but averages one every 1–2 years for the first 5–10 years of the illness. About 50% of patients who begin with relapsing-remitting MS will develop secondary-progressive MS 10-15 years after disease onset. During this phase of illness, patients progressively worsen year to year and do not have prolonged periods of stabil-

ity. Patients may continue to have relapses superimposed on their progressive course or more commonly cease to have clinical relapses. About 10% of patients have primary-progressive MS, in which they have a progressive course from onset. Occasionally, patients with primary-progressive MS will have one or more relapses later in their disease course, and these are referred to as having progressive-relapsing MS.

Signs and symptoms of MS reflect the various white matter tracts involved in the disease and vary among patients. Common signs and symptoms include decreased vision, impaired color vision and optic disc pallor from optic neuritis; diplopia, internuclear ophthalmoplegias, nystagmus, dysarthria, ataxia, tremors, and trigeminal neuralgia from brainstem and cerebellar lesions; weakness, spasticity, and pyramidal tract signs of the legs and arms, numbness, dysesthesias and impaired sensation in the extremities, Lhermitte's sign, urinary urgency and incontinence, urinary retention, sexual dysfunction, and

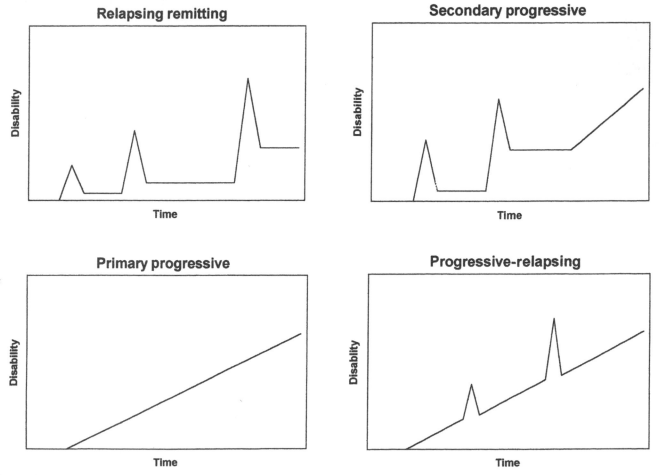

Figure 20.4 Clinical patterns of multiple sclerosis (MS). About 90% of MS patients start with a relapsing remitting course. Forty to fifty percent of patients with relapsing remitting MS will eventually enter a phase of illness called secondary-progressive MS, in which there is progressive worsening with or without superimposed relapses. Ten percent of patients never have relapses and have primary-progressive MS, in which there is continuous progression from onset. Progressive-relapsing MS affects 1–2% of patients and is characterized by an initial course like that of primary-progressive MS, with subsequent occurrence of one or more relapses.

▼

Box 20.2 Diagnostic criteria for multiple sclerosis

▶ Temporal criterion: The patient must have had at least two episodes of neurologic dysfunction consistent with a demyelinating disorder or have had a progressive course for 1 year or more.

▶ Anatomic criterion: The patient must have objective evidence of at least two anatomically separate white matter lesions within the central nervous system (CNS) demonstrated by neurologic examination, magnetic resonance imaging (MRI) scan or evoked potentials.*

▶ Exclusionary criterion: There must be no other explanation for the patient's problems.

* One objectively demonstrated lesion is permitted if the patient's cerebrospinal fluid has IgG abnormalities (elevated IgG index and synthesis rate; oligoclonal bands).

gait impairment from spinal cord lesions; and cognitive impairment and depression from cerebral hemisphere involvement. Excessive fatigue typically accompanies the illness and probably reflects the increased energy demand for conduction of action potentials along demyelinated axons. Demyelinated axons are also sensitive to ambient temperature, and patients often note that their symptoms are transiently worsened with fever, hot weather, or taking a hot shower or bath.

Multiple sclerosis is a clinical diagnosis (Box 20.2). No laboratory test or imaging study makes the diagnosis. Although criteria (McDonald et al.) have recently been revised, diagnosis continues to require a careful history, neurologic examination, and appropriate ancillary tests. The diagnosis of MS rests on the objective demonstration of CNS white matter lesions that are disseminated in time and space, for which there is no other explanation. Patients must have had two or more neurologic events separated in time or a progressive course extending over 1 year, with objective demonstration of two or more affected parts of the CNS by neurologic examination, appropriate MRI, or evoked potentials. Cerebrospinal fluid abnormalities help to confirm the inflammatory nature of the disorder but do not substitute for objective demonstration of lesions disseminated in time. Finally, as mentioned, there must be no other explanation, such as cerebrovascular disease or nutritional deficiency, for the patient's problems. The 2005 revised McDonald criteria permit one to use ancillary testing, most notably MRI, to demonstrate dissemination in time and space, thus allowing earlier diagnosis of clinically definite MS. For example, if a patient has a CIS and then develops a new T2 white matter lesion on MRI (obtained at least 3 months after the first MRI), the requirement for

dissemination in time would be fulfilled, eliminating the need for a second clinical attack.

Ancillary studies are often useful for objectively demonstrating multiple lesions and excluding other explanations for the patient's symptoms. Brain and spinal cord MRI are the most useful of the ancillary tests. Brain MRI often demonstrates white matter lesions within the cerebral hemispheres and less frequently within the brainstem and cerebellum (Figure 20.5). It is important to realize, however, that white matter lesions similar to those seen in MS may occur as a consequence of aging and in other disorders, including cerebrovascular disease, migraine, monophasic demyelinating disorders, and other immune-mediated diseases that affect the CNS. In addition, not all patients with MS will have an abnormal brain MRI. At least 10% of patients with clinically definite MS will have normal brain MRI scans because their MS spares the brain and involves only the spinal cord and optic nerves. Spinal MRI is useful in excluding the presence of compressive lesions, such as spondylosis, herniated discs, and tumors, and may reveal MS lesions within the spinal cord. Performing MRI with gadolinium is helpful in assessing for active lesions since these will enhance (Table 20.5).

Evoked potentials offer another means of electrophysiologically demonstrating the presence of lesions

Table 20.5 Multiple sclerosis

Discriminating features
▶ Relapsing remitting course
▶ Signs and symptoms of multifocal white matter disease of the central nervous system
▶ Age of onset between 20 and 55
▶ Absence of other diseases to explain neurologic problems
▶ Multiple white matter abnormalities on cerebral magnetic resonance imaging (MRI) scan
▶ Elevated cerebrospinal fluid (CSF) IgG index and synthesis rate; CSF oligoclonal bands
▶ Generalized fatigue or lassitude
▶ Worsening of symptoms with fever, hot weather or exertion

Consistent features
▶ Optic neuritis
▶ Upper motor neuron type weakness of one or more extremities
▶ Cerebellar ataxia
▶ Sensory abnormalities of one or more extremities
▶ Neurogenic bladder
▶ Internuclear ophthalmoplegia

Variable features
▶ Progressive course from onset
▶ Family history of MS
▶ Lhermitte's sign
▶ Trigeminal neuralgia

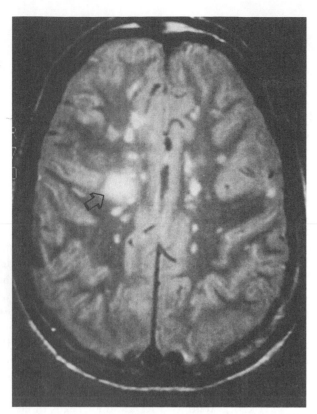 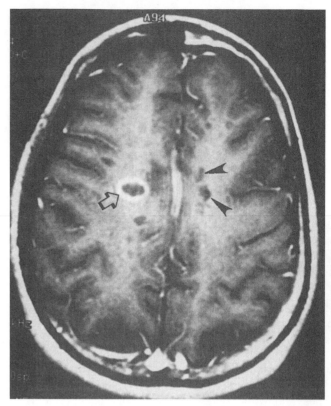

Figure 20.5 Multiple sclerosis (MS). A: T2-weighted brain magnetic resonance imaging (MRI) in a patient with MS during a relapse reveals multiple areas of increased signal in the white matter of both cerebral hemispheres, including an acute lesion within the right hemisphere (*arrow*). B: The acute lesion has ring enhancement (*arrow*) on a T1-weighted brain MRI with gadolinium, indicating increased permeability in the blood–brain barrier because of active inflammation. In addition, several chronic MS lesions do not enhance and appear as areas of decreased signal (*arrowheads*).

within the CNS. Visual, auditory, and somatosensory evoked potentials detect MS lesions within the optic nerves, brainstem, and spinal cord, respectively. Evoked potentials are most useful in detecting clinically silent lesions and therefore are of use in objectively establishing anatomically disseminated lesions. However, diseases other than MS can cause evoked potential abnormalities. Abnormal evoked potentials thus help to establish the presence of an electrophysiologic abnormality in a given neurologic pathway, but do not identify the nature of that abnormality.

Cerebrospinal fluid analysis is frequently useful in MS. Cerebrospinal fluid in MS is typically clear and colorless with a cell count usually less than 5/mm3 and rarely greater than 50/mm³. Cerebrospinal fluid total protein is typically normal or slightly elevated and rarely exceeds 100/dL. Glucose is normal. IgG abnormalities are the most important CSF finding in MS. Up to 90–95% of patients with clinically definite MS have some identifiable abnormality of CSF IgG. Total CSF IgG is elevated in a majority of patients. Measurements of intra-blood–brain barrier IgG synthesis, either IgG index or IgG synthesis rate, are abnormal in 80–90% of patients. Oligoclonal bands, a qualitative IgG abnormality seen on gel electrophoresis of CSF, occur in up to 90–95% of patients. These IgG abnormalities result from the presence of activated plasma cells within the CNS and reflect the inflammatory nature of MS. Cerebrospinal fluid IgG abnormalities are not present in about 10% of cases of clinically definite MS, and plasma cells appear to be absent from the pathologic inflammatory response in some patients with MS. In addition, CSF IgG abnormalities may not be seen in patients who are early in the course of their illness. It is important also to note that oligoclonal bands and elevated IgG index and synthesis rates occur in inflammatory diseases other than MS, including viral infections, systemic lupus erythematosus, vasculitis, Lyme disease, syphilis, and sarcoidosis.

A few diseases may mimic MS and should be considered in the differential diagnosis. These include systemic lupus erythematosus; Sjögren disease; Lyme disease; isolated CNS angiitis; cerebrovascular disease; syphilis; vitamin B$_{12}$, vitamin E, or copper deficiency; neurologic complications of human immunodeficiency virus and human T-lymphotropic virus-I; sarcoidosis; and compressive lesions of the spinal cord, including cervical spondylosis, tumors, arteriovenous malformations, herniated discs, and Arnold Chiari type I malformations.

Knowledge about the protean clinical presentations of MS and disorders that can mimic MS is critical to guiding the clinician in performing appropriate testing and ultimately in diagnosing MS. This generally requires the expertise of a neurologist.

Multiple sclerosis is a treatable condition. Corticosteroids shorten the course of MS relapses and are given for the treatment of optic neuritis and ATM. Treatment of relapsing-remitting MS with human recombinant β-interferon or glatiramer acetate reduces the frequency and severity of relapses of MS and decreases long-term disability from disease. β-interferon has also been studied in the treatment of secondary-progressive MS. The results of several trials have been mixed. To date, definitive evidence of benefit from β-interferon in the treatment of secondary-progressive MS has not been reproduced in clinical trials. However, there may still exist a modest benefit in slowing the progression of disease in this patient population and in decreasing relapses. For those with aggressive relapsing-remitting disease or secondary-progressive disease, mitoxantrone has been shown to be effective in reducing the relapse rate and slowing progression of disease. However, mitoxantrone is also associated with an important dose-dependent risk of cardiac toxicity and a possible increased risk of leukemia.

Natalizumab is currently the most effective proven treatment for breakthrough relapsing disease. It is a monoclonal antibody that was specifically designed to target the immune mechanism in MS and block leukocyte trafficking into the CNS. Based on promising early trial results, it was approved by the U.S. Food and Drug Administration (FDA) for use in MS in 2004. By 2005, natalizumab was temporarily removed from use due to the occurrence of a rare, often fatal viral infection of the brain, progressive multifocal leukoencephalopathy (PML). This complication occurred in two patients with MS receiving the drug in combination with interferon-β1a and a third receiving it alone for Crohn's disease. The reason for PML with natalizumab is unknown, and the exact risk of PML is also not established. The estimated incidence of PML with natalizumab was found to be approximately 1 case per 1,000 patients. Since being re-released for use in MS, three additional cases of PML have been reported. The risks of long-term use of natalizumab remain uncertain. Currently, the authors reserve this treatment for patients with relapsing MS who have failed treatment with β-interferon and glatiramer acetate. Other potential targeted monoclonal antibody therapies, such as rituximab, daclizumab, and alemtuzumab, are currently under clinical investigation. Oral treatments for relapsing MS are also being tested in clinical trials.

Off-label treatment with pulse methylprednisolone (1 g IV once a month), methotrexate (7.5 mg orally once a week), or azathioprine (2–2.5 mg/kg/day orally) may slow progression in some patients with primary or secondary-progressive MS. However, there remains no consistent, controlled evidence of significant benefit from any current therapy in slowing primary or secondary progression. In general, these treatments should only be used by physicians familiar with the management of MS and the use of these medications. A large number of treatments also may help manage neurologic symptoms resulting from MS, including baclofen and tizanidine for spasticity; oxybutynin, tolterodine, and hyoscyamine for detrusor hyperreflexia; intermittent catheterization for urinary retention; amantadine and modafinil for fatigue; carbamazepine and gabapentin for trigeminal neuralgia; and antidepressants for depression.

▼

Pearls and Perils

Multiple sclerosis

▶ Multiple sclerosis (MS) is a clinical diagnosis, highly dependent on a knowledgeable physician's ability to appropriately interpret the patient's history, neurologic examination, and results of laboratory and imaging studies.

▶ Definite MS cannot be diagnosed following a single episode of neurologic dysfunction; MS is a chronic illness, and the clinical course must show that the patient has a chronic illness.

▶ Cerebral magnetic resonance imaging (MRI) scans can be normal in patients with MS, and other conditions can cause white matter abnormalities similar to that of MS.

▶ Cerebrospinal fluid (CSF) IgG abnormalities (elevated IgG index and synthesis rate; oligoclonal bands) may be absent in patients with MS and can occur in other inflammatory diseases of the central nervous system.

▶ Although patients may have normal neurologic examinations during remissions, MS cannot be diagnosed without objective evidence of neurologic dysfunction.

▶ Early in the course of MS, physicians may mistakenly attribute the patient's symptoms to a psychologic etiology, thereby delaying diagnosis.

Neuromyelitis Optica (Devic Disease)

Neuromyelitis optica (NMO) is a severe relapsing and progressive demyelinating disease of the CNS that predominantly affects the optic nerves and the spinal cord. The disease is characterized by attacks of blindness affecting one or both eyes in addition to attacks of severe longitudinally extensive transverse myelitis. When acute bilateral optic neuritis is recognized, it should at least raise clinical suspicion for the diagnosis of NMO. Although NMO is significantly more rare than MS in Europe and North America, NMO appears to be over-represented in Asian and African populations, and NMO or "opticospinal MS" may be their more typical form of demyelinating disease.

Because optic neuritis and transverse myelitis may occur in both NMO and MS, it may be challenging to distinguish one diagnosis from the other. However, key features distinguish NMO from MS. In contrast to MS, NMO typically spares the remainder of the brain. There remain none to few brain lesions in NMO even many years after the onset of symptoms. In NMO, spinal cord lesions are also more longitudinally extensive than in MS. The spinal cord lesions often traverse over three or more vertebral segments in a contiguous fashion (Figure 20.6). Finally, CSF studies are typically normal, with an absence of oligoclonal bands. Unfortunately, another important difference is that the relapses in NMO tend to be more severe, with less complete recovery. The higher rate of permanent injury and disability progression in NMO is most likely explained by neuropathologic differences. Although the lesions in MS are more purely demyelinating, the lesions in NMO are more often also necrotizing.

The cause of NMO is unknown but is believed to have a pathogenesis that differs from that of MS. Like MS, NMO is believed to have an autoimmune patho-

> ### Consider Consultation When...
>
> ▶ There is acute or subacute loss of vision in a patient who is not known to have multiple sclerosis (MS).
> ▶ The patient has signs and symptoms of a myelopathy and has a spinal magnetic resonance imaging (MRI) scan that does not reveal the cause.
> ▶ The diagnosis of MS or acute disseminated encephalomyelitis (ADEM) is suspected based on the patient's history, examination, or MRI scan results.
> ▶ The patient has a diagnosis of MS and is having one or more disabling relapses per year or a progressive course.

genesis. In fact, MS and NMO were once believed to be variant presentations of the same disease. However, the neuropathologic differences and the recent identification of an IgG antibody against aquaporin-4 in NMO suggest that they are pathologically distinct. Testing for this NMO antibody is now commonly performed to support and distinguish a diagnosis of NMO. The best treatment for NMO is unknown, but there is general agreement that recombinant β-interferon and glatiramer acetate are ineffective. The most commonly used treatments for NMO are immunosuppressive and have included corticosteroids, plasma exchange, and intravenous immunoglobulin (IVIg) for acute exacerbations, as well as azathioprine with or without prednisone, mycophenolate mofetil, rituximab, and cyclophosphamide for disease modification. Evidence suggests that combination therapy with azathioprine and long-term prednisone may slow the disease. In an open-label study of seven patients, treatment with azathioprine and long-term prednisone resulted in no relapses over 18 months of observation. A more recent open-label study of eight patients supported the potential use of rituximab, an anti-CD 20 monoclonal antibody that eliminates circulating B cells. Results showed that rituximab may reduce relapse rate and even improve Expanded Disability Status Scale (EDSS) scores. Another small open-label study of five patients suggested that mitoxantrone may reduce relapses and MRI activity in NMO.

Annotated Bibliography

Cook SD, ed. *Handbook of multiple sclerosis*, 4th ed. New York: Taylor & Francis, 2006.
  Contains reviews of the pathophysiology, clinical manifestations, and treatment of multiple sclerosis.
Compston A, McDonald I, Noseworthy J, et al., eds. *McAlpine's multiple sclerosis*, 4th ed. New York: Churchill Livingstone, 2005.
  Provides a detailed review of the clinical manifestations, epidemiology, and immunopathology of multiple sclerosis.

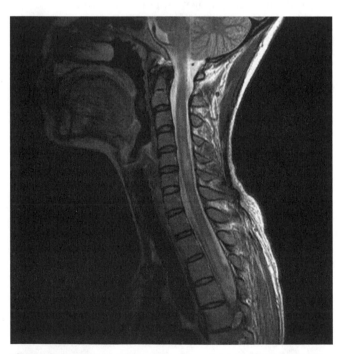

Figure 20.6 Neuromyelitis optica. T2-weighted spinal magnetic resonance imaging (MRI) in a patient with neuromyelitis optica reveals two separate longitudinally extensive areas of increased signal that each extend across three or more spinal cord segments in a contiguous fashion.

Frohman EM, Racke MK, Raine CS. Multiple sclerosis: The plaque and its pathogenesis. *N Engl J Med* 2006;354(9):942–955.
Discusses the pathogenesis of the inflammatory and neurodegenerative elements of the multiple sclerosis plaque.

Polman CH, Reingold SC, Edan G, et al. Diagnostic criteria for multiple sclerosis: 2005 revisions to the "McDonald criteria." *Ann Neurol* 2005;58:840–846.
Discusses the updated diagnostic criteria for multiple sclerosis.

Schapiro R. *Managing the symptoms of multiple sclerosis*, 5th ed. New York: Demos Publications, 2007.
Discusses approaches to managing a variety of symptoms resulting from MS.

Neoplastic Diseases

Marc C. Chamberlain

Neuro-oncology is an evolving subspecialty in neurology. Patients with neuro-oncologic problems include those with primary brain tumors, metastatic tumors to the nervous system, and with treatment-related complications affecting both the peripheral and central nervous system (CNS). This chapter discusses several components of neuro-oncology. However, conspicuously absent are discussions of several less common primary brain tumors (such as ependymomas) and primitive neuroectodermal tumors (such as medulloblastoma). Many of these tumors are more common in the pediatric age group and are discussed in another volume in this series, *Diagnosis-based Pediatric Neurology*.

This chapter is divided into eight sections and discusses, in sequence, glial neoplasms, meningiomas, pituitary adenomas, intracranial nerve sheath tumors, brain metastases, epidural spinal cord compression, leptomeningeal metastasis and, finally, paraneoplastic disorders. Although not comprehensive, sufficient information is presented in each section to assist in obtaining a basic understanding with regards to incidence, presenting signs and symptoms, and treatment of these various disorders.

Glial Neoplasms

The incidence of primary brain tumors in the United States is approximately 18,500 new cases per year or 10 per 100,000 adults. This represents 2% of the estimated 800,000 new cases of cancer occurring in adults per year in the United States. Of the estimated 18,500 primary tumors of brain occurring annually in the United States in adults, approximately 60% are gliomas. Among the infiltrative gliomas, 40–50% are glioblastomas; 30–35% are anaplastic astrocytomas; and 15–20% are well-differentiated gliomas.

Neurologic symptoms and signs affecting patients with glial neoplasms reflect the location of the tumor and the rapidity of glioma growth. General symptoms include headache, gastrointestinal upset including nausea and vomiting, personality changes, and slowing of psychomotor function. Because the brain parenchyma does not have pain-sensitive structures, headache has been attributed to local swelling and distortion of pain-sensitive nerve endings associated with blood vessels in the meninges. Although some tumors grow without headache as a prominent symptom, others rapidly produce headache that can vary in severity and quality but frequently occurs in the early morning hours. Some patients complain of an uncomfortable feeling in the head rather than headache.

Gastrointestinal symptoms such as loss of appetite, nausea, and occasionally vomiting occur in all patients but are more common in children and in patients harboring tumors in the infratentorial space.

Changes in personality, mood, mental capacity, and concentration can be noted early and can be the only abnormalities observed. In general, patients with brain tumors tend to sleep longer at night and nap during the day. These symptoms, although not unique to brain tumors, could easily be confused with depression or other psychiatric problems.

Focal symptoms can be episodic (for example, seizures) or progressive. Seizures are an important harbinger of brain tumors. Although only 1% of patients presenting with seizures are diagnosed with a brain tumor, the association increases with increasing patient age. Seizures are a presenting symptom in approximately 20% of patients with supratentorial brain tumors. Rapidly growing malignant gliomas are likely to produce complex partial motor or sensory seizures. However, secondarily generalized seizures are also common. In patients with slowly growing astrocytomas, such as gangliogliomas and oligodendrogliomas, seizures may antedate the clinical diagnosis by months to years. Focal seizures in patients older than 40 years of age should alert one to consider a tumor as a possible cause until proven otherwise. All adult patients presenting with seizures should undergo diagnostic contrast-enhanced magnetic resonance (MRI) or computed tomograph (CT) brain imaging.

The distribution of gliomas in the brain has a direct relationship to the size of the brain region or lobe. The most frequent locations are, in decreasing order of frequency, the frontal, parietal, temporal, and occipital lobes. Frontal lobe tumors may be asymptomatic or may produce slowing of contralateral hand movements, contralateral spastic hemiparesis, marked elevation in mood, or loss of initiation (frontal lobe executive functions) and dysphasia. Bifrontal disease is, unfortunately, common and can cause bilateral hemiparesis, spastic paraparesis, urinary incontinence, and severe impairment of the intellect, personality, and mood. Temporal lobe tumors may be clinically silent or may produce impairment of recent memory, homonymous quadrantanopsia, auditory hallucinations, and even aggressive behavior. Involvement of the nondominant temporal lobe can lead to minor perceptual problems and spatial disorientation. Dominant temporal lobe involvement can cause dysnomia, impaired perception of verbal commands, and aphasia. Parietal lobe tumors affect sensory and perceptional functions more than motor functions, although minor hemiparesis frequently coexists. In addition, homonymous hemianopsia and visual inattention or perceptual abnormalities may occur with parietal lobe tumors. Occipital lobe tumors produce contralateral homonymous hemianopsia or nonformed visual hallucinations. Thalamic and basal ganglia tumors result in nonspecific headaches (due to either hydrocephalus or raised intracranial pressure [ICP]), aphasic syndromes, or contralateral sensory abnormalities.

Several considerations regarding brain tumor therapy are unique to brain neoplasms. The resident organ, brain, is vital to the patient. Approximately 15 different cell types can give rise to a primary brain tumor, and the World Health Organization (WHO) recognizes over 100 varieties of brain tumors. The margins between tumor

and normal brain are frequently obscure. The concept of brain adjacent to tumor (BAT) is important, as tumor cell infiltration frequently precedes endothelial changes such that a substantial volume of tumor exists outside of the region indicated by contrast-enhanced imaging. A relatively intact blood–brain barrier exists in this region due to the limited tumor-induced neoangiogenesis and therefore limits drug access. Many classes of anticancer drugs are toxic to the CNS if the blood–brain barrier is extensively breached by either cerebrospinal fluid (CSF) drug administration or by blood–brain barrier modification.

Several variables affect survival in patients with primary brain tumors. These include tumor histology, age of the patient, neurologic deficit and ability to perform activities of daily living, proliferative capacity of the tumor, extent of surgery, dose of radiation therapy, and chemotherapy.

The classification of astrocytomas is confusing in that a number of systems have been used. Kernohan introduced a system in 1949 that grades tumors from I through IV, with grade IV (often called glioblastoma multiforme), being the most malignant. The WHO introduced a system with four grades (i.e., well-differentiated gliomas or grade I; low-grade gliomas or grade II; anaplastic astrocytomas or grade III; and glioblastoma multiforme or grade IVI), and this is the classification system most often used today. In general, median survival for well-differentiated gliomas (also called low-grade astrocytomas) is 5–8 years; for anaplastic astrocytoma is 2–3 years; and for glioblastoma multiforme is 1+ year. Oligodendrogliomas, a subset of glial neoplasms, representing 5–20% of all glial neoplasms, are characterized as either low-grade (median survival 10+ years) or anaplastic (median survival 7+ years), and as either pure oligodendroglial or mixed tumors (most often both oligodendroglial and astrocytic components).

Age independently affects survival in patients with primary brain tumors. Median survival is longer in

---

Pearls and Perils

Glial neoplasms

▶ Focal neurologic deficits due to neuroradiographically documented mass lesions may be either a primary brain tumor or a metastatic brain tumor.

▶ Glial tumors typically present subacutely as solitary lesions and most often with seizures, symptoms of raised intracranial pressure, or hemiparesis.

▶ Metastatic tumors typically present acutely as single (20%) or multiple (80%) lesions and most often with headache, seizures, or confusion.

younger compared to older patients with a similar tumor type. An explanation for this phenomenon is suggested by laboratory studies demonstrating increased tumor cell cytotoxicity to radiation and chemotherapy in tumors from younger patients. These data suggest that, with increasing age, tumors may acquire various treatment-resistance mechanisms, making them inherently less responsive to therapy.

The proliferative capacity of brain tumors may also impact survival. A variety of methods are available for estimating proliferative capacity and, within the astrocytoma series, higher DNA labeling indices are seen with glioblastoma multiforme relative to well-differentiated gliomas. In addition, within a glioma grade, it appears that tumors with higher proliferative capacity result in shorter survivals as compared to those with low proliferative capacity.

Another variable affecting survival is the extent of surgery. A number of studies have compared biopsy versus subtotal to total resection for malignant gliomas. For example, data from the Japanese Brain Tumor Registry show an improvement in 5-year survival rates in patients with well-differentiated gliomas who have undergone near or gross total resection compared to patients who have undergone biopsy or partial resection. Amarati has presented data regarding higher-grade gliomas that demonstrates a 2-year survival of 19% with gross total resection versus a 2-year survival of 0% with subtotal resection. Recently, the Glioma Outcome Project, a national consortium constructed to evaluate outcome in high-grade gliomas, also demonstrated improved survival in patients undergoing resective surgery as compared to biopsy.

The Brain Tumor Study Group has looked at the dose–response relationship of radiation therapy as an independent variable affecting survival in patients with malignant gliomas. These studies demonstrate that a radiation dose less than 4,500 cGy in grade III and IV gliomas results in a median survival of approximately 13 weeks, compared to a median survival of 42 weeks with a dose of 6,000 cGy. In addition, the Brain Tumor Study Group has shown that the addition of radiation therapy to surgery is beneficial relative to surgical therapy only. This effect is seen for both grade III and IV gliomas.

The preliminary report of Stupp, and the recently published randomized European and Canadian trial, has substantially altered the algorithm for initial treatment of glioblastoma. These studies clearly demonstrated a benefit for chemotherapy (temozolomide) in the initial treatment of patients with glioblastoma by showing an improvement in median (14.6 versus 12 months) and 2-year survival (27% versus 10%) in patients receiving or not receiving temozolomide. As a consequence, this treatment regimen (temozolomide given concurrently with radiotherapy followed by 6 monthly cycles of temozolomide) has become the new standard of care for patients with newly diagnosed glioblastoma. As a study correlative, methylguanine methyltransferase expression was evaluated. Methylguanine methyltransferase analysis (by promoter methylation status) is relevant, as prior studies had indicated that methylguanine methyltransferase is the predominant repair enzyme of alkylator-based chemotherapy-induced DNA injury and that methylguanine methyltransferase gene silencing (by promoter methylation) was correlated with improved response and survival. Outcome was significantly improved in patients treated with temozolomide and, additionally, in patients with methylated methylguanine methyltransferase promoter treated with temozolomide (median survival 21.7 months versus 15.3 months). Notably, in patients with unmethylated methylguanine methyltransferase promoter, no difference was seen between patients treated with temozolomide or radiotherapy only (median survival 12.7 versus 11.8 months). Recently, an analysis of a secondary end-point of this trial, health-related quality of life, revealed no negative effect on quality of life with the addition of temozolomide to radiotherapy.

The treatment of gliomas is predicated on accurate histologic diagnosis. This can be achieved for essentially all tumors either with an attempt at gross total removal or by stereotactic biopsy techniques using either CT or MRI. Malignant gliomas in adults are predominantly supratentorial and unifocal. The standard approach to malignant supratentorial glioma is complete resection followed by irradiation therapy and alkylator- based chemotherapy in glioblastoma. Most advocate as complete a resection as possible, since there appears to be no increase in surgical morbidity. The extent of surgical resection is best evaluated within 3 days of surgery by contrast-enhanced neuroimaging since, to this point, only minimal granulation tissue is present, and visible enhancement accurately reflects residual tumor.

Because a dose–response relationship exists with respect to tumor control and dose of radiation, brain tolerance doses of 6,000–6,500 cGy are recommended. With doses greater than this amount, there is an increase in the incidence of radiation injury to brain including both radiation necrosis and vasculopathy, obviating the survival benefits of higher doses of radiation therapy. To minimize delayed-late radiation injury to normal brain (which is often manifested as progressive intellectual decline and an extrapyramidal parkinsonian syndrome), smaller volumes of brain are generally irradiated. A 2–3 cm penumbra surrounding the contrast-enhancing tumor margin, as defined by preoperative neuroimaging, is suggested.

Chemotherapy, as indicated, now has an established role in patients with glioblastoma. In addition, it is likely that, based on tumor content of the DNA repair enzyme methylguanine methyltransferase, patients with newly diagnosed glioblastoma can be stratified into those who likely will respond to temozolomide (low content of methylguanine methyltransferase) and those who will not (high content of methylguanine methyltransferase). However, the assay that determines methylguanine methyltransferase tumor content is not yet commercially available, but likely will be in the near future. Another prognostic marker indicative of improved outcome and response to therapy is loss and translocation of the 1p and 19q chromosomes (the so-called 1p19q co-deletion), a genotype seen in oligodendroglial gliomas. Two recently reported cooperative group randomized trials, one performed by the Radiation Therapy Oncology Group (RTOG) and the other by the European Organization for Research and Treatment of Cancer (EORTC), evaluated adjuvant chemotherapy in the treatment of anaplastic oligodendrogliomas. Both trials utilized procarbazine, CCNU, and vincristine, although administration of chemotherapy was both neoadjuvant and dose-intense in the ROTG trial, and adjuvant (standard dose and schedule) in the EORTC trial. In neither study was chemotherapy associated with improved overall survival. A benefit was seen with respect to progression-free survival in the RTOG trial, but only in patients with 1p19q co-deleted anaplastic oligodendroglioma. In addition, both trials demonstrated by molecular analysis that 25% (EORTC) to 50% (RTOG) of histologically defined anaplastic oligodendrogliomas contained the 1p19q co-deletion. This group of patients (1p19q co-deleted) had substantially improved overall and progression-free survival irrespective of treatment (median overall survival >7 years). In contrast, partially or non-1p19q deleted anaplastic oligodendrogliomas behave like anaplastic astrocytoma or glioblastoma, with median survivals ranging from 2 to 3 years. Both cooperative group trials concluded that 1p19q co-deleted anaplastic oligodendrogliomas is a distinct tumor type, separable from other anaplastic gliomas and deserving of histology- and molecular biology-specific clinical trials. The studies also concluded that genotyping of anaplastic oligodendroglioma is not recommended outside of clinical trials, since therapy does not differ based on genotype results. Overall, these trials failed to provide compelling evidence in support of adjuvant chemotherapy in the treatment of newly diagnosed anaplastic gliomas, and the evidence-based standard of care remains maximal safe resection followed by involved-field radiotherapy.

Either brachytherapy or stereotactic radiosurgery may be useful in the treatment of recurrent gliomas. By contrast, two randomized trials have established that neither brachytherapy nor stereotactic radiotherapy is of benefit in the adjuvant treatment of glioblastoma. The limitations of stereotactic radiotherapy are based on the necessity to meet well-defined criteria including a definable target by CT or MR imaging, a unifocal lesion, supratentorial noneloquent brain location, absence of corpus callosum or deep nuclei involvement, a surgically accessible location, and no dimension of the tumor exceeding 5–6 cm (brachytherapy) or 3 cm (stereotactic radiosurgery). These criteria mean that only 10–15% of patients with recurrent high-grade gliomas will be eligible. Approximately 50% of patients treated with brachytherapy require reoperation for radiation necrosis with or without evidence of tumor recurrence. Evaluating radiation necrosis is difficult using conventional anatomic imaging studies such as cranial MR and CT. As such, positron emission tomography (PET), functional brain MR (spectroscopy, perfusion), and single photon emission computerized tomography (SPECT) have been utilized to differentiate between recurrent tumor and necrosis. Recurrent malignant tumors, in appropriate patients, are best managed by reoperation followed by chemotherapy or treated by stereotactic radiotherapy techniques. A variety of chemotherapeutics have been utilized; however, treatment intent in patients with recurrent malignant gliomas is palliative, as long-term survivors (defined as survival greater than 2 years) are rare. Increasingly, the role of targeted therapies for the treatment of gliomas (for example the epidermal growth factor receptor inhibitor, erlotinib) is being explored and, of particular note, the antiangiogenic agent bevacizumab appears to show significant antiglioma activity.

Meningiomas

Meningiomas are the most frequently encountered nonglial primary intracranial brain tumor, with an incidence of between 13% and 19%. Additionally, meningiomas are diagnosed in 12% of tumors arising in the spinal canal. The majority of patients with symptomatic meningiomas present in their fifth to seventh decade of life. Intracranial meningiomas are found twice as often in women as in men. Their size may increase during pregnancy, and they occasionally are associated with breast cancer. Using various biochemical techniques, meningiomas have been found to have high levels of progesterone receptors and low to absent levels of estrogen receptors on their surface. Little is known about the natural history and growth rate of asymptomatic meningiomas. As many as 2% of people over 60 years of age harbor incidental meningiomas at autopsy, with larger tumors more common as age increases.

In the classic monograph by Cushing, meningiomas were divided into nine major morphologic types. Seven of these were further divided into a total of 20 subtypes. Subsequent recognition of the lack of prognostic significance for most of these subtypes led to a widely adopted simplified scheme of three commonly encountered classic patterns: meningothelial, fibrous, and transitional. In addition to these basic patterns, the newly revised WHO classification includes eight morphologically distinct variants. However, no prognostic difference exists among these morphologic variants and those that exhibit a classic pattern. Malignant meningiomas are uncommon, making up 5–10% of all meningiomas, and they are the most aggressive with respect to clinical behavior. Brain invasion, when present, is the most reliable criteria for determining malignancy. At time of reoperation, up to 20% of meningiomas appear malignant. In the majority of patients with meningiomas, an etiologic explanation is lacking. However, meningiomas may be encountered in several cancer-predisposing familial syndromes (such as neurofibromatosis type 2) and, occasionally, they are radiation induced.

The clinical problems that result from the growth of meningiomas occur over months to years. This is in contrast to the deficits resulting from an intracranial metastasis or malignant glial neoplasm, which progress over days or weeks. This gradual progression of symptoms or decline in neurologic function caused by meningiomas parallels the slow rate of growth that is typical for most of these tumors. The locations of meningiomas correlate with the known distribution of the arachnoid villi, the presumed cell of origin. These sites are, in order of decreasing frequency the parasagittal region, cavernous sinus, tuberculum sella, lamina cribrosa, foramen magnum, and the torcular region. For each location, a characteristic neurologic deficit is produced.

Parasagittal meningiomas arise from the inner hemispheric falx and the dura adjacent to the superior sagittal sinus. They are classified according to location as anterior, middle, or posterior, and result in chronic headaches, memory difficulties, and personality changes. Occasionally, obstructive hydrocephalus may develop with resulting dementia, urinary incontinence, and gait difficulties. Additionally, posterior tumors can result in evolving leg weakness, either symmetric or asymmetric, giving rise to a cerebral cause of paraparesis. On occasion, focal seizures may occur with tumors in this location. Tumors that compress the superior sagittal sinus or venous outflow may result in raised ICP accompanied by headaches, papilledema, nausea, and vomiting.

Convexity meningiomas arise from the dura overlying the cerebral hemisphere. Headaches are the most common symptom although, not infrequently, seizures or focal neurologic deficits may result from tumors in this location. Sphenoid ridge meningiomas occur either medially or laterally in relationship to the sphenoid bone. Medial sphenoid ridge meningiomas may trap the internal carotid artery and optic nerve or invade the cavernous sinus. Consequently, stroke, visual loss, loss of facial sensation in the ophthalmic division of the trigeminal nerve, and disturbance of functioning of cranial nerves III, IV, and VI may occur. Lateral sphenoid ridge meningiomas displace the frontal and temporal lobes and give rise to headaches, seizures and, occasionally, speech and motor deficits.

Subfrontal meningiomas include those that originate from the olfactory groove and parasellar regions. Parasellar meningiomas include tumors of the tuberculum sella and cavernous sinus. Olfactory groove meningiomas displace the frontal lobes, resulting in personality changes, memory difficulties, and often loss of smell. Headaches and seizures may also occur. Tumors that arise from the dura above the tuberculum sella present with visual loss that is usually accompanied by headache. Bilateral visual field deficits are most common. Tumors that invade the cavernous sinus affect cranial nerves III, IV, V, and VI. In addition, headaches with retro-orbital pain are not infrequent.

Meningiomas located in the posterior fossa are located either anterior to the brainstem in the clivus, over the posterior aspect of the cerebellar hemisphere, in the cerebellopontine angle, or at the foramen magnum. Tumors in the cerebellopontine angle present with hearing loss, tinnitus, and facial paresis. Meningiomas involving the foramen magnum cause sensory loss and spasticity due to compression of the lower brainstem. Most tumors in this location also cause cerebellar deficits in addition to cranial nerve disturbances.

Cranial CT scans are adequate for detecting all but the smallest symptomatic meningiomas. However, because cranial MRI scans are far more accurate in defining specific types of tumors, when a patient is suspected of having a brain tumor, the initial diagnostic study of choice is a cranial MRI with contrast. Cerebral angiography, once the standard investigative method used to diagnose meningiomas, now has relatively few indications in the diagnosis of meningiomas. Angiograms are performed today if preoperative endovascular techniques are planned to occlude the blood supply to the meningioma to reduce operative blood loss. The typical radiographic appearance of a meningioma is of a dural-based mass of variable size that enhances in a uniform manner after infusion of a contrast agent. Because most meningiomas are benign, they tend to have a distinct interface with the

---

▼

Pearls and Perils

Meningiomas

▶ Meningiomas are common tumors and in general do not invade brain but rather are found in the compartment separating brain and skull.

▶ Standard therapy is surgical resection in patients with symptomatic meningiomas.

▶ Stereotactic radiotherapy is an alternative treatment in patients with inoperable tumors or in whom comorbid medical conditions prevent surgery.

brain and, as they grow, compress and displace rather than invade, nearby structures.

The conservative approach to therapy is to document growth of the tumor with serial cranial MRI scans and closely monitor the patient's condition. This strategy may be appropriate for small, asymptomatic tumors that are incidentally discovered and for patients who are judged to be poor candidates for surgery because of underlying medical problems. The problem with this approach is determining how often to repeat the cranial images. Under these conditions, and because the radiographic appearance of most meningiomas does not reliably predict behavior, an initial follow-up image should be obtained at 3–6 months. Intervals between successive images should be increased if the tumors size is unchanged.

The goal of surgical treatment for intracranial meningiomas is twofold: (1) complete removal of the tumor and (2) preservation or improvement of neurologic function. Surgery is still the mainstay of treatment because most meningiomas are well-circumscribed, benign tumors that can be removed without causing permanent neurologic deficits. For a patient with newly diagnosed meningiomas in a favorable location, there is a reasonable expectation that surgery will be curative. Multiple studies report a recurrence rate of approximately 10% at 20 years after complete removal of a histologically benign meningioma. When the resection is subtotal, however, the long-term outlook is less favorable, with a 50% recurrence at 10 years.

Extensive experience suggests that radiation therapy is effective in controlling the growth of subtotally resected meningiomas and is associated with a very low rate of complications. Following radiation therapy, reduction in the volume of visible tumor is infrequent, usually less than 15%, and often delayed over many years. Although these irradiated tumors continue to enhance on cranial imaging, they may remain stable for years following radiotherapy.

Other modalities used to treat meningiomas include stereotactic radiosurgery (a technique in which a large dose of radiation therapy is delivered with great precision to a target identified by neuroimaging), which is particularly applicable in locations where tumor resection is not possible or in the patient who has medical contraindications to surgery. Increasingly, stereotactic radiotherapy is utilized for frail elderly patients and in tumors where location precludes surgery (for example, the cavernous sinus) and often without pathologic confirmation. Long-term survival and outcomes are comparable to those achieved with conventional fractionated radiotherapy.

The benefit of chemotherapy for newly diagnosed and nonirradiated meningiomas is uncertain, as few data exist. Chemotherapy has been utilized for recurrent meningiomas, particularly meningiomas refractory to surgery and radiotherapy, or in patients who decline radio-

therapy. Although the literature is limited, oral hydroxyurea, α-interferon, and somatostatin analogues may be applicable in such circumstances. The treatment of aggressive or malignant meningiomas is more problematic, as standard therapies, surgery, and radiotherapy have a limited impact on overall survival.

Pituitary Adenomas

Pituitary adenomas account for 10–15% of all intracranial neoplasms. Although most are histologically benign, some behave aggressively because of their critical location and associated endocrine disorders. The choice of treatment for symptomatic pituitary tumors vary with the particular type of adenoma and can include pharmacologic treatment, surgery, or radiotherapy.

The reported annual incidence of pituitary tumor in the United States ranges from 0.2 to 2.8 per 100,000 population. The estimated current prevalence of symptomatic pituitary tumors is approximately 24,000. Clinically unapparent pituitary adenomas are even more common. At the University of Iowa hospital, McCormick found such tumors in 9.1% of 1,600 consecutive autopsies.

In the past, pituitary adenomas were classified by light microscopy into acidophil, chromophobe, and basophil types. Electron microscopy, radioimmunoassay, and immunocytochemistry have expanded our knowledge of these tumors, so that better correlation of morphology and function has become possible. A contemporary classification system taken from Kovacs distinguishes several types and subtypes of pituitary adenomas. The major types identified correspond to either the presence or absence of specific hormones in tumor cells. The five main types are the prolactin cell, growth hormone cell, mixed growth hormone/prolactin cell, adrenocorticotropic hormone (ACTH) cell, and undifferentiated cell adenomas.

The mechanisms by which pituitary tumors cause signs and symptoms include: (a) mechanical compression of surrounding adjacent structures, including the optic chiasm and cavernous sinus; (b) endocrine disturbances, including hypo- and hypersecretory states; and (c) acute pituitary apoplexy, a syndrome that results from infarction or hemorrhage into the pituitary, usually into an undiagnosed tumor. Similar to pituitary apoplexy is Sheehan syndrome. This results from pituitary necrosis secondary to infarction following postpartum hemorrhage and hypovolemia. It results in hypopituitarism, which may present either acutely or subacutely. The signs and symptoms of a pituitary mass include headache, visual loss, cranial nerve palsy (cranial nerves III, IV, V or VI or any combination thereof), and an alteration in level of consciousness.

Headache is a frequent symptom in patients with pituitary tumors, occurring in 50% of patients with macroadenomas (tumors greater than 10 cm in size), it and is the primary presenting symptom in 14% of patients. Although bifrontal, retro-orbital, or bitemporal location of pain is found most frequently, headache associated with pituitary neoplasms may occur anywhere in the head. The cause of headache is unknown but may relate to pressure on the diaphragma sella. The optic chiasm, located superior to the sella turcica, is particularly susceptible to pressure damage from a pituitary macroadenoma with suprasellar extension. Patients classically present with either bitemporal hemianopsia or a superior bitemporal defect. Because red perception is generally lost first with optic nerve and chiasm injury, peripheral field-testing should be done with a small red object to uncover subtle defects. Large invasive adenomas may extend to the hypothalamus and result in disturbances in temperature regulation, food intake, thirst and fluid balance, sleep cycle, behavior, and autonomic nervous system function. Diabetes insipidus, somnolence, and hyperphagia with obesity are the commonest manifestations of hypothalamic involvement. Encroachment into the cavernous sinus by lateral invasion of pituitary tumors may affect the III, IV, and VI cranial nerves in addition to the ophthalmic and maxillary divisions of the V cranial nerve. Clinically, ptosis, diplopia, ophthalmoplegia, and decreased facial sensation are usually found. Lateral extension may also affect the temporal lobes, leading to uncinate (mesial temporal lobe) partial seizures. Anterior extension, with involvement of frontal lobes, results in alterations of personality and occasionally in defects in smell.

Excessive secretion of one or more of the pituitary trophic hormones leads to the development of specific clinical syndromes, such as acromegaly, amenorrhea, galactorrhea, or Cushing disease, whereas loss of normal trophic hormone secretion may result in hypogonadism, hypothyroidism, or hypoadrenalism. Some patients, usually those with large tumors, will have manifestations of both hypersecretion of one hormone and hyposecretion of others. Thus, in each patient, the clinician must determine whether and to what extent the tumor has involved structures in close proximity to the sella turcica, the bony structure within which the pituitary resides, and evaluate the state of pituitary hormones.

The commonest functional tumor of the pituitary, prolactinoma, is diagnosed most frequently in women, which may be a reflection of the differences in the clinical manifestations of hyperprolactinemia in men and women. Women generally present at a younger age (second through fourth decade) with menstrual disturbances, with or without galactorrhea, and pathologically have a predominance of microadenomas (tumors defined as less than 10 cm in size). Conversely, men present at a later age than that of women, with larger tumors, and decreased libido and impotence as the major endocrine-related symptoms. Because the tumors in men are generally large, visual field abnormalities and secondary hypogonadism, hypothyroidism, and adrenal insufficiency are more often encountered. The serum concentration of prolactin roughly correlates with tumor size, and therefore the mean prolactin concentration in men with prolactin-secreting tumors is higher than that in women. The diagnosis of prolactin-secreting pituitary tumors is relatively straightforward. Two or three basal serum prolactin concentrations should be measured on separate days. A patient with persistent hyperprolactinemia should have either cranial CT or MR of the pituitary-hypothalamic region.

Therapeutic considerations depend on the associated symptoms and the size of the lesion on cranial imaging. An important consideration in the treatment of microprolactinomas is the natural history of untreated hyperprolactinemia. A number of reports indicate that neither tumor size nor prolactin levels change over a number of years in the majority of women with microprolactinomas. Therefore, in patients with untreated microadenomas, clinical symptoms, serum prolactin levels, and the appearance of the pituitary gland must be carefully monitored. Despite the relative stability in tumor size, therapy may be necessary because of reproductive dysfunction (including infertility, menstrual abnormalities, and galactorrhea) in women and sexual dysfunction in men. The treatment of microadenomas is primarily pharmacological and utilizes a dopamine agonist such as bromocriptine. Resection by transsphenoidal hypophysectomy is frequently not curative, and recurrences are seen in up to 40% of patients. In addition, a 16% rate of biochemical recurrences has been reported in the absence of radiographic evidence of tumor recurrence. Radiation therapy has been abandoned for microprolactinomas because of the associated hypopituitarism and the proven efficacy of drug therapy. Bromocriptine rapidly lowers serum prolactin levels, restores normal gonadal function, and decreases tumor size. Discontinuance of bromocriptine therapy leads to the re-emergence of hyperprolactinemia in most patients, however. In a small group of patients treated with a dopamine agonist, hyperprolactinemia can spontaneously remit, allowing discontinuation of therapy. Therefore, dopamine agonist therapy should be discontinued every 2 years on a trial basis to determine the need for continued therapy. Bromocriptine is also the initial therapy for the majority of patients with macroprolactinomas, including those with visual loss, because surgical cure is unlikely, and the risk of tumor recurrence is high. Most patients require bromocriptine indefinitely because discontinuation of therapy may be associated with rapid enlargement of tumor.

Excessive secretion of growth hormone by pituitary tumors in a child or adolescent, before fusion of the epiphyseal growth centers of long bones, results in gigantism, whereas in adults, it becomes clinically manifest as acromegaly. Acromegaly occurs with equal frequency in men and women, and the clinical features develop slowly.

Excessive growth of soft tissue results in the characteristic coarsening of facial features, enlargement of hands, feet, tongue, and skin tags around the neck and axilla, and entrapment of the median nerve, which results in the carpal tunnel syndrome. Stimulation of cartilage and bone growth leads to prognathism, dental malocclusion, frontal bossing, and hypertrophic osteoarthropathy. Organomegaly with enlargement of the liver, spleen, kidney, and heart are often found at autopsy in patients with acromegaly.

Echocardiographic abnormalities such as septal hypertrophy and left ventricular hypertrophy are common, as is hypertension. These manifestations of growth hormone excess are not directly due to growth hormone but rather to tissue growth factors, especially somatomedins, which are secreted under the influence of growth hormone. Growth hormone itself has direct anti-insulin effects and induces insulin resistance and hyperinsulinism. Thus, impaired glucose tolerance is frequently seen in patients with acromegaly. Clinically, however, diabetes is seen in only 10–15% of patients.

The diagnosis of acromegaly requires biochemical evidence of excessive growth hormone secretion or activity. The *sine qua non* of diagnosis has been the lack of adequate suppression of growth hormone during an oral glucose tolerance test. As noted earlier, the growth-promoting activity of growth hormone is actually due to somatomedins. Insulin-like growth factor 1 (somatomedin C) is elevated in patients with active acromegaly and correlates better with clinical activity than do fasting or glucose-suppressed growth hormone levels. A normal result effectively rules out acromegaly.

Neurosurgical therapy of pituitary adenomas may be required in several groups of patients, including patients whose tumors are unresponsive to dopamine agonist therapy, patients with rapidly progressive visual loss, patients who are unable to tolerate dopamine agonist therapy, and patients whose tumors grow during dopamine agonist treatment. No study has reported a higher complete surgical resection rate following preoperative treatment with a dopamine agonist. Radiation therapy (and increasingly stereotactic radiotherapy) should be considered primarily in patients with macroadenomas who require additional treatment and cannot tolerate dopamine agonist therapy. In those with acromegaly or Cushing disease, the majority of patients are discovered to have macroadenomas, and neurosurgical treatment is the initial treatment of choice in all such patients. In the event that complete surgical resection is not possible, radiation therapy is typically required. However, the disadvantage of radiation therapy is the delayed therapeutic effect, particularly in patients with Cushing disease, and the development in all patients of radiation-induced hypopituitarism. Radiation therapy is delivered using conventional once-per-day fractionation schedules to a total dose of 45–50 Gy or, as mentioned earlier, single-fraction stereotactic radiotherapy.

Intracranial Nerve Sheath Tumors

Intracranial nerve sheath tumors constitute 4–8% of all intracranial tumors. Most are acoustic neuromas or cranial nerve VIII tumors, recently renamed *vestibular schwannomas*. Nerve sheath tumors also occur in the extraocular motor nerves (cranial nerves III, IV, and VI), the trigeminal cranial nerve (V), the facial cranial nerve (VII), the nerves of the jugular foramen (cranial nerves IX, X, and XI), and the hypoglossal cranial nerve (XII), although all these tumors are uncommon.

Vestibular schwannomas comprise 6% of all intracranial tumors. Surveys in the United States have demonstrated incidences of 10 tumors per 1 million populations, yielding a total of 2,000 new vestibular schwannomas annually in the United States. Spontaneous, sporadic vestibular schwannomas account for 95% of these tumors, with patients having a mean age of 50 years at time of presentation. The remaining 5% of patients with vestibular schwannomas have neurofibromatosis type 2 and present earlier, with an average age of presentation of 31 years. Vestibular schwannomas are rare in patients with neurofibromatosis type 1.

Unilateral hearing loss, seen in over 90% of patients, is the most common presenting complaint, often accompanied by tinnitus. Some patients note vertigo (20%), imbalance (50%), facial numbness (50%), or weakness (10%), particularly when tumors become large. Headache frequency and tumor size increase together, and lower cranial nerve abnormalities are rare in the absence of multiple tumors, as is common in neurofibromatosis type II.

Extraocular nerve schwannomas, although uncommon, typically cause diplopia, and can arise along the III, IV, and VI cranial nerves, within the cavernous sinus, or within the subarachnoid space.

Trigeminal schwannomas usually present with facial numbness or dysesthesias, or trigeminal neuralgia, but occasionally cause cavernous sinus compression and diplopia. They are located either within or posterior to the Meckel cave on the temporal floor.

Facial nerve schwannomas arise within the temporal bone, usually in the geniculate ganglion or the vertical portion of the VII cranial nerve. They most often cause hearing loss but can also cause facial weakness or hemifacial spasm. Because vestibular schwannomas can also cause hearing loss and facial spasm or weakness, distinguishing between these two tumors by clinical or radiographic studies can be problematic.

Schwannomas of the jugular foramen arise within the posterior fossa, expand the jugular foramen, and extend extracranially below the skull base. They typically cause focal dysfunction of one or more of the IX, X, or XI cranial nerves, resulting in hoarseness, swallowing difficulty, or shoulder weakness.

Hypoglossal schwannomas are rare and can arise at any point along the course of the XII cranial nerve from the brainstem parenchyma, to the subarachnoid space, or extracranially. Isolated tumors produce tongue hemiatrophy and weakness.

If a tumor is very large, causing substantial brain or brainstem compression with neurologic symptoms, surgery is needed to reduce the tumor bulk or remove it entirely. However, as most tumors are benign, in selected cases, patients may be followed with serial cranial imaging studies. This is primarily true in elderly patients, particularly those with minimal symptoms. For vestibular schwannomas, older patients (65 years) often do not undergo surgery when deafness or mild gait instability are the only clinical problems. In elderly patients with large vestibular schwannomas presenting with severe gait disturbances and multiple falls, surgery is recommended, using either subtotal or complete tumor resection. Most often, surgery is performed translabyrinthine with resulting deafness. Stereotactic radiosurgery, a procedure not infrequently used for smaller vestibular schwannomas, has not been effective in treating patients with brainstem compression and gait instability, as its benefit is delayed for months to years. In general, surgery is recommended if the intracranial schwannomas are large enough to cause neurologic deficits other than in the nerve of origin, or if they enlarge on sequential radiographs. As most nerve sheath tumors present symptomatically during the fifth and sixth decades, patients with these tumors remain at risk for 20–30 years, a long time during which a tumor is likely to grow. In the overwhelming majority of these patients, surgical removal of tumor is recommended.

Radiosurgery, utilizing either the gamma knife or with specially modified linear accelerators, has been practiced for at least two decades, but few data are available for long-term follow-up of patients treated with this procedure. In the last several years, an increasing number of patients in the United States have been treated with this modality. Approximately 40% of patients' tumors appear to be reduced by radiation, another 40% remain unchanged, and 15–20% continue to grow following irradiation. Essentially all patients treated with stereotactic radiation become deaf on the tumor side within 2–3 years after surgery. In addition, nearly a third of patients develop facial weakness or numbness, which often improves over time.

Brain Metastases

Metastatic cancer may affect the skull, the dura, or the brain. Metastases to the skull vault are most common and

particularly likely to affect patients with cancer of the breast and prostate, although most patients so affected are asymptomatic. Occasionally, dural metastases may compress the sagittal sinus, raising ICP and causing a pseudo-tumor-like syndrome. Metastases to the base of the skull are likely to cause cranial nerve abnormalities before compressing or invading the brain. Tumors arising in the skin of the head or neck can invade cranial nerves and grow centripetally to involve the brain. This is particularly common with melanoma, head and neck cancers, and basal cell skin cancers. Tumors metastasizing to the dura can also secondarily invade the brain. The most common cause of symptomatic brain dysfunction in cancer patients is when a distant neoplasm, such as a lung cancer, hematogenously metastasizes to the brain substance.

In the United States, approximately 1 million patients will develop a new cancer each year. Of these, approximately 150,000 will develop symptomatic intracranial metastases during life, and over half of these will represent spread from cancer of the lung. Approximately 20% of patients with intracranial metastases will have a breast primary, 13% melanoma, 4% renal, and 1% an unknown primary.

Symptoms and signs of brain metastasis are similar to those of primary brain tumors. Headache (24%), weakness (20%), cognitive and behavioral disturbances (14%), seizures (12%), and ataxia (7%) are the most common presenting signs and symptoms.

The symptoms of brain metastasis arise from one of several pathophysiologic mechanisms. The tumor itself, by occupying space, can cause direct damage to brain structures or pathways located at the site where the tumor grows. Once the metastasis has reached a size of 5 cm or more, neovascularization of the tumor disrupts the blood–brain barrier, raising tissue pressure in the metastasis and leading to brain edema. Current evidence suggests that substances made by the tumor, or the brain's response to the tumor, also disrupts the blood–brain barrier in the normal brain surrounding the tumor. Brain edema, by its mass effect and probably by its content of cytokines, causes brain dysfunction in the area surrounding the tumor. The mass effect sometimes becomes large enough to lead to cerebral herniation, which, in turn, compresses and damages brain structures distant from the tumor. Obstruction of spinal fluid pathways causes hydrocephalus, thus compounding the problem of elevated ICP.

The symptoms and signs of a brain metastasis are usually slowly progressive. Sudden changes may occur when the tumor bleeds or becomes cystic. Episodic alterations of neurologic function in patients with metastatic brain cancer are usually the result of either seizures (with or without postictal abnormalities) or cerebral *plateau waves*. Plateau waves often occur in a patient with otherwise asymptomatic increased ICP due to brain or leptomeningeal metastases. They are particularly likely to be precipitated by assuming the upright posture after having been recumbent for a time.

The therapy of brain metastases has two major components, symptomatic or supportive and definitive. Because many of the important symptoms of the brain metastases result from brain edema or from seizures, antiedemic agents such as corticosteroids, and anticonvulsants are considered important aspects of the treatment of brain metastases. In addition, patients with cancer are often hypercoagulable and thus at increased risk for deep vein or other thromboses. Accordingly, anticoagulants are also part of the supportive care in selected patients.

Several definitive therapies are available including surgery, radiation, and chemotherapy or biologic therapy. Approximately 20% of patients who present with brain metastases have a single lesion in the brain, and in another 20–30% there are two lesions. Only about a third of patients have three or more lesions in the brain. Thus, approximately two-thirds of patients (those with one to three metastases) are potential candidates for some focal therapy. Prospective analysis of single brain metastases indicate that surgery followed by irradiation is superior to brain irradiation alone for prolonging and enhancing the quality of life. Surgery for a single and accessible brain metastasis has become the gold standard against which other therapies must be measured.

It is established that radiation therapy following surgical removal of a brain metastasis prolongs or increases the quality of life and inhibits intraparenchymal brain recurrence. However, most studies involving surgical resection utilize whole-brain radiotherapy. The role of stereotactic radiotherapy, either following or in lieu of surgical resection, has increasingly become an alternative treatment option. For patients with multiple brain metastases, whole-brain external beam irradiation has long been the standard treatment. The treatment is usually delivered as 10 fractions at 300 cGy per dose. Other dose fractionation schedules appear to give equal results. The higher the dose per fraction, the more likely that long-term survivors will develop late-delayed radiation brain damage. Accordingly, in patients with a good prognosis, protracted radiation therapy of 200 cGy fraction in 20 fractions may be desirable. Recently, focal radiation, administered either by gamma knife or radiosurgically by linear accelerator, has been given in preference to whole-brain irradiation, especially for patients with single or few metastases. Focal radiotherapy has the advantage of being able to deliver high doses of radiation to a tumor and spare surrounding normal brain. In these studies, local control of metastatic brain disease was similar to that achieved by surgical resection and whole-brain radiotherapy; however, distant control of non-locally treated metastatic brain disease was inferior to surgery followed by whole-brain irradiation. The adjuvant role of stereotactic focal radiotherapy in the

treatment of solitary or oligometastatic brain metastases (two to three brain metastases) remains controversial, as a recent randomized trial suggested that oligometastatic brain disease treated with gamma knife followed by whole-brain radiotherapy had no improvement in survival relative to whole-brain radiotherapy alone. Another method to manage solitary brain metastasis is by interstitial implantation of radioactive sources (such as the Glia-Site device) into a metastatic tumor, often called *brachytherapy*. This permits a high and continuous dose of radiation therapy to the tumor, sparing the surrounding normal tissues. This method may enhance survival in highly selected patients. However, selection criteria remain to be established. Lastly, surgical resection of a solitary metastasis followed by implantation of carmustine polymers (Gliadel), followed by whole-brain radiotherapy, may have a role in the treatment of solitary brain metastasis. Whole-brain radiotherapy was originally designed with two purposes in mind. The first was to treat established metastatic tumors in the brain, and the second was to treat micrometastases that might not be identifiable by currently available imaging techniques. The issue of late cognitive effects of whole-brain radiotherapy have been clarified in that metastatic tumor volume and response to CNS-directed therapy appear to be the primary determinants of cognitive outcome, and not whole-brain radiotherapy as was once believed.

Most evidence suggests that brain metastases, once established, respond about as well as a systemic tumor to chemotherapeutic agents. Accordingly, for small and relatively asymptomatic metastases that have arisen from chemosensitive primaries such as breast cancer or small-cell lung cancer, one might consider chemotherapy before using other approaches. This is particularly true when other systemic tumor is present and requires treatment. Another instance in which systemic chemotherapy has proven useful is in patients who have failed surgery or radiotherapy and remain candidates for further therapy. In this special situation, there is evidence that the CNS-active oral chemotherapy agent temozolomide may provide modest benefit.

Brain metastases are a serious and often devastating complication of systemic cancer. Various techniques, including stereotactic radiosurgery and high-dose chemotherapy, give a promise of better control. The more aggressive approach to brain metastases not only increases survival of patients with even widespread systemic disease, but also substantially enhances the quality of that individual's life.

Epidural Spinal Cord Compression

The vertebral column is the most frequent site for skeletal metastases. Typically, the vertebral body is affected first, with the posterior elements involved only one-seventh as often as the anterior elements. In patients examined post mortem, approximately 70% of patients have demonstrable vertebral metastases. Nearly one-half of these patients require treatment for symptomatic pain from spinal bony metastases. It has been estimated that approximately 5% of patients with cancer who come to autopsy have epidural spinal cord compression, and approximately 18,000 cases of spinal cord compression occur annually in the United States.

In decreasing order of incidence, primary tumors causing epidural spinal cord compression are breast (20%), lung (13%), lymphoma (11%), prostate (9%), sarcoma (9%), kidney (7%), head and neck (6%), miscellaneous (5%), myeloma (4%), gastrointestinal (4%), melanoma (3%), germ cell (2%), gynecologic (2%), neuroblastoma (2%), and unknown primary tumors (2%). Although the lumbar vertebra is most commonly affected by tumor metastases, it is the thoracic spine that compromises the spinal cord more frequently. Approximately 15% of all epidural spinal cord compression involves the cervical spine, 68% the thoracic spine, and 16% the lumbosacral spine. Pathologically, three stages of epidural spinal cord compression are seen. In the earliest stages, white matter edema occurs with preserved spinal cord blood flow. In the mid stage, mechanical compression of the spinal cord is added to increasing white matter edema. In the final stage, spinal cord blood flow decreases below a critical flow level, producing irreversible ischemic spinal cord damage.

Several modes of tumor spread to the epidural spinal cord space are evident. Most often, direct extension occurs from a direct vertebra, as in carcinoma of the breast, lung, or prostate. Lymphomas and neuroblastomas more commonly migrate through intervertebral foramina into the epidural space from adjacent perivertebral lymph nodes. Hematogenous spread from the venous plexus of Batson or radicular arteries rarely occurs. Several factors probably contribute to the high incidence of metastatic

deposition and growth in vertebral bodies. These include the valveless epidural venous plexus of Batson, the fact that vertebral bodies contain vascular bone marrow (red marrow) throughout life, and the fact that red marrow, because of its greater vascularity, appears to be a nutritive environment for the establishment of metastases.

There is striking similarity in the clinical presentation of patients with epidural spinal cord compression regardless of the origin of the primary tumor. Pain is almost always the earliest and most significant symptom, seen in 95% of patients. The discomfort is typically gradual and onset is progressive over weeks or months. It may be focal, radicular, or referred. It is most often marked at night and aggravated by movement. Local pain is localized, aching, and continuous. Radicular pain is often intermittent, shooting in quality, and unilateral or bilateral. Referred pain occurs at a distal site without a radiating component. The pain of epidural spinal cord compression may be accompanied by evidence of motor, sensory, or autonomic dysfunction. Because a metastatic tumor typically invades the canal from the vertebral body, the motor functions of the anterior part of the spinal cord are usually compromised first, with sensory disturbances following as the cord are displaced posteriorly and impinges on the laminae. The sensory level is not a reliable indicator of the level of cord compression, since it is often several segments below the actual site of compromise. Loss of anal or urethral sphincter control, with associated incontinence, is usually a late sign. In one large series, 87% of patients presented with weakness at time of diagnosis, of which 15% were paraplegic and 50% were paraparetic. A sensory deficit was noted in approximately three-quarters of patients, and bladder and bowel dysfunction occurred in nearly half. Various classification schemata have been proposed for epidural spinal cord compression. Portenoy's classification defines three groups: group I, patients having signs or symptoms of new or progressive spinal cord conus medullaris or cauda equina disease; group II, patients having mild, stable symptoms or signs of epidural spinal cord compression or either radiculopathy or plexopathy without evidence of epidural spinal cord compression; and group III, patients having isolated back pain without neurologic signs or symptoms.

Many diagnostic studies are utilized for imaging the spine in patients with epidural spinal cord compression, including plain radiographs, bone scans, CT (usually with intrathecal enhancement, i.e., myelography), and MRI with contrast. Approximately 30–50% of the vertebral body density must be destroyed before any changes can be recognized on plain spine films, making them a relatively insensitive test. However, the degree of abnormality seen on plain films often correlates with the degree of epidural spinal cord compression. In patients with greater than 50% collapse of the vertebral body, three-quarters

---

▼

Pearls and Perils

Epidural spinal cord compression

▶ Pain in a cancer patient, either local, referred or radiating, suggests symptomatic vertebral body metastases and possible spinal cord compression.

▶ All cancer patients with back pain require spinal imaging—initially plain films and, if sufficient concern exists, spinal magnetic resonance imaging.

▶ Early treatment with radiotherapy prevents disease progression and, in particular, motor impairments.

will have epidural spinal cord compression. In general, bone scan has a very limited role for predicting the presence or absence of epidural spinal cord compression. Magnetic resonance imaging of the spine has proved to be the most useful study.

In patients without known cancer, biopsy is performed either percutaneously or by open methods. In the majority of patients with epidural spinal cord compression, as mentioned earlier, the epicenter of metastatic disease is in the vertebral body. In these cases, laminectomy fails to decompress the cord, and potentially exacerbates spinal instability by compromising the load-bearing posterior bony spine elements. In such patients, vertebrectomy may be the preferred approach. Furthermore, in patients with vertebral body collapse and spinal instability (i.e., extrusion of bony elements into the spinal canal, significant kyphosis, or subluxation), radiotherapy is unlikely to decompress the spinal cord. As a result, these patients are best considered for vertebral body resection and spinal reconstruction. Furthermore, patients clinically failing radiotherapy, either during initial treatment or subsequently, may be considered for surgery. Vertebrectomy and spine instrumentation should be considered in all patients with epidural spinal cord compression based on a recent randomized clinical trial in which the inclusion criteria included a single site of ESCC, adult age, histology not showing lymphoma or myeloma, absence of paraplegia, primary tumor not posterior spine element–based, and expected survival less than 3 months. There is, in addition, a subset of patients with posterior element-based disease who benefit from laminectomy and spine instrumentation. Nonetheless, the majority of patients with epidural spinal cord compression are best treated with radiotherapy to all sites identified radiographically. Furthermore, radiotherapy is administered to all patients following surgery (typically 6 weeks from time of surgery), most often as 10 fractions with 300 cGy per fraction (total dose 30 Gy).

Otherwise, surgical intervention, in particular laminectomy, has not been shown to be more effective than medical treatment. With respect to medical treatment, chemotherapeutics have a very limited role in the primary treatment of epidural spinal cord compression. However, steroids in conjunction with involved-field radiotherapy are the preferred treatment modality in the majority of patients. Most patients are treated with conventional, standard once-per-day fractionated radiotherapy schedules, up to a total dose of approximately 3,000 cGy given in 10 fractions.

Leptomeningeal Metastasis

In clinical studies, leptomeningeal metastasis (LM) has been estimated to occur in 4–15% of patients with solid tumors, 7–15% of patients with lymphomas, 5–15% of patients with leukemia, and 1–2% of patients with primary brain tumors. In patients with solid tumors, breast (range of occurrence: 22–54%), lung (10–26%), melanoma (17–25%), and gastrointestinal (4–14%) cancers are most frequently encountered. Carcinomas of unknown primary origin constitute 1–7% of all cases of LM, a range similar to that of patients with other metastatic complications of the CNS. Autopsy studies of patients with cancer demonstrate a very high incidence of LM, exceeding that seen in clinical studies. In a Memorial-Sloan Kettering study, an 8% incidence of LM was demonstrated in patients with cancer and post mortem CNS analysis.

Leptomeningeal metastases are pleomorphic in their clinical presentation because they affect all levels of the CNS. In general, LM affects three domains of neurologic disturbance including (1) the central hemispheres, (2) the cranial nerves, (3) the spinal cord and roots. The common symptoms of cerebral hemispheric dysfunction in decreasing order of occurrence are: headache, mental status change, nausea and vomiting, weakness, and seizures. Signs found in patients with LM and cerebral hemisphere disturbance include mental status changes (confusion and dementia), seizures, papilledema, and hemiparesis. Symptoms referable to disturbance of cranial nerve function in decreasing order of occurrence are: double vision, hearing loss, facial numbness, and loss of vision. Signs of cranial nerve dysfunction include ophthalmoplegia with abducens palsy, oculomotor dysfunction, trochlear palsies, trigeminal sensory or motor loss, cochlear dysfunction, and optic neuropathy. Spinal symptoms are referable to either the spinal cord or exiting nerve roots and spinal meninges. These symptoms include in decreasing order of occurrence, weakness, pain, limb numbness, pain (neck, back or in radicular patterns), and bladder or bowel dysfunction. Common signs of spinal cord dysfunction are extremity weakness, which may be caused by either lower motor neuron dysfunction (e.g., cauda equina involvement) or upper motor neuron dysfunction (e.g., with myelopathy or conus medullaris involvement), dermatomal or segmental sensory loss, asymmetries in deep tendon reflexes, gait ataxia, nuchal rigidity, and pain on straight leg raising.

With progression of LM, new signs and symptoms appear that often affect CNS domains not previously involved and, in addition, preexisting findings often worsen. As in the initial examination, neurologic findings in patients with progressive disease exceed patient symptoms. Clinicians should recognize the pleomorphic clinical manifestations of LM and maintain a high clinical suspicion of LM in an appropriate clinical context.

The single most useful laboratory test in diagnosing LM is CSF examination, usually by lumbar puncture. In nearly all patients with LM, the CSF is abnormal regardless of the results of CSF cytology. A CSF cytology result that is positive for malignant cells is a standard method by which LM is diagnosed in most clinical series. The variable results of CSF analysis in patients with LM are partially explained by the multifocal nature of LM. Cerebrospinal fluid obtained from a site distant from pathologically involved meninges may yield misleading results regarding disease presence or response to therapy. Repeated taps may be necessary. In a large study from Sloan Kettering, the initial lumbar CSF examination results were cytologically positive in only 50% of patients, and these increased to 75% following a second CSF examination. In the only autopsy study of LM, 50–60% of patients with LM established post mortem had negative antemortem CSF cytology.

A variety of neuroradiographic methods are available to evaluate patients with suspected LM including cranial CT, brain and spine MR, CT myelography, and radionuclide CSF flow studies. Abnormalities are common on brain and spinal neuroimaging (approximately 40% of all patients with LM), which, importantly, also reveal areas of bulky disease. In addition, hydrocephalus may be demonstrated. Bulky disease is most responsive to radiotherapy, as opposed to regional chemotherapy. Radioisotope CSF flow studies, or so-called *radionuclide ventriculography*, best assesses functional anatomy of the CSF spaces. These radioisotope CSF flow studies are superior in detecting interruption of CSF flow in patients with LM when compared to cranial or spine CT or MR and are seen in 30% of all patients with LM due to solid cancers. Therefore, flow studies provide the best radiographic assessment of CSF circulation.

Patients with suspected LM should undergo a sequential method of evaluation including: (a) CSF analysis for pathologic confirmation, (b) contrast-enhanced cranial CT or MR for detection of bulky disease, (c) CT myelography or spine MR to define bulky disease, and (d) radioisotope CSF flow studies.

The treatment of LM varies because there are no well-accepted therapies. Furthermore, all established and published treatments are palliative. Because LM involves the entire neuraxis, treatment is designed to accompany the entire subarachnoid space, including the ventricular system, cisterns, and spinal subarachnoid space.

Only three chemotherapeutic agents are currently used for intra-CSF drug administration in patients with LM. These include methotrexate, cytosine arabinoside (or the depot formulation liposomal cytarabine), and thioTEPA. At present, no compelling data suggest an improved response when using multiple agents versus single agent intra-CSF drug therapy in the treatment of LM. Notwithstanding the pharmacokinetic advantages of intraventricular CSF drug administration as compared with intralumbar CSF drug administration, only two studies document that this method of administration results in improved patient survival when compared with intralumbar drug administration.

In patients with LM, the response to treatment is a function primarily of clinical improvement of LM-related neurologic signs and symptoms and secondarily of CSF cytology (in patients with positive cytology). In general, only pain-related neurologic symptoms improve with treatment. Neurologic symptoms such as confusion, cranial nerve deficits, ataxia, and segmental weakness minimally improve or stabilize with successful treatment.

Because progression of systemic cancer accounts for 50–60% of LM deaths, and treatment-related complications for another 5%, it is difficult to assess response rates for patients with truly progressive LM. Given these constraints, the treatment of LM is palliative and rarely curative, with a range of overall survival of 2–6 months (median 3 months) and with only 10–15% of patients alive at 1 year.

Paraneoplastic Disorders

Paraneoplastic syndromes have practical clinical importance despite the fact that they affect only a very small percentage (1–2%) of cancer patients. For patients with a known cancer diagnosis, the treating physician needs to differentiate paraneoplastic syndromes from the more common neuro-oncological disorders such as metastases or the various neurologic complications of cancer treatment. Paraneoplastic syndromes are an important consideration in patients without a known neoplasm, since, in most patients, the neurologic symptoms are the presenting feature of their tumor. Prompt recognition of a paraneoplastic syndrome in such a patient should lead to a careful search for an otherwise occult tumor.

A variety of paraneoplastic syndromes due to remote effects of cancer on the nervous system have been defined (Table 21.1). The majority of these syndromes are uncommon, and only some of the more frequently presenting syndromes will be discussed.

▼

Pearls and Perils

Leptomeningeal metastasis

▶ Leptomeningeal metastasis may present with brain, cranial nerve, or spinal cord symptoms.

▶ Coexistent brain metastases or hydrocephalus is not uncommon and requires evaluation.

▶ Cerebrospinal fluid cytology is false-negative in 40% or more of patients.

Table 21.1 Paraneoplastic or remote effects of cancer on the nervous system

Brain and cranial nerves
- ▶ Paraneoplastic cerebellar degeneration
- ▶ Opsoclonus-myoclonus
- ▶ Limbic encephalitis
- ▶ Optic neuritis
- ▶ Retinal degeneration

Spinal cord
- ▶ Necrotizing myelopathy
- ▶ Myelitis
- ▶ Subacute motor neuropathy
- ▶ Motor neuron disease

Peripheral nerves and ganglia
- ▶ Subacute or chronic sensorimotor peripheral neuropathy
- ▶ Acute polyradiculoneuropathy (Guillain-Barré syndrome)
- ▶ Mononeuritis multiplex
- ▶ Brachial neuritis
- ▶ Sensory neuronopathy
- ▶ Autonomic neuronopathy

Neuromuscular junction and muscle
- ▶ Lambert-Eaton myasthenic syndrome
- ▶ Myasthenia gravis
- ▶ Dermatomyositis, polymyositis
- ▶ Acute necrotizing myopathy
- ▶ Neuromyopathy
- ▶ "Stiff man" syndrome

Encephalomyeloradiculitis

Three distinct classes of paraneoplastic autoantibodies have been identified:

1. Tumor and neuron-/muscle-restricted autoantibodies reactive with plasma membrane constituents. These antibodies are potentially pathogenic for the nervous system; the best characterized are the antinicotinic acetylcholine receptor antibodies (associated with thymoma resulting in myasthenia gravis) and the anti–calcium channel antibodies (associated with small-cell lung cancer resulting in the Lambert-Eaton myasthenic syndrome).

2. Tumor and neuron-/muscle-restricted autoantibodies reactive with cytoplasmic and nuclear constituents. Antibodies of this class are valuable as markers of specific underlying tumors but have not been demonstrated to be pathogenic. Examples include anti-Purkinje cell cytoplasmic antibodies (called anti-Yo) and antineuronal nuclear antibodies type 1 (called anti-Hu) and type 2 (called anti-Ri).

3. Non organ–specific autoantibodies. Antibodies of this class (for example, antinuclear, antismooth muscle, and antimitochondrial) are frequently associated with thymoma, small-cell lung cancer, hepatoma, and melanoma.

The major diagnostic challenge presented by neurologic paraneoplastic disorders occurs when the physician is confronted with a patient who has serious and often disabling neurologic symptoms for which no cause is apparent. Certain features, however, should suggest consideration of a paraneoplastic syndrome. Most paraneoplastic syndromes evolve subacutely over days or weeks and then stabilize. In general, most neurologic paraneoplastic syndromes are usually severe. The majority of patients have substantial neurologic disability, which is acquired in a relatively short period of time. Additionally, neurologic paraneoplastic syndromes are clinically characteristic. Cerebellar degeneration, limbic encephalitis, opsoclonus-myoclonus, and the Lambert-Eaton myasthenic syndrome suggest that the disorder is paraneoplastic. However, none of these syndromes, even the most characteristic, is invariably associated with cancer (Table 21.2). Cerebrospinal fluid pleocytosis, elevated protein, and increased immunoglobulin levels often accompany paraneoplastic syndromes. In addition, paraneoplastic syndromes frequently affect one particular region of the nervous system, with additional subtle or minor findings suggesting dysfunction outside that area. Finally, some patients, as mentioned earlier, with neurologic paraneoplastic syndromes have distinctive autoantibodies in their serum and CSF. A variety of specific syndromes can be encountered and, in decreasing order of prevalence, are discussed below.

Paraneoplastic Cerebellar Degeneration

Paraneoplastic cerebellar degeneration is the most common paraneoplastic syndrome that affects the brain. This disorder may complicate any malignant tumor but is most

---

Table 21.2 Estimated incidence of neurologic disorders that are paraneoplastic syndromes

Syndrome	% paraneoplastic
Lambert-Eaton myasthenic syndrome	60
Subacute cerebellar degeneration	50
Subacute sensory neuronopathy	20
Opsoclonus-myoclonus (children)	50
Opsoclonus-myoclonus (adults)	20
Sensory motor peripheral neuropathy	10
Encephalomyelitis	10
Dermatomyositis	10

common with lung tumors (especially small-cell), gynecologic neoplasms (especially ovarian), and Hodgkin disease. Neurologic manifestations precede detection of associated tumor in more than half of patients. Cerebellar signs predominate, beginning with gait instability, progressing to severe truncal and appendicular ataxia, and often associated with dysarthria and nystagmus. Cerebellar dysfunction usually stabilizes, by which time, however, the patient is usually severely incapacitated. Several different antibodies react with Purkinje cells, the target cells of this disorder, in the cerebellum. The best characterized is an antibody designated as anti-Purkinje cell antibody or anti-Yo. This antibody is found in high titers in the serum and CSF of affected patients.

Opsoclonus-Myoclonus

Another paraneoplastic disorder is that of opsoclonus-myoclonus, which complicates neuroblastoma in children and a variety of tumors in adults. Opsoclonus may be isolated but is often associated with myoclonus affecting the trunk, limbs, and head, in addition to ataxia in varying combinations. In general, no autoantibody is detected, however, anti-Ri (or antineuronal antibody type 2) has occasionally been demonstrated.

Retinal Degeneration

Paraneoplastic retinal degeneration is usually associated with small-cell lung cancer; however, other tumors have been reported. Visual symptoms precede the detection of the underlying tumor, and the characteristic triad of affected patients includes severe photosensitivity, scotomatous visual loss, and attenuation of the retinal arteriole caliber. The electroretinogram is abnormal. However, visual evoked potentials are usually normal. Characteristic of this disorder is widespread degeneration and loss of photoreceptor cells. Often, anti-Ri (or antineuronal antibody type 2) antibodies are detected in serum and CSF.

Sensory Neuronopathy/Encephalitis

Sensory neuronopathy/encephalitis is characterized by a variety of clinical abnormalities including sensory neuropathy; autonomic neuropathy, myelopathy, including motor neuronopathy; cerebellar degeneration; brainstem abnormalities; and dementia (limbic encephalitis). Most patients with this disorder have small-cell lung cancer, although occasional patients have Hodgkin disease or other neoplasms. The sensory neuropathy is severe, begins with pain and paresthesias in the distal extremities, and rapidly ascends, often involving the trunk and face. All sensory modalities are lost, as are deep tendon reflexes, and patients are incapacitated by a severe sensory ataxia. Motor strength remains normal. The autonomic

neuropathy is manifested by postural hypotension, sexual impotence, and severe disabling constipation. The myelopathy is clinically characterized by lower motor neuron weakness, sometimes with upper motor neuron dysfunction (thereby resembling amyotrophic lateral sclerosis). The cerebellar degeneration is identical to that of paraneoplastic cerebellar degeneration discussed earlier. The clinical presentation of brainstem encephalitis is quite variable, with some patients having opsoclonus, others, cerebellar signs, and still others, central autonomic dysfunction. In addition, parkinsonian or other movement disorders have been described. Limbic encephalitis is characterized by severe loss of recent memory often associated with behavioral abnormalities, hallucinations, and seizures. In all patients, an antibody variously called anti-Hu or antineuronal antibody type 1 may be detected in serum or CSF.

Subacute Motor Neuronopathy

Subacute motor neuronopathy is a paraneoplastic disorder associated with Hodgkin disease or other malignant lymphomas. Characteristically, neurologic symptoms begin after diagnosis of the tumor and typically when the tumor is in remission. Subacute, progressive, painless lower motor neuron weakness affects the legs more than the arms. Sensory loss is mild despite profound weakness. No consistent antibody has been demonstrated.

Subacute or Chronic Sensorimotor Peripheral Neuropathy

Subacute or chronic sensorimotor peripheral neuropathy may be associated with any cancer but especially lung cancer. Signs are predominantly distal, symmetric, and more marked in the lower extremity with weakness, gait instability, sensory impairment, and loss of deep tendon reflexes.

Lambert-Eaton Myasthenic Syndrome

The Lambert-Eaton myasthenic syndrome is characterized by muscle weakness, particularly in the pelvic girdle. On occasion, patients complain of muscle pain and only rarely are extraocular muscle weakness or dysarthria encountered. Dysphagia, however, is a common finding. Symptoms of cholinergic dysautonomia, including dry mouth and impotence, occur in 50% of patients. Unexplained paresthesias are also commonly seen, as are absent deep tendon reflexes. Physiologically, the Lambert-Eaton myasthenic syndrome is characterized by a specific abnormality of the cholinergic presynaptic junction. Limited release of acetylcholine occurs due to a recently recognized antibody directed against presynaptic calcium channels.

Polymyositis-Dermatomyositis

Approximately 10% of patients with polymyositis or dermatomyositis have an underlying paraneoplastic syndrome. Most patients are older than 40 years of age, and breast, lung, ovarian, and gastric malignancies are most common in this population. As in noncancer-related polymyositis-dermatomyositis, clinical features involve proximal muscle weakness, characteristic skin changes, and typical abnormalities seen on muscle biopsy.

In general, treatment of neurologic paraneoplastic syndromes is unsuccessful. Exceptions are the Lambert-Eaton myasthenic syndrome, which responds well to plasmapheresis and often resolves after the tumor is successfully treated. However, most paraneoplastic syndromes affecting the nervous system run a course independent of the underlying cancer. In a few instances, successful treatment of the underlying neoplasm has yielded resolution of the paraneoplastic syndrome, but enthusiastic reports of other treatments, including plasmapheresis and immunosuppression with steroids, have not generally been borne out.

Annotated Bibliography

Cairncross G, Berkey B, Shaw E, et al. Phase III trial of chemotherapy plus radiotherapy compared with radiotherapy alone for pure and mixed anaplastic oligodendroglioma: Intergroup Radiation Oncology Group trial 9402. *J Clin Oncol* 2006;24(18):2707–2714.
A randomized trial of anaplastic oligodendrogliomas showing no benefit (except with respect to patients with co-deleted tumors showing an improvement in PFS) to neoadjuvant PCV chemotherapy in either nondeleted or co-deleted tumors.

Chamberlain MC. Neoplastic meningitis. *J Clin Oncol* 2005; 23(15):3605–3615.
A contemporary review of the diagnosis and management of leptomeningeal disease.

Chang SM, Parney IF, Huang W, et al. Patterns of care for adults with newly diagnosed malignant glioma. *JAMA* 2005;293: 557–564.
An overview of the Glioma Outcome Project.

Dalmau J, Graus F, Rosenblum MK, Posner JB. Anti-Hu-associated paraneoplastic encephalomyelitis/sensory neuronopathy. A clinical study of 71 patients. *Medicine* 1992; 71(2):59–72.
The best overview of the paraneoplastic disorder anti-Hu.

Dropcho EJ. Autoimmune central nervous system paraneoplastic disorders: Mechanisms, diagnosis, and therapeutic options. *Ann Neurol* 1995;37(S1):S102–S113.
The most recent and comprehensive review of paraneoplastic disorders.

Klibanski A, Zervas NT. Diagnosis and management of hormone-secreting pituitary adenomas. *N Engl J Med* 1991; 324(12):822–831.
Management of patients with hormone-producing pituitary adenomas.

Levin VA, ed. *Cancer in the nervous system*. New York: Churchill Livingstone, 1996.
An excellent monograph on cancer in the nervous system.

Loblaw DA, Perry J, Chambers A, et al. Systemic review of the diagnosis and management of malignant extradural spine cord compression: The Cancer Care Ontario Practice Guidelines Initiative's Neuro-Oncology Disease Site group. *J Clin Oncol* 2005;23:2028–2037.
A contemporary overview of metastatic epidural spinal cord compression.

Patchell RA, Tibbs PA, Walsh JW, et al. A randomized trial of surgery in the treatment of single metastases to the brain. *N Engl J Med* 1990;322(8):494–500.
The best phase III trial comparing surgery to radiotherapy in patients with solitary brain metastasis

Patchell R, Tibbs PA, Regine F, et al. Direct decompressive surgical resection in the treatment of spinal cord compression caused by metastatic cancer: A randomized trial. *Lancet* 2005;366;20:643–648.
The best phase III trial comparing radiotherapy with or without surgery in patients with epidural spinal cord compression.

Posner JB. Paraneoplastic syndromes. *Neurologic Clin* 1991; 9(4):919–939.
An excellent review of paraneoplastic disorders.

Rockhill J, Mrugala M, Chamberlain MC. Intracranial meningiomas: An overview. *J Neurosurg Neurosurg Focus* 2007; 23(4):E1.
An excellent overview of meningiomas

Stewart LA. Chemotherapy in adult high-grade glioma: A systemic review and meta-analysis of individual patient data from 12 randomized trials. *Lancet* 2002;359:1011–1018.
One of two meta-analyses demonstrating a 5-6% improvement in overall survival with the inclusion of adjuvant chemotherapy in malignant gliomas.

Sundaresan N, Steinberger AA, Moore F, et al. Indications and results of combined anterior-posterior approaches for spine tumor surgery. *J Neurosurg* 1996;85:438–446.
An overview of surgical approaches in patients with metastatic epidural spinal cord metastases.

Stupp R, Mason WP, van den Bent M, et al. Radiotherapy plus concomitant and adjuvant temozolomide for glioblastoma. *N Eng J Med* 2005;352,987–996.
A randomized trial by the EORTC defining a new standard of care for patients with newly diagnosed GBM.

van den Bent MJ, Carpentier AF, Brandes AA, et al. Adjuvant procarbazine, lomustine and vincristine improves progression free survival but not overall survival in newly diagnosed anaplastic oligodendrogliomas and oligoastrocytomas: A randomized European Organization for Research and Treatment of Cancer Phase III trial. *J Clin Oncol* 2006;24(18): 2715–2722.
A randomized trial of anaplastic oligodendrogliomas showing no benefit to neoadjuvant PCV chemotherapy in either nondeleted or co-deleted tumors (i.e., regardless of genotype).

Wasserstrom WR, Glass JP, Posner JB. Diagnosis and treatment of leptomeningeal metastases from solid tumors: Experience with 90 patients. *Cancer* 1982;4:759–772.

The most frequently quoted review of carcinomatous meningitis, a classic paper.

Wong ET, Hess KR, Gleason MJ, et al. Outcomes and prognostic factors in recurrent glioma patients enrolled onto phase II clinical trials. *J Clin Oncol* 1999;17:2572–2578.

A retrospective evaluation of eight clinical trials in patients with recurrent malignant gliomas demonstrating the value of progression-free survival at 6 months and establishing benchmarks for subsequent trials.

Wrouski M, Arbit E, Burt M, Galicich JH. Survival after surgical treatment of brain metastases from lung cancer: A follow-up study of 231 patients treated between 1976 and 1991. *J Neurosurg* 1995;83:605–616.

The surgical management of patients with solitary brain metastasis.

Young Jr. WF, Scheithauer BW, Kovacs KT, et al. Gonadotroph adenoma of the pituitary gland: a clinicopathologic analysis of 100 cases. *Mayo Clin Proc* 1996;71:649–656.

A recent review of pituitary adenomas and their treatment.

CHAPTER 22

Dementing and Degenerative Disorders

Michael S. Rafii, Ronald J. Ellis, and Jody Corey-Bloom

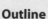

Outline

- ▶ Epidemiology of the dementias
- ▶ Dementias associated with neurodegenerative disorders
- ▶ Dementias associated with cerebrovascular disease
- ▶ Dementias associated with infectious, inflammatory, and immune disorders
- ▶ Dementias associated with systemic disorders
- ▶ Dementias associated with structural disorders of the brain
- ▶ Treatment and management issues in dementing disorders
- ▶ Summary

Dementia is a syndrome characterized by acquired impairments in multiple domains (including cognition, behavior, and functioning) that can be caused by over 70 disease entities or disorders. Of these, the three most common are Alzheimer disease (AD), dementia with Lewy bodies (DLB), and vascular dementia (VaD) (Figure 22.1). Although the diagnosis of dementia in clinically symptomatic patients is often straightforward at present, it is important to note that only 20 years ago there was considerable uncertainty about this syndrome. Patients followed-up after an initial diagnosis of dementia were later found to have other disorders in as many as 25–50% of cases. A majority of these had syndromal depression. More recently, agreement upon operational definitions has resulted in specific criteria, which have improved the diagnosis of dementia in modern clinical series. Most criteria, such as that of the *Diagnostic and Statistical Manual of Mental Disorders* (4th edition) (DSM-IV), require that the cognitive decline be severe enough to impair social or occupational activities.

Dementia represents a social burden of enormous magnitude. Three factors contribute to this burden. First, dementing illnesses are becoming increasingly prevalent as aging occurs in the population. Second, dementia is a functionally disabling disorder that endures for many years in affected individuals. Finally, dementia appears to interact with other illnesses to produce excess disability. Thus, dementia affects individuals with age-related disabilities from stroke, heart disease, and musculoskeletal disorders, for example. Dementia may unmask latent illnesses, such as depression and nutritional deficiency. With treatment of these concurrent conditions, clinical improvement may occur, but progressive decline due to the underlying neurodegenerative dementing illness resumes eventually. This does not diminish the importance of treatment for these concurrent illnesses, which can greatly improve the quality of an individual's life.

Because it is not possible in the space provided to give a detailed discussion of every disease entity capable of producing dementia, we will focus on the more common disorders, and on those for which the primary clinical presentation is a dementia syndrome. Less common disorders, and those for which dementia is a secondary clinical manifestation, will be addressed only briefly in the text and in tables. Treatments specific to pathophysiologically defined disease processes will be discussed in appropriate sections. The final section will address general management strategies for selected clinical problems that may be seen in any of the various dementing disorders.

Epidemiology of the Dementias

Community surveys have generated widely varying estimates of dementia prevalence, ranging from 5% to 15% in persons over age 65 years. The differences in these estimates are determined in part by the criteria used by investigators to identify dementia cases. Nevertheless, even when consistent guidelines are used, a certain level of disagreement remains. Another source of variability is real

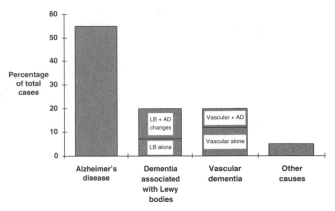

Figure 22.1 Relative frequencies of the common dementing illnesses. *AD,* Alzheimer disease; *LB,* Lewy bodies.

differences between communities in risk factors for disease (e.g., gene frequencies, cerebrovascular risk factors, and education) and in age distributions. Subjects over age 85 are probably underrepresented in most community surveys. In part, this is because such subjects are reluctant to participate in studies, or because they reside in residential facilities or nursing homes that are not distributed uniformly throughout the communities and may not be sampled adequately.

Although uncertainty remains as to the precise population frequency of dementia, all studies agree that advancing age is the single most important determinant of risk. Thus, the age-specific prevalence of dementia rises exponentially, doubling with every 5-year increase in chronological age between 65 and 85 (Figure 22.2). To a great extent, these figures reflect age-related increases in the prevalence of AD itself. Estimates of the prevalence of dementia in those over the age of 85 range from 25% to 47%, the latter figure obtained in the seminal but controversial East Boston study by Evans. During the next several decades, the continuing rapid increase in the proportion of individuals over age 85 in the United States will contribute to a precipitous rise in the absolute numbers of patients with dementia.

Dementias Associated with Neurodegenerative Disorders

Alzheimer Disease

Alzheimer disease, the most prevalent cause of dementia in the elderly, is defined both by its clinical features and by its unique pathology. In 1907, Alois Alzheimer described the presence of neuritic plaques (he termed these "miliary bodies") and neurofibrillary tangles in the neocortex, hippocampus, and other regions in the brain of a patient who died in her fifties with a progressive dementia. During the first half of the 20th century, this disease

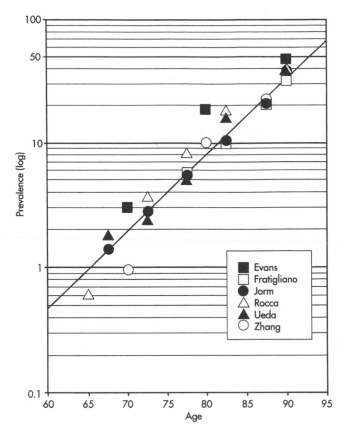

Figure 22.2 Semilog plot of dementia prevalence versus age.

was considered to be a disorder of the presenium. However, as cases of dementia in older individuals were studied systematically, it became apparent that the clinical and pathologic features observed in presenile and senile patients were identical. It was finally appreciated that AD is one of the most prevalent and malignant disorders of aging.

Risk factors

Advancing age. As noted previously, age is the single most important risk factor for AD. Alzheimer disease increases dramatically in both prevalence and incidence after the age of 65, and doubles approximately every 5 years in persons between 65 and 95 years of age. More than 14% of individuals older than 65 years have AD, and the prevalence increases to at least 40% in individuals older than 80 years.

Genes and family history. Next to age, the most important risk factor for AD is a positive family history. Individuals with a first-degree relative (mother, father, sibling) with AD show a three- to fourfold, age-corrected increase in risk. The relative risk increases to 7.5 in persons who have two or more first-degree relatives with AD.

In families with early (ages 40–60) disease onset, AD is inherited in an autosomal dominant manner. Investigators have now identified and sequenced three genes responsible for more than 90% of these early-onset familial cases. In order of frequency, these mutations involve the presenilin-1 (PS-1) gene on chromosome 14, the presenilin-2 (PS-2) gene on chromosome 1, and the amyloid precursor protein (APP) gene on chromosome 21. Over 120 different point mutations on these three genes have been identified.

Apolipoprotein E. The story is different in late-onset (after age 65) AD. The e4 allele of apolipoprotein E (APOE e4) is now recognized as a major susceptibility risk factor for the development of sporadic AD. The e4 allele is present in 26% of the general population, with the other principal allelic variants being e2 and e3. Subjects homozygous for APOE e4 have an 85% chance of developing AD by age 85, whereas those heterozygous for the allele have a 45–50% chance, and those with no e4 alleles have a 5–15% chance. Overall, the risk of developing AD is increased five- to tenfold in subjects homozygous for the APOE e4 allele, and two- to fourfold in subjects who are heterozygous. Thus, the e4 allele is the major susceptibility gene for sporadic late-onset AD and is responsible for about 40% of cases. An additional effect of the e4 allele is to decrease the age of onset of AD. In one study, the mean age of AD onset was 68 years for e4/e4 homozygotes, 76 years for e4 heterozygotes, and 86 years for persons lacking an e4 allele.

The identification of these genetic determinants and susceptibility factors is likely to play a major role in the eventual development of methods to prevent or delay the onset of AD. At a more practical level, however, physicians need to deal with the question of whether to do genetic testing in specific patients and their families. Since up to 50–60% of late-onset AD patients do not possess an e4 allele, genotyping is currently not recommended for predictive risk assessment except within specific research environments.

Education. Several studies indicate that lack of education is a risk factor for AD. Uneducated persons have a twofold increase in risk when compared with those who have more than 6 years of education. Both the prevalence and incidence of dementia, especially AD, are lower among persons with higher degrees of education.

Gender. Alzheimer disease occurs in about twice as many women as men. The mechanisms responsible for this are unclear. However, some factors that may account for this include an abrupt decline in estrogen production in postmenopausal women, differential longevity of women, and differences in education.

Head injury. Head injury, sufficient to produce loss of consciousness, has been reported to be a significant risk factor for AD in some studies but not others. There is now evidence that head injury in a person with at least one APOE e4 allele markedly increases the risk of developing AD.

Mild cognitive impairment

Mild cognitive impairment (MCI) is a clinical transitional state between the cognitive changes of aging and the earliest clinical features of dementia. As such, it does not represent an extreme of normal aging but should be considered an incipient stage of dementia. Early detection is the key to delaying progression to dementia. The prevalence of MCI is about 12–15% among nondemented individuals over the age of 65 years. The original Petersen criteria for MCI centered on memory impairment: (a) memory complaint, preferably corroborated by an informant; (b) memory deficit for age and education; (c) preserved general cognitive function; (d) intact activities of daily living; (e) not demented. The construct of MCI has since been expanded to encompass a wider range of early cognitive symptomatology. The new criteria include any cognitive complaint by a patient or informant. A determination must then be made as to whether a true definable deficit is present. This is typically done through a detailed history, mental status examination and, often, formal neurocognitive testing. There must be a decline in cognitive function with preservation of most activities of daily living, such that the individual does not meet criteria for dementia. The clinician must then decide whether memory impairment is part of the clinical picture. If so, the patient is categorized as amnestic MCI; if not, the patient is characterized as nonamnestic MCI. It is then determined if a single cognitive domain or multiple domains are involved. Domains typically include memory, language, executive function, or visuospatial skills. The potential subtypes of MCI thus include: amnestic MCI, single domain; amnestic MCI, multiple domain; nonamnestic MCI, single domain; and nonamnestic MCI, multiple domain.

Patients with MCI, especially those with amnestic MCI, often have similar pathology to those with AD. In fact, patients with amnestic MCI typically have pathologic changes intermediate between normal aging and AD. Pathology in amnestic MCI usually consists of medial temporal lobe atrophy, medial temporal lobe intracellular neurofibrillary tangles composed of phosphorylated protein, and sparse diffuse extracellular neocortical amyloid plaques.

With regard to progression to dementia, MCI patients typically progress at a rate of 10–15% per year (as compared to normal elderly, who progress at a rate of 1–2% per year). Severity of symptoms, including greater memory impairment at baseline or involvement of multiple cognitive domains, predicts a faster rate of progression to dementia. Hippocampal, ventricular, and whole-brain atrophy on magnetic resonance imaging (MRI), in addition to hypometabolism in the parietal and temporal lobes on functional imaging using 2-[^{18}F] fluoro-2-deoxy-D-glucose (FDG) and positron emission tomography (PET) scan (the FDG-PET scan), predict progression to dementia. The presence of one or more APOE e4 alleles also predicts faster conversion to AD. Finally, certain biomarkers in the cerebrospinal fluid (CSF), including elevated τ and reduced amyloid β, predict more rapid progression to AD.

The American Academy of Neurology recommends the following evaluations for all individuals suspected of having MCI: noncontrast brain computed tomography (CT) or MRI, screening for depression, vitamin B$_{12}$ and thyroid function testing, with screening for syphilis in high-risk populations only. To date, no drug has convincingly demonstrated symptomatic or disease-delaying effects in MCI.

Protective factors

Several epidemiologic studies have suggested that anti-inflammatory drugs, including both steroids and nonsteroidal anti-inflammatory drugs (NSAIDs), may delay the onset and progression of AD. Persistent engagement in social and leisure activities (both cognitive and physical), in addition to effortful mental activities, may also reduce the risk of AD. Finally, fish consumption and higher dietary intake of antioxidants has been associated with a lower risk of developing AD in several prospective studies.

Pathogenesis

The pathologic hallmarks of AD include brain atrophy, neuronal death, synaptic loss, and the presence of neurofibrillary tangles (NFT) and senile (neuritic) plaques. A significant loss of large neurons occurs in association areas of the cerebral cortex and in the hippocampal formation, particularly the entorhinal cortex. Cholinergic neurons in the basal forebrain nucleus of Meynert are lost as well. Decrements in cortical choline acetyltransferase due to degeneration of this system may play a major role in the memory deficits of AD, although perhaps not as early as had previously been suggested. Even more marked is the loss of presynaptic endings in these regions of the brain, the severity of which shows a high correlation with the extent of cognitive loss in the year prior to autopsy.

Consensus with regard to the pathologic course of AD has only recently been achieved. Plaques and tangles are found in the entorhinal cortex in many cognitively normal older individuals. As AD develops, however, these changes spread to the neocortex, with their highest concentrations in the parietal and temporal association cortices. There is relative sparing of the primary visual, auditory, somatosensory, and motor cortices.

Neurofibrillary tangles contain numerous paired helical filaments (PHF) composed of hyperphosphorylated τ protein, a protein normally present in axons, stabilizes the microtubular transport system. In AD, hyperphosphorylation of τ leads to detachment of τ from microtubules and formation of insoluble PHF, which aggregate in the body of the neuron.

The neuritic plaque consists of a collection of abnormal nerve endings surrounding a core of amyloid. This amyloid is derived from soluble β-amyloid peptides (mostly Aβ40 and Aβ42), which complex with a variety of other proteins to form highly insoluble β-pleated fibrils. In vitro, β-amyloid is neurotoxic. The β-amyloid peptide is a minor cleavage product of APP, which is secreted by neurons. The gene for APP is located on chromosome 21 and is triplicated in individuals with Down syndrome, all of whom develop the pathologic features of AD by age 40.

An additional important pathologic finding in many Alzheimer brains is the presence of β-amyloid in cerebral and meningeal blood vessels. When the concentration of vascular β-amyloid is particularly high, cerebral hemorrhages or ischemic strokes may result. It is possible that many of the cases of mixed vascular and Alzheimer dementia represent strokes due to superimposed vascular amyloidosis rather than arteriosclerotic disease.

Clinical features

The course of AD has been described as "tri-linear." Early on, the progression of the disease is often slow—in some cases so slow that the diagnosis becomes suspect. Later, as progression accelerates and dramatic changes are apparent on mental status examination, the diagnosis becomes evident (Table 22.1). Finally, a period of severe cognitive impairment occurs during which even basic activities of daily living are lost, eventually culminating in death.

Inability to recall recently learned information such as lists, telephone numbers, or appointments is a typical early symptom of AD. Although memory difficulties are a widely recognized feature of the disease, other behavioral and mental disturbances may occur concurrently. Patients who are actively employed may experience difficulty in organizing their work activities or in problem solving, leading to crucial business mistakes. Individuals who are in retirement may experience difficulty in pursuing hobbies, especially intellectual pursuits or games that require mnemonic and associative mental abilities, such as bridge. Family members report that patients ask the same questions repeatedly. Spontaneous speech is interrupted by word-finding pauses, and circumlocutions may replace the names of people, objects, or locations. As dementia progresses, many patients become more recognizably aphasic. Visuospatial impairment in AD results in symptoms such as misplacing objects or getting lost, difficulty with recognizing and drawing complex figures, and impaired driving. Difficulty with calculation (affecting skills such as handling money), apraxia, and agnosia are further problems that develop in AD. Apraxia may impair

---

Table 22.1 Alzheimer disease

Discriminating features

Early

► Early impairment of recent memory
► Normal motor, sensory and cerebellar function
► Relatively preserved social comportment

Later

► Gradually, progressive deterioration in language, visuospatial abilities, and other cognitive abilities

Consistent features

Early

► Inability to recall recent events
► Depression
► Delusions (stealing, jealousy)
► Loss of driving abilities

Later

► Increasing dependence in activities of daily living
► Agitation, anxiety
► Sleep disturbance
► Weight loss
► Delusions, hallucinations

Variable features

Early

► Progressive aphasia
► Visual agnosia
► Hallucinations (visual)
► Mild Parkinsonism (bradykinesia, facial masking, gait abnormality)

Later

► Progressive Parkinsonism
► Rigidity with contractures
► Myoclonus
► Seizures

---

activities such as operating appliances or dressing. As might be expected, more complex skills tend to break down first, while highly overlearned motor tasks (e.g., playing a musical instrument, using tools) may be retained until relatively late in the course. Agnosia develops in middle to late stages of AD and includes features such as failing to recognize family members or spouses. Deficits in problem solving, abstraction, reasoning, decision-making, and judgment may become apparent. Patients may have difficulty with organizing complex tasks such as a vacation trip, large family meal, or financial and other business deals. Impaired judgment may lead to unusual susceptibility to requests or solicitations and difficulty driving. On the other hand, social comportment and interpersonal skills are often strikingly preserved in AD, and may remain relatively intact long after memory and insight have been lost.

Behavioral or psychiatric symptoms occur frequently in AD. Over and above a general decline of activity and interest in virtually all patients with AD, depressive symptoms occur in as many as 50% of patients, although major depression is uncommon. Delusions are frequently encountered in AD, although they are rarely as systematized as in schizophrenia. They often have a paranoid flavor, with fears of personal harm, theft of personal property, and marital infidelity. Hallucinations, primarily visual, are much less common than delusions, occurring in up to 20% of patients. In addition to depressive and psychotic symptoms, patients with AD show a wide range of behavioral abnormalities including agitation, wandering, and sleep disturbances, especially as the disease progresses.

These disturbances of cognition and behavior stand in marked contrast to the relative preservation of basic motor and sensory skills, as well as personality and social comportment, seen especially early in AD. Thus, to the casual observer, many early Alzheimer patients appear normal. Clinically, there is a lack of focal findings on detailed neurologic examinations. One exception is mild parkinsonism—bradykinesia, facial masking, and gait abnormalities, sometimes accompanied by a postural tremor—which may develop in a substantial number of patients. The bedside mental status examination in early

---

▼

Pearls and Perils

Alzheimer disease

► Alzheimer disease (AD) is the most frequent type of dementia in elderly persons.
► Age is the single most important risk factor for AD. Prevalence of AD doubles approximately every 5 years in persons between 65 and 95.
► Neuropathologic hallmarks of AD are brain atrophy, neurofibrillary tangles, neuritic plaques, neuronal death, and synaptic loss.
► Apolipoprotein E allele status is a major susceptibility risk factor for the development of sporadic AD.
► Memory loss is the cardinal and typically earliest symptom of AD. Deficits in memory and at least one other domain of cognitive functions with impairments in social and occupational functioning are required for the diagnosis of AD.
► Mental status examination is critical and neuropsychological tests are important in difficult cases. Blood chemistries and brain imaging are essential to rule out other causes of dementia.
► Current U.S. Food and Drug Administration (FDA)-approved AD treatments include four cholinesterase inhibitors and one N-methyl-D-aspartate (NMDA) receptor channel blocker.

AD reveals difficulty with delayed recall of word lists, stories, and similar material—for example, the phrase "John Brown, 42 Market Street, Chicago." Although patients have no difficulty with immediate repetition of this name and address (demonstrating that they have adequate registration), they are nevertheless unable to recall the material after just a few minutes, even when provided with cues. Impairment in category fluency is another important early finding. Given 60 seconds to produce as many animal names as possible, patients are able to generate only a short list, usually fewer than 10 names.

As the disease progresses, other areas of cognition become involved in addition to memory and verbal fluency. These areas include language, spatial and constructional skills, and conceptual or semantic knowledge. The "draw a clock" test is particularly useful in demonstrating a loss of complex concepts (the idea of a clock and how its parts interrelate to signify the time) and ability to reconstruct these concepts in the form of a drawing (Figure 22.3).

Diagnosis

Autopsy studies have shown that the accuracy of the clinical diagnosis of probable AD using NINCDS-ADRDA (National Institute of Neurological and Communicative Diseases and Stroke-Alzheimer's Disease and Related Disorders Association) criteria (Table 22.2) can reach 90%.

The diagnosis requires historical evidence of an insidious onset and functional decline (e.g., loss of ability to handle money). Mental status examination is critical, and neuropsychological tests are very important in difficult cases. Blood chemistries and brain imaging are essential to rule out metabolic disorders, vascular disease, and space-occupying brain lesions that may be mistaken for AD. These tests may include thyroid function studies, vitamin B_{12} levels, and brain CT or MRI. With positron emission tomography (PET) or single photon emission computed tomography (SPECT) imaging, a pattern of biparietal decrease in cerebral blood flow is sometimes helpful in diagnosis, although functional imaging is not routinely used in clinical practice. Cerebrospinal fluid tests for τ and β-amyloid peptide may be of research interest, but definitive diagnosis is still based upon autopsy findings. Table 22.3 lists some of the circumstances in which specialist consultation may be worthwhile.

Treatment

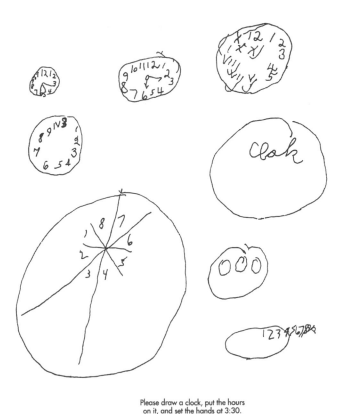

Please draw a clock, put the hours
on it, and set the hands at 3:30.

Figure 22.3 Clock drawings created by patients with Alzheimer disease. Instructions read to the patient are printed at the bottom.

Table 22.2 Summary of NINCDS-ADRDA criteria for the clinical diagnosis of Alzheimer disease (AD)

Level of diagnostic certainty	Required features
Definite AD	Neuropathologic tissue diagnosis by autopsy or biopsy
	Clinical dementia, as defined below
Probable AD	Deficits in memory and at least one other domain of cognitive functioning, such as language or visuospatial abilities documented by mental status examination and preferably detailed neuropsychological testing
	Absence of delirium or sensory impairments accounting for the cognitive deficits
	Insidious onset between ages 40 and 90 years
	Progressive course with no focal neurologic findings
	Absence of other conditions capable of producing dementia, such as stroke
Possible AD	Meets first two criteria under "Probable AD," and
	a) course is atypical – e.g. subacute onset, isolated progressive aphasia, right parietal syndrome
	or
	b) another illness capable of producing dementia is present (most commonly stroke or depression), but is not judged to be the primary cause of the dementia syndrome

Table 22.3 When specialists can be helpful

Clinical presentation	Differential diagnosis	Evaluation or intervention	Appropriate specialist
Depressive symptoms plus cognitive change	Alzheimer's disease versus depressive pseudodementia	Trial of antidepressant	Psychiatrist
Mild cognitive and functional complaints but normal mental status examination	Normal versus early Alzheimer's disease	Neuropsychological testing	Neurologist and neuropsychologist
Motor changes in a patient with mild or moderate dementia	Alzheimer's disease vs. Lewy body variant, vascular disease, normal pressure hydrocephalus	Detailed neurological evaluation	Neurologist
Significant cognitive slowing in a patient with mild or moderate dementia	Alzheimer's disease vs. Lewy body variant, progressive supranuclear palsy, subcortical vascular disease	Neurological and neuropsychological evaluation	Neurologist and neuropsychologist

To date, the United States Food and Drug Administration (FDA) has proved four acetylcholinesterase (AChE) inhibitors and one N-methyl-D-aspartate (NMDA) receptor antagonist for the treatment of AD (Table 22.4). AChE inhibitors, through inhibition of AChE, the enzyme that breaks down acetylcholine (ACh), prolong the action of ACh at postsynaptic receptors by preventing its hydrolysis.

Tacrine (Cognex). Tacrine (Cognex), a noncompetitive AChE inhibitor, was the first drug approved by the FDA in 1993 for the treatment of AD. It is generally of historical interest only since it is no longer being actively marketed.

Donepezil (Aricept). Donepezil (Aricept), a second-generation, reversible noncompetitive AChE inhibitor, was the second drug approved by the FDA for treatment of mild to moderate AD. The efficacy and safety of donepezil have been demonstrated in several double-blind, placebo-controlled, randomized clinical trials of both mild to moderate and more severe AD. In mild to moderate AD, donepezil was associated with a 2.5–2.9-point treatment effect on the Alzheimer's Disease Assessment Scale-Cognitive Section (ADAS-Cog). In addition, about 25% of mild to moderate AD subjects treated with donepezil showed noticeable clinical improvement on the Clinician's Interview Based Impression of Change-Plus Caregiver Input (CIBIC-Plus), compared with 11–14% of subjects

Table 22.4 Alzheimer disease (AD) treatments

	Tacrine	Donepezil	Rivastigmine‡	Galantamine	Memantine
Trade name	Cognex	Aricept	Exelon	Reminyl	Namenda
Mechanisms of actions	AChE inhibition Noncompetitive Reversible	AChE inhibition Noncompetitive Reversible	AChE inhibition Pseudo irreversible	AchE inhibition Competitive Reversible	NMDA receptor Antagonist Noncompetitive
Indication	Mild to moderate AD	Mild to moderate AD	Mild to moderate AD	Mild to moderate AD	Moderate to severe AD
Treatment effects (ADAS-Cog scores)	1.4–2.2	2.5–2.9	2.3–3.8	3.1–3.9	N/A
Dosage	80–160mg	5–10mg	3–12mg	8–24mg	10–20mg
Frequency	Four times per day	Daily	Twice daily	Twice daily	Twice daily
Titration period	Every 6 weeks	After 4–6 weeks	Every 4 weeks	Every 4–8 weeks	Every week
Half-life (hours)	3	70	1.5	7	60–80
Route of elimination	Hepatic (cytochrome P450 1A2)	Hepatic (cytochrome P450 2D6 and 3A4)	Hepatic/AChE	Hepatic (cytochrome P450 2D6 and 3A4)	Renal/hepatic
Typical side-effects	Cholinergic GI, hepatotoxicity	Cholinergic GI, muscle cramps	Cholinergic GI, anorexia	Cholinergic GI, anorexia	Confusion, agitation

‡The recently approved rivastigmine patch is available in two doses, 4.6 and 9.5 mg, and is applied once daily.

in placebo groups. In more severe AD patients (average Mini-Mental State Examination (MMSE) score at baseline of 12), significant treatment effects in favor of donepezil were observed on the MMSE, CIBIC-Plus, and Neuropsychiatric Inventory (NPI) in one 24-week study. Several studies have shown long-term benefit (more than 1 year) of donepezil in AD.

Generally speaking, donepezil is easy to use (once daily dosing with elimination half-life of 70 hours) and well tolerated, with relatively limited side effects. The major side effects are primarily gastrointestinal (nausea, vomiting, and diarrhea). In some patients, leg cramps and sleep disturbances (vivid dreams) have been occasionally reported with long-term use.

Rivastigmine (Exelon). Rivastigmine (Exelon), a pseudo irreversible AChE inhibitor that also inhibits butyrylcholinesterase, was the third drug approved by the FDA for the treatment of mild to moderate AD. Rivastigmine is metabolized primarily by AChE itself, with minimal involvement of the major cytochrome P450 isozymes. It also has relatively low plasma protein binding, with an elimination half-life of 1.5 hours. Rivastigmine is administrated twice daily.

The safety and efficacy of rivastigmine in the treatment of AD have been evaluated in three large double-blind, placebo-controlled, multicenter trials with over 2,100 mild to moderate AD patients. The 26-week U.S. study with 699 AD patients demonstrated an ADAS-Cog treatment–placebo difference of 3.8 points for high-dose and 2.1 points for low-dose rivastigmine. The other two studies also demonstrated a clinically and statistically significant benefit on cognition. However, 30–40% of patients in these trials suffered cholinergic side effects of nausea, vomiting, and diarrhea, in some cases due to rapid forced titration (weekly dosage increases). Weight loss and anorexia were observed occasionally. Long-term benefit (more than 1 year) of rivastigmine in AD was observed in one U.S. trial. In 2007, the FDA approved the Exelon Patch for the treatment of mild to moderate Alzheimer disease. The Exelon Patch is also approved to treat mild to moderate Parkinson disease dementia. The patch, applied once daily to the back, chest, or upper arm, circumvents issues with oral ingestion of pills, maintains steady blood levels of the drug, and reduces its gastrointestinal side effects.

Galantamine (Reminyl). Galantamine (Reminyl), a tertiary alkaloid, is a selective, reversible, and competitive AChE inhibitor, which was approved by the FDA in 2001 for symptomatic treatment of mild to moderate AD. In addition to its AChE inhibitory effect, galantamine may also enhance CNS cholinergic function through modulation of nicotinic ACh receptors, but the clinical significance of this is unknown. Like donepezil and rivastigmine, the major side effects are cholinergic, affecting primarily the gastrointestinal system.

Galantamine has been evaluated in four large clinical trials of 3 to 24 months' duration. Significant treatment effects were observed in mild to moderate AD patients treated with galantamine on cognitive performance, global function, behavior, and activities of daily living. In the 5-month and 6-month U.S. studies, about 34–35% of patients treated with galantamine achieved clinically meaningful (≥4 points) improvements in ADAS-Cog score, as compared to placebo (18–20%). In the 6-month study, the difference on ADAS-Cog score between galantamine and placebo groups was 3.9 points.

Thus, current AChE inhibitors have modest beneficial effects for mild to moderate AD patients. They are generally safe and easy to use, and have not been associated with significant drug–drug interactions. In addition to cholinergic side effects, AChE inhibitors could, in theory, exacerbate stomach ulcers, asthma, and cardiac arrhythmias.

Memantine (Namenda). Memantine (Namenda), a low to moderate affinity, noncompetitive NMDA receptor antagonist, is the latest drug approved by the FDA for the treatment of AD. Unlike AChE inhibitors, memantine is approved for moderate to severe AD and acts as an NMDA receptor open-channel blocker. It has been suggested that excessive activation of NMDA receptors may contribute to AD pathogenesis. Memantine is given twice daily, with a terminal elimination half-life of about 60–80 hours. It has no significant drug–drug interaction since it undergoes minimal metabolism and does not require CYP450 enzymes. Importantly, memantine has no significant effect on the action of AChE inhibitors and can be used concurrently with them.

Several large, multicenter, double-blind, placebo-controlled clinical trials in Europe and the United States have been conducted to study the safety and efficacy of memantine in the treatment of AD. To date, all published data come from trials with moderate to severe AD patients. In one U.S. trial, memantine treatment was associated with delay in both global (CIBIC-Plus) and functional deterioration. In addition, mean scores on the Severe Impairment Battery (a cognitive test for advanced AD patients) were also significantly better in the memantine-treated group. Similar results were observed in another U.S. trial in which the AD patients were already receiving donepezil.

Dementia with Lewy Bodies

Although still debated, DLB is perhaps the second most common cause of dementia in the elderly. Lewy bodies (LB), the neuronal inclusions classically associated with idiopathic Parkinson disease (PD), have been recognized as important in late-life dementia only within the past decade. Clinicopathologic correlation studies have identified three primary groups of patients in whom LB likely play a causal role in the development of dementia. These are (a) patients with PD who become demented (PD with dementia or PDD); (b) demented patients with both neocortical LB and Alzheimer-type neuropathologic changes (Lewy body variant of AD or LBV—the most common form of LB disease; and (c) patients with progressive dementia and diffuse neocortical LB pathology in isolation (diffuse Lewy body disease or DLBD).

Prevalence and risk factors

Despite the absence of cognitive changes in James Parkinson's original account of the disease, it is now clearly recognized that dementia occurs in as many as half of PD cases prior to death. In one community prevalence survey, 41% of patients with PD met neuropsychological and functional criteria for dementia. Patients most likely to develop dementia include those older than 70 years with severe motor impairment. The prevalence of dementia associated with cortical Lewy bodies, on the other hand, remains a subject of debate. The immunocytochemical stains necessary for reliable identification of cortical Lewy bodies were developed only recently. Thus, relatively few centers have published prevalence figures. Nevertheless, among the available data from neuropathologic case series, cortical Lewy bodies have been reported in 15–30% of clinically demented elderly. The vast majority of these brains show accompanying Alzheimer-type changes.

Pathogenesis

The classical LB of PD are eosinophilic cellular inclusions located in monoaminergic and cholinergic neurons of the locus ceruleus, substantia nigra, and basal nucleus of Meynert. They have a dense core surrounded by a lucent halo and require no special staining techniques for adequate visualization. In comparison, neocortical LB, the type most strongly linked to dementia, are smaller and lack a halo. They are reliably visualized with ubiquitin immunocytochemistry, although ∝-synuclein immunohistochemistry staining is more sensitive, visualizes more Lewy bodies, and also demonstrates Lewy neurites. The major component of the Lewy body is ∝-synuclein, a 140-amino acid protein, which is encoded by SNCA, a gene located on chromosome 4. The function of ∝-synuclein is unknown. Brains of patients with LBs demonstrate severe depletion of both cholinergic and dopaminergic markers.

Clinical features

Core clinical features of DLB include fluctuating cognition, prominent visual hallucinations, and parkinsonism. Cognitive decline occurs late in the course of PD, often 10 years after disease onset. It is characterized by impairment in executive functions, visuospatial skills, free-recall memory, and verbal fluency, consistent with a pattern of frontal/subcortical dementia. Patients with DLB, on the other hand, typically present with symptoms of memory impairment and mild extrapyramidal features. Bradykinesia, facial masking, and rigidity are the most frequent signs of parkinsonism in these patients. Resting tremor is distinctly uncommon. Formed visual hallucinations are frequent and may be elicited or exacerbated by levodopa treatment. In addition, rapid eye movement (REM) sleep disorder and autonomic dysfunction (orthostatic hypotension and carotid-sinus hypersensitivity) are common. The clinical presentation of DLBD is often indistinguishable from that of LBV, although the memory loss may be less severe.

Diagnosis

As with AD, definitive diagnosis of DLB rests on brain biopsy or autopsy. Generally speaking, the accuracy of the clinical diagnosis of DLB is relatively low based on the Consortium for DLB diagnostic criteria. Using these criteria against neuropathology, several studies have reported specificities of 71–100% but sensitivities of only 22–75%. The diagnosis of DLB is suspected clinically in patients who present with an AD-like dementia and manifest signs of mild parkinsonism or early and prominent visual hallucinations. Neuropsychological testing may help to distinguish pure AD from DLB. Matched for overall dementia severity, patients with LB show relatively more deficits in attention and executive function, verbal fluency, and visuospatial functions. Recognition memory and basic language functions are generally preserved until later in the course of disease. The importance of distinguishing so-called pure AD from DLB is that patients in the latter group may progress more rapidly and develop severe parkinsonism in response to treatment with neuroleptics.

Treatment

The treatment of DLB generally parallels that for AD. No controlled clinical trials have evaluated the treatment of parkinsonism in DLB, although case reports and small series of patients whose motor impairments were successfully treated with levodopa have been published. Clinical experience suggests that levodopa is probably less effective in treating motor impairments in DLB than in idiopathic PD patients. If anti-parkinsonism drugs are necessary, the lowest effective dose of levodopa should be used. Traditional neuroleptics and other dopamine blockers such as metoclopramide are probably best avoided. If necessary, the newer atypical antipsychotic medications can be used in the lowest effective dose with caution.

Although it has been suggested that AChE inhibitors may be more effective in treating DLB due to early and prominent CNS cholinergic dysfunction in these patients, only one double-blind, placebo-controlled, multicenter trial has evaluated the safety and efficacy of

AChE inhibitors in the treatment of DLB. A 5-month study of rivastigmine in DLB showed a significant benefit of treatment on behavioral symptoms as assessed by the NPI despite no significant benefit on cognition.

Frontotemporal Degenerative Dementias

Frontotemporal dementia (FTD) is a term applied to a group of clinical and pathologic disorders with significant heterogeneity but sharing a predilection for the frontal and anterior temporal cortices. As a group, they are thought to constitute about 5–10% of the degenerative dementias, but up to 50% of cases presenting before age 60; however, the literature on FTD is confusing since different terms and schemes have been used to describe this entity. As an overall clinical syndrome, authors often refer to FTD, Pick complex, Pick disease, or frontotemporal lobar degeneration. Although Kertesz and Munoz proposed the designation the *Pick complex of diseases* in 1998, most investigators appear to prefer the classification of frontotemporal lobar degeneration (FTLD) used by Neary and colleagues (1998), based on an international consensus conference, to recognize three clinical syndromes: behavioral variant of FTD (bvFTD), progressive nonfluent aphasia (PNFA), and progressive fluent aphasia/semantic dementia (SD).

Clinical features

Table 22.5 contrasts the clinical features of FTLD and other dementias with those of AD. The clinical features typical of FTLD include early onset; family history of dementia; changes in social demeanor, behavior, and personality; language difficulties; and impairments in planning, attention, and problem solving. Patients with bvFTD comprise about 50% of all FTLD cases. There is a 2:1 male predominance, and mean age at diagnosis is 58 years. Early decline in social interpersonal conduct, emotional blunting, and loss of insight are common. There may be a decline in personal hygiene and grooming, mental rigidity and inflexibility, distractibility, stereotyped behavior, hyperorality, and dietary changes. It can be fairly rapidly progressive with only about 3–4 years from diagnosis to death. Approximately 20% show an autosomal dominant inheritance pattern, and about 15% of FTD patients develop amyotrophic lateral sclerosis (ALS). This syndrome is referred to as FTD associated with motor neuron disease (FTD-MND). Progressive nonfluent aphasia (PNFA) or primary progressive aphasia (PPA) comprises about 25% of FTLD cases and shows a moderate rate of disease progression. The cognitive symptoms include changes in verbal fluency and pronunciation, in addition to word-finding difficulties, agrammatism, and phonemic paraphasias. Patients may have stuttering, impaired repetition, apraxia of speech, and may develop impaired executive function and working memory. Semantic dementia comprises slightly less than 20% of FTLD cases and has the slowest rate of disease progression (approximately 5 years from diagnosis to death). Most cases are sporadic without any clear pattern of heritability. Although patients can demonstrate behavioral symptoms such as emotional withdrawal, depression, mental rigidity, and compulsions, the characteristic hallmark is loss of word meaning, in addition to poor word recognition, naming, and word recall. There may also be agnosia for faces and objects. Clinical features of corticobasal syndrome (apraxia, cortical sensory loss, myoclonus, rigidity, bradykinesia, tremor, hemidystonia) and progressive supranuclear palsy (PSP; supranuclear gaze problems, axial rigidity, parkinsonism) can sometimes be seen as well.

Table 22.5 Discriminating features of dementias

Feature	Alzheimer Disease	Dementia with Lewy bodies	Frontotemporal dementia	Vascular dementia
Age at onset	Most 65 years or older	Most 65 years or older	Often 40–65 years	Most 65 years or older
Onset	Insidious with slowly progressive worsening	Insidious with slowly progressive worsening	Insidious with slowly progressive worsening	Sudden with stepwise deterioration
Presenting symptom	Memory	Memory	Language difficulties with anomia and paraphasias	Depends on the lesion site
Social skills	Typically preserved until dementia is advanced	Typically preserved until dementia is advanced	Often lost early	Depends on the lesion site
Other presenting symptoms	Depression Decline in category fluency	Visual hallucinations Parkinsonism REM sleep disorder	Impaired planning Disorganized behavior Apathy Lack of initiative Disinhibition	Focal neurologic symptoms or signs MRI or CT findings Other vascular events

Neuropathology

The neuropathologic findings in FTD are quite heterogeneous. On gross examination of the brain, FTD patients may have varying degrees of atrophy of the frontal and temporal lobes. The atrophy may be asymmetric and, in some cases, extend into the parietal lobes. Microscopically, there may be neuronal loss, microvacuolation, astrocytic gliosis and, in some cases, characteristic lesions such as ballooned neurons and Pick bodies. Using immunocytochemistry, however, the pathologist can evaluate for τ and ubiquitin inclusions. The presence or absence of τ-positive inclusions simplifies the classification into a tauopathy or a non-tauopathy.

Diagnosis and treatment

Except in cases with a clear family history, diagnosis rests on obtaining brain tissue at biopsy or autopsy. In some cases, brain MRI (frontal atrophy) or PET (anterior hypometabolism) may aid with diagnosis. No specific treatments are available, although symptomatic therapy can ameliorate some of the behavioral problems (see last section of this chapter). Consultation with a dementia specialist is helpful when a frontotemporal dementia is suspected, and particularly when there is a history of a similar disorder in family members.

Other Neurodegenerative Dementias

In several additional neurodegenerative diseases, dementia may be a prominent, although usually secondary, manifestation. In all of these, clinical diagnosis is best coordinated through consultation with a neurologist specializing in dementia.

Huntington disease is an autosomal dominant disorder characterized by behavioral changes and chorea at onset. Difficulties with complex mental activities may be seen early in the course of the illness. In patients with advanced disease, dementia is universal. The cause is an unstable trinucleotide repeat on chromosome 4, and genetic testing is widely available. Age at onset decreases as the length of the abnormal triplet repeat increases.

Progressive supranuclear palsy, or the Steele-Richardson-Olszewski syndrome, is a degenerative disorder of unknown etiology characterized neuropathologically by atrophy of the midbrain with neuronal loss, gliosis, and globose tangle formation in subcortical and brainstem nuclei. The prototypical presentation involves loss of volitional vertical eye movements, rigidity, and frequent falls, with gait instability and retropulsion. The earliest complaints are of cognitive difficulty in more than one-quarter of cases. Progressive supranuclear palsy accounts for some misdiagnoses of AD in large clinicopathologic series. The diagnosis in living patients is based on the history and neurologic examination. The cognitive impairment of PSP is typically "subcortical," which is in contrast to the "cortical" pattern of deficits observed in AD. Rostral midbrain atrophy in PSP is detected by mid-sagittal plane MRI. The shape of the atrophy looks like the bill of a hummingbird (hence, "hummingbird sign").

Other uncommon neurodegenerative disorders in which dementia may be a prominent manifestation are the multiple system atrophies, Guamanian ALS-parkinsonism-dementia complex (also known as Lytico-Bodig), and dentatorubropallidoluysian atrophy, a genetic disorder due to an unstable trinucleotide repeat on chromosome 12.

Dementias Associated with Cerebrovascular Disease

The designation *vascular dementia* implies the presence of a dementia syndrome accompanied by evidence from the clinical history, neurologic examination, and neuroimaging studies of cerebrovascular lesions causally connected to the dementia. This definition encompasses a variety of clinical presentations and pathophysiologies. Brain infarctions differ in location, size, and extent across patients, producing many different constellations of localizing signs and symptoms. Use of the plural, "dementias," emphasizes this heterogeneity.

Prevalence and Risk Factors

As a group, the vascular dementias are uncommon. However, in population-based studies, about 29–41% of dementia cases have some vascular pathology. Less than one-third of these represent "pure" vascular dementia syndromes, whereas the remainder are mixed disorders, with both cerebrovascular disease and other etiologies (most commonly AD) contributing to the clinical picture. The prevalence of the vascular dementias mirrors the prevalence of stroke. Almost half a million persons suffer stroke each year in the United States. Of these, 7–20% are demented with the first stroke, and 5% per year will become demented thereafter. In other industrialized countries, where the incidence of stroke is higher than in the United States, vascular dementias are also more common.

One of the biggest changes that has occurred in the field of vascular dementia is a name change that has evolved out of a sense that the prevalence of cognitive impairment caused by vascular disease is probably underestimated. Current criteria for vascular dementia emphasize the sequelae of strokes—putting the focus on the development of dementia. The new term *vascular cognitive impairment* (VCI) recognizes an important earlier stage and the notion of risk factors in a susceptible host, so-called "brain at risk."

Knowledge of stroke risk factors can be useful both for the diagnosis and management of patients with VCI.

Risk factors vary according to the pathophysiology of the underlying vascular lesions (Table 22.6). Broadly, the principal modifiable risk factors are hypertension, heart disease including atrial fibrillation, cigarette smoking, diabetes mellitus, and heavy alcohol consumption. Nonmodifiable risk factors include advancing age, gender, race, and ethnicity. Specific stroke subtypes are associated more or less strongly with individual risk factors. For example, lacunar strokes are related to hypertension and smoking, but not to heart disease.

Pathogenesis

Because the specific mechanisms by which cerebrovascular disease is produced may influence the manner in which patients present, it is useful to be familiar with some of the more common and classical of these pathogenic mechanisms. Table 22.6 lists several of these. Generally, VCI can be divided into large-vessel dementia (multi-infarct dementia and strategic infarct dementia), small-vessel dementia (lacunar state, Binswanger disease, and CADASIL [cerebral autosomal dominant arteriopathy with subcortical infarcts and leukoencephalopathy]), and hemorrhagic vascular dementia (lobar hemorrhage, subarachnoid hemorrhage, and subdural hematoma). Large-vessel thromboembolic disease and cardiogenic embolization are widely recognized by primary care physicians. Lacunar stroke and Binswanger disease are less familiar and may be confused with one another. CADASIL is a common form of hereditary arteriopathy affecting small to medium-sized arteries and causing subcortical infarcts, cognitive decline, and dementia. The pathognomonic changes are specific granular osmiophilic material (GOM) within the media adjacent to degenerated smooth muscle cells of the blood vessel wall. It is caused by mutations in the *Notch3* gene. Cerebral amyloid angiopathy is an underrecognized cause of both hemorrhagic and ischemic stroke. Risk factors include advancing age and the presence of concomitant AD. Granulomatous angiitis of the CNS (GACNS) may produce multifocal infarctions due to spasm and thrombosis of small cerebral vessels. The clinical presentation of GACNS may mimic that of hypertensive lacunes or Binswanger disease. Cerebral angiography and meningeal-cortical biopsy are necessary for reliable diagnosis. Another less common entity whose pathogenesis is poorly understood is granular cortical atrophy, in which microinfarctions are diffusely distributed in cortical layers.

The causal attribution of dementia to cerebrovascular disease in individual patients can be a source of disagreement among clinicians. Patients with AD, for example, frequently have infarcts that are causally unrelated to the dementia—that is, incidental strokes. In many cases, however, accompanying cerebrovascular disease may be pathophysiologically related to the dementia. In AD, parenchymal amyloid deposition results in plaques, whereas vascular amyloid deposition results in hemorrhages and infarcts. Conversely, patients with histories strongly suggestive of vascular dementia commonly have contributing medical or degenerative conditions that are sufficient to produce dementia in themselves. At issue is whether, in a specific case, the cerebrovascular lesions occupy a sufficient volume, hence damaging the particular brain structures necessary to impair multiple domains of cognition. In the case of isolated strokes of the cerebellum or lower brainstem structures, causal relationships are not tenable. However, when lesions affect the subcortical cerebral white matter, basal ganglia, or frontal lobes, for example, there is considerable room for debate.

Some general guidelines can clarify issues of causation in most cases. The likelihood that vascular lesions

---

Table 22.6 Pathogenesis of vascular cognitive impairment

Identifying lesions	Primary stroke mechanisms	Pathophysiology
Multiple cortical-subcortical infarcts in the distribution of large cerebral vessels (MCA, ACA, PCA)	• Large vessel thromboembolism • Cardiogenic embolism	• Atherosclerotic vascular disease • Atrial fibrillation, transmural myocardial infarction (MI), congestive heart failure
Strategic infarct – specific locations for higher functions	• Large vessel thromboembolism • Cardiogenic embolism	• Atherosclerotic vascular disease • Atrial fibrillation, transmural MI, congestive heart failure
Multiple small to medium-sized infarcts of subcortical gray and white matter ("lacunes")	• Thrombosis of small, penetrating arteries • CADASIL	• Microangiopathy, lipohyalinosis, fibrinoid necrosis • Granular osmiophilic material and thickening of the arterial wall
Multiple lobar hemorrhages and infarcts	• Weakening of small vessel walls with thrombosis and hemorrhage	• Cerebral amyloid angiopathy • Amyloid deposition in superficial cortical and meningeal vessels

MCA, middle cerebral artery; ACA, anterior cerebral artery; PCA, posterior cerebral artery.

are the primary cause of a dementia syndrome increases with the volume of tissue infarcted. Volumes of 100 cm^3 or more are virtually always associated with dementia; 50–100 cm^3 of infarcted tissue will very likely produce dementia. In comparison, less than 10 cm^3 of infarcted tissue rarely, if ever, results in dementia. When total infarct volume measures between 10 cm^3 and 50 cm^3, location becomes important. Small, strategically placed lesions of the medial thalamus, caudate, angular gyrus, basal forebrain, and hippocampus can cause dementia. In addition, there is an increasing probability that lesions will produce dementia if strokes have occurred in both cerebral hemispheres.

Clinical features

The spectrum of clinical manifestations of VCI is protean. Rapidity of onset and the tempo of progression of symptoms are important. Many patients become acutely symptomatic at the time of a diagnosed stroke and show subsequent stepwise accumulation of cognitive, motor, and sensory deficits. However, because some patients with Binswanger disease show an insidious, gradually progressive dementia, the diagnosis of vascular dementia is supported by, but does not require, abrupt onset and stepwise progression. Specific clinical signs commonly occur in patients with VCI. Pseudobulbar palsy is a condition in which dysarthria and dysphagia (with increased risk of aspiration pneumonia) are accompanied by an increase in the jaw jerk and snout reflex. This is frequently associated with pseudobulbar affect—an enhanced tendency to laugh or cry with only slight provocation. Spastic hemiparesis, paraparesis, or quadriparesis, and focal sensory loss, hemianopsia, or quadrantopia occur in varying combinations. In the absence of frank weakness, the gait may be impaired from deficits in the initiation or execution of movement, and incontinence frequently accompanies this. Table 22.7 relates some of these clinical signs and symptoms to the character of the underlying lesions and their pathophysiology.

In CADASIL, most patients present with one or several of the following clinical syndromes: migraine with aura (30%), ischemic events (transient ischemic attacks [TIAs] or subcortical infarcts, 85%), cognitive impairments (60%), and mood disorders (20%). Migraine with aura usually presents early (mean age of onset = 25 years). The mean age of onset of ischemic events is 46 years. Most of the ischemic events are recurrent subcortical TIAs or lacunar infarcts.

Diagnosis

Diagnosis of the VCI syndromes requires clinicians to integrate information from the medical history, presenting symptoms, neurologic examination, and laboratory and neuroimaging studies. The Hachinski Ischemic Score (HIS) has been widely used by neurologists in daily practice with relatively good sensitivity and specificity. Research diagnostic criteria such as those of the DSM-IV, the National Institute of Neurologic Disorders and Stroke and the Association Internationale pour la Recherche et l'Enseignement en Neurosciences (NINDS-AIREN), and State of California AD Diagnostic and Treatment Centers (ADDTC) criteria were designed to operationalize and systematize the integration of this information. They can be applied with reasonable reliability by experienced practitioners, but may be somewhat cumbersome for routine clinical use. All require the presence of a dementia syndrome as well as evidence of etiologically related cerebrovascular disease. Because of the high rate of misdiagnosis observed, consultation with a dementia specialist may be useful.

Table 22.7 Clinical presentations of some prototypical* vascular dementias

Identifying lesions	Clinical presentation	Risk factors
Multiple[†] cortical and subcortical infarcts in the distribution of major cerebral vessels (MCA, ACA, PCA)	• Abrupt onset in association with clinically diagnosed stroke • Stepwise progression • Focal neurologic signs including visual field defect, hemiparesis	CHF, CAD Atrial fibrillation Hypertension Diabetes mellitus
Multiple small to medium-sized infarcts of subcortical gray and white matter (lacunar state)	• Abrupt onset and stepwise progression‡ • Pseudobulbar palsy • Early incontinence without urologic cause • Gait disorder characterized as "magnetic," Parkinsonian or apractic	Hypertension Diabetes
Lobar hemorrhages or infarcts due to cerebral amyloid angiopathy	• Abrupt onset and stepwise progression • Neuroimaging showing multiple lobar cerebral hemorrhages	Age over 70 years Concomitant AD

*Individual patients are likely to demonstrate features from more than one of these categories.
†In unusual cases, a strategically placed single infarct—for example, involving the midline thalamus or the dominant caudate—may produce sufficient impairments in multiple cognitive domains to permit a diagnosis of dementia.
‡In so-called "Binswanger disease," onset may be insidious and progression gradual.

Pearls and Perils

Vascular cognitive impairment

▶ Mixed dementias are common, frequently resulting from combinations of neurodegenerative disorders, such as Alzheimer disease, and superimposed vascular disease.

▶ Onset of cognitive difficulties in association with a documented stroke represents strong evidence for vascular dementia. In cases in which this temporal connection is lacking, follow-up evaluations will often clarify the diagnosis by revealing additional strokes associated with stepwise cognitive decline.

▶ Avoid diagnosing vascular dementia in patients with isolated cognitive decline. Focal, noncognitive neurologic signs such as hemiparesis, visual field loss, or gait disorder should be sought.

▶ T2-weighted magnetic resonance (MRI) brain scans often detect abnormal white matter hyperintensities of nonvascular origin and unclear clinical significance. Computed tomography (CT) and T1-weighted MRI scans should be relied upon instead to make a diagnosis of cerebral infarction. CT and MR are supportive, but not diagnostic, as incidental strokes are common in Alzheimer disease and other dementias.

Treatment

The principal goals of therapy in VCI patients are prevention of recurrent strokes, management of associated functional and behavioral changes, and treatment of related medical and neurologic conditions. Secondary stroke prophylaxis will vary according to the pathophysiology of stroke in individual patients. Some special considerations apply in those with dementia. Warfarin anticoagulation is more effective than aspirin for stroke prophylaxis in patients with atrial fibrillation (AF) of valvular origin, and in those with nonvalvular AF plus another risk factor such as hypertension, left ventricular hypertrophy, or atrial enlargement. Some vascular dementia patients are at increased risk for falls due to gait impairment, leading to concerns about intracranial hemorrhage. Treatment should therefore be individualized. Aspirin is effective stroke prophylaxis for patients with a prior stroke or TIA and none of the previously addressed risk factors. Clopidogrel (Plavix) and dipyridamole-aspirin (Aggrenox) are alternatives to aspirin and warfarin used, for example, in cases of aspirin failure or intolerance.

Modifiable stroke risk factors should be specifically addressed. For example, aggressive control of hypertension can clearly diminish the risk of recurrent stroke in the elderly and may potentially prevent vascular dementia. Several antihypertensive trials have demonstrated a reduction in the rate of cognitive decline. β-Adrenergic blockers and central α-adrenergic inhibitors frequently exacerbate sedation and cognitive impairment in demented individuals. Better choices are diuretics, angiotensin-converting enzyme inhibitors, and calcium channel blockers. Cessation of smoking also decreases stroke risk.

Finally, several clinical trials have evaluated the safety and efficacy of AChE inhibitors and the NMDA receptor antagonist memantine in the treatment of mild to moderate vascular dementia. However, use of these agents would be considered "off-label" since they have not been approved by the FDA for this indication. Nevertheless, in randomized, placebo-controlled studies of fairly large numbers of vascular dementia and mixed dementia subjects, modest but significant benefit in favor of active drug have been demonstrated with regard to cognition at 6 months.

Dementias Associated with Infectious, Inflammatory, and Immune Disorders

Human Immunodeficiency Virus–Associated Dementia

Human immunodeficiency virus-type 1 (HIV-1) infection is the most common preventable and treatable cause of neurocognitive impairment in individuals under age 50 years. In many Western countries, combination antiretroviral therapy has not only significantly reduced overall morbidity and mortality due to HIV but also has substantially altered the types and severity of neurologic manifestations of HIV infection. In recognition of these changes, an international consensus working group recently published updated clinical research diagnostic criteria for HIV-1–associated neurocognitive disorders. As in previous classification systems, the diagnosis of HIV-1–associated neurocognitive disorders (HAND) is made on the basis of clinical criteria; there is no single diagnostic test or marker. The recently revised criteria identify three levels of cognitive disorder: HIV-associated asymptomatic neurocognitive impairment (ANI), HIV-1–associated mild neurocognitive disorder (MND), and HIV-1–associated dementia (HAD). Although each of these disorders is related to HIV, together they do not describe the natural history of this disease, as is the case with mild cognitive impairment as an incipient form of Alzheimer disease. Instead, they are three separate disorders that a given patient may transition between in either direction. Thus, for example, some patients remain stably in the MND category, others may worsen to become demented, and still others may improve to become unimpaired. These three categories of neurocognitive disorder have in common that delirium must be absent in order to make the diagnosis, and that any contributing causes other than HIV

Key Clinical Questions

HIV-associated dementia

▶ What are the patient's current and nadir CD4 count, viral load (plasma HIV RNA) and antiretroviral treatment status?

Knowing the answer to this questions is essential to ascertain the conditions for which the patient is at risk. The current CD4+ lymphocyte count is a marker of the integrity of cellular immune responses at the time the test is performed. The nadir CD4 indexes the maximum degree of prior immune suppression. The plasma viral load measures the extent of ongoing viral replication. Combination anti-retroviral therapy is variably effective, but typically reduces viral replication and substantially benefits cellular immunity, thereby protecting patients from death and halting or slowing disease progression. Frank dementia and serious central nervous system opportunistic diseases, such as toxoplasmo-sis and progressive multifocal leukoencephalopathy, are generally seen only among patients with CD4 counts <200. By comparison, mild cognitive impairment and non-HIV related neurologic morbidities are more likely to occur in patients with higher CD4 counts.

must be judged not to be the principal cause of the cognitive impairment. At times, this can present considerable diagnostic difficulty, since comorbidities such as substance abuse, depressive disorders, and head injury are quite common among HIV-infected patients. Classifying the severity of the disorder depends in part on the degree of measurable cognitive impairment, as assessed by neuropsychological testing, and also on the degree of impact on daily functioning, as assessed by history taking, both self-report and informant-based. In a setting in which neuropsychological testing is not available, the diagnosis of ANI, by definition, cannot be made.

Prevalence and risk factors

In the United States, HIV infection affects nearly 1 million persons. Worldwide, the prevalence is approximately 40 million. The number of HIV-infected individuals over age 50 years is growing rapidly, and incident cases are accelerating fastest among women, intravenous drug users, and ethnic minorities.

Early in the HIV epidemic, dementia was a common sequela of advanced disease, affecting more than 50% of patients prior to death. Subsequently, widespread treatment with zidovudine (AZT) reduced the incidence of HIV dementia dramatically. With the later introduction of combination therapy and highly active antiretroviral therapies (HAART), further improvement was seen. The incidence of most HIV-related opportunistic infections,

including those affecting the CNS, has dropped markedly. Changes in diagnosis and clinical management have altered the face of HIV, such that what was once an almost uniformly fatal illness is now—at least for those in developed countries where antiretroviral drugs are available—a chronic disease requiring long-term medical management. Survival has been greatly prolonged among patients with dementia. Very recently, however, the appearance of dementia in persons whose CD4 counts have rebounded with HAART, and the relative increase of dementia as a proportion of AIDS-defining opportunistic illnesses, has suggested to some that the CNS is not being treated as effectively as the lymphatic tissues. Table 22.8 lists important risk factors for HIV dementia and cognitive impairment. The prevalence of these disorders increases in concert with systemic disease progression. Low hemoglobin concentrations are an additional independent risk factor.

Neuropathogenesis

It has become clear that HIV enters the CNS early after infection, and is present throughout the course of disease. Entry into the CNS is via a "Trojan horse" mechanism, likely involving infected cells of the macrophage-monocyte lineage, and perhaps lymphocytes as well. In the adult brain, only macrophages and microglia are productively infected. HIV does not effectively enter or replicate in neurons, suggesting that dementia occurs through indirect mechanisms.

HIV encephalitis is a diagnosis made by neuropathologic evaluation of brain tissue. It is characterized by a number of features that are individually nonspecific (white matter pallor, microglial nodules, multinucleated giant cells, and gliosis), but when they occur as a constellation in the setting of known HIV infection, produce a characteristic neuropathologic signature. The pathologic findings are typically mild, even in cases in which dementia is severe. Further, encephalitis is neither necessary nor sufficient for dementia. Thus, although frequently the two coexist, each may be present independent of the other. Immunocytochemical staining using antibodies directed against the HIV envelope protein gp41 are helpful in delineating the extent of brain infection. Some degree of neuronal loss can be demonstrated, but

---

Table 22.8 Risk factors for AIDS dementia

▶ Older age at diagnosis of AIDS

▶ Elevated plasma viral load (>50,000 copies per mL)

▶ Elevated cerebrospinal fluid (CSF) viral load (>200 copies/mL)

▶ CD4 count less than 100/μL

▶ Low hemoglobin concentration (less than 15 mg/dL)

▶ Systemic disease progression

this correlates only modestly with cognitive status. Instead, severe damage to dendrites and synapses is readily evident. The sparsity of infected cells and the imprecise correlation between the severity of pathology and the degree of dementia indicates that host factors are likely to play a role in neuropathogenesis. Alterations in the balance of cytokines, neurotrophic factors, and neurotoxins, including glutamate receptor active compounds, have been found. An important unanswered question is why some patients with HIV infection develop dementia before death while others do not.

Clinical features and course

HIV-associated dementia should be suspected when a patient presents with insidiously progressive cognitive decline occurring over a period of weeks or months. The classical triad is cognitive, behavior, and motor symptoms. In early stages, the neurologic examination is typically normal or shows only slowing of repetitive movements or increased tendon reflexes. Focal cortical signs such as hemianopia, agnosia, or paraphasic language disturbance are absent. Patients are not able to learn new information—such as word lists—as well as previously, but they do not show the rapid forgetting that is commonly seen in AD. Also affected are patients' abilities to maintain and shift attention, and to sustain a line of reasoning to solve a problem. These features are characteristic of executive cognitive dysfunction.

In advanced stages of HIV dementia, now rarely seen, patients are apathetic, indifferent, and may be confined to bed due to motor impairment and incontinence. The neurologic examination will show frontal release signs, spasticity, and hyperreflexia, particularly in the legs.

Diagnosis

The diagnoses of HIV dementia and milder cognitive impairment are made by clinical criteria, after exclusion of other potential causes. No single laboratory test estab-

lishes the diagnosis, but ancillary studies are useful for supporting or refuting it. Neuropsychological evaluation may be particularly helpful in cases where impairment is mild.

Differential diagnostic considerations

The principal differential diagnostic considerations in HIV patients with cognitive changes are encephalopathies (delirium) due to drugs and metabolic derangements, chronic brain syndromes due to substance use and head injury, CNS opportunistic disease, and severe primary psychiatric disturbances. Renal and hepatic insufficiencies are capable of causing encephalopathy directly, or through diminished clearance of CNS-active drugs. In toxic and metabolic encephalopathies, delirium with variable attention and arousal represents the most typical presentation. Occasionally, however, chronic use of medications such as narcotic analgesics, anticholinergics, and antipsychotics, can result in an insidious cognitive deterioration that may mimic dementia. An attempt should be made to remove or reduce the dose of any potentially offending agents.

Although less common nowadays, it remains important to differentiate encephalopathies due to opportunistic diseases from those that are attributable to HIV infection of the CNS directly or indirectly. Opportunistic CNS conditions still occur in patients who fail antiretroviral drug therapy. To estimate the likelihood that neurologic dysfunction is related to CNS opportunistic disease, one must know the CD4 count.

The principal brain opportunistic diseases in AIDS are toxoplasmosis, primary CNS lymphoma, cryptococcal meningitis, cytomegalovirus (CMV) encephalitis, and progressive multifocal leukoencephalopathy (PML) (Table 22.9). All of these conditions may produce cognitive deterioration. Patients with intellectual decline due to toxoplasmosis, lymphoma, and PML almost always manifest focal, noncognitive neurologic signs, such as hemiparesis, ataxia,

Table 22.9 Clinical characteristics differentiating frequent neurologic complications in AIDS

	Evolution, time course	Impaired consciousness	Fever	Focal signs
AIDS dementia	Months	−	−	−
Toxoplasmosis	<2 weeks	+	+	+++
Lymphoma[1]	2–8 weeks	+/−	−	+
PML[2]	<2 weeks	−	−	++
Cryptococcal meningitis[3]	<2 weeks	+	+++	−
CMV[4]	<4 weeks	+/−	+	+ (brainstem)

CMV, cytomegalovirus; PML, progressive multifocal leukoencephalopathy.
[1,2,4]Search for specific virus PCR in CSF (EBV, JC, CMV, respectively).
[3]Search for specific cryptococcus neoformans antigen in CSF.

Table 22.10 Radiologic characteristics distinguishing common neurologic complications in AIDS

	Principal location	Number	Appearance	Contrast enhancement	Mass effect
HIV dementia	White matter	Diffuse	Ill-defined, confluent	–	–
Toxoplasmosis	Basal ganglia	1 to many	Abscess	++	+/++
Lymphoma	Periventricular	1 to several	Mass	+++	+
PML	Subcortical white matter	1 to several	Multifocal	–	–
Cryptococcosis	Gray matter	1 to multiple	Multicystic	–	–
CMV	Periventricular or diffuse	0 to several	Patchy or confluent	++	–

or cranial nerve dysfunction. In addition, focal cerebral lesions are evident on imaging studies (Table 22.10). Occasionally, a nonfocal encephalopathy may be caused by a midline lymphoma affecting deep structures of both cerebral hemispheres, by diffuse PML, or by multifocal cerebral toxoplasma lesions. Cryptococcal meningitis can produce cognitive changes, but these changes typically resolve with treatment. Magnetic resonance imaging scans with and without gadolinium enhancement are optimally sensitive and specific for imaging opportunistic processes in AIDS. There is debate as to whether neurosyphilis is more aggressive and more resistant to treatment in HIV-infected individuals, but dementing presentations (that is, paretic neurosyphilis) are rare and are overshadowed by meningeal and vascular syndromes.

Cytomegalovirus brain infection in particular, because of its clinical similarity to HIV dementia in some cases, is clearly the most important of these conditions in the differential diagnosis of dementia. In cases of CMV encephalitis, the CD4 lymphocyte count is almost always below 50. Distinguishing characteristics include the pace of onset, which is usually more rapid (weeks) in CMV encephalitis, the presence of cranial nerve deficits (particularly eye movement abnormalities), and the occurrence of electrolyte imbalances, which are probably due to CMV adrenalitis or the syndrome of inappropriate antidiuretic hormone. Routine CSF studies may be normal and do not differentiate between CMV and HIV encephalitis. However, use of rapid culture assays (shell vial antigen detection) or DNA amplification using polymerase chain reaction techniques on CSF may be helpful. In some patients, brain MRI demonstrates ependymal enhancement, a finding highly suggestive of CMV ventriculoencephalitis.

Useful tests

When available, neuropsychological testing is very helpful in diagnosis. It provides clear documentation of cognitive impairment and assists in differentiating HIV dementia from other disorders that may cause impairment. Useful screening neuropsychological tests are those that examine psychomotor speed, such as the Trailmaking Tests, Grooved Pegboard, and Digit-Symbol. Also useful are tests of verbal and nonverbal learning (e.g., the Hopkins Verbal Learning Test) and sustained attention (Paced Auditory Serial Addition Test). Such tests should be administered by an experienced examiner and interpreted by comparison to normative data with appropriate demographic corrections, including age, gender, education, and in some cases, ethnicity. The influence of premorbid conditions, including previous head trauma and learning disability, as well as the effects of systemic illness and substance abuse, need to be considered carefully when interpreting results from neuropsychological testing.

Treatment

Antiretroviral medications. The number of agents in the armamentarium of drugs available to be used in combination antiretroviral therapy continues to expand rapidly. These include agents from well-established classes and from newer classes. The established classes are the nucleoside reverse transcriptase inhibitors (e.g., zidovudine, stavudine, Epivir), the non-nucleoside reverse transcriptase inhibitors (e.g., nevirapine, efavirenz), and the HIV protease inhibitors (e.g., atazanavir, indinavir, lopinavir). Newer drug classes include agents that inhibit viral fusion with the cell membrane; inhibitors of the HIV-specific enzyme, integrase; and competitive inhibitors of CCR5, one of the major coreceptors for HIV cellular entry. Typically, three drugs from at least two different classes are combined as HAART. Monotherapy (a single antiretroviral drug) and dual therapy (a combination of two antiretroviral drugs) have been clearly shown to be inferior to combinations of three or more drugs. The overall goal, in addition to suppressing plasma viral load below the limits of detection, is to exert selective pressure on multiple viral genes, reducing the likelihood that drug resistance will arise. Although many different variations on this strategic theme are used clinically, not all combinations are effective and safe. Therefore, the drugs should be prescribed only by a physician with expertise and experience in treating patients with HIV infection. Numerous case reports and series document dramatic improvement in individuals who previously met criteria for frank dementia due to HIV. Data continue to accumulate suggesting that antiretroviral drugs that more effectively penetrate the blood–brain barrier may enhance viral suppression in the CNS and optimize the recovery of cognitive function and in patients starting antiretroviral therapy (Letendre et al., 2008). An ongoing clinical trial is testing a strategy for combining medications to maximize cognitive recovery (May et al., 2007).

Other Infectious Causes of Dementia

Prion disease

Prion diseases are caused by genetically coded modifications of an endogenous protein called the prion protein (PrP). These modifications may be vertically inherited, or may be transmitted horizontally to other hosts by means such as corneal transplants. The resulting subacute spongiform encephalopathies present as neurologic disorders, including dementia. Gerstmann-Straussler-Scheinker disease is a familial, dominantly inherited prion disorder due to a point mutation. Its manifestations include presenile dementia and prominent spinocerebellar dysfunction. In Creutzfeldt-Jakob disease (CJD), which is sporadic and transmissible, a rapidly progressive dementia is typically accompanied by stimulus-induced myoclonus. Other neurologic features are nonspecific and include extrapyramidal signs, cerebellar ataxia, pyramidal signs, and cortical blindness. Many CJD cases are iatrogenic. More than 300 cases of iatrogenic CJD have been reported since the first evidence of iatrogenic transmission in 1974. The mechanisms include corneal transplant, neurosurgical instruments, human dura mater grafts, depth electrodes, and human pituitary hormones.

The first case of new variant CJD (vCJD) was reported in 1996. Thought to be linked to bovine spongiform encephalopathy, vCJD manifests with unusual clinical and neuropathologic features. The early clinical symptoms are frequently psychiatric, although a minority presents with memory impairment and persistent pain. Neurologic function deteriorates and, by 6 months, most patients have ataxia, cognitive impairment, and involuntary movements. Eventually, they become mute, incontinent, and die, with a mean duration of illness of about 13 months.

The definite diagnosis of CJD is dependent on biopsy or autopsy findings. However, certain laboratory tests can support the diagnosis. In conjunction with history and clinical examination, detection of 14-3-3 and other proteins (PrPsc, NSE, and S-100) in CSF, brain MRI, and electroencephalogram (EEG) have significantly improved the sensitivity and specificity of the clinical diagnosis of CJD.

There is no disease-specific treatment currently available for prion diseases. However, advances in our understanding of their pathogenesis have provided treatment strategies, several of which are already in clinical development.

Neurosyphilis

Once common, the general paresis of late neurosyphilis (a progressive dementia with psychotic features) has become quite rare in the antibiotic era, even as other forms of neurosyphilis have resurged due to HIV coinfection. Criteria for diagnosis are the presence of an appropriate clinical syndrome, a reactive fluorescent treponemal antibody-absorbed (FTA-ABS) or microhemagglutination test for treponema pallidum (MHA-TP) in blood, a positive CSF VDRL, and CSF pleocytosis. A positive CSF VDRL result is specific for the diagnosis of neurosyphilis, but the sensitivity, ranging from 30 to 70%, is relatively low. Cerebrospinal fluid FTA-ABS, on the other hand, is very sensitive, but has relatively low specificity. However, the diagnosis of neurosyphilis can be excluded by a negative CSF FTA-ABS test. The current recommended treatment regimen for neurosyphilis includes intravenous aqueous crystalline penicillin G 18–24 million units per day or 3–4 million units every 4 hours for 10–14 days. Alternatively, procaine penicillin G can be given intramuscularly at 2.4 million units per day with oral probenecid for 10–14 days. The treatment will usually arrest the progress of dementia. Although there is evidence that HIV-infected patients may relapse neurologically after standard treatment regimens, neurosyphilis occurs in only about 1% of HIV patients.

Dementias Associated with Systemic Disorders

Systemic disorders can contribute to cognitive impairments, whether or not they constitute the primary cause of dementia. Acquired metabolic disorders, such as those due to organ failure or endocrine dysfunction, intoxications, nutritional deficiencies, and inherited metabolic abnormalities may all lead to dementia. Likely contributors should be investigated in all patients. Chapter 23 provides additional discussion of these issues.

Acquired Metabolic and Endocrine Disorders

Blood chemistry studies are usually sufficient to screen for likely metabolic sources of cognitive dysfunction. Serum electrolytes, including calcium and magnesium; renal function measurements; glucose; liver function studies; and sometimes an arterial blood gas should be performed early in the evaluation of any new patient, and repeated whenever abrupt clinical changes occur. Normal individuals with acute systemic disorders such as hepatic or renal failure develop delirium, rather than dementia. It is well known, however, that delirium in a patient with a minor systemic disorder such as fever may be the presenting manifestation of a progressive dementing illness.

Hematologic studies and thyroid function tests provide additional information about possible malignancies, nutritional deficiency states, and endocrine dysfunction that may be etiologically linked to cognitive deterioration. An EEG demonstrating triphasic waves is highly suggestive of an underlying metabolic abnormality, and is the most compelling rationale for obtaining this study in the evaluation of dementia patients.

Toxic encephalopathies

Intoxications are similar to metabolic abnormalities in their frequency and propensity to exacerbate cognitive impairment due to other causes. Table 22.11 lists some common medications that can cause reversible cognitive dysfunction in the context of a dementia syndrome, or even in cognitively normal individuals. Elderly individuals with or without dementia demonstrate alterations in drug distribution volume, metabolism, and elimination that can predispose to elevated drug levels.

Alcohol

In addition to acute effects, long-term exposure to toxins such as alcohol can cause or contribute to dementia. Alcoholic dementia is reported to develop after decades of consistent heavy consumption. It is characterized by mild global intellectual dysfunction with preserved language abilities and relative sparing of memory, but diagnosis in individual cases is often difficult. In patients with severe dementia and those with prominent deficits in learning new information, other diagnoses should be considered. The Korsakoff amnestic syndrome, which is also alcohol-related in most cases, might easily be considered in the context of a discussion of nutritional deficiencies. It represents a failure of cellular metabolism due to a lack of thiamine, and it frequently emerges with the resolution of a Wernicke encephalopathy. Nevertheless, a prior history of Wernicke may be absent. Korsakoff syndrome is characterized by an inability to learn new information that is out of proportion to all other cognitive difficulties. Apathy and mild to moderate executive dysfunction are common as well.

Nutritional deficiencies

Deficiency of vitamin B_{12} (cobalamin) is unique among the nutritional deficiencies in its capacity to produce a dementia syndrome in isolation from other characteristic neurologic and systemic signs. Why some patients with B_{12} deficiency become demented while others develop myelopathy, peripheral neuropathy, or combinations of these disorders is not known. Cognitive loss may be mild and noted only on neuropsychological testing, or severe, resulting in dementia. Eighty percent of adult-onset cases of pernicious anemia are attributable to lack of intrinsic factor due to atrophic gastritis. Other causes of deficiency include malabsorption due to surgical resection of the stomach or ileum, jejunal diverticulitis, tropical sprue, and bacterial overgrowth. With advancing age, there is a general loss of absorptive capacity for the vitamin. Acute development of B_{12} deficiency syndromes has been noted to occur with nitric oxide exposure during anesthesia. The diagnosis in suspected cases is made by demonstration of a low serum B_{12} level (<200 pg/mL). If the value falls in the indeterminate range (200–250 pg/mL), high serum methylmalonic acid and homocysteine levels confirm the diagnosis. Vitamin B_{12} replacement arrests progression of the dementia.

Inherited Metabolic Disorders and Storage Diseases

Inherited metabolic and storage diseases typically present with neurologic syndromes in infants and children. However, certain disorders may come to medical attention as dementias occurring in adulthood. Additional neurologic abnormalities are usually present, such as movement disorders or peripheral neuropathy. Table 22.12 lists some of these disorders. Additional information and differential diagnoses may be obtained by consulting primary sources (see Bibliography).

Dementias Associated with Structural Disorders of the Brain

Structural brain disorders can cause potentially reversible dementia syndromes in some patients. As a group, these

---

Table 22.11 Examples of commonly used medications that may produce cognitive impairment

Drug type	Specific examples	Risk factors for cognitive side effects
Antiarrhythmics, inotropics	Digoxin	Decreased lean body mass resulting in increased levels of water soluble drugs
Antihypertensives	Propranolol Clonidine	
Anticholinergics	Amitriptyline	Alzheimer disease and other dementing illnesses
	Diphenhydramine Oxybutynin	
Sedatives	Diazepam	Use of drugs with long half-lives
	Triazolam Phenobarbital	
Antipsychotics	Haloperidol Fluphenazine	Older age

Table 22.12 Examples of rare inherited metabolic disorders in which dementia may be a clinical feature

Disease	Clinical features	Pathophysiology
Familial idiopathic cerebral calcification (Fahr's disease)	Parkinsonism, dystonia or chorea with pyramidal tract signs and ataxia, in addition to dementia Autosomal dominant or recessive inheritance	Dense ferrocalcific deposits in basal ganglia
Adrenoleukodystrophy	Progressive spastic paraparesis, visual agnosia, occasional dementia X-linked recessive inheritance	Accumulation of very long chain fatty acids; dysmyelinating lesions
Late-onset neuronal ceroid lipofuscinosis (Kufs disease)	Slowly progressive ataxia, spasticity, choreoathetosis, dementia Autosomal recessive inheritance	Abnormal accumulation of lipopigments in lysosomes

disorders constitute the principal indication (besides cerebrovascular disease) for obtaining a neuroimaging study in the evaluation of patients with dementia.

Idiopathic Adult Hydrocephalus

In the idiopathic adult hydrocephalus syndrome, so-called "normal pressure" hydrocephalus, CT and MR studies demonstrate a disproportionate enlargement of the cerebral ventricles and evidence of transependymal CSF leakage. Cortical sulci, in contrast, may be only minimally dilated or even effaced. Although the pathophysiology is incompletely understood, the designation "normal pressure" has been dropped because there is evidence that high CSF pressures occur at least transiently. Typically, however, opening pressures are normal on routine lumbar puncture (LP). The clinical presentation consists of an insidious, gradually progressive dementia with gait ataxia and urinary incontinence. Headache and papilledema are absent, while diffuse corticospinal tract signs (Babinski signs and hyperreflexia) may be present. Patients may have a historical risk factor, such as head trauma, previous subarachnoid hemorrhage, or meningitis, but the majority of cases are idiopathic. Obvious clinical improvement in gait or mental status after removal of 30–50 mL of CSF by high-volume LP strongly suggests the diagnosis. Radionuclide cisternography may sometimes help with diagnosis, but it cannot reliably predict outcome from shunt surgery. More than 50% of patients treated with ventriculo- or lumboperitoneal CSF shunting show stabilization or reversal of their clinical deficits. However, surgical treatment has substantial morbidity that includes bacterial infections (meningitis, ependymitis), subdural hemorrhage from stretching of cortical bridging veins, seizures, and shunt malfunction. The best surgical candidates appear to be patients with known risk factors such as prior meningitis or subarachnoid hemorrhage.

Other Structural Disorders

Dementia may be caused by certain brain tumors, subdural hematomas, and as a late complication of multiple sclerosis or repetitive head trauma in boxers. Lateralizing signs on neurologic examination are a tip-off, and neuroimaging is useful in suspected cases. Midline lesions and multifocal cerebral pathology may present problems in differential diagnosis. Astrocytomas infiltrating both cerebral hemispheres, often glioblastoma multiforme, can occasionally present as progressive cognitive impairment without focal neurologic signs. A similar presentation may occur with large midline tumors, such as subfrontal meningiomas. Chronic subdural hematomas, particularly when bilateral, have been known to mimic AD, although typically patients show prominent fluctuations in arousal. Importantly, the atrophy associated with AD can predispose to the occurrence of subdural bleeding, so that the presence of a subdural hematoma does not exclude underlying AD. Although CT can sometimes miss an isodense subdural hematoma, MRI provides reliable visualization.

Dementia pugilistica is a delayed syndrome occurring in former career boxers, usually those with several hundred bouts fought. Motor manifestations typically precede cognitive deterioration by one or two decades. These include gait ataxia and pseudobulbar dysarthria with varying combinations of parkinsonism, cerebellar, and pyramidal signs. Neuropathologic features include a large and fenestrated septum cavum, depigmentation and degeneration of the substantia nigra and basal ganglia, extensive neurofibrillary tangles, diffuse β-amyloid plaques in cerebral cortex, and marked loss of Purkinje cells in the cerebellum.

Treatment and Management Issues in Dementing Disorders

General Management Issues

We have previously discussed treatments specifically designed to address the pathophysiology of specific dementing disorders. Such treatments include, for example, AChE inhibitors and memantine for AD, anticoagulants for vascular dementia, and antiretroviral agents for HIV-associated dementia. In addition to these disease-specific treatments, clinicians should familiarize themselves with management strategies for issues and problems common to all of the dementia syndromes. These include functional decline, such as impaired driving, as well as behavioral changes, such as depression, agitation, anxiety, wandering, sleep disturbance, and hallucinations. Appropriate interventions depend upon the specific issues that confront a patient and his or her caregiver at the time of referral. Patients' needs change over the course of disease, and none of these interventions is applicable to all individuals. Many centers employ a multidisciplinary team approach including, for example, a neurologist, social worker, psychologist, and occupational therapist to evaluate and provide for these varying needs.

Table 22.13 lists some difficulties that arise frequently in dementia patients, and for which patients and families may be unprepared. The Alzheimer's Association provides attorney referrals for setting up conservatorships and designating surrogates for health care decision-making (Alzheimer's Association, National Chapter, Suite 1000, 919 North Michigan Avenue, Chicago, IL 60611–1676; telephone 800–272–3900). Local chapters can also give information on patient and caregiver support groups, day care centers, and respite services. Various publications also provide much useful and up-to-date information on management strategies. An example is the book *Understanding Difficult Behaviors: Some Practical Suggestions for Coping with Alzheimer's Disease and Related Illnesses.* (For copies, write to: Alzheimer's Care and Training Center, Senior Health Building, 5401 McAuley Drive, P.O. Box 994, Ann Arbor, MI 48106. Telephone: 313–712–4334.) In addition, many families find *The 36-Hour Day* to be a very useful guide for day-to-day coping.

Behavioral Management

Behavioral symptoms common to dementia patients include agitation, wandering, hallucinations, delusions, depression, anxiety, and sleep disturbance. Although drug therapy may be helpful in selected cases, simple nonpharmacologic interventions may obviate the need for pharmacologic treatment. If medications are necessary, it is good practice to use the minimal effective dose and to choose the drug with the fewest and mildest side-effects (Table 22.14).

Agitation and psychosis

Agitated behaviors are often distressing to caregivers and are potentially dangerous to patients themselves. Demented patients may engage in purposeless, stereotyped activities such as tearing up tissue paper. Verbal agitated behaviors include arguing, shouting, swearing, moaning, and worrying out loud in a compulsive, repetitive fashion. Infrequently, patients can become physically assaultive. Since the causes of agitation are multifactorial, its treatment and management should be multidisciplinary. Agitation may be provoked by a variety of remediable pre-

---

Table 22.13 Special issues in the management of dementia patients

Problem area	Appropriate management or intervention
Healthcare decisions	Power of attorney for healthcare decisions; living will
Financial matters	Power of attorney; conservatorship
Driving	Physicians are required to report the diagnosis of dementia to state authorities in California and some other states
General safety	Identification bracelet; home safety measures

Table 22.14 Psychotropic treatments in dementia

Depression
▶ Selective serotonin reuptake inhibitors
▶ Fluoxetine (Prozac)
▶ Paroxetine (Paxil)
▶ Sertraline (Zoloft)
▶ Fluvoxamine (Luvox)
▶ Citalopram (Celexa)
▶ Venlafaxine (Effexor)
▶ Escitalopram (Lexapro)
▶ Tricyclics
▶ Nortriptyline (Pamelor)
▶ Trazodone (Desyrel)
▶ Nefazodone (Serzone)
▶ Mirtazapine (Remeron)

Agitation
▶ Risperidone (Risperdal)
▶ Olanzapine (Zyprexa)
▶ Quetiapine (Seroquel)
▶ Trazodone

Anxiety
▶ Buspirone (BuSpar)
▶ Lorazepam (Ativan)
▶ Alprazolam (Xanax)

Delusions
▶ Risperidone (Risperdal)
▶ Olanzapine (Zyprexa)
▶ Quetiapine (Seroquel)

Insomnia
▶ Trazodone (Desyrel)
▶ Zolpidem (Ambien)
▶ Short-acting benzodiazepine

cipitants and situational factors. For example, pain should be treated with analgesics, and recurrent urinary urgency should be eliminated by relieving obstructive prostatism. Distraction is a highly effective and readily available technique for interrupting such behaviors. Patients with a propensity to wander should wear an identification safety bracelet. Special door locks and barriers may be necessary as well. Patients usually respond well when allowed to wander in a safe, supervised area.

When other interventions for agitation have failed, or when resources to implement them are unavailable, pharmacologic therapy may be tried. Trazadone (Desyrel) is an inhibitor of serotonin reuptake that has shown promise in ameliorating agitated behaviors. Typical neuroleptic medications are a last resource because of the high frequency of adverse side effects in elderly demented patients. But the newer "atypical" neuroleptics such as risperidone, olanzapine, and quetiapine may be useful for controlling agitation in demented patients with lesser risk of side effects. Several placebo-controlled, double-blind trials have demonstrated the safety and efficacy of the "atypical" neuroleptics in treatment of agitation. Severe behavioral disorders sometimes require inpatient hospitalization.

Psychosis

More than one-third of dementia patients experience hallucinations, sensory misperceptions, or delusions at some point in the course of their illness. In many, particularly those with PD, nonthreatening visual hallucinations occur. These, as well as delusions, are best ignored if they do not cause particular distress to the patient or caregivers. When problematic, they may be treated with *small* doses of newer atypical neuroleptics since higher doses may, like the typical neuroleptics, be associated with parkinsonism (rigidity, akinesia, parkinsonian gait), akathisia, tardive dyskinesia, orthostatic hypotension, sedation, and exacerbation of cognitive impairment. Patients with mild parkinsonian features prior to treatment may develop severe stiffness and bradykinesia following initiation of neuroleptics.

Depression

Except in patients with very early dementia, where cognition and insight are relatively preserved, psychotherapy for depression does not appear to be particularly beneficial. On the other hand, depression is typically quite responsive to pharmacologic therapy. Drug classes that may be tried include the selective serotonin reuptake inhibitors (SSRIs) and the tricyclic antidepressants. In general, the safety profile of the SSRIs is excellent. Sertraline may have some metabolic advantages over the other SSRIs, since it has few drug–drug interactions. The dose is 50–100 mg/day. Adverse effects of the SSRIs include insomnia, tremor, weight loss, and ejaculatory dis-

turbance. Among the tricyclic antidepressants, desipramine and nortriptyline are commonly chosen because they are the least anticholinergic. Relative contraindications to tricyclics include pretreatment postural hypotension, narrow-angle glaucoma, and clinically significant heart disease or conduction abnormalities. Nortriptyline (Pamelor) is administered 25–100 mg/day in divided doses. The dosing for desipramine (Norpramin) is 50–150 mg/day. Monoamine oxidase (MAO) inhibitors are generally avoided because of the difficulty in managing the necessary dietary restrictions.

Anxiety

Anxiety, like agitation, often results from pain, discomfort, and distressing circumstances. Addressing these conditions may ameliorate symptoms. When medically necessary, pharmacologic agents can be of help. Benzodiazepines are problematic because of their increased half-lives and concentrations of active metabolites in the elderly. Repeated dosing leads to high blood levels, sedation, habituation, and, ultimately, dependence. Withdrawal signs (increased anxiety) may occur on cessation of the drug. Intermittent, rather than daily use, is generally recommended. Buspirone, an azapirone derivative with 5HT1A receptor agonist activity, is an alternative to the benzodiazepine anxiolytics for long-term, daily use. This drug acts through nonbenzodiazepine mechanisms, is less habituating, and has a good safety profile in the elderly. It is administered 15–30 mg/day in divided doses.

Sleep disturbance

Sleep disturbances in demented patients have diverse etiologies, including structural and functional changes in the midbrain-diencephalic systems that subserve wakefulness and sleep. Also, in many cases, drugs contribute to the problem. Reversals of the diurnal sleep cycle, insomnia, and frequent awakenings may respond to conservative environmental and behavioral manipulations. Affected patients should be kept awake as much as possible during the day, and evening fluids should be avoided so as to minimize sleep interruption. Warm milk at bedtime may be all that is needed to promote sleep onset. Light therapy and melatonin have received considerable attention of late, but their usefulness in AD is not yet established.

When pharmacologic therapy is needed, trazodone has the particular advantage of acting on the serotonergic systems thought to be involved in sleep induction and maintenance. Benzodiazepines are probably best avoided, although oxazepam and temazepam have been used because they are short acting and have fewer active metabolites. Triazolam (Halcion) has prominent amnesiogenic effects, mitigating against its use in dementia. Chloral hydrate, 500–1,000 mg at bedtime is an option, and its rapid onset of action may be useful, although its duration of action is quite short. Barbiturates should not be used in the elderly because of their long half-lives and tendency to cause falls and fractures.

Summary

Greater public and medical awareness has resulted in a more widespread appreciation of the clinical syndrome of dementia and its differentiation from other disorders such as delirium, depression, and normal aging. Considerable advances have been made in our understanding of the pathogenesis of AD, the most common cause of dementia in the elderly. Furthermore, these advances have resulted in the emergence of new treatments. An area of particular interest concerns the discovery of both genetically determined forms of AD and inherited factors that increase susceptibility to the disease. Lewy bodies, once thought to be synonymous with PD, are now recognized as an important contributor to late-life dementia, even though a full understanding of their pathogenetic role has yet to be achieved. Cerebrovascular disease remains common not only as a primary cause of dementia, but also as a contributing cause in many patients with concomitant AD. This is true in part because cerebral amyloid angiopathy predisposes to the occurrence of stroke in AD. HIV-associated dementia remains a substantial source of morbidity and disability in younger adults, despite the rapidly expanding repertoire of anti-HIV drugs available to clinicians. Although dementia remains a difficult clinical problem, it appears that currently available treatments can substantially benefit, if not ameliorate, many of its cognitive and behavioral manifestations.

Annotated Bibliography

Chung JA, Cummings JL. Neurobehavioral and neuropsychiatric symptoms in Alzheimer's disease: Characteristics and treatment. *Neurol Clin* 2000;18:829–846.
Review of neuropsychiatric symptoms and their treatment in AD.

Corey-Bloom J, Thal LJ, Galasko D, et al. Diagnosis and evaluation of dementia. *Neurology* 1995;45:211–218.
Early practice parameter from the American Academy of Neurology on the diagnosis and evaluation of dementia.

Cummings J, Vinters H, Cole G, Khachaturian Z. Alzheimer's disease: Etiologies, pathophysiology, cognitive reserve, and treatment opportunities. *Neurology* 1998;51(Suppl 1):S2–S17.
Authoritative review of the pathology, pathophysiology, epidemiology, and management of AD.

Doody RS, Stevens JC, Beck C, et al. Practice parameter: Management of dementia (an evidence-based review). Report of the Quality Standards Subcommittee of the American Academy of Neurology. *Neurology* 2001;56:1154–1166.
Recently published practice parameter from the American Academy of Neurology (AAN) on key issues in the management of dementia.

Knopman DS, DeKosky ST, Cummings JL, et al. Practice parameter: Diagnosis of dementia (an evidence-based review). Report of the Quality Standards Subcommittee of the American Academy of Neurology. *Neurology* 2001;56:1143–1153.
Recently published practice parameter from the AAN examining issues related to the diagnosis of dementia.

Morris JC. Clinical presentation and course of Alzheimer disease. In: Terry RD, Katzman R, Bick KL, Sisodia SS, eds. *Alzheimer disease*, 2nd ed. Philadelphia: Lippincott Williams & Wilkins, 1999:11–24.
Good discussion of the clinical features of AD.

Petersen RC. Mild cognitive impairment. *Lancet* 2006; 367(9527):1979.
Review of the mild cognitive impairment syndrome.

Selkoe DJ. Translating cell biology into therapeutic advances in Alzheimer's disease. *Nature* 1999;399:A23–A31.
Review of progress in our understanding of the molecular biology of AD and potential therapeutic interventions.

Terry RD, Katzman R, Bick KL, Sisodia SS, eds. *Alzheimer Disease*, 2nd ed. Philadelphia: Lippincott Williams & Wilkins, 1999.
Authoritative review of all aspects of AD and other dementias, from clinical features and diagnosis to neuropathological findings, molecular biology, and genetics.

CHAPTER 23

Systemic Diseases

Stephanie Lessig and Jody Corey-Bloom

Endocrine Disorders

Neurologic complications are commonly associated with hyper- and hypo-function of different endocrine glands. Although each gland will be considered separately, many interactions also occur between glands, hormones, and their control mechanisms that may have profound effects on the functioning of the nervous system.

Thyroid

Hypothyroidism

Thyroid hormone has a critical influence on cellular metabolic activity and is also integrally involved in the growth, development, and function of the central nervous system (CNS). Low thyroid hormone levels cause slowing of various metabolic processes. Adult-onset hypothyroidism is usually caused by primary thyroid gland disorders like autoimmune thyroiditis, surgical or radiologic ablation of the thyroid gland, iodine deficiency, thyroid gland tumors, or as a result of various medications such as para-amino salicylates, iodides, and thiocyanates. Hypothyroidism can also be secondary to pituitary dysfunction, causing impaired release of thyroid stimulating hormone.

Hypothyroidism may clinically present with marked psychomotor retardation, weight gain, fatigue, cold intolerance, bradycardia, or subnormal temperature. Other features include headache, weakness, dry skin, brittle hair, constipation, and lipid abnormalities. Examination of these patients will often demonstrate "hung-up" reflexes, due to a prolonged relaxation time of muscles after reflex elicitation.

Severe hypothyroidism, referred to as *myxedema*, has prominent neurologic involvement. In myxedema, psychomotor retardation, lethargy, impaired attention and concentration, and dementia are not unusual. Seizures may occur, and psychosis or other psychiatric syndromes are common. "Myxedema madness" has been used to describe the symptoms of irritability, paranoia, hallucinations, and delusions that accompany this state. With severe hypothyroidism, a state of hypothermia, bradycardia, hypotension, and respiratory failure ("myxedema coma") may develop and is associated with high mortality.

Other neurologic complications of hypothyroidism include myopathy, which is usually mild and associated with increased levels of creatinine phosphokinase (CPK). Electromyogram (EMG) examination of proximal muscles may reveal short-duration, low-amplitude, polyphasic motor unit action potentials (myopathic units) without spontaneous activity. Muscle biopsy often demonstrates only nonspecific changes such as type II muscle fiber atrophy and glycogen accumulation. Percussion of muscles in the setting of hypothyroidism may show the phenomenon of local mounding called "myoedema." Mononeuropathies are also frequently seen with hypothyroidism. The most common mononeuropathy is carpal tunnel syndrome, which occurs in up to 10% of hypothyroid patients and is often bilateral. Hypothyroidism may rarely be associated with a large-fiber peripheral polyneuropathy with reduced vibration and proprioception. Re-

▼

Pearls and Perils

Thyroid dysfunction

▶ Both hypothyroidism and hyperthyroidism can cause proximal muscle weakness.

▶ Certain drugs (e.g., lithium) can produce abnormal thyroid levels on laboratory testing.

▶ There is an increased incidence of myasthenia gravis in patients with thyroid disease and vice versa.

▶ Slowed relaxation time of deep tendon reflexes ("hung-up reflexes") is seen in hypothyroidism but is not specific for it. Hung-up reflexes can also be seen in diabetes, hypothermia, and in the presence of certain drugs.

▶ Cerebrospinal fluid protein may be elevated, sometimes to >100/dL, in patients with hypothyroidism.

▶ Neuropathy is so uncommon in hyperthyroidism that another cause should be sought when it is found in association with it.

Table 23.1 Hypothyroidism

Discriminating features
▶ Decreased serum levels of thyroid hormones
▶ Increased serum TSH
▶ "Myoedema"
▶ Reversible sensorineural hearing loss

Consistent features
▶ Headache, weight gain, periorbital edema
▶ Psychomotor retardation
▶ Forgetfulness, inattention, apathy, and slowing of speech, movement, and mentation
▶ Increase in serum cholesterol
▶ Elevated cerebrospinal total protein
▶ Reduced amplitude electroencephalogram

Variable features
▶ "Hung up" reflexes
▶ Dementia
▶ Seizures
▶ Psychiatric syndromes ("myxedema madness")
▶ "Myxedema coma"
▶ Myopathy
▶ Mono- and polyneuropathies

versible sensorineural hearing loss, with or without tinnitus, develops in 75% of hypothyroid patients.

Diagnosis of hypothyroidism is based on finding decreased serum levels of thyroid hormones. Cerebrospinal fluid (CSF) examination is generally normal, although total protein may be elevated. The electroencephalogram (EEG) shows generalized slowing and, with severe disease, reduced amplitude may be present.

Treatment of hypothyroidism consists of thyroid replacement, which should be instituted cautiously in patients with heart disease. Most of the neurologic complications of hypothyroidism, including carpal tunnel syndrome, respond to replacement therapy, and may revert completely by 6–8 weeks following institution of treatment (Table 23.1).

Hyperthyroidism

Thyroid hormones increase the basal metabolic rate and skeletal muscle heat production. Thyrotoxic patients are insulin-resistant at the post receptor level, and have increased muscle protein catabolism along with increased fat oxidation and lipoprotein lipase activity. The most important cause of hyperthyroidism is diffuse toxic goiter (Graves disease). General features include hyperactivity, insomnia, heat intolerance, sinus tachycardia, and weight loss. Personality changes, irritability, and even mania and psychosis may accompany hyperthyroidism. Seizures are infrequently seen. Delirium may be observed as a manifestation of thyroid storm (Table 23.2).

Most patients have neuromuscular complaints, and more than 50% have muscle weakness. Weakness is primarily proximal and usually out of proportion to the

amount of muscle wasting. However, severe wasting may also occur. Myalgia, fatigue, and exercise intolerance are common. Occasionally, respiratory, bulbar, and esophageal involvement may occur. Mild CPK elevation is not uncommon. On EMG, myopathic units without spontaneous activity are seen, although rarely an inflammatory myopathy can occur. Treatment with thyroid-blocking agents such as propylthiouracil and methimazole restores euthyroid function and reverses most of the neurologic deficits of thyrotoxicosis. Adrenergic blocking agents may improve muscle strength acutely, as may glucocorticoids that block the peripheral conversion of T4 to T3. Weakness usually resolves within 4 months of treatment, and persistent weakness is rare. The tremor of hyperthyroidism is that of an exaggerated physiologic tremor, and usually responds well to β-blockade.

An association exists between myasthenia gravis and thyroid disorders. Hyperthyroidism is seen in approximately 5.7% and hypothyroidism in approximately 5.3% of myasthenic patients. Thyrotoxic periodic paralysis is another thyroid-associated disorder. Paralytic attacks are triggered by carbohydrate load, cold, or rest after exercise. Weakness may be limited to exercised muscles or may be generalized. Hypokalemia is consistently present in these patients.

Ophthalmopathy of hyperthyroidism is a chronic inflammatory condition of the orbit that is associated with autoimmune thyroiditis. The orbital tissues surrounding the globe become infiltrated with lymphocytes

Table 23.2 Hyperthyroidism

Discriminating features
▶ Increased serum levels of thyroid hormones
▶ Presence of thyroid stimulating immunoglobulins in Graves disease

Consistent features
▶ Hyperactivity, weight loss, insomnia
▶ Tremor
▶ Decreased serum cholesterol and triglycerides

Variable features
▶ Dysthyroid orbitopathy; ocular abnormalities
▶ Proximal muscle weakness
▶ Hyperactive reflexes
▶ Personality changes,
▶ Irritability, delirium
▶ Seizures

Pearls and Perils

Parathyroid dysfunction

▶ Seizures occur in 50% or more of patients with hypoparathyroidism but rarely occur in hyperparathyroidism.
▶ Psychiatric symptoms are common in both hypoparathyroidism and hyperparathyroidism.
▶ Myopathy, which may be severe, is a common finding in hyperparathyroidism, not hypoparathyroidism.

and plasmacytes. Edematous swelling of the extraocular muscles results in proptosis that may be unilateral or bilateral. The patient has a "staring" appearance and, frequently, diplopia, as a result of limitation of eye movements. Unlike other neurologic manifestations of thyroid disease that resolve with a return to the euthyroid state, severe thyroid ophthalmopathy does not resolve with medical treatment and may require surgical decompression.

Parathyroid: Disorders Associated with Calcium and Vitamin D Metabolism

Hyperparathyroidism

Disorders associated with primary and secondary hyperparathyroidism and osteomalacia are grouped together because of clinical similarities. Parathyroid hormone (PTH) functions to maintain extracellular calcium (Ca^{2+}) concentration. The commonest cause of parathyroid hormone oversecretion is a solitary adenoma of the parathyroid glands. Elevated serum alkaline phosphatase and calcium levels with depressed serum phosphate levels are useful markers of hyperparathyroidism. Hypercalciuria is common, and osteopenia is seen on bone radiographs. Levels of PTH are usually elevated but may be normal. Primary hyperparathyroidism usually affects patients between the third and fifth decades and is more common in women. Polyuria, constipation, nausea, and renal stones are primary manifestations. Mental status changes are also frequent, including irritability, impaired short-term memory, and psychiatric complaints. Neuromuscular complaints of weakness, wasting, and fatigue are variably associated. One series reported muscle cramps in 45% of patients with primary hyperparathyroidism. Severely affected patients have proximal weakness with a waddling gait. Bulbar and sphincter muscles are usually spared. Electromyographic studies may reveal myopathic units, like those seen in other endocrinopathies. Muscle histology generally shows no abnormality, although type 2 fiber grouping with internal nuclei and group atrophy may be seen.

Hypoparathyroidism

Hypoparathyroidism occurs as a result of decreased secretion of parathyroid hormone. Although it can occur idiopathically, hypoparathyroidism is most often seen following surgical excision or infarction. It can also occur as a result of reduced peripheral action of the hormone. Serum calcium is low and phosphorous may be elevated. Decreased serum calcium produces a state of neuromuscular hyperexcitability ("tetany") that comprises carpopedal spasm, cramps, twitching, and paresthesias. Latent tetany can be evoked by mechanical stimulation of the facial nerve (Chvostek sign) and by occlusion of venous return from an arm, producing carpopedal spasm (Trousseau sign). Neuroimaging may reveal intracranial calcifications, especially in the basal ganglia (Table 23.3).

The neurologic manifestations of hypoparathyroidism result primarily from hypocalcemia and consist of neuromuscular hyperexcitability, mental status changes (including dementia), and seizures. Florid psychiatric syndromes, including psychosis, are not uncommon. Seizures secondary

Table 23.3 Hypoparathyroidism

Discriminating features
▶ Decreased serum levels of parathyroid hormone and calcium
▶ Increased serum levels of phosphorus

Consistent features
▶ Neuromuscular hyperexcitability ("tetany")
▶ Generalized seizures poorly responsive to anticonvulsants

Variable features
▶ Mental status changes and psychiatric symptoms
▶ Myopathy
▶ Basal ganglia calcifications on neuroimaging

to hypocalcemia are well recognized and are usually generalized. Anticonvulsants are generally not required, and correction of the serum calcium is usually sufficient.

Adrenal

Cushing syndrome

Cushing syndrome results from excess circulating adrenal corticosteroids. The commonest etiology is hypersecretion of adrenocorticotrophic hormone (ACTH) by the pituitary. Most cases of Cushing syndrome are caused by benign pituitary adenomas (Cushing disease), which are significantly more common in women than in men. Truncal obesity, hirsutism, and hypertension are general features of Cushing syndrome. The neurologic manifestations include primarily mental status changes and muscle weakness. The mental status changes can range from irritability to prominent psychosis and affective disorders. Most patients have frank proximal weakness with demonstrable myopathic findings on EMG. Muscle biopsy typically shows type II atrophy. Myalgias may accompany the weakness, which affects the lower extremities to a greater degree than the upper extremities.

Iatrogenic glucocorticoid-induced neuromuscular disorders

Chronic treatment with iatrogenic glucocorticoids can also produce significant muscle weakness in up to 60% of patients. The dose and duration of steroid treatment required to induce chronic steroid myopathy is unclear. Treatment involves reducing the steroid dose as much as possible or switching to an alternate-day regimen.

An acute myopathy following treatment with steroids, especially in patients with status asthmaticus, has been well documented in the literature in recent years. It has been described frequently in the setting of use of muscle relaxants like vecuronium in combination with steroids. The myopathy is severe and frequently requires prolonged ventilatory support. Flaccid quadriparesis is noted long after the discontinuation of the muscle relaxants, and the weakness may take months to recover. Muscle biopsy shows nonspecific myopathic changes on light microscopy and selective loss of myosin filaments in muscle fibers on electron microscopy (Table 23.4).

Addison disease

Addison disease results from adrenal insufficiency due to either pituitary (lack of ACTH) or adrenal failure. Adrenal insufficiency is often missed because the clinical presentation can be quite nonspecific. Key clinical features include weakness, fatigue, anorexia, nausea/vomiting, weight loss, and symptoms of volume depletion. The most important neurologic manifestations are mental status changes and muscle weakness. Mental status changes, including psychiatric symptoms, are seen in 35–70% of pa-

Table 23.4 Frequency of clinical features of primary adrenal insufficiency

Symptoms	Signs	Laboratory findings
Weakness/ fatigue (100%)	Weight loss (100%)	Hyponatremia (90%)
Anorexia (100%)	Hyperpigmentation (97%)	Hyperkalemia (66%)
Nausea and diarrhea (56%)	Hypotension (91%)	Hypoglycemia (40%)
	Vitiligo (rare)	Hypercalcemia (6%)

tients with Addison disease, ranging from irritability and depression to acute confusional states and even coma. Approximately 25–50% of patients with adrenal insufficiency have significant muscle weakness secondary to a myopathy that is associated with muscle cramping.

Treatment of Addison disease includes oral replacement with hydrocortisone and, if aldosterone is also deficient, treatment with fludrocortisone acetate, a mineralocorticoid.

Pancreas (Diabetes)

Involvement of the peripheral and autonomic nervous systems is probably the most common neurologic complication of diabetes. Diabetic polyneuropathy is the most common neuropathy in developed countries. Its prevalence estimates vary, depending upon diagnostic criteria and the patient populations examined. Several large studies indicate that approximately 80% of patients with diabetes will eventually develop clinical neuropathy. It is important to remember that, in diabetes, the prevalence of neurologic involvement depends on the duration and severity of hyperglycemia. The Diabetes Control and Complications Trial (DCCT) demonstrated the importance of strict glycemic control in decreasing the incidence and slowing the progression of diabetic neuropathy. Diabetic neuropathy is categorized into distinct syndromes according to the predominant pattern of neurologic involvement, however, many overlap syndromes occur.

Distal symmetrical polyneuropathy

The most common form of diabetic neuropathy, distal symmetric polyneuropathy, begins insidiously and progresses slowly. It may be associated with a variety of symptoms such as burning, stinging, allodynia, hypersensitivity, or loss of sensation in the lower extremities that progress to involve the upper extremities. On neurologic examination, distal symmetrical sensory loss is usually present with diminution of deep tendon reflexes. Classic "stocking–glove" sensory loss is typical in this disorder. It may involve small- or large-fiber neurons, and may also be associated with autonomic involvement.

Pathologically, this is characterized predominantly by loss of nerve axons, initially sensory, followed by motor axonal loss that results in weakness in severe cases. Nerve conduction studies typically show slowing, especially distally, and needle electrode examination of muscle shows distal changes indicative of chronic partial denervation with reinnervation.

Autonomic neuropathy

Autonomic neuropathy is common in diabetes. Some autonomic abnormalities may be asymptomatic, such as pupillary size and response to light and accommodation. Other organ involvement, especially when severe, may have significant morbidity, including postural hypotension, gastroparesis, impaired bladder and sexual function, and enteropathy with constipation or diarrhea. Cardiovascular involvement due to autonomic dysfunction can result in resting tachycardia, hypotension, silent myocardial infarction, prolonged QT interval, or sudden death. Up to one-quarter of diabetic men are believed to have cardiovascular autonomic involvement, and the prevalence increases with advancing age. Treatment of autonomic hypotension involves increased fluid intake, supplementary salt, and pressure stockings. Resistant cases may require fludrocortisone (a mineralocorticoid) or midodrine (an adrenergic agent).

Lumbar polyradiculopathy (diabetic amyotrophy)

Radiculopathy or polyradiculopathy, often overlapping with plexopathy in the lumbar region, may be seen in diabetics. The terms *diabetic amyotrophy*, *diabetic femoral neuropathy*, and *diabetic polyradiculoneuropathy* have all been used to explain this entity. The most common type of diabetic polyradiculopathy is high lumbar radiculopathy involving the L2, L3, and L4 roots. It usually evolves quickly over days to weeks, involving significant pain and weakness of the anterior thigh. Severe weakness accompanied by atrophy of the quadriceps muscle is seen on neurologic examination along with occasional weakness of other L3- and L4-innervated muscles. Sensory loss is generally only mild and patchy, but the patellar reflex is reduced or absent. Symptoms usually reach a plateau within 6 months. The prognosis for recovery is good and continues for months to years. The diagnosis is made on the basis of history, clinical examination, and EMG studies. The same process can occur in the contralateral leg, either within days or months to years after the initial attack (Box 23.1).

Peripheral and cranial mononeuropathies

Acute and subacute neuropathies are also common in diabetes, often presenting in a distinctive fashion. Two types of focal neuropathy are seen: mononeuropathies occurring at pressure points, and spontaneously occurring neuropathies believed to be vascular in origin. The most

▼

Box 23.1 Diabetic neuropathy

Symmetric distal neuropathy
▶ Small-fiber (painful/anesthetic)
▶ Large-fiber (ataxic)
▶ Autonomic

Asymmetric neuropathy
▶ Compression mononeuropathies (median, ulnar, peroneal)
▶ Vascular neuropathies
▶ Plexopathy/polyradiculopathy (including amyotrophy)
▶ Cranial neuropathies

common compression neuropathies include median neuropathy at the wrist (carpal tunnel syndrome), ulnar neuropathy at the elbow, and peroneal neuropathy at the fibular head. Spontaneous vascular insults may also occur at the level of the root, plexus, or individual nerve. Root lesions or radiculopathies are common in diabetics and can occur at any spinal level. Pain is a prominent symptom, and unilateral trunk involvement is a frequent complaint. Characteristically, thoracic and upper lumbar roots are involved. On EMG examination, fibrillation potentials are found at multiple levels in the paraspinal musculature. The root symptoms often persist for several months before resolving completely, only to recur again at a different level. Involvement of one or more of the cranial nerves is not uncommon in diabetes. The third and sixth nerves are the most frequently affected. The third-nerve palsy in diabetes is typically "pupillary sparing" due to selective infarction of the nerve and sparing of the parasympathetic fibers, which are circumferentially arranged at the surface. Onset is usually abrupt, with an associated ptosis. Complete recovery within 3–6 months is the rule (Table 23.5).

Table 23.5 Diabetes

Discriminating features
▶ Elevated fasting plasma glucose
▶ Elevated serum glycosylated hemoglobin
▶ Association with diabetic retinopathy and nephropathy

Consistent features
▶ Distal symmetric polyneuropathy
▶ Increased risk of stroke

Variable features
▶ Autonomic neuropathies
▶ Compression mononeuropathies
▶ Lumbar plexopathy or polyradiculopathies
▶ Cranial neuropathies, especially 3rd and 6th cranial nerves
▶ Coma associated with ketoacidosis or hyperosmolarity

<table>
<tr><td>

▼

Pearls and Perils

Diabetes

▶ Potential causes of altered sensorium in diabetes are myriad: nonketotic hyperglycemic coma, diabetic ketoacidosis, stroke, uremia, hypophosphatemia, iatrogenic hypoglycemia, infection, etc.

▶ Focal signs or seizures are extremely uncommon in diabetic ketoacidosis and should prompt a search for an underlying structural cause.

▶ Early in its course, a third-nerve palsy due to aneurysmal compression may appear to be pupillary sparing.

</td><td>

▼

Pearls and Perils

Sickle cell disease

▶ Stroke is the most common presenting neurologic complication of sickle cell disease.

▶ Stroke may result from:
  – proximal larger vessel disease with hypoperfusion
  – distal small vessel disease due to sludging
  – arterial embolism

▶ Stroke recurrence in sickle cell disease is prevented by prophylactic transfusion.

</td></tr>
</table>

Diabetes is also associated with a two- to fourfold increased risk of stroke. Diabetes appears to accelerate atherogenesis in both small and large arteries and is, along with hypertension, an important cause of lacunar infarction. There is some evidence that hyperglycemia at the time of a stroke may be associated with increased morbidity and mortality. Therefore, it may be important to maintain patients in a euglycemic state in the setting of stroke.

Nonketotic hyperosmolar coma (NKC) and diabetic ketoacidosis can be important causes of coma in diabetics. Infection may be a significant precipitating factor in both. Unlike diabetic ketoacidosis, focal neurologic signs (such as aphasia, visual field cut, hemiparesis) are common with NKC, as are seizures. The mechanism of these focal neurologic deficits remains unclear, however.

Hematologic Disorders

Sickle Cell Anemia

Sickle cell disease (SCD) is a group of genetic disorders characterized by production of hemoglobin S. Stroke is the most devastating complication of SCD, and SCD is the most common cause of stroke in children. Convulsions can occur either independently or in association with acute stroke. Disorders of consciousness (most often due to intracranial hemorrhage) and meningitis (due to functional asplenia) can also occur, albeit less often. Headaches and visual loss may also occur.

The pathogenesis of stroke in SCD is unclear. Previously thought to be due to small-vessel obstruction by sickled erythrocytes, it now appears that lesions in major vessels, particularly the internal carotid and anterior and middle cerebral arteries, are important in the pathogenesis of stroke in SCD. In most patients, stroke occurs without warning. However, approximately 25% occur in the setting of a sickling or aplastic crisis. Approximately 75% of strokes are ischemic and 25% hemorrhagic. Ischemic

strokes are more frequent in patients younger than 20 and hemorrhagic strokes in older patients.

Computed tomography (CT) and magnetic resonance imaging (MRI) are the initial tests of choice for stroke assessment and transcranial Doppler (TCD) ultrasound is the imaging tool of choice for stroke prediction. Recent studies utilizing cranial MRI suggest that the frequency of cerebral infarction (up to 25%) is approximately twofold higher than that of clinically evident stroke in these patients. However, the clinical significance of silent infarction in SCD remains unclear. Risk factors for stroke include low steady-state hemoglobin, prior clinical stroke, and history of priapism. Risk for ischemic stroke recurrence in SCD patients can be lowered by chronic prophylactic transfusions aimed at maintaining the level of sickle hemoglobin lower than 30%. It is not clear if silent infarcts predispose to subsequent clinical stroke or give rise to cognitive deficits.

Myeloproliferative Disorders

Thrombosis and, paradoxically, bleeding are major causes of morbidity and mortality in the myeloproliferative disorders. These are a group of bone marrow hematopoietic stem cell disorders that include polycythemia vera (PV), essential thrombocythemia, chronic myelogenous leukemia, and myeloid metaplasia. Polycythemia vera is characterized by an increase in red blood cells. Essential thrombocythemia is characterized by a marked elevation of platelet count. Thrombosis is a major cause of mortality and morbidity in the myeloproliferative disorders. There are likely multiple factors involved, including thrombocytosis, increased whole blood viscosity, and abnormal platelet function.

Neurologic manifestations occur in approximately 13–25% of patients with myeloproliferative disorders and include stroke, transient ischemic attacks, sinus vein thrombosis, seizures, chronic headache, tinnitus, lightheadedness, and mononeuritis multiplex. A preponderance of subcortical or basal ganglia lacunar infarcts has been demonstrated in an autopsy series of patients with PV. Lacunes result from the occlusion of small penetrating arteries, which are particularly susceptible to thrombosis. Aseptic cavernous sinus thrombosis is an extremely rare phenomenon that has been reported in patients with PV. It has been suggested that patients found to have this symptom complex without known infectious predisposing causes should be carefully evaluated to rule out myeloproliferation.

In all patients with polycythemia, cerebral blood flow is reduced due to increased blood viscosity. Improvement in cerebral blood flow occurs with a reduction of the hematocrit. The primary method of treatment of these patients is venesection ("blood letting"), which is typically performed periodically to maintain the patient's hematocrit at less than 45. Comorbid risk factors for stroke, for example, smoking and hypertension, should additionally be addressed and treated in an attempt to decrease stroke in polycythemic patients.

The pathophysiology of essential thrombocythemia remains poorly understood. Abnormalities of platelet function have been described, including evidence of both hyper- and hypoaggregability. Whether the qualitative disturbances of platelet function are primarily responsible for the clinical manifestations of the disease is uncertain, as reduction in platelet number often results in clinical improvement despite persistence of functional platelet abnormalities. Several varieties of therapy are available for treating essential thrombocythemia including antiplatelet agents, plasmapheresis, and cytotoxic agents such as melphalan and hydroxyurea. In general, most neurologic symptoms respond to antiplatelet agents.

Certain other hematologic disorders also produce an increased blood viscosity and are frequently associated with similar neurologic manifestations. These disorders include increased white blood cells (hyperleukocytosis, occurring primarily in the context of leukemia), or increased serum proteins (multiple myeloma and Waldenstrom macroglobulinemia).

Thrombotic Thrombocytopenic Purpura

Thrombocytopenic purpura (TTP) is a rare syndrome of microangiopathic hemolytic anemia, thrombocytopenia, neurologic abnormalities, fever, and renal dysfunction (the pentad). Thrombocytopenic purpura is characterized by platelet aggregates in the microvasculature, resulting in blood vessel occlusion that gives rise to tissue ischemia and end-organ damage. An understanding of the pathogenesis of TTP is still evolving, and evidence accumulated over recent years suggests that the abnormal processing of Von Willebrand factor (VWF) plays a central role in the etiology of platelet aggregation in TTP. Clinical features and laboratory evaluation help in establishing the diagnosis. Thrombocytopenia, moderately severe anemia. and

a peripheral blood smear with numerous fragmented erythrocytes (schistocytes), nucleated red blood cells, and basophilic stippling are often present. Coagulation studies are very helpful in differentiating TTP from disseminated intravascular coagulation (DIC). Unlike DIC, the prothrombin time, partial thromboplastin time, and fibrinogen values are all normal in TTP. This is important, as both entities can have a similar morphologic picture on peripheral smear.

Neurologic symptoms include confusion, generalized headaches, altered mental status, focal deficits in the motor or sensory systems, seizures, visual disturbance, and even coma. These symptoms tend to be waxing and waning in nature, possibly because of microhemorrhagic and microocclusive vascular changes in the brain. Visual complaints may occur from retinal choroidal or vitreous hemorrhage and, rarely, retinal detachment (Table 23.6).

Thrombocytopenic purpura was almost universally fatal until the introduction of plasma exchange therapy in the 1970s, which improved the outcome to 82% survival. A number of other therapeutic modalities have been utilized with only modest success including corticosteroids, splenectomy, and antiplatelet drugs. Early treatment usually results in remission. However, relapse can be seen in up to 10%. Treatment with vincristine along with plasma exchange has been reported to be successful in recurrent or refractory cases.

Neurologic Complications of Hepatic Disease

Neurologic impairment is a frequent concomitant of liver disease, both acute hepatic failure and chronic liver dys-

---

Table 23.6 Thrombotic thrombocytopenic purpura

Discriminating features
▶ Pentad of hemolytic anemia, thrombocytopenia, fever, uremia, and neurologic dysfunction

Consistent features
▶ Normal coagulation tests
▶ Hyperbilirubinemia
▶ Fluctuating neurologic disturbances that may resemble transient ischemic attacks

Variable features
▶ Changes in mental status
▶ Seizures
▶ Hemiparesis
▶ Aphasia
▶ Visual field defects
▶ Permanent neurologic complications
▶ Coma

function (usually cirrhosis). In addition, certain viral infections that primarily affect the liver (e.g., hepatitis C) also have specific neurologic complications. Other primarily hepatic diseases with neurologic manifestations include Wilson disease, the porphyrias, and ALA-dehydrase deficiency.

Hepatic Failure

Acute or fulminant hepatic failure, with a mortality rate of 85%, is associated with an encephalopathy. As with other encephalopathies, there are attentional disturbances and a reduced level of consciousness. Distinct clinical stages of hepatic encephalopathy have been described, as noted in Box 23.2. On physical examination, cranial nerves are usually intact. Motor examination may reveal a flapping tremor or asterixis, increased tone, hyperreflexia, and an extensor plantar response (Table 23.7).

As might be expected, laboratory tests of liver function are abnormal, and evidence of a coagulopathy is usually present. Although no single cause has been identified for hepatic encephalopathy, ammonia appears to be either an important culprit or at least a marker of encephalopathy severity. The blood ammonia level, if done on arterial blood, correlates well with the severity of liver disease, the patient's clinical state, and the level of brain dysfunction. The gastrointestinal tract normally produces ammonia. It is detoxified in the liver by conversion to urea, which is then eliminated by the kidney. Studies have shown that a good relationship also exists between the degree of ammonia elevation and CSF glutamine in patients with hepatic encephalopathy. The mechanism by which ammonia affects neuronal function remains unclear. However, toxin hypersensitivity and possibly toxic endogenous benzodiazepine ligands have been implicated. Other studies, which may be helpful in evaluating a patient with hepatic encephalopathy, include the EEG, which typically shows abnormalities ranging from mild θ-wave slowing to more severe δ-wave slowing or triphasic waves. Brain MRI may show increased T1 hyperdensities in the basal ganglia, particularly in the globus pallidus.

Table 23.7 Hepatic encephalopathy

Discriminating features
▶ Acute hepatic failure or chronic liver dysfunction
▶ Abnormalities of tests of liver function
▶ Elevated serum ammonia levels
▶ Elevated cerebrospinal fluid glutamine

Consistent features
▶ Coagulopathy
▶ Attentional disturbances
▶ Reduced level of consciousness
▶ Electroencephalographic slowing

Variable features
▶ Asterixis
▶ Increased muscle tone
▶ Hyperreflexia
▶ Extensor plantar responses
▶ Seizures
▶ Coma

The management of hepatic encephalopathy includes general supportive measures plus methods to reduce the burden of ammonia, including elimination of dietary protein, control of gastrointestinal bleeding if present, and purgatives and enemas to decrease nitrogenous compounds in the colon. Lactulose is a synthetic disaccharide cathartic that has become a mainstay of treatment of hepatic encephalopathy because of its efficacy in reducing arterial ammonia. Unfortunately, treatment of fulminant hepatic failure has not been very successful and, in some cases, the availability of a donor liver for transplantation is the only true opportunity for a good recovery.

Patients with chronic hepatic failure may also develop a clinical picture similar to hepatic encephalopathy. This usually occurs in the setting of intercurrent infection, excessive dietary protein intake, or gastrointestinal hem-

---

Box 23.2 Clinical stages of hepatic encephalopathy

▶ Stage 1: Mild alterations in cognition and behavior; slight incoordination and postural tremor
▶ Stage 2: Reduced attention, lethargy; asterixis, paratonia, ataxia
▶ Stage 3: Delirium, somnolence; hyperreflexia, myoclonus, seizures
▶ Stage 4: Decorticate or decerebrate posturing; coma

Pearls and Perils

Hepatic encephalopathy

▶ Although asterixis can be seen in hepatic encephalopathy, it is by no means specific for this entity and may be encountered in other metabolic encephalopathies associated with uremia, severe pulmonary disease, and malnutrition.
▶ Triphasic waves are an abnormal electroencephalogram pattern that may accompany hepatic, uremic, anoxic and other metabolic encephalopathies.

Table 23.8 Diseases of the heme pathway

Disease	Chromosome	Enzyme	Inheritance
Sideroblastic anemia	Xp11.21	ALA synthase erythroid	X-linked recessive
delta-aminolevulinic acid dehydratase-deficient porphyria (ADP)	9q34	ALA dehydratase	Autosomal recessive
Acute intermittent porphyria (AIP)	11q24.1—> q24.2	Porphobilinogen deaminase	Autosomal dominant
Congenital erythropoietic porphyria (CEP)	10q25.2—> q26.3	Uroporphyrinogen III cosynthase	Autosomal recessive
Porphyria cutanea tarda	1p34	Uroporphyrinogen decarboxylase (PCT)	Autosomal dominant
Hereditary coproporphyria (HCP)	3q12	Coproporphyrinogen oxidase	Autosomal dominant
Variegate porphyria (VP)	1q22 or 23	Protoporphyrinogen oxidase	Autosomal dominant
Erythropoietic protoporphyria (EPP)	18q21.3 or 22	Ferrochelatase	Autosomal dominant

orrhage. The encephalopathy resolves as the offending crisis is treated. In general, patients with chronic hepatic disease fare much better than patients with fulminant hepatic failure.

Porphyrias

Porphyrias are inherited or acquired disorders due to deficiencies of specific enzymes of the heme biosynthetic pathway. When clinically expressed, they are associated with striking accumulations of heme pathway intermediates. Heme is synthesized predominantly in the liver and bone marrow, where it is used primarily to make cytochrome P-450 enzymes and hemoglobin, respectively. δ-Aminolevulinate synthase (also known as δ-aminolevulinic acid [ALA] synthase, ALAS), is the rate-limiting first step of heme synthesis. The heme synthesis pathway subsequently involves seven other enzymes. Mutations of the erythroid-specific form of δ-ALAS are found in X-linked sideroblastic anemia. Mutations in genes for the other seven enzymes are found in the porphyries (Table 23.8).

Two major types of clinical manifestations are characteristic of porphyrias (Table 23.9). Cutaneous photosensitivity occurs in the types of porphyria in which porphyrins accumulate. Neurologic manifestations occur in porphyrias characterized by accumulation of the porphyrin precursors δ-ALA and porphobilinogen (PBG). These "acute porphyrias" share many clinical features and are similarly managed. Neurologic complaints occur with δ-ALA dehydratase-deficient porphyria (ADP), acute intermittent porphyria (AIP), hereditary coproporphyria (HCP), and variegate porphyria (VP). Acute intermittent porphyria, the most common porphyria with neurologic manifestations, will be discussed in further detail.

The mechanism of neural damage in AIP is unknown. ALA is structurally analogous to γ-aminobutyric acid (GABA) and can interact with GABA receptors. However, ALA and other heme pathway products have not been convincingly shown to be neurotoxic. Symptom onset is typically after puberty and may recur intermittently, with attacks lasting days followed by complete recovery. Poorly localized abdominal pain is the most common symptom. Tachycardia, hypertension, restlessness, fine tremors, and excessive sweating due to sympathetic overactivity have been noted. Other manifestations include nausea and vomiting; constipation or diarrhea; pain in the limbs, head, neck, abdomen or chest; muscle weakness; and sensory loss.

A motor axonal polyneuropathy can develop in AIP. Weakness commonly begins in the proximal muscles and occurs more often in the arms than in the legs. It can also be asymmetric and focal. Cranial and sensory nerves can

Table 23.9 Major differentiating features of the most common human porphyrias

Disorder	Initial symptoms	Exacerbating factors	Most important screening tests	Treatment
Acute intermittent porphyria	Acute neurologic and visceral symptoms	Drugs (mostly P-450 inducers), progesterone, low calorie intake	Urinary porphobilinogen	Heme, glucose
Porphyria cutanea tarda	Chronic blistering skin lesions	Iron, alcohol, estrogens, hepatitis C virus, halogenated hydrocarbons	Plasma (or urine) porphyrins	Phlebotomy, low-dose chloroquine
Erythropoietic protoporphyria	Painful skin and swelling (mostly acute)		Plasma (or erythrocyte) porphyrins	Beta-carotene

be affected. Sudden death, presumably from cardiac arrhythmia, may also occur. Neuropsychiatric manifestations of AIP include anxiety, insomnia, hallucinations, paranoia, depression, and disorientation that can be especially severe during acute attacks. These may be mistaken for a primary mental disorder. Seizures may also occur as an acute neurologic manifestation of AIP.

Recognition of precipitating factors is most important in management. Avoidance of drugs that are hepatic heme pathway and ALAS inducers (such as barbiturates, steroid hormones, and sulfonamides among several others) remains key to preventing attacks. Reduced caloric intake, usually instituted in an effort to lose weight, is also a common precipitant. Intercurrent infections, major surgery, and cigarette smoking may also provoke attacks. The diagnosis of AIP is confirmed by measuring urinary PBG, which is increased during an acute attack.

Treatment of acute attacks usually requires hospitalization for the administration of intravenous (IV) glucose and heme in addition to management of nausea, vomiting, and pain. Observation for neurologic complications, electrolyte imbalances, and nutritional status, as well as investigation of precipitating factors is required. Heme therapy and carbohydrate loading are specific therapies, as they repress hepatic ALAS and overproduction of ALA and PBG. Heme therapy is effective, and should be initiated early after confirmation of the diagnosis. Seizure treatment can be difficult, as almost all antiseizure drugs can exacerbate AIP. However, gabapentin and vigabatrin may be given safely.

Neurologic Complications of Renal Failure

Uremic Encephalopathy

Early uremic features include subtle encephalopathic symptoms such as inability to concentrate, drowsiness, and insomnia. Mild behavioral changes, loss of memory, and errors in judgment may occur. Associated neuromuscular irritability is often present, manifest as hiccoughs, cramps, and fasciculations/twitching of muscles. A "flapping tremor" due to loss of tone (asterixis), as noted in hepatic encephalopathy, may also be seen with uremia. Myoclonus that is multifocal, primarily involving the facial and proximal musculature, and chorea are common as uremia progresses. Terminal uremia leads to seizures, stupor, and coma.

Diagnosis obviously relies on the demonstration of abnormal renal function tests in the setting of an encephalopathy. However, EEG may show encephalopathic changes of excessive θ- and δ-wave activity especially frontally, in addition to bilateral spike-and-wave complexes (triphasic waves) in a modest number of patients. Treatment of the underlying uremia will most often re-

verse the encephalopathy, although nonspecific changes on the EEG may persist. Rarely, convulsions may accompany uremic encephalopathy and may require treatment. It is important to remember that plasma anticonvulsant levels measured by the laboratory include both bound and free levels. Measured levels, even with adequate therapeutic dosing, are always reduced in uremic individuals due to decreased protein binding. However, as there is a higher fraction of free, unbound drug, ordinary dosing is usually sufficient despite low plasma levels.

Chronic Renal Failure

Polyneuropathy

Polyneuropathy is frequently seen in advanced chronic renal failure (CRF) and initially involves sensory more than motor nerves. The lower extremities are more involved than the upper, and distal portions of the extremities more than proximal. If dialysis is not instituted soon after onset of sensory abnormalities, motor involvement follows. This includes loss of deep tendon reflexes, weakness, peroneal nerve palsy (foot drop) and, eventually, flaccid quadriplegia. Accordingly, evidence of peripheral neuropathy is a firm indication for the initiation of dialysis or transplantation. Some of the CNS and neuromuscular complications of advanced uremia resolve with dialysis. Successful transplantation may reverse the peripheral neuropathy.

Restless legs

Restless legs is a common complaint in CRF patients. The restless leg syndrome is characterized by an ill-defined sensation of discomfort in the lower legs requiring frequent leg movement. Symptomatic improvement can usually be achieved with small doses of dopamine agonists or levodopa.

Dialysis Disequilibrium Syndrome

Dialysis disequilibrium most often occurs during the initiation of treatment of CRF with dialysis. It is presumed to be due to rapid reduction of blood urea levels with raised intracranial pressure (ICP), resulting in cerebral edema secondary to rapid (dialysis-induced) shifts of osmolality and pH between extracellular and intracellular fluids. Clinical manifestations are nausea, vomiting, drowsiness, headache and, rarely, seizures. The symptoms may occur up to 8–24 hours after dialysis, and can persist for hours to days. Using a dialysis regimen that produces slower solute removal can prevent the syndrome.

Dialysis Dementia

Dialysis dementia is a distinctive syndrome that can occur in patients who are chronically dialyzed for several years.

▼

Pearls and Perils

Renal disease

▶ Uremic neuropathy is almost invariably present by the time patients require dialysis.
▶ Mononeuritis multiplex and autonomic neuropathies reflect other conditions that predispose to renal disease (e.g., diabetes).
▶ Metabolic disturbances such as hypocalcemia, hyperkalemia, hypernatremia, and hyperphosphatemia may contribute to uremic encephalopathy.
▶ Anticoagulation during dialysis and associated hypertension may increase the risk of intracranial hemorrhage in patients with renal disease.

It is a progressive, usually fatal, encephalopathy that develops over months to years. Dialysis dementia is characterized by cognitive deterioration, speech apraxia, myoclonus, behavioral abnormalities including psychosis and, occasionally, focal abnormalities on neurologic examination. Aluminum accumulation has been implicated as the cause of dialysis dementia, as incidence of the syndrome has declined dramatically since aluminum has been eliminated from dialysate fluid. The most effective treatment is deferoxamine, a chelating agent that binds aluminum in plasma. A year of treatment or more is often required to see improvement.

Complications of Organ Transplantation

Neurologic complications following organ transplantation almost invariably result from infections related to immunosuppression, complications of medications used for immunosuppression, or cerebrovascular disease. Infections of the CNS develop in about 9% of patients and cerebrovascular lesions in 3%. The two most common infections are segmental herpes zoster and cryptococcal meningitis. *Listeria monocytogenes*, *Aspergillus*, and cytomegalovirus are other important causes of CNS infection in these patients. Progressive multifocal leukoencephalopathy caused by JC virus is manifest by progressive focal neurologic dysfunction. Infectious complications of the immunocompromised host are further discussed in Chapter 19. The high prevalence of cerebrovascular disease in transplanted patients also likely reflects the disease processes (e.g., diabetes and hypertension) that necessitated the transplantation in the first place.

Encephalopathy can result from a number of risks linked to organ transplant such as the procedure itself, immunosuppressive medications, systemic infections, microangiopathic thrombopathy, and complications induced by graft versus host disease. "Minor" neurologic symptoms resulting from immunosuppressants include tremor, headache, paresthesias, and insomnia. Diffuse encephalopathies and other neurologic complications such as seizures have been noted to occur at a higher rate in liver transplant patients as compared to other organ transplants, along with akinetic mutism, central pontine myelinolysis, and neuromuscular symptoms. Diffuse encephalopathy has an incidence of about 11% in liver transplant recipients. Transplant patients who experience neurologic complications appear to require longer hospitalizations and have a poorer outcome overall. In addition, the risk of developing malignancies, such as primary CNS lymphomas (PCNSL) and possibly gliomas, is higher in immunologically suppressed patients. The overall risk of cancer has been noted to be 100-fold greater in renal transplant recipients than in age-matched, nonimmunosuppressed cohorts.

Posterior reversible encephalopathy syndrome

Neurotoxicity is a significant complication of the use of immunosuppressive medications, especially tacrolimus and cyclosporine, both of which have been associated with posterior reversible encephalopathy syndrome (PRES). Posterior reversible encephalopathy syndrome is characterized clinically by mental status changes, seizures, and cortical blindness that are usually reversible with discontinuation of the offending medication. Posterior reversible encephalopathy syndrome is also characterized by specific findings on neuroimaging: posteriorly predominant hyperintensity of the white matter on T2-weighted and fluid-attenuated inversion recovery (FLAIR) images.

Nutritional Disorders Affecting the Nervous System

Neurologic disorders due to nutritional deprivation in the United States may be seen in certain populations who are at higher risk of inadequate intake or absorption of several vitamins. These include the elderly, vegans, alcohol-dependent individuals, and patients with malabsorption. Inadequate folate status, for example, is associated with neural tube birth defects. Folate and vitamins B_6 and B_{12} are required for homocysteine metabolism, and deficiencies are associated with increased risk of stroke. Excessive doses of vitamins may also result in adverse neurologic outcomes.

Retinol (Vitamin A, B-Carotene)

Deficiency of vitamin A is associated with a variety of ophthalmic disorders, including night blindness, corneal ulceration, and keratomalacia. Night blindness occurs because retinol insufficiency impedes production of rhodopsin, the primary chemical photoreceptor for the retinal rods. Since the rods sustain vision in conditions of low illumination, deficiency of retinol results in reduced visual acuity at night.

Excessive intake of most carotenoids causes a benign, yellowish discoloration of the skin. Large doses of canthaxanthin, a carotenoid, can induce a retinopathy. In adults, ingestion of over 500,000 IU of vitamin A may cause acute toxicity, manifest by skin changes, liver necrosis, and acute intracranial hypertension. Chronic toxicity, occurring with chronic daily intake of over 25,000 IU, is marked by alopecia, dermatitis, hepatocellular necrosis, and hyperlipidemia, in addition to pseudotumor cerebri and ataxia.

The neurologic syndrome of pseudotumor cerebri is characterized clinically by increased ICP associated with chronic headache and visual symptoms, in the absence of an intracranial mass lesion. Visual symptoms include transient visual obscurations, diplopia, scintillation, pulsating halos, black spots, and reduced visual acuity. On neurologic examination, patients have papilledema and, occasionally, sixth-nerve palsies. Cerebrospinal fluid pressure is extremely elevated, but the fluid itself is normal. Neuroimaging of the brain may demonstrate small or slit-like ventricles. The greatest threat from this condition is to vision, since sustained elevated pressures can result in progressive visual loss. Management begins with correcting any underlying precipitating factors such as hypervitaminosis A and encouraging weight loss. Acetazolamide is the initial drug of choice to decrease CSF formation. Occasionally, furosemide is needed. Serial lumbar punctures have been used to reduce CSF pressure. Regular ophthalmologic evaluation is warranted and, in some cases, optic nerve decompression may be necessary to relieve the papilledema and preserve vision.

Thiamine (Vitamin B₁)

Thiamine pyrophosphate, the coenzyme form of thiamine, is required for branched-chain amino acid and carbohydrate metabolism. Recommended Dietary Allowance (RDA) for thiamine is 1.2 mg/day for males and 1.1 mg/day for females. The median intake of thiamine in individuals residing in the United States from food alone is 2 mg/day. In Western countries, the primary causes of thiamine deficiency are poor nutritional intake associated with alcoholism, cancer, and other chronic illnesses. Alcohol is also known to interfere directly with the absorption of thiamine and with the synthesis of thiamine pyrophosphate. Thiamine deficiency is associated with many neurologic disorders including beriberi, Wernicke encephalopathy, and Korsakoff psychosis.

Thiamine deficiency

Beriberi. Thiamine deficiency in its early stage induces anorexia, irritability, apathy, and generalized weakness.

Prolonged thiamine deficiency causes beriberi, which is classically categorized as wet or dry, although considerable overlap occurs. In either form of beriberi, patients may complain of pain and paresthesias. Wet beriberi presents primarily with cardiovascular symptoms, marked by high-output congestive heart failure due to impaired myocardial energy metabolism and dysautonomia. Patients with dry beriberi present with a symmetric ascending polyneuropathy of the motor and sensory systems with diminished reflexes. The neuropathy is axonal and affects the legs most markedly. Variable sensory deficits, including paresthesias, dysesthesias, burning, even lancinating pains, are common. Sensory examination demonstrates vibratory and proprioceptive impairment, in addition to reduced pain and light touch sensation in a glove-and-stocking distribution. Tendon reflexes are either lost or reduced, and there may be distal weakness with foot drop. Upper extremity involvement is usually delayed. Since other vitamins may perhaps play a role in the development of this polyneuropathy, many authors suggest daily supplementation with vitamins of the B group in addition to 25 mg of thiamine.

Wernicke encephalopathy and Korsakoff psychosis. The Wernicke-Korsakoff syndrome is probably best thought of as two phases of the same disease: that is, the acute stage, Wernicke encephalopathy; and the more chronic, later-evolving stage, Korsakoff syndrome or psychosis.

Precipitation of the acute encephalopathy occurs against the backdrop of longstanding inadequate nutritional intake of thiamine such as in chronic alcohol abuse, malignancy, chronic dialysis, or acquired immune deficiency syndrome (AIDS). More recently, Wernicke encephalopathy has been described in obese patients following bariatric surgery. A carbohydrate load may be the precipitating factor for the acute encephalopathy. Therefore, IV glucose should never be given without thiamine.

Wernicke encephalopathy presents as an acute or subacute triad of mental impairment, ocular motor disturbance (ophthalmoplegia, ocular palsies, nystagmus), and cerebellar ataxia. The mental confusion can include primarily an amnestic disorder, apathy, reduced attention span, and in some cases, perceptual distortions. Bilateral sixth-nerve palsies are the most common ocular motor disturbance, but conjugate gaze palsies, internuclear ophthalmoplegia, and vertical and horizontal nystagmus may also be encountered. The ataxia tends to be primarily midline, affecting the trunk and lower extremities. It may be mild and reflected only as difficulty with tandem walking, or quite severe, evidenced by severe truncal titubation (Table 23.10).

Korsakoff syndrome or psychosis is the more chronic condition, characterized by a profound amnestic syndrome with relative preservation of other cognitive abilities. Patients display anterograde amnesia (i.e., an inability to form new memories) and a variable degree of retrograde amnesia. Confabulation is a frequent con-

Table 23.10 Thiamine deficiency

Discriminating features
▶ Precipitation with carbohydrate load
▶ Cardiac disease associated with beriberi

Consistent features
▶ Inadequate nutrition secondary to alcohol abuse or other chronic illness

Variable features
▶ Wernicke encephalopathy: mental confusion, ocular motor disturbance, ataxia
▶ Korsakoff' psychosis: profound amnestic syndrome
▶ Beriberi polyneuropathy

comitant of the disorder, although by no means specific to it. On careful physical examination, persistent features of Wernicke encephalopathy may also be found, including horizontal nystagmus and gait ataxia.

The neuropathologic lesions are essentially identical to those of Wernicke encephalopathy. Spongy degeneration of astrocytes is found in midline structures of the brain, such as the medial thalamic nuclei, mammillary bodies, periaqueductal gray area of the midbrain, and tegmentum of the pons. Degeneration of the superior cerebellar vermis is usually present. The lesions in the thalami and mammillary bodies probably account for the confusion, memory loss, and confabulation. The pontine tegmental lesions likely cause the oculomotor palsies, and the midline cerebellar degeneration causes the truncal ataxia.

The evaluation of patients with thiamine deficiency begins with a high index of suspicion and recognition that the disorder is not restricted to alcoholics. Serum thiamine levels lack sufficient sensitivity and specificity to be used alone in detecting thiamine deficiency. Red blood cell transketolase activity assay is a more accurate assessment of thiamine deficiency and, thus, more useful.

Treatment of acute thiamine deficiency is 100 mg/day of thiamine given parenterally for 7 days, followed by 10 mg/day orally until there is complete recovery. Ophthalmologic improvement occurs within days. Other manifestations gradually clear, although psychosis in the Wernicke-Korsakoff syndrome is frequently permanent or may persist for several months. Parenteral thiamine should be given prophylactically to all chronic alcoholic patients in the emergency room to prevent precipitation of thiamine deficiency upon the provision of glucose-containing solutions.

Thiamine-responsive disorders

Several inherited enzyme deficiency disorders, although not accompanied by a vitamin deficiency, may nonetheless be vitamin responsive, because of defects in metabolic pathways requiring thiamine. Maple syrup urine disease, a

branched-chain aminoaciduria, for example, is responsive to high-dose thiamine, which induces the enzyme -ketoacid decarboxylase and promotes the metabolism of branched-chain amino acids. Leigh syndrome (subacute necrotizing encephalopathy due to thiamine triphosphate deficiency in the brain), and thiamine-responsive lactic acidosis, are other disorders that may respond to thiamine therapy.

Niacin (Nicotinic Acid and Nicotinamide)

Over 200 niacin-dependent enzymes carry out oxidation and reduction reactions in the body and are involved in the synthesis and breakdown of all carbohydrates, lipids, and amino acids.

Niacin nutritional deficiency

Deficiency of nicotinic acid causes pellagra, which affects the skin, gastrointestinal system, and CNS. Pellagra is thus known by the classic triad of the "three Ds"—dermatitis, diarrhea, and dementia. Dementia and confusion are the most constant findings, followed by diarrhea (50%) and dermatitis (30%). In industrialized countries, particularly among alcoholics, niacin deficiency may present with only encephalopathy. Other features of CNS involvement include irritability, depression, insomnia, and cognitive deterioration. Patients may have altered sensorium, diffuse rigidity of the limbs, with positive grasp and sucking reflexes. Optic neuropathy, vertigo, extrapyramidal signs, spastic dysarthria, long-tract signs, and ataxia can also develop. Involvement of the peripheral nervous system (PNS) is often evident by the development of a painful peripheral neuropathy. Loss of vibratory sense and proprioceptive ability may reflect either the neuropathy or posterior column deficits.

Treatment consists of administration of 40–250 mg of niacin daily, which is adequate to reverse most of the signs and symptoms of niacin deficiency. Coexisting deficiencies of thiamine and pyridoxine are common, especially in alcoholics, and their replacement is well warranted.

Non-nutritional niacin deficiency

Carcinoid syndrome can also produce niacin deficiency, as tryptophan (amino acid precursor of niacin) is diverted to the production of serotonin, leaving little available for the production of nicotinic acid. Hartnup disease, an autosomal recessive defect in tryptophan absorption by the gut and kidney, can present identically to pellagra and is responsive to niacin administration.

Pyridoxine (Vitamin B$_6$)

Pyridoxine is unique in that both the deficiency and toxic states result in neurologic symptoms. Pyridoxal phosphate is the active biochemical form of pyridoxine. It is a

▼

Pearls and Perils

Nutritional deficiencies

▶ Nicotinic acid, thiamine (B$_1$), and cyanocobalamin (B$_{12}$) deficiencies may all present with cognitive disturbances.

▶ Pyridoxine (B$_6$) deficiency is associated with seizures in infants but a sensorimotor neuropathy in adults.

coenzyme of amino acid metabolism, particularly tryptophan and methionine. Deficiency of pyridoxine inhibits nerve lipid and myelin synthesis. Pyridoxine is also involved in neurotransmitter synthesis, with dopamine, serotonin, epinephrine, norepinephrine, and GABA all in need of pyridoxine for their production.

Pyridoxine deficiency is usually dietary but may accompany treatment with certain medications such as isoniazid and hydralazine and, very rarely, valproate. Deficiency of pyridoxine affects the blood, skin, and nervous system. A mixed (motor and sensory) distal symmetric polyneuropathy and, less frequently, an optic neuropathy have been reported in patients with pyridoxine deficiency. The polyneuropathy is characterized by sensory loss or pain and paresthesias in distal limbs, weakness, and loss of reflexes. Irritability, insomnia, psychiatric disturbances, confusion, and other intellectual impairment may also occur.

Urinary assays for xanthurenic acid and other pyridoxine metabolites may be performed following tryptophan loading in patients suspected of having pyridoxine deficiency. Daily intake of vitamin B$_6$ (150–450 mg) prevents the deficiency associated with isoniazid and should be used by patients on this drug. Once the neuropathy is established, it may improve, but does not entirely resolve, with replacement. Infants born to pyridoxine-deficient mothers may develop neonatal seizures as part of their vitamin deficiency state, a condition that is distinct from an inherited disorder of pyridoxine-responsive seizures.

Excess pyridoxine also results in an axonal sensory polyneuropathy. Mega-doses of pyridoxine, generally in excess of 2 g/day, are known to be toxic. However, toxicity with longstanding use of as little as 200 mg/day has been reported. Symptoms of paresthesias, ataxia, and burning feet may occur 1 month to 3 years after starting megadoses of pyridoxine. Posterior column function is involved earlier and to a greater degree than the spinothalamic pathway. Therefore, sensory ataxia may be prominent early. After stopping pyridoxine, the majority of patients improve, but the condition rarely resolves completely.

Cobalamin (Vitamin B$_{12}$)

Recognition of cobalamin deficiency is of particular importance because it not only causes macrocytic anemia,

but also a wide variety of neurologic and psychiatric abnormalities that are preventable or reversible if diagnosed early. The etiology of cobalamin deficiency in adults is usually decreased ingestion, impaired absorption, or impaired utilization of the vitamin. Cobalamin is not present in plants. Thus, extreme vegetarian diets can result in its deficiency. Animal cobalamin is tightly bound to proteins and requires the concerted action of HCl and pepsin for release in the stomach. Intrinsic factor is required for the absorption of cyanocobalamin by the intestine. Malabsorption due to lack of sufficient intrinsic factor is specifically called *pernicious anemia*. Vitamin B$_{12}$ malabsorption may also occur in a number of other settings, including chronic gastritis, post-gastrectomy, celiac disease, pancreatic insufficiency, and intestinal bacterial overgrowth. The resultant macrocytic anemia usually occurs before neurologic signs and symptoms are manifest. However, occasionally, neurologic symptoms parallel or even precede the anemia.

The most widely known neurologic disorder resulting from B$_{12}$ deficiency is subacute combined degeneration of the spinal cord, which reflects involvement of its lateral and dorsal columns. Clinical manifestations include tingling paresthesias of the feet with prominent vibration and proprioceptive deficits on examination. Weakness and stiffness of the legs may develop in addition to a spastic gait. Because of corticospinal involvement, there may be hyperreflexia and extensor plantar responses. With time, the hyperreflexia may be replaced by hyporeflexia as a peripheral polyneuropathy becomes superimposed (Table 23.11).

A variety of mental status changes may occur in B$_{12}$ deficiency, including a progressive dementia with impairment of memory and other intellectual abilities, in addi-

---

Table 23.11 Vitamin B$_{12}$ deficiency

Discriminating features
▶ Decreased serum vitamin B$_{12}$
▶ Pernicious anemia
▶ Abnormal Schilling test
▶ Antibodies to intrinsic factor and to gastric parietal cells

Consistent features
▶ Megaloblastic anemia with basophilic stippling
▶ Hypersegmented neutrophils
▶ Malabsorption states or other gastrointestinal disease

Variable features
▶ Subacute combined degeneration of the spinal cord with posterior column loss, spasticity, hyperreflexia and extensor plantar responses
▶ Superimposed peripheral neuropathy
▶ Mental status changes including progressive dementia
▶ Visual disturbances

tion to psychiatric disturbances ranging from depression to paranoid states. Visual disturbances, reflecting involvement of the optic nerves, may also occur.

Neuropathologically, patchy demyelination with swelling of myelin layers and vacuoles is encountered initially in the thoracic cord. Later, the demyelination spreads to include much of the white matter of the cord in addition to the deep white matter of the cerebral hemispheres and optic nerves. With time, axons degenerate in both the ascending tracts of the posterior columns and the descending pyramidal tracts. The combined degeneration of both ascending and descending tracts of the spinal cord is characteristic of vitamin B_{12} deficiency and has led to the designation of the disorder as *subacute combined degeneration of the spinal cord.*

Plasma B_{12} concentration is an accurate indication of B_{12} status, and the normal range has been considered to be 150–900 pg/mL. However, some observations suggest that up to 10% of individuals who have plasma B_{12} values between 150 and 400 pg/mL may have neuropsychiatric complications of B_{12} deficiency in the absence of megaloblastic anemia. Such persons can be identified by an elevated level of methylmalonic acid in the blood, which can be corrected with parenteral B_{12} administration. An elevation in serum methylmalonic acid is a sensitive and specific indicator of cellular B_{12} deficiency. Homocysteine elevation is also noted in B_{12} deficiency but is not specific, as it is also seen with deficiency of folic acid.

Treatment consists of 1 g of intramuscular (IM) B_{12} daily for several doses, followed by 1 g weekly for several months, while neurologic symptomatology is monitored. This should be followed by 1 g IM on a monthly basis and continued indefinitely. Improvement is usually seen within 3–6 months, especially if replacement is begun early.

Vitamin E (α-Tocopherol, Tocotrienols)

Vitamin E is an antioxidant that reduces peroxide production, thus preventing free radical injury of cell membranes. It is a lipid soluble vitamin that is absorbed in the small intestine and ultimately incorporated in the liver into low-density and very low-density lipoproteins for transfer to the cells of the body (Table 23.12).

Vitamin E deficiency

Vitamin E deficiency can result from reduced intake, fat malabsorption syndromes, inhibition of enterohepatic circulation, hereditary disorders, and abetalipoproteinemia. Neurologically, vitamin E deficiency can cause areflexia, ataxia, cutaneous sensory impairment, position and vibratory sense abnormalities and, less commonly, ophthalmoplegia, nystagmus, dysarthria, muscle weakness, and extensor plantar responses. A familial disorder of iso-

---

Table 23.12 Neurologic findings in vitamin E deficiency

▶ Truncal and appendicular ataxia
▶ Areflexia
▶ Abnormal vibration sense and proprioception
▶ Ophthalmoplegia
▶ Retinitis pigmentosa and acanthocytosis (in patients with abetalipoproteinemia)
▶ Dysarthria
▶ Generalized weakness
▶ Extensor plantar responses

---

lated vitamin E deficiency (due to a defect in α-tocopherol transfer protein) produces a syndrome that is clinically indistinguishable from Friedreich ataxia. Abetalipoproteinemia (Bassen-Kornzweig syndrome) is marked by retinitis pigmentosa and acanthocytosis of red blood cells. There is a decreased serum level of cholesterol and triglycerides. Neuropathologically, vitamin E deficiency leads to axonal membrane injury. There is resultant axonal degeneration of peripheral nerve, dorsal root ganglia, and posterior columns.

Diagnosis of vitamin E deficiency relies on serum α-tocopherol, which is a reliable indicator of body vitamin E content. Treatment is vitamin E supplementation. Administration of α-tocopherol (400 mg daily) may reverse or prevent progression of the effects of a vitamin E deficiency. However, doses of up to 100 IU/kg/day are required in those with familial vitamin E deficiency syndrome or abetalipoproteinemia. Injectable vitamin E can be used for those who cannot absorb oral medication. Prognosis for recovery depends on the duration of symptoms prior to initiation of treatment.

Vitamin E toxicity

Toxic symptoms related to excessive intake of vitamin E are often not recognized. Depressed levels of vitamin K–dependent procoagulants and potentiation of oral anticoagulants have been reported, as has impaired leukocyte function with delayed wound healing. Toxic doses also cause increased bleeding and may slightly increase the incidence of hemorrhagic stroke. Additional neurologic symptoms of vitamin E toxicity include headache, fatigue, and muscle weakness.

Systemic Autoimmune Diseases

A variety of disorders comprise the systemic autoimmune diseases or collagen vascular diseases. These disorders differ from organ-specific diseases in that autoimmune pathologic lesions may be found in multiple organs and

---

Pearls and Perils

Systemic lupus erythematosus (SLE)

▶ Neuropsychiatric signs and symptoms are common in SLE.
▶ Three pathogenetic mechanisms account for most
  neuropsychiatric syndromes in SLE:
   – antiphospholipid antibodies
   – antineuronal antibodies
   – vasculitis
▶ Secondary causes of neurologic disturbance in patients
  with SLE include:
   – steroid-induced psychosis or myopathy
   – opportunistic infection(s)
   – metabolic derangements

---

tissues. Systemic lupus erythematosus (SLE) is one such disorder with protean manifestations. It serves well as a prototype of systemic autoimmune disorders because of its abundant autoimmune manifestations. However, other collagen vascular diseases with CNS involvement will also be discussed.

Systemic Lupus Erythematosus

Systemic lupus erythematosus is a disease of unknown etiology in which tissues and cells are damaged by pathogenic autoantibodies and immune complexes. Neurologic and psychiatric manifestations of SLE are both frequent and varied, occurring in 33–75% of SLE patients. In approximately 15%, neurologic dysfunction is the first manifestation of the illness. The neurologic manifestations of SLE can be classified as those directly related to immunologic CNS involvement and those occurring as secondary manifestations; that is, related to complications of the disease and its treatment. Secondary neurologic complications are more frequent than primary ones and include those related to infections (associated with immunosuppression) in addition to those related to metabolic (e.g., uremia) or treatment (e.g., corticosteroid) complications.

Pathophysiology

Three pathophysiologic mechanisms account for the majority of direct manifestations of SLE in the nervous system: noninflammatory vasculopathy, vasculitis, and antibody-mediated processes. Lupus patients may have a bland vasculopathy with perivascular accumulation of mononuclear cells without necrosis. The vasculopathy causes small infarcts due to luminal occlusion, and also may cause indirect injury by affecting the blood–brain barrier and allowing antibodies to enter the CNS. True vasculitis in the brain and spinal cord is rare in SLE.

When CNS vasculitis does occur, it is frequently associated with intracranial hemorrhage. In contrast to the rarity of CNS vasculitis in patients with SLE, the PNS is commonly (approximately 10% of patients) affected by systemic vasculitis. This causes mononeuritis multiplex and may play a role in the distal symmetric polyneuropathy that affects SLE patients. A number of autoantibodies have been demonstrated in SLE patients with neurologic involvement. Many of the neurologic manifestations, specifically the nonfocal symptoms, are probably antineuronal autoantibody-mediated. Antineuronal antibodies (ANeA) are found in up to half of patients with CNS involvement, and are thought to play a role in SLE-associated dementia, neuropsychiatric disorders, and seizures.

Antiphospholipid antibodies (APA) refer to a group of circulating antibodies against negatively charged phospholipids including cardiolipin. Antiphospholipid antibodies can be detected by various methods including prolonged coagulation tests, presence of the lupus anticoagulant, and a biologic false-positive test for syphilis or anticardiolipin antibody. If a suspicion of APA exists, all four tests should be performed. Lupus is the disease most commonly associated with APA, as reflected by lupus anticoagulant and anticardiolipin antibodies occurring in 34% and 44%, respectively, of patients with SLE. Antiphospholipid antibodies (and particularly lupus anticoagulant) appear to increase the risk of stroke syndromes in SLE, and have also been implicated in symptoms of chorea and seizures.

Stroke

Strokes occur in SLE via a variety of mechanisms including cardiogenic emboli, large-vessel stenosis, small-vessel occlusion, and intracranial hemorrhage. Estimated frequency of strokes or transient ischemic attacks ranges from 5–16% of patients with lupus. The incidence of stroke is also increased in SLE patients with hypertension, renal or cardiac disease, and coagulopathy.

Antiphospholipid syndrome

Antiphospholipid syndrome (APS), as mentioned earlier, is a risk factor in patients with SLE. Antiphospholipid antibodies are associated with venous and arterial thrombosis, spontaneous abortion (probably caused by placental thrombosis), and thrombocytopenia. Patients with APA may be at particular risk for recurrent strokes and multi-infarct dementia. Lupus chorea is strongly associated with the presence of APA. A number of mechanisms have been proposed to explain how APA produce thromboembolic phenomena in patients with SLE. The effects of APA on platelets, circulating factors of both the intrinsic and extrinsic clotting systems, and components of vessel walls promoting thromboembolic phenomenon have all been demonstrated. Additionally, APA may play a critical role in the development of verrucous endocarditis (Libman-Sacks endocarditis), a common postmortem finding in patients with lupus. The presence of Libman-Sacks endocarditis predisposes to endocardial thrombosis and subsequent embolic phenomenon responsible for strokes.

Well-designed therapeutic trials in patients with APS are not available. However, clinical experience suggests that anticoagulation with or without aspirin may prevent further thrombotic complications. Corticosteroids, immunosuppressants, and plasmapheresis have also been used with mixed results.

Neuropathy

About 10–15% of patients with SLE develop a peripheral neuropathy, which is thought to be due to a vasculopathy of the small arteries supplying the affected nerves. Autonomic neuropathy has also been reported, resulting in gastrointestinal, bladder, cardiac, and pupillary abnormalities. Neuropathy due to SLE is frequently asymmetrical (mononeuritis multiplex). It usually affects the sensory more than the motor nerves. The neuropathy generally responds to steroid treatment. However, not all patients improve, and a complete response may take weeks to months because of the slow pace of nerve regeneration.

Neuropsychiatric manifestations

Neuropsychiatric manifestations of SLE are common, occurring in up to 60% of patients. Neuropsychiatric disturbances include psychosis, dementia, acute confusional states, cognitive impairment, depression, and anxiety. A number of antibodies, especially ANeA, have been associated with neuropsychiatric disturbances in patients with SLE. ANeA levels often fluctuate with disease activity, and assays can be performed both on serum and CSF. Whether ANeAs are neurocytotoxic, however, remains to be established. In general, neuropsychiatric disturbances in patients with lupus are corticosteroid responsive.

Other neurologic presentations

Seizures, stroke, headache, cranial nerve abnormalities, chorea, Guillain-Barré syndrome, and transverse myelopathy are among various neurologic syndromes that may complicate SLE. The etiology of these disorders is unclear. Seizures occur in 14% or more of patients with SLE and are more often generalized than partial. Chorea, seen in 2% of patients with SLE, is typically of sudden onset, either unilateral or bilateral, and improves gradually. Pseudotumor cerebri is a rare but recognized complication of SLE, which presents with raised ICP, papilledema, and headache. Dural venous sinus thrombosis can also occur in SLE patients and should be considered in those presenting with raised ICP.

Corticosteroids with or without cyclophosphamide are the most useful agents in treating lupus-associated vasculitis. A variety of neurodiagnostic tests are available and often performed in patients with SLE and neurologic disturbance. However, in general, clinical acumen provides the most significant diagnostic information, and laboratory studies are by and large supportive. Serologic studies (assays of APA or ANeA), CSF analysis, neuroimaging (especially MRI), and EEG are most frequently utilized. Cerebral angiography has been used to evaluate for vasculitis, but is of limited value. Laboratory studies should be individualized for any given patient.

Rheumatoid Athritis

Neurologic complications of rheumatoid arthritis (RA), although not common early in the disease course, can result in major symptoms and disability as the disease progresses. The PNS is more commonly targeted than the CNS, including compressive neuropathies, distal sensory neuropathies, and mononeuritis multiplex. Compressive neuropathies result from underlying arthropathies, whereas mononeuritis multiplex and sensory polyneuropathies occur secondary to an arteritis. Carpal tunnel syndrome is the most common neurologic manifestation of RA. Headache and neck pain are other prominent complaints of RA patients. When these complaints are accompanied by structural abnormalities, the most common finding is disease of the C1–C2 lateral facet joints, in association with radicular pain in the C2 dermatome.

The most devastating complication, however, is destructive disease of the cervical spine, with attendant myelopathy. Spinal instability at the atlantoaxial joint due to subluxation develops particularly in patients with advanced RA. The risk of neurologic complications and choice of appropriate therapy varies with the direction of subluxation.

Masses of inflammatory granulation tissue called *rheumatoid nodules* can develop in up to 20–30% of RA patients and are usually subcutaneous in location. Very infrequently, such rheumatoid nodules can develop in the meninges, involving the dura, with associated mass effect or rheumatoid pachymeningitis. They may also involve the spinal cord with associated myelopathy. Treatment is corticosteroids with or without cyclophosphamide.

Muscle involvement in RA may be multifactorial. Muscle biopsy specimens commonly reveal type II fiber atrophy that is likely related to disuse and steroid treatment. Focal myositis may also occur in muscles immediately adjacent to involved joints. In some patients, a disseminated nodular myositis is observed. Approximately 4–6% of patients with RA have superimposed polymyositis or dermatomyositis, which can be distinguished from the more common nodular myositis by their more malignant course, marked muscle enzyme elevation, and diffuse inflammatory infiltrates on muscle biopsy.

Finally, vasculitic myopathy can occur and may also contribute to weakness in some patients.

Progressive Systemic Sclerosis

Progressive systemic sclerosis (PSS), formerly termed *scleroderma*, is an uncommon rheumatic disease characterized by excessive fibrosis of a variety of tissues, microvascular abnormalities, and autoimmune phenomena. Nearly all patients with PSS, or its more limited variant, the CREST (calcinosis, Raynaud phenomena, esophageal hypomotility, sclerodactyly, and telangiectasia) syndrome, experience Raynaud phenomenon. The most common neurologic manifestations of PSS are headache, cranial neuropathies or peripheral neuropathy, and myopathy. Trigeminal nerve sensory dysfunction is the most common cranial nerve manifestation, affecting up to 4% of patients. Trigeminal motor function is not impaired. Numbness may be accompanied by dysesthesia in the trigeminal distribution. Peripheral neuropathy also occurs in PSS, and is a distal axonal sensorimotor polyneuropathy. Patients with PSS often also have a variety of subclinical manifestations of autonomic neuropathy. The most common neurologic manifestation of PSS is myopathy, which occurs in 17% of patients and is associated with type II fiber atrophy on muscle biopsy. This is a noninflammatory myopathy with minimal elevation of CPK and aldolase. The myopathy, usually nonprogressive, rarely requires immunosuppressive therapy. However, on occasion, it meets the criteria for polymyositis. In this instance, there may be concurrent cardiac involvement and a substantial risk of congestive heart failure and sudden death.

Mixed Connective Tissue Disease

Mixed connective tissue disease (MCTD) is an overlap syndrome of SLE, PSS, and polymyositis that is associated with antibodies against ribonucleoprotein. Neuropsychiatric manifestations are common, occurring in up to 55% of patients with MCTD. In general, the neuropsychiatric symptoms parallel those found in patients with lupus. Aseptic meningitis (seen in 25% of patients) and transverse myelitis (seen in 10% of patients), appear more commonly than in lupus. Furthermore, patients with MCTD are notable for the conspicuous absence of thromboembolic phenomena.

Sjögren Syndrome

Sjögren syndrome (SS) is characterized by keratoconjunctivitis sicca (dry eyes) and xerostomia (dry mouth). It is most commonly associated with rheumatoid arthritis. Neuromuscular complications may affect up to 10% of SS patients and generally resemble the extraspinal manifestations of RA, even in the absence of associated RA. A myopathy characterized by patchy, focal inflammatory infiltrates is common but rarely symptomatic, and polymyositis is rare. Several forms of neuropathy have been described including a slowly progressive sensory polyneuropathy, a minimally disabling sensorimotor polyneuropathy and, occasionally, more rapidly progressive mononeuritis multiplex. A number of patients have been described with a sensory neuronopathy that is caused by inflammation of selected dorsal root ganglia. Over weeks to years, these patients developed progressive sensory loss (primarily affecting vibratory and position sense), which ultimately became a disabling sensory ataxia. Pain and paresthesias were common. In addition, many patients exhibited severe autonomic impairment with pupillary involvement, orthostatic hypotension, and generalized anhydrosis. Trigeminal sensory neuropathy, identical to that observed in PSS, can also occur either in isolation or in association with the sensory neuronopathy.

Laboratory manifestations of SS include elevated ANA titers, positive rheumatoid factor, an elevated erythrocyte sedimentation rate, and polyclonal hypergammaglobulinemia, in addition to the more specific SSA (anti-Ro) and SSB (anti-La) antibodies. Cyclophosphamide and prednisone are the treatments of choice for the vasculitis of SS. Treatment of the neuronopathies has been less encouraging. However, recently, some favorable response to IV immunoglobulin, in conjunction with corticosteroids, has been reported.

The Vasculitides

Classically, the vasculitic syndromes have been categorized by the predominant size and type of blood vessels most commonly affected among patients with the disorder. Large-sized arteries are affected in Takayasu and giant cell (temporal) arteritis. Medium- and small-sized arteries are affected in polyarteritis nodosa, granulomatous angiitis, Wegener granulomatosis, lymphomatoid granulomatosis, Cogan syndrome, and isolated CNS vasculitis. Small-sized arteries are affected in Henoch-Schönlein purpura, vasculitis secondary to connective tissue diseases, essential cryoglobulinemia, hypersensitivity vasculitis, and drug-induced vasculitis. Temporal arteritis, Cogan syndrome, amphetamine-induced angiitis, and isolated angiitis of the nervous system typically present with CNS complaints, whereas evidence of generalized vasculitis is usually observed in the other vasculitides prior to CNS involvement. In addition, a number of infectious diseases may cause neurologic dysfunction as a result of vasculitis, including syphilis, Lyme disease, tuberculosis, hepatitis, and trigeminal herpes zoster.

The presence of vasculitis should be considered in patients who present with systemic symptoms in combination with evidence of single and/or multiorgan dysfunction. Although neither sensitive nor specific, common complaints and signs of vasculitis include fatigue, fever, arthralgias, abdominal pain, renal insufficiency, and neurologic dysfunction. The presence of certain signs, such as mononeuritis multiplex, palpable purpura, and pulmonary-renal involvement, is strongly suggestive of vasculitis.

From a neurologic perspective, any CNS or PNS symptom or sign can be produced by a vasculitis. A common presentation of vasculitis of the CNS is headache, with or without superimposed delirium, and multifocal neurologic deficits. Diffuse CNS involvement is characterized by the acute or subacute onset of headache, behavioral or personality change, memory impairment, psychiatric symptoms, and occasionally alterations in consciousness. Generalized seizures may occur but are more common in patients with focal disease. Focal CNS involvement may be marked by single or multiple cranial nerve palsies, ophthalmoplegia, and movement disorders. Visual loss due to vasculitic involvement of the optic nerve (ischemic optic neuritis) is seen in up to 50% of patients with temporal arteritis, but can also be seen in patients with Wegener granulomatosis and occasionally polyarteritis nodosa. An isolated myelopathy is sometimes seen in patients with either isolated CNS angiitis or drug-induced vasculitis, but is uncommon in other types of vasculitic disease.

Peripheral nerves as well as muscles can be affected in vasculitis. The most distinctive presentation is that of mononeuritis multiplex, although this appears to be the least prevalent form. A much more common presentation is a distal symmetric/asymmetric "stocking–glove" sensorimotor polyneuropathy that appears to be a consequence of ischemic damage or infarction of peripheral nerve vasa vasorum. Regardless of the pattern of neuropathy, PNS vasculitis not infrequently presents as severe burning pain in the distribution of the involved nerves. Involvement of skeletal muscle may lead to a symmetric proximal weakness that is indistinguishable from that seen in polymyositis or dermatomyositis.

The clinical course of vasculitic disease is extremely variable. When the vasculitis affects primarily the CNS or PNS, the course is usually subacute or chronic, with a stuttering progression of deficits. An acute, fulminant monophasic picture has also been reported. It is important to note that most of the vasculitic syndromes can produce disturbances in both the CNS and PNS, and often simultaneously. Exceptions would include isolated CNS angiitis and Takayasu arteritis, which are restricted to the CNS, and temporal arteritis and Behçet disease, which affect the PNS only rarely.

Similar to the evaluation of patients with SLE, multiple laboratory tests are utilized to evaluate and diagnose the vasculitic syndromes. Cranial CT or MRI, cerebral arteriography, nerve conduction studies, electromyography and, in particular, brain meningeal or arterial biopsy are most often useful. As with SLE, the laboratory workup of patients with vasculitis must be individualized, with particular attention to the patient's clinical presentation and sites of CNS and PNS involvement.

Because of the relative rarity of the vasculitic syndromes, few controlled, randomized, prospective therapeutic trials have been performed. In the vast majority of patients with CNS or PNS manifestations, some form of immunosuppressive therapy, with combined corticosteroids and cytotoxic agents (usually cyclophosphamide), is indicated. This combination has been shown to be effective in series of patients with Wegener granulomatosis and polyarteritis nodosa. For isolated CNS angiitis, recent data suggest that cytotoxic agents may not be necessary in all cases. Thus, the decision to add a cytotoxic agent should be based upon the clinical severity of the CNS vasculitis. The optimal duration of therapy is not known. Some investigators suggest that treatment be continued for 6–12 months following clinical remission, a regimen similar to that used in systemic vasculitis.

Alcohol and Drugs of Abuse

Neurologic Complications of Alcohol Abuse

Alcohol is one of the most widely used psychoactive drugs and is associated with a wide variety of complications affecting every level of the nervous system. In some instances, the disorders represent a direct cytotoxic action of alcohol. In others, they are the result of systemic effects of alcohol, including metabolic disturbances, nutritional deficiencies, and the like.

Alcohol intoxication

Alcohol is a CNS depressant whose toxic effects can be produced in any individual who ingests sufficient quantities of the substance. Blood levels of 100 mg/dL typically

---

▼

Pearls and Perils

Vasculitis

▶ Vasculitis may mimic any primary neurologic disorder.
▶ Central nervous system vasculitis is characterized by either diffuse or focal patterns of involvement.
▶ Peripheral nervous system vasculitis results in three patterns including:
 – mononeuritis multiplex
 – symmetric distal sensorimotor polyneuropathy (DSPN)
 – overlapping mononeuritis multiplex and DSPN.

cause drunkenness in occasional imbibers. Chronic alcohol abusers can tolerate levels up to 500 mg/dL without apparent effects. The phenomenon of acute intoxication depends on the blood alcohol concentration, the rate at which it has been attained, and the time during which it has been maintained. Intoxication with alcohol produces dysfunction of the cerebellar and vestibular systems in addition to higher cognitive abilities. Diffusion of alcohol into the cupula of the inner ear can produce intense positional vertigo. With increasing blood alcohol levels, more significant central nervous depression occurs, including hyporeflexia, cardiac and respiratory compromise, and ultimately coma.

Alcohol withdrawal

The manifestations of alcohol withdrawal occur when a person decreases or stops a high level of alcohol intake, either after a binge lasting a matter of days or after the regular ingestion of alcohol sustained over many months. The earliest findings of alcohol withdrawal may occur within 6–8 hours of alcohol cessation. However, typically, symptoms of alcohol withdrawal occur approximately 12–24 hours after abrupt cessation of intake. Initially, there is tremulousness, which is associated with hyperacuity of all sensory modalities, hyperreflexia, hypervigilance, anxiety, tachycardia, hypertension, and insomnia. Withdrawal seizures can occur in approximately 3–4% of untreated patients. These are characteristically generalized seizures occurring within 6–48 hours of alcohol withdrawal. Focal seizures are not typical for withdrawal and warrant evaluation for a structural etiology. Most patients have more than one seizure, but usually less than five. Status epilepticus is uncommon in the setting of alcohol withdrawal but can occur. Epileptic status is a medical emergency and should be treated with anticonvulsants in the same manner as status due to any other etiology. For patients with seizures without status epilepticus, treatment of seizures is more controversial. Although patients can be loaded with anticonvulsants acutely, it is usually not necessary to continue anticonvulsants. There is some suggestion that treatment with tapering doses of long-acting benzodiazepines is more efficacious, especially if continued abstinence from alcohol is expected. Alcohol withdrawal itself may also potentially aggravate any preexisting seizure disorder unrelated to the alcohol abuse. Thiamine must be given and electrolyte abnormalities, especially hypomagnesemia, should be corrected.

Delirium tremens comprises a combination of psychic and autonomic hyperactivity, usually occurring after 3–5 (but occasionally as late as 14) days of alcohol abstinence. Only 5–6% of untreated patients withdrawing from alcohol develop this life-threatening syndrome. Its features include confusion, agitation, hallucinations, tremor, and autonomic hyperactivity (tachycardia, fever, sweating). The hallucinations are primarily visual but may be kinesthetic. Effective sedation with benzodiazepines remains the mainstay of treatment. In addition, IV hydration, thiamine and multivitamins, correction of electrolyte abnormalities (usually hypomagnesemia and hypokalemia), and supportive care are essential.

Alcoholism-associated cognitive impairment

Cognitive impairment occurs from a variety of causes in alcoholic patients. The Wernicke-Korsakoff syndrome, due to a deficiency of vitamin B_1 (thiamine), has been previously described in this chapter as an important cause of confusion and memory disturbances in alcoholics and chronically malnourished patients. Deficiency of nicotinic acid (niacin), also previously described in this chapter, may result in confusion and intellectual deterioration. Cognitive impairment in alcoholics can also occur in the setting of hepatic encephalopathy, subdural hematoma, traumatic brain injury, or anoxic encephalopathy. In addition, alcoholic brain disease, unrelated to the Wernicke-Korsakoff syndrome, has been recognized as an important cause of dementia in chronic alcoholics. The symptoms are usually mild, but involve impairment in psychometric test performance of frontal and temporal lobe function.

Marchiafava-Bignami disease

This is a rare toxic disease seen in some chronic alcoholics that results in progressive demyelination and necrosis of the corpus callosum. The process may extend laterally into the neighboring white matter and occasionally as far as the subcortical regions. The exact mechanism responsible for this demyelination is not known. Clinically, this entity presents with depressed consciousness, confusion, dysarthria, and seizures. There is no treatment for Marchiafava-Bignami disease, which is frequently fatal (Table 23.13).

Pearls and Perils

Alcohol abuse

▶ Focal seizures in alcoholics imply a structural lesion and should not be attributed to withdrawal.

▶ Alcoholics should never be given glucose without thiamine because of the risk of precipitating a Wernicke encephalopathy.

▶ A subset of patients with alcohol withdrawal seizures will have epilepsy and require long-term anticonvulsant therapy.

▶ Delirium tremens is a life-threatening condition and should be treated as a medical emergency.

Table 23.13 Chronic alcohol abuse

Discriminating features
▶ Symptoms of alcohol withdrawal after abrupt cessation of drinking often with generalized seizures
▶ Development of delirium tremens 3–5 days after ethanol withdrawal

Consistent features
▶ Hypomagnesemia, hypokalemia
▶ Chronic cerebellar syndrome
▶ Alcoholic polyneuropathy
▶ Alcoholic brain disease

Variable features
▶ Acute or chronic alcoholic myopathy
▶ Wernicke-Korsakoff syndrome
▶ Central pontine myelinolysis

Cerebellar degeneration

Many alcoholics develop a chronic cerebellar syndrome that may represent a direct toxic effect of alcohol on the Purkinje cells of the cerebellum. It appears to involve the anterior vermis and paravermian regions of the cerebellum, producing a truncal and gait ataxia. The ataxia is usually gradually progressive and typically involves the lower extremities to a greater degree than the upper extremities. It may be associated with a mild dysarthria. Treatment consists of cessation of alcohol intake and chronic thiamine and multivitamins, which can often preclude further deterioration.

Alcoholic polyneuropathy

Peripheral polyneuropathy secondary to excessive alcohol use is extremely common. Like other peripheral neuropathies, it is a distal, symmetric, axonal sensorimotor neuropathy that appears gradually and is accompanied by symptoms of pain, burning, dysesthesias, and numbness. Patients often complain of muscle cramps, especially distally. On physical examination, there is usually decreased vibratory sense in addition to deficits of light touch, reduced or absent deep tendon reflexes, and weakness. Cessation of alcohol intake may halt further progression of the neuropathy. Treatment of the pain usually consists of low doses of tricyclic antidepressants (e.g., amitriptyline) or anticonvulsants (e.g., carbamazepine or gabapentin).

Alcoholic myopathy

Both an acute and a chronic form of alcoholic myopathy exist. The acute form typically occurs with binge drinking and is associated with muscle pain, weakness and, often, rhabdomyolysis. Serum CPK can be moderately to severely elevated. Acute alcoholic myopathy should be distinguished from acute weakness due to hypokalemia and hypophosphatemia. The chronic form of alcoholic myopathy is common, occurring in up to 50% of alcoholics. It is characterized by slowly evolving proximal weakness of the lower extremities. Unlike the acute form, there is usually no muscle pain and no elevation of serum CPK.

Central pontine myelinolysis

Central pontine myelinolysis (CPM) is a rare syndrome characterized by subacute to acute quadriparesis, conjugate gaze palsies, pseudobulbar palsy, and obtundation. It is usually seen in the setting of overzealous correction of hyponatremia and, although most often described in alcoholics, can also been seen in patients with liver disease from any cause, malnutrition, malignancy, and burns. Central pontine myelinolysis typically develops over several days to a week after correction of the serum sodium. Pathologically, characteristic lesions of demyelination are seen symmetrically in the ventral pons. The syndrome generally carries a poor prognosis. However, some patients have improved over weeks to months.

Neurologic Complications of Drug Abuse

Various neurologic complications arise from the use of nonmedical, recreational drugs such as cocaine, methamphetamine, hallucinogens, and heroin. Complications of some of the commonly used recreational drugs will be discussed in the following section.

Cocaine

Cocaine ("coke," "snow," "c," "flake," "blow") is extracted from the leaf of the shrub *Erythroxylum coca* and is a fine, white, odorless substance with a bitter taste. Since the early 1970s, cocaine use had grown dramatically in popularity. Estimates suggest that the number of Americans who have tried cocaine at least once rose from 5.4 million in 1974 to 21.6 million in 1982. However, the

---

▼

Pearls and Perils

Drug abuse

▶ Cocaine and amphetamines are the two drugs of abuse most commonly associated with seizures.
▶ Patients presenting with an initial seizure should be screened for the presence of illicit drugs.
▶ Withdrawal from illicit drugs, particularly benzodiazepines and barbiturates, can be associated with seizures.
▶ Cocaine and amphetamines increase the risk of intraparenchymal and subarachnoid hemorrhage.
▶ Many over-the-counter diet aids contain sufficient amounts of sympathomimetics to cause stroke.

use of cocaine has declined in recent years from an estimated 5.7 million current users in 1985 to an estimated 1.2 million current users in 2000. Nevertheless, the epidemic of cocaine use, with its associated medical and neurologic sequelae, make it a major public health concern. Cocaine can be smoked or taken intranasally, intravenously, or intramuscularly. It has a very brief plasma half-life. It is a stimulant drug that blocks the reuptake of monoamines into presynaptic terminals. This blockade increases dopamine, norepinephrine, and serotonin in the synaptic cleft, causing overstimulation of postsynaptic receptors acutely.

Amphetamines

The amphetamines are a large class of synthetic stimulants that include dextroamphetamine, methamphetamine (Methedrine, "speed," "crank," "crystal meth"), methylphenidate (Ritalin), methylene-dioxyamphetamine (MDA), and methylene-dioxy-methamphetamine (MDMA, "ecstasy"). Amphetamines are indirect-acting sympathomimetics. They affect the CNS by blocking reuptake of dopamine and promoting the release of dopamine and norepinephrine. Amphetamines have a much longer duration of action compared to cocaine. They can be taken orally or intravenously. Additionally, methamphetamine crystals can be smoked ("smoking ice").

Acute effect of cocaine and stimulant intoxication. Typical signs of acute cocaine and other stimulant intoxication include anxiety, paranoia, tremor, mydriasis, tachycardia, diaphoresis, hypertension, and hypothermia. Psychosis, formication, and transient signs of delirium may be present and may be difficult to distinguish from primary psychiatric disorders. With cocaine use, these signs generally resolve within 24 hours. However, because of the long half-life of methamphetamine and other amphetamine derivatives, toxic psychosis resulting from the use of these substances may last for several days.

Stimulant-associated neurologic complications. Neurologic complications of cocaine use include strokes that may be ischemic or hemorrhagic. Although the exact mechanisms of cocaine-related strokes are not fully understood, it appears that direct vasoconstriction may play an important role in ischemic stroke. Myocardial infarction, cardiac arrhythmia, and cardiomyopathy associated with cocaine use also carry a high risk of embolism. In addition, acute hypertension may predispose to intracranial hemorrhage, especially in those with underlying aneurysms or vascular malformations.

Neurologic complications of methamphetamine abuse, like cocaine, include stroke, both ischemic and hemorrhagic, in addition to a choreiform movement disorder that usually resolves within several days of cessation of drug intake. An "amphetamine-induced vasculitis" or

---

Table 23.14 Cocaine and amphetamine abuse
Discriminating features
▶ Positive urine toxicology screen for cocaine or amphetamines
Consistent features
▶ Hyperactivity, tremor, anorexia
▶ Tachycardia, increased blood pressure
▶ Dilated pupils
Variable features
▶ Generalized seizures
▶ Hemorrhagic stroke
▶ Paranoia, delusions of crawling bugs with amphetamine
▶ Choreiform movement disorder with amphetamine
▶ Amphetamine-induced vasculitis

---

necrotizing arteritis has been described that appears to involve both small and medium-sized arteries. It remains to be clarified, however, whether this occurs as a direct effect of the drug or secondary to an adulterant (Table 23.14).

Hallucinogens

There are two basic groups of hallucinogens: the natural hallucinogenic substances such as mescaline (from the peyote cactus), psilocybin ("magic mushrooms"), and marijuana, and the synthetic hallucinogens, including LSD, phencyclidine (PCP), and STP. Mescaline and psilocybin are taken orally with an onset of action of 30–40 minutes. The main effects appear to be a distorted sense of space and time, in addition to enhancement of colors and sounds.

Marijuana ("grass," "weed," "pot") is a mixture of the flowers and small leaves of a species of hemp called *Cannabis sativa* whose preferred route of administration in Western countries is by smoking. The most potent psychoactive alkaloid in marijuana is tetrahydrocannabinol (THC). Early on, there is euphoria, depersonalization, an alteration of time sense, and impaired coordination and gait. With longer use and higher doses, there may be difficulty concentrating, confusion, disorientation, frank psychosis, and flashbacks. Intoxication does not usually require treatment.

Phencyclidine (PCP, "angel dust") is a synthetic agent that is somewhat difficult to classify, as it affects most neurotransmitter systems. Its primary use is to obtain hallucinogenic effects. PCP can be taken orally, intravenously, "snorted" intranasally, or smoked (by mixing it with tobacco). Its effects include distortions of body image, detachment, disorientation, decreased sensation (anesthetic effects), and violent behavior. At higher doses, one typically sees nystagmus, ataxia, dysarthria, an acute confusional state, and sometimes self-mutilation, stupor, or coma. Movement disorders and generalized seizures are not uncommon. The "triad" of PCP toxicity is nystagmus, hypertension, and acute behavioral changes. Occasionally, a patient on PCP becomes unresponsive while awake and alert, which can be mistaken for akinetic mutism or catatonia. The toxic effects of PCP may last days, and overdosage has been fatal.

In general, the adverse psychologic consequences of hallucinogenic drugs include panic reactions ("bad trips"), acute psychotic (especially PCP) or depressive reactions, and flashbacks. They are probably best managed with "talking down" or sedation with a benzodiazepine. Psychotic behavior should be controlled with neuroleptics, and seizures should be treated with IV diazepam.

Opioids

Natural opiates are derived from the opium poppy that contains several active compounds. Commonly abused synthetic and naturally derived opioids include heroin, hydromorphone, codeine, meperidine, butorphanol, and hydrocodone. The abuse of heroin, a synthetic opiate ("smack," "skag," "H," "brown," "horse"), in particular, has risen significantly. Heroin has a shorter duration of action than morphine and is three to five times more potent. Like all narcotics, it is thought to exert its effects through opiate receptors in the CNS and elsewhere. It can be sniffed, smoked, and injected subcutaneously ("skin popping") or intravenously.

Acute opioid intoxication. Severe intoxication or overdose with opioids is a medical emergency. Miosis or pinpoint pupils seen with most opioids can be used to identify intoxication. The most concerning effect is respiratory depression from direct suppression of respiratory centers in the midbrain and medulla. Anoxia and hypotension can result in neurologic complications of postanoxic encephalopathy, cerebral infarction, and acute transverse myelopathy.

For severe cases, the administration of the pure opioid antagonist naloxone in combination with general supportive measures is indicated. Naloxone has a shorter half-life than most opiates and usually requires repeated dosing. Naloxone administration to an opioid-dependent individual, however, can result in a severe withdrawal syndrome (Table 23.15).

Common medications used in the treatment of acute opioid withdrawal include the α_2-adrenergic agonist clonidine to decrease tremor, diaphoresis, and agitation; cyclobenzaprine for muscle cramps; and dicyclomine for gastrointestinal symptoms. Another option is to convert the patient to an equivalent dose of another opioid, then gradually reduce the dose to minimize withdrawal. When a patient has been detoxified completely from opioids, naltrexone may be used to help prevent relapse. Decreased illicit opioid use has been found with using naltrexone in highly motivated patients. An alternative approach for treatment of opioid addiction is to substitute

the abused opioid with a long half-life opioid to prevent withdrawal symptoms from emerging. The most commonly used medication for this purpose is methadone. With a half-life of 24–36 hours and good oral bioavailability, methadone can prevent the onset of opioid withdrawal syndrome for 24 hours or more. Methadone has been shown to reduce or eliminate opioid craving, and to block the effects of illicitly used opioids. A summary of the neurologic signs and symptoms of drug abuse is shown in Table 23.16.

Table 23.15 Opiate overdose

Discriminating features
- Positive urine toxicology screen for heroin or morphine
- Reversal by naloxone, a specific opiate antagonist

Consistent features
- Pinpoint pupils
- Respiratory depression
- Coma

Variable features
- Postanoxic encephalopathy
- Infectious complications including AIDS
- Ischemic infarction

Table 23.16 Summary of neurologic signs and symptoms of drug abuse

Signs or symptoms	Drugs
Pupils	
Pinpoint	Opiates
Dilated	Stimulants
Slow reactive	Hallucinogens
Extraocular movement	
Nystagmus	Depressants, phencyclidine (PCP)
Speech	
Slow	Opiates
Slurred	Depressants, opiates
Rapid	Stimulants
Motor	
Tremor (fine)	Hallucinogens, stimulants
Tremor (coarse)	Depressants
Reflexes	
Brisk	Stimulants
Depressed	Depressants
Seizures	Opiates, stimulants, over-the-counter drugs

Volatile hydrocarbon abuse

The main neurologic disorders associated with chronic volatile hydrocarbon abuse are peripheral neuropathy, cerebellar disease, chronic encephalopathy, and dementia. Apart from the peripheral neuropathy, the clinical features may be nonspecific, and evidence for solvent-related toxicity is, in most cases, circumstantial without clear dose–response relationship. However, peripheral neuropathy has been associated with n-hexane and methyl n-butyl ketone. Toluene exposure causing neurologic disease has also been well documented and will be discussed here as a prototype of volatile substance abuse.

Toluene abuse. Toluene is a volatile hydrocarbon used as a gasoline additive, but also in an extensive number of ways as a solvent in the paint, rubber, printing, adhesive, and cosmetic industries. Toxicity can occur from accidental or deliberate inhalation of fumes, in addition to ingestion and absorption through the skin. Toluene abuse or glue sniffing (also "huffing," "bagging") has become widespread, especially among children and adolescents, because it is readily available and inexpensive. Acute intoxication with toluene from inhalation primarily affects the CNS, causing headache, euphoria, dizziness, confusion, vertigo, tinnitus, hallucinations, seizures, ataxia, stupor, and coma.

Chronic exposure with toluene has devastating and multifocal sequelae for the CNS. These include cerebral cortex atrophy, cerebellar degeneration and ataxia, optic and peripheral neuropathies, psychosis, decreased cognitive ability, blindness, and deafness. Pathologic changes occurring in the brain consist of prominent degeneration and gliosis of the ascending and descending long tracts, in addition to diffuse demyelination and atrophy. Brain imaging may reveal cerebral, cerebellar, and brainstem atrophy. Magnetic resonance imaging shows loss of gray–white matter differentiation and increased periventricular signal intensity on T2-weighted sequences.

γ-Hydroxybutyrate

Several new recreational drugs gained in popularity in the 1990s and continue to be widely used today. Among them, γ-hydroxybutyrate (GHB) has been most notorious. GHB has been purported to enhance sociability and reduce inhibition, which has led to its use in all-night dance raves. It has also been dubbed a "date-rape" drug because its sedative effect has been used to facilitate nonconsensual sex. GHB intoxication can present with a spectrum of neurologic effects from mild nystagmus, ataxia, dizziness, and sedation to severe respiratory depression, apnea, coma, and death. Several reports have described patients with marked agitation or stimulation in the face of prolonged apnea and hypoxia. Treatment is supportive, including aspiration precautions because of nausea and vomiting. Atropine, neostigmine, and physostigmine have been used to treat the bradycardia. For more complicated ingestions, airway protection or ventilatory support may be necessary.

Annotated Bibliography

Alshekhlee A, Kaminski HJ, Ruff RL. Neuromuscular manifestations of endocrine disorders. *Neurol Clin* 2002;20(1):35–58, v–vi.
Comprehensive review of the neuromuscular disorders associated with many endocrine disturbances.

Berlit P. Neuropsychiatric disease in collagen vascular diseases and vasculitis. *J Neurol* 2007;254 [Suppl 2]: II/87–II/89.
Review of neuropsychiatric symptoms associated with various collagen vascular diseases and vasculitis.

Brust JCM. Acute neurologic complications of drug and alcohol abuse. *Neurol Clin* 1998;16(2):503–519.
Excellent review of the neurologic emergencies encountered in recreational users of drugs and ethanol.

Harati Y. Diabetic peripheral neuropathies. *Ann Intern Med* 1987;107(4):546–559.
Review of the group of heterogeneous syndromes known as the diabetic peripheral neuropathies.

McRae AL, Brady KT, Sonne SC. Alcohol and substance abuse. *Med Clin North Am* 2001;85(3):779–801.
Excellent review of substance use disorders.

Sigal LH. The neurologic presentation of vasculitic and rheumatologic syndromes. A review. *Medicine (Baltimore)* 1987; 66(3):157–180.
Comprehensive review of the rheumatologic and vasculitic syndromes affecting the CNS.

Ropper AH, Brown RH, eds. Diseases of the nervous system due to nutritional deficiency. In: *Adams & Victor's principles of neurology.* New York: McGraw-Hill, 2005.
Excellent review of nervous system manifestations of nutritional deficiency.

Ropper AH, Brown RH, eds. Alcohol and alcoholism. In: *Adams & Victor's principles of neurology.* New York: McGraw-Hill, 2005.
Excellent review of nervous system manifestations of alcoholism.

Bibliography

Chapter 1

Blessed G, Tomlinson BE, Roth M. The association between quantitative measures of dementia and of senile change in the cerebral grey matter of elderly individuals. *Br J Psychiatry* 1968;114:797–811.

Folstein MF, Folstein SE, McHugh PR. 'Mini-Mental State:' a practical method for grading the cognitive state of patients for clinicians. *J Psychiatr Res* 1975;12:189–198.

Jozefowicz, Ralph F. The Neurologic History. In Goldman L, et al., eds. *Cecil's textbook of medicine*, 21st ed. Philadelphia: Saunders, 2000.

Mayo Clinic and Mayo Foundation. *Clinical examinations in neurology*. Philadelphia: WB Saunders, 1976.

Tinetti ME, Ginter SF. Identifying mobility dysfunctions in elderly patients. *JAMA* 1988;259:190–1193.

Chapter 2

Binnie CD. Ambulatory diagnostic monitoring of seizures in adults. *Adv Neurol* 1987;46:169–182.

Blum D. Prevalence of bilateral partial seizure foci and implications for electroencephalographic telemetry monitoring and epilepsy surgery. *Electroencephalogr Clin Neurophysiol* 1994;91:329–336.

Blume WT. Generalized sharp and slow wave complexes. *Brain* 1973:289–306.

Bortone E, Bettoni L, Giorgi C, et al. Post-anoxic theta and alpha pattern coma. *Clin Electroencephalogr* 1994;25:156–159.

Delgado-Escueta AV, Treiman DM. Focal status epilepticus: Modern concepts. In: Luders H, Lesser RP, eds. *Epilepsy: Electroclinical Syndromes*. London: Springer-Verlag; 1987: 346–391.

Dinner DS, Luders H, Morris HM, et al. Juvenile myoclonic epilepsy. In: Luders H, Lesser RP, eds. *Epilepsy: Electroclinical Syndromes*. London: Springer-Verlag;1987:131–150.

Drazkowski JF. Using EEG in a consultative role. *Semin Neurol* 2003;23:295–305.

Ebersole JS. Ambulatory EEG: Telemetered and cassette-recorded. *Adv Neurol* 1987;46:139–155.

Engel J Jr., Henry TR, Risinger MW, et al. Presurgical evaluation for partial epilepsy: Relative contributions of chronic depth-electrode recordings versus FDG-PET and scalp-sphenoidal ictal EEG. *Neurology* 1990;40:1670–1677.

Engel J. Surgery for seizures. *New Engl J Med* 1996;334(10): 647–652.

Fisher RS, Raudzens P, Nunemacher M. Efficacy of intraoperative neurophysiological monitoring. *J Clin Neurophysiol* 1995;12(1):97–109.

French J. Pseudoseizures in the era of video-electroencephalogram monitoring. *Curr Opin Neurol* 1995;8(2):117–120.

Frost JD Jr. Automatic recognition and characterization of epileptiform discharges in the human EEG. *J Clin Neurophysiol* 1985;2:231–249.

Gotman J. Seizure recognition and analysis. *Electroencephalogr Clin Neurophysiol Suppl* 1985;37:133–145.

Gutrecht JA. Clinical implications of benign epileptiform transients of sleep. *Electroencephalogr Clin Neurophysiol* 1989; 72:486–490.

Hirsch L, Klassen J, Mayer SA, Emmerson RG. Stimulus-induced rhythmic or period ictal discharges (SIRPIDS): A common EEG phenomenon in the critically ill. *Epilepsia* 2004; 45(2):109–123

Hughes JR, Schlagenhauff RE, Magoss M. Electroclinical correlates in the six per second spike and wave complex. *Electroencephalogr Clin Neurophysiol* 1965:71–77.

Klass DW, Brenner RP. Electroencephalography of the elderly. *J Clin Neurophysiol* 1995;12(2):116–131.

Klass DW, Westmoreland BF. Nonepileptogenic epileptiform electroencephalographic activity. *Ann Neurol* 1985;18:627–635.

Kubicki S, Scheuler W, Wittenbecher H. Short-term sleep EEG recordings after partial sleep deprivation as a routine procedure in order to uncover epileptic phenomena: An evaluation of 719 EEG recordings. *Epilepsy Res Suppl* 1991;2:217–230.

Loftus CM, Traynelis VC. *Intraoperative Monitoring Techniques in Neurosurgery*. New York: McGraw Hill, Inc., 1994.

Morris GL 3rd, Galezowska J, Leroy R, et al. The results of computer-assisted ambulatory 16-channel EEG. *Electroencephalogr Clin Neurophysiol* 1994;91(3):229–231.

Raroque HG Jr., Wagner W, Gonzales PC, et al. Reassessment of the clinical significance of periodic lateralized epileptiform discharges in pediatric patients. *Epilepsia* 1993;34: 275–278.

Tassinari CA, Michelucci R, Forti A, et al. The electrical status epilepticus syndrome. *Epilepsy Res Suppl* 1992;6:111–115.

van Donselaar CA, Schimsheimer RJ, Geerts AT, et al. Value of the electroencephalogram in adult patients with untreated idiopathic first seizures. *Arch Neurol* 1992;49(3):231–237.

Williamson PD. Frontal lobe epilepsy. Some clinical characteristics. *Adv Neurol* 1995;66:127–150; discussion 150–152.

Yamashita S, Morinaga T, Ohgo S, et al. Prognostic value of electroencephalogram (EEG) in anoxic encephalopathy after cardiopulmonary resuscitation: Relationship among anoxic period, EEG grading and outcome. *Intern Med* 1995;34(2): 71–76.

Chapter 3

Albers JW, Kelly JJ. Acquired inflammatory demyelinating polyneuropathies: Clinical and electrodiagnostic features. *Muscle Nerve* 1989;12:435–451.

Albers JW. Clinical neurophysiology of generalized polyneuropathy. *Clin Neurophysiol* 1993;10:149–166.

American Association of Electrodiagnostic Medicine, American Academy of Neurology, and American Academy of Physical Medicine and Rehabilitation. Practice parameter for electrodiagnostic studies in carpal tunnel syndrome: Summary statement. *Muscle Nerve* 1993;16:1390–1391.

American Association of Electrodiagnostic Medicine. Recommended policy for electrodiagnostic medicine. At http://www. aaem.net/aaem/practiceissues/RecPolicy/recommended_policy_1.cfm. Accessed 26 June 2008.

Barry DT. AAEM minimonograph #36: Basic concepts of electricity and electronics in clinical electromyography. *Muscle Nerve* 1991;14:937–946.

Benatar M, Kaminski HJ. Evidence report: The medical treatment of ocular myasthenia (an evidence-based review). Report of the Quality Standards Subcommittee of the American Academy of Neurology. *Neurology* 2007;68(24):2144–2149. Epub 2007 Apr 25.

Benatar M. A systematic review of diagnostic studies in myasthenia gravis. *Neuromuscul Disord* 2006;16(7):459–467.

Bodensteiner JB. Congenital myopathies. *Muscle Nerve* 1994;17:131–144.

Bromberg MB, Feldman EL, Albers JW. Chronic inflammatory demyelinating polyradiculoneuropathy: Comparison of patients with and without an associated monoclonal gammopathy. *Neurology* 1992;42:1157–1163.

Bromberg MB. The role of electrodiagnostic studies in the diagnosis and management of polymyositis. *Compr Ther* 1992;18:17–22.

Cornblath DR, Kuncl RW, Mellits ED, et al. Nerve conduction studies in amyotrophic lateral sclerosis. *Muscle Nerve* 1992;15:1111–1115.

Daube JR. Electrophysiologic studies in the diagnosis and prognosis of motor neuron disease. *Neurol Clin* 1985;3:473–493.

Denys EH. AAEM minimonograph #14: The influence of temperature in clinical neurophysiology. *Muscle Nerve* 1991;14: 795–811.

Donofrio PD, Albers JW. AAEM minimonograph #34: Polyneuropathy: Classification by nerve conduction studies and electromyography. *Muscle Nerve* 1990;13:889–903.

Feldman EL, Bromberg MB, Albers JW, et al. Immunosuppressive treatment of multifocal motor neuropathy. *Ann Neurol* 1991;30:397–401.

Fisher MA. AAEM minimonograph #13: H reflexes and F waves: Physiology and clinical indications. *Muscle Nerve* 1992;15:1223–1233.

Gitter AJ, Stolov WC. AAEM minimonograph #16: Instrumentation and measurement in electrodiagnostic medicine: Part II. *Muscle Nerve* 1995;18:812–824.

Gitter AJ, Stolov WC. AAEM minimonograph #16: Instrumentation and measurement in electrodiagnostic medicine: Part I. *Muscle Nerve* 1995;18:799–811.

Griffin JW, Cornblath DR, Alexander E, et al. Ataxic sensory neuropathy and dorsal root ganglionitis associated with Sjögren's syndrome. *Ann Neurol* 1990;27:304–315.

Griggs RC, Mendell JR, Miller RG. *Evaluation and Treatment of Myopathies*. Philadelphia: F.A. Davis, 1995.

Hoogendijk JE, de Visser M, Bolhuis PA, et al. Hereditary motor and sensory neuropathy type I: Clinical and neurographical features of the 17p duplication subtype. *Muscle Nerve* 1994; 17:85–90.

Howard JF, Sanders DB, Massey JM. The electrodiagnosis of myasthenia gravis and the Lambert-Eaton myasthenic syndrome. *Neurol Clin* 1994;12:305–330.

Ionasescu VV. Charcot-Marie-Tooth neuropathies: From clinical description to molecular genetics. *Muscle Nerve* 1995; 18:267–275.

Miller RG. AAEM case report #1: Ulnar neuropathy at the elbow. *Muscle Nerve* 1991;14:97–101.

Nobile-Orazio E, Meucci N, Barbieri S, et al. High-dose intravenous immunoglobulin therapy in multifocal motor neuropathy. *Neurology* 1993;43:537–544.

Olafsson E, Jones HR, Guay AT, et al. Myopathy of endogenous Cushing's syndrome: A review of the clinical and electromyographic features in 8 patients. *Muscle Nerve* 1994;17:692–693.

Olney RK. AAEM minimonograph #38: Neuropathies in connective tissue disease. *Muscle Nerve* 1992;15:531–542.

Pourmand R. Metabolic myopathies. A diagnostic evaluation. *Neurol Clin* 2000;18(1):1–13.

Ross MA, Kimura J. AAEM case report #2: The carpal tunnel syndrome. *Muscle Nerve* 1995;18:567–573.

Saguil A. Evaluation of the patient with muscle weakness. *Am Fam Physician* 2005;71(7):1327–1336.

Singleton JR, Smith AG, et al. Increased prevalence of impaired glucose tolerance in patients with painful sensory neuropathy. *Diabetes Care* 2001;24(8):1448–1453.

Trontelj JV, Stalberg E. Single fiber electromyography in studies of neuromuscular function. *Adv Exp Med Biol* 1995;384: 109–119.

Wertsch JJ. AAEM case report #25: Anterior interosseous nerve syndrome. *Muscle Nerve* 1992;15:977–983.

Wolfe GI, Baker NS, et al. Chronic cryptogenic sensory polyneuropathy: Clinical and laboratory characteristics. *Arch Neurol* 1999;56: 540–547.

Yuen EC, So YT, Olney RK. The electrophysiologic features of sciatic neuropathy in 100 patients. *Muscle Nerve* 1995;18: 414–420.

Chapter 4

Bonneville F, et al. Imaging of cerebellopontine angle lesions: An update. Part 2: Intra-axial lesions, skull base lesions that may invade the CPA region, and non-enhancing extra-axial lesions. *Eur Radiol* 2007;17(11):2908–2920.

Buchpiguel CA, et al. PET versus SPECT in distinguishing radiation necrosis from tumor recurrence in the brain. *J Nucl Med* 1995;36:159–164.

Chalijub G, et al. MR imaging of clival and paraclival lesions. *Am J Roentgenol* 1992;159:1069–1074.

Chong VF, et al. Imaging of the nasopharynx and skull base. *Magn Reson Imaging Clin N Am* 2002;10(4):547–571.

Davis PC, et al. The brain in older persons with or without dementia: Findings on MR, PET, SPECT Images. *AJR Am J Roentgenol* 1994;162:1267–1278.

Erlemann R. Imaging and differential diagnosis of primary bone tumors and tumor-like lesions of the spine. *Eur J Radiol* 2006;58(1):48–67.

Fine MJ, et al. Spinal cord ependymomas: MR imaging features. *Radiology* 1995;197:655–658.

Foerster BR, et al. Intracranial infections: Clinical and imaging characteristics. *Acta Radiol* 2007;48(8):875–893.

Forrester DM. Infectious spondylitis. *Semin Ultrasound CT MR* 2005;25(6):461–473.

Gallagher CN, et al. Neuroimaging in trauma. *Curr Opin Neurol* 2007;20(4):403–409.

Gallucci M, et al. Degenerative disease of the spine. *Neuroimaging Clin N Am* 2007;17(1):87–103.

Grimme JD, et al. Congenital anomalies of the spine. *Neuroimaging Clin N Am* 2007;17(1):1–16.

Isaacson B, et al. Lesions of the petrous apex: Diagnosis and management. *Otolaryngol Clin North Am* 2007;40(3):479–519.

Khanna AJ, et al. Use of magnetic resonance imaging in differentiating compartmental location of spinal tumors. *Am J Orthop* 2005;34(10):472–476.

Köhrmann M, et al. Acute stroke imaging for thrombolytic therapy: An update. *Cerebrovasc Dis* 2007;24(2–3):161–169.

Kucharcyk W, et al. Detection of pituitary microadenomas: Comparison of keyhole fast spin echo, unenhanced, and conventional contrast enhanced MR imaging. *AJR Am J Roentgenol* 1994;163:671–679.

Leonardi M, et al. Neuroradiology of spine degenerative diseases. *Best Pract Res Clin Rheumatol* 2002;16(1):59–87.

Mhuircheartaigh NN, et al. MR imaging of traumatic spinal injuries. *Semin Musculoskelet Radiol* 2006;10(4):293–307.

Mielke R, et al. HMPAO SPET and FDG PET in Alzheimer's disease and vascular dementia's comparison of perfusion and metabolic pattern. *Eur J Nucl Med* 21:1052–1060.

Olson EM, et al. Extraspinal abnormalities detected on MR images of the spine. *AJR Am J Roentgenol* 1994;162:679–684.

Olson EM, et al. MR detection of white matter disease of the brain in patients with HIV infection: Fast spin echo vs. conventional spin echo pulse sequences. *AJR Am J Roentgenol* 1994;162:1199–1204.

Rennert J, et al. Imaging of sellar and parasellar lesions. *Clin Neurol Neurosurg* 2007;109(2):111–124.

Rooney WD, et al. Recent advances in the neuroimaging of multiple sclerosis. *Curr Neurol Neurosci Rep* 2005;5(3):217–224.

Schellinger PD, et al. Noninvasive angiography (magnetic resonance and computed tomography) in the diagnosis of ischemic cerebrovascular disease. Techniques and clinical applications. *Cerebrovasc Dis* 2007;24[Suppl 1]:16–23.

Siewert B, et al. Brain lesions in patients with multiple sclerosis: Detection with echo-planar imaging. *Radiology* 1995;196:765–771.

Som PM, et al. Inflammatory lesions and tumors of the nasal cavities and paranasal sinuses with skull base involvement. *Neuroimaging Clin N Am* 1994;4(3):499–513.

Sundgren PC, et al. Spinal trauma. *Neuroimaging Clin N Am* 2007;17(1):73–85.

Tali ET, et al. Spinal infections. *Eur Radiol* 2005;15(3):599–607.

Taylor A, Patz F, eds. *Clinical Practice of Nuclear Medicine.* New York: Churchill Livingstone, Inc., 1991.

Tien RO, et al. Herpes virus infections of the CNS: MR findings. *AJR Am J Roentgenol* 1993;161:167–176.

Yetkin EZ, et al. Multiple sclerosis: Specificity of MR for diagnosis. *Radiology* 1991;178:447–451.

Young GS. Advanced MRI of adult brain tumors. *Neurol Clin* 2007;25(4):947–973.

Chapter 5

Brophy C, et al. Defecation syncope secondary to functional inferior vena caval obstruction during a Valsalva maneuver. *Ann Vasc Surg* 1993;7(4):374–377.

Coplan NL, et al. Carotid sinus hypersensitivity: Case report and review of the literature. *Am J Med* 1984;77(3):561–565.

Critchley EM, et al. Evaluation of syncope. *Br Med J* 1983;286(6364):500–501.

Day SC, et al. Evaluation and outcome of emergency room patients with transient loss of consciousness. *Am J Med* 1982;73(1):15–23.

Eagle K, et al. Evaluation of prognostic classifications for patients with syncope. *Am J Med* 1985;79(4):455–460.

Editorial. Explaining syncope. *Lancet* 1991;338(8763):353–354.

Esaki T, et al. Surgical management of glossopharyngeal neuralgia associated with cardiac syncope: Two case reports. *Br J Neurosurg* 2007;21(6):599–602.

Fouad F. A strategy for the syncope workup. *Cleve Clin J Med* 1993;60(3):184–185.

Gambardella A, et al. Late-onset drop attacks in temporal lobe epilepsy: A reevaluation of the concept of temporal lobe syncope. *Neurology* 1994;44(6):1074–1078.

Gastaut H, et al. Electro-encephalographic study of syncope: Its differentiation from epilepsy. *Lancet* 1957;273(7004):1018–1025.

Grubb BP, et al. Orthostatic hypotension: Causes, classification, and Treatment. *Pacing Clin Electrophysiol* 2003;26[4 Pt 1]:892–901.

Haimovic I, et al. Transient unresponsiveness in the elderly: Report of five cases. *Arch Neurol* 1992;49(1):35–37.

Heaven DJ, et al. Syncope. *Crit Care Med* 2000;28[10 Suppl]:N116–N120.

Jansen R, et al. Postprandial hypotension in elderly patients with unexplained syncope. *Arch Intern Med* 1995;155(9):945–952.

Kapoor WN, et al. Prolonged electrocardiographic monitoring in patients with syncope: Importance of frequent or repetitive ventricular ectopy. *Am J Med* 1987;82(1):20–28.

Kapoor WN, et al. Using a tilt table to evaluate syncope. *Am J Med Sci* 1999;317(2):110–116.

Kaufmann H. Treatment of patients with orthostatic hypotension and syncope. *Clin Neuropharmacol* 2002;25(3):133–141.

Khan IA, et al. Long QT syndrome: Diagnosis and management. *Am Heart J* 2002;143(1):7–14.

Lempert T, et al. Mass fainting at rock concerts. *N Engl J Med* 1995;332(25):1721.

Lewis DA, et al. Specificity of head-up tilt testing in adolescents: Effect of various degrees of tilt challenge in normal control subjects. *J Am Coll Cardiol* 1997;30(4):1057–1060.

Linzer M, et al. Cardiovascular causes of loss of consciousness in patients with presumed epilepsy: A cause of the increased sudden death rate in people with epilepsy? *Am J Med* 1994; 96(2):146–154.

Marine JF. Catheter ablation therapy for supraventricular arrhythmias. *JAMA* 2007;298(23):2768–2778.

Metheetrairut C, et al. Glossopharyngeal neuralgia and syncope secondary to neck malignancy. *J Otolaryngol* 1993;22(1):18–20.

Odeh M, et al. Glossopharyngeal neuralgia associated with cardiac syncope and weight loss. *Arch Otolaryngol Head Neck* 1994;120(11):1283–1286.

Palma V, et al. Hindbrain hernia headache and syncope in type I Arnold-Chiari malformation. *Acta Neurol (Napoli)* 1993; 15(6):457– 461.

Sagrista-Sauleda J, et al. Reproducibility of sequential head-up tilt testing in patients with recent syncope, normal ECG and no structural heart disease. *Eur Heart J* 2002;23(21):1706–1713.

Schuele SU, et al. Video-electrographic and clinical features in patients with ictal asystole. *Neurology* 2007;69(5):423–424.

Thomas J, et al. Orthostatic hypotension. *Mayo Clin Proc* 1981;56(2):117–125.

van Leishout JJ, et al. The vasovagal response. *Clin Sci* 1991;81(5):575–586.

Wayne HH. Syncope: Physiological considerations and an analysis of the clinical characteristics in 510 patients. *Am J Med* 1961;30:418–438.

with syncope. *Ann Emerg Med* 2001;37:771–776.

Chapter 6

Afzelius L-E, Henriksson NG, Wahlgren L. Vertigo and dizziness of functional origin. *Laryngoscope* 1980;90:649–656.

Aita JF. Why patients with Parkinson's disease fall. *JAMA* 1982;247:515–516.

Baloh RW, Honrubia V, Jacobson K. Benign positional vertigo: Clinical and oculographic features in 240 cases. *Neurology* 1987;37:371–378.

Brandt T, Daroff RB. Physical therapy for benign paroxysmal positional vertigo. *Arch Otolaryngol* 1980;106:484–485.

Brandt T, Steddin S, Daroff RB. Therapy for benign paroxysmal positioning vertigo, revisited. *Neurology* 1994;44:796–800.

Brandt T, Steddin S. Current view of the mechanism of benign paroxysmal positioning vertigo: Cupulolithiasis or canalolithiasis? *J Vestib Res* 1993;3:373–382.

Caliman E, Gurgel JD, Costa KV, et al. Dizziness associated with panic disorder and agoraphobia: Case report and literature review. *Rev Bras Otorrinolaringol (Engl Ed)* 2007;73:569–572.

Cawthorne T. Vestibular injuries. *Proc R Soc Med* 1945;39:270–273.

Chiu KY, Pun WK, Luk KDK, Chow SP. Sequential fractures of both hips in elderly patients: A prospective study. *J Trauma* 1992;32:584–587.

Cooksey FS. Rehabilitation in vestibular injuries. *Proc R Soc Med* 1945;29:273–275.

Droller H, Pemberton J. Vertigo in a random sample of elderly people living in their homes. *J Laryngol Otol* 1953;67:689–694.

Duncan GW, Parker SW, Fisher CM. Acute cerebellar infarction in the PICA territory. *Arch Neurol* 1975;32:364–368.

Eggers SD. Migraine-related vertigo: Diagnosis and treatment. *Curr Pain Headache Rep* 2007;11:217–226.

Ekman A, Mallmin H, Michaëlsson K, Ljunghall S. External hip protectors to prevent osteoporotic hip fractures. *Lancet* 1997;350:563–564.

Epley JM. The canalith repositioning procedure: For treatment of benign paroxysmal positioning vertigo. *Otolaryngol Head Neck Surg* 1992;107:399–404.

Freeman R. Neurogenic orthostatic hypotension. *N Engl J Med* 2008;358:615–624.

Grad A, Baloh RW. Vertigo of vascular origin: Clinical and electronystagmographic features in 84 cases. *Arch Neurol* 1989;46:281–284.

Grisso JA, Kelsey JL, Strom BL, et al. Risk factors for falls as a cause of hip fracture in women. *N Engl J Med* 1991;324:1326–1331.

Haines TP, Bennell KL, Osborne RH, Hill KD. Effectiveness of targeted falls prevention programme in subacute hospital setting: Randomized controlled trial. *BMJ* 2004;328:676–679.

Herdman SJ, Tusa RJ, Zee DS, et al. Single treatment approaches to benign paroxysmal vertigo. *Arch Otolaryngol Head Neck Surg* 1993;119:450–454.

Herdman SJ. Treatment of benign paroxysmal positional vertigo. *Phys Ther* 1990;70:381–388.

Huang GY, Yo Y. Small cerebellar strokes may mimic labyrinthine lesions. *J Neurol Neursurg Psychiatry* 1985;48:263–265.

Jensen J, Lundin-Olsson L, Nyberg L, Gustafson Y. Fall and injury prevention in older people living in residential care facilities. A cluster randomized trial. *Ann Intern Med* 2002;136:733–741.

Johnell O, Melton LJ, Atkinson EJ 3rd, et al. Fracture risk in patients with parkinsonism: A population-based study in Olmsted County, Minnesota. *Age Aging* 1992;21:32–38.

Kallin K, Lundin-Olsson L, Jensen J, et al. Predisposing and precipitating factors for falls among older people in residential care. *Public Health* 2002;116:263–271.

Kao CH, Chen CC, Wang SJ, et al. Bone mineral density in patients with Parkinson's disease measured by dual photon absorptiometry. *Nucl Med Commun* 1993;14:173–177.

Keim RJ. Evaluating the patient with disequilibrium. *Geriatrics* 1978;33:87–92.

Kienzle MG. Syncope: Pursuing the common and prognostically important causes. *Heart Dis Stroke* 1992;1:123–127.

Lanska DJ, Remler B. Benign paroxysmal positioning vertigo: Classic descriptions, origins of the provocative positioning technique, and conceptual developments. *Neurology* 1997;48:1167–1177.

Lauritzen JB, Peterson MM, Lund B. Effect of external hip protectors on hip fractures. *Lancet* 1993;341:11–13.

Leveque M, Labrousse M, Seidermann L, Chays A. Surgical therapy in intractable benign paroxysmal positional vertigo. *Otolaryngol Head Neck Surg* 2007;136:693–698.

Linzer M. Syncope. *South Med J* 1987;80:545–553.

Munoz JE, Miklea JT, Howard M, et al. Canalith repositioning maneuver for benign paroxysmal positional vertigo: Randomized controlled trial in family practice. *Can Fam Physician* 2007;53:1049–1053.

Newman-Toker DE, Cannon LM, Stofferahn ME, et al. Imprecision in patient reports of dizziness symptom quality: A cross-sectional study conducted in an acute care setting. *Mayo Clin Proc* 2007;82:1329–1340.

Noble RJ. The patient with syncope. *JAMA* 1977;237:1372–1376.

Nordell E, Jarnlo GB, Jetsen C, et al. Accidental falls and related fractures in 65–74 year olds: A retrospective study of 332 patients. *Acta Orthop Scand* 2000;71:175–179.

Norre ME, Beckers A. Benign paroxysmal positional vertigo in the elderly: Treatment by habituation exercises. *JAGS* 1988;36:425–529.

Onrot J, Goldberg MR, Hollister AS, et al. Management of chronic orthostatic hypotension. *Am J Med* 1986;80:454–464.

Ross RT. *Syncope*. London, WB Saunders Co., 1988.

Sato Y, Iwamoto J, Kanoko T, Satoh K. Alendronate and vitamin D2 for prevention of hip fracture in Parkinson's disease: A randomized controlled trial. *Mov Disord* 2006;21:924–929.

Sato Y, Kaji M, Tsuru T, Oizumi K. Risk factors for hip fracture among elderly patients with Parkinson's disease. *J Neurol Sci* 2001;82:89–93.

Sato Y, Kikuyama M, Oizumi K. High prevalence of vitamin D deficiency and reduced bone mass in Parkinson's disease. *Neurology* 1997;49:1273–1278.

Schuknecht HF. Cupulolithiasis. *Adv Otorhinolaryngol* 1973;22:434–443.

Semont A, Freyss E, Vitte P. Curing the BPPV with a liberatory maneuver. *Adv Otorhinolaryngol* 1988;42:290–293.

Stanton VA, Hsieh YH, Camargo CA Jr., et al. Overreliance on symptom quality in diagnosing dizziness: Results of a multicenter survey of emergency physicians. *Mayo Clin Proc* 2007;82:1319–1328.

Thomas JE, Schirger A, Fealey RD, Sheps SG. Orthostatic hypotension. *Mayo Clin Proc* 1981;56:117–125.

Tinetti ME. Preventing falls in elderly persons. *N Engl J Med* 2003;348:42–49.

Venosa AR, Bittar RS. Vestibular rehabilitation exercises in acute vertigo. *Laryngoscope* 2007;117:1482–1487.

Williams DR, Watt HC, Lees AJ. Predictors of falls and fractures in bradykinetic rigid syndromes: A retrospective study. *J Neurol Neurosurg Psychiatry* 2006;77:468–473.

Chapter 7

Alexander NB. Gait disorders in older adults. *J Am Geriatr Soc* 1996;44:434–451.

Barr ML, Kiernan JA. *The Human Nervous System: An Anatomical Viewpoint*, 8th ed. Philadelphia: Lippincott Williams & Wilkins, 2004.

Brook MH. The symptoms and signs of neuromuscular diseases. In: *A Clinician's View of Neuromuscular Diseases*, 2nd ed. Baltimore: Williams & Wilkins;1986:1–35.

Chan CW, Rudins A. Foot biomechanics during walking and running. *Mayo Clin Proc* 1994;69:448–461.

Elble RJ, Moody C, Leffler K, Sinha R. The initiation of normal walking. *Mov Disord* 1994;9:139–146.

Hoppenfeld S, Hutton R, eds. *Examination of Gait, Physical Examination of the Spine and Extremities*. New York: Prentice Hall;1995:133–141.

Jankovic J, Nutt JG, Sudarsky L. Classification, diagnosis, and etiology of gait disorders. *Adv Neurol* 2001;87:119–133.

Keane JR. Hysterical gait disorders: 60 cases. *Neurology* 1989;39:586–589.

Knutsson E, Lying-Tunell U. Gait apraxia in normal-pressure hydrocephalus: Patterns of movement and muscle activation. *Neurology* 1985;35:155–160.

Krawetz P, Nance P. Gait analysis of spinal cord injured: Effects of injury level and spasticity. *Arch Phys Med Rehabil* 1996;77:635–638.

Lechtenberg R, ed. Signs and symptoms of cerebellar disease. In: *Handbook of Cerebellar Diseases. Neurological Disease and Therapy*, Vol. 16. New York: Marcel Dekker;1993:31–42.

Leibovitz A, Schwartz J, Rosenfeld V, et al. Acute stooped position in elderly with Alzheimer's disease. *J Am Geriatr Soc* 1993;41:468.

Nutt JG. Classification of gait and balance disorders. *Adv Neurol* 2001;87:135–141.

Ondo W. Gait and balance disorders. *Med Clin North Am* 2003;87(4):793–801, viii.

Ounpuu S. The biomechanics of walking and running. *Clin Sports Med* 1994;13:843–863.

Richardson JK, Ashton-Miller JA. Peripheral neuropathy: An often-overlooked cause of falls in the elderly. *Postgrad Med* 1996;99:161–172.

Schiller F. Staggering gait in medical history. *Ann Neurol* 1995;37:127–135.

Sorock GS, Labiner DM. Peripheral neuromuscular dysfunction and falls in an elderly cohort. *Am J Epidemiol* 1992;136:584–591.

Sudarsky L, Ronthal M. Gait disorders among elderly patients: A survey study of 50 patients. *Arch Neurol* 1983;40:740–743.

Sudarsky L, Simon S. Gait disorder in later-life hydrocephalus. *Arch Neurol* 1987;44:263–267.

Sudarsky L. Neurologic disorders of gait. *Curr Neurol Neurosci Rep* 2001;1(4):350–356.

Terry JB, Rosenberg RN. Frontal lobe ataxia. *Surg Neurol* 1995;44:583–588.

Tinetti ME. Preventing falls in elderly persons. *N Engl J Med* 2003;348:42–49.

Wagner EH, LaCroix AZ, Grothaus L, et al. Preventing disability and falls in older adults: A population-based randomized trial. *Am J Pub Health* 1994;84:1800–1806.

Woo J, Ho SC, Lau J, et al. Age-associated gait changes in the elderly: Pathological or physiological? *Neuroepidemiology* 1995;14:65–71.

Zatsiorky VM, Werner SL, Kaimin MA. Basic kinematics of walking: Step length and step frequency. A review. *J Sports Med Phys Fitness* 1994;34:109–134.

Chapter 8

Ahmed SV, et al. Post lumbar puncture headache: Diagnosis and management. *Postgrad Med J* 2006;82:713–715.

Armon C, Evans RW. Addendum to assessment: Prevention of post-lumbar puncture headaches. Report of the Therapeutics and Technology Assessment Subcommittee of the American Academy of Neurology. *Neurology* 2005;65:510–512.

Ayata C, et al. Suppression of cortical spreading depression in migraine prophylaxis. *Ann Neurol* 2006;59:652–661.

Barnat MR. Post-traumatic headache patients I: Demographics, injuries, headache and health status. *Headache* 1986;26:271–277.

Bolay H, et al. Intrinsic brain activity triggers trigeminal meningeal afferents in a migraine model. *Nat Med* 2002;8:136–142.

Brew BJ, Miller J. Human immunodeficiency virus-related headache. *Neurology* 1993;43:1098–1100.

Bussone G, et al. Frovatriptan for the prevention of postdural puncture headache. *Cephalalgia* 2007;27:809–813.

Cady RK. The convergence hypothesis. *Headache* 2007;47[Suppl 1]: S44–S51.

Cao Y, et al. Functional MRI-BOLD of visually triggered headache in patients with migraine. *Arch Neurol* 1999;56:548–554.

Chronicle EP, Mulleners WM. Anticonvulsant drugs for migraine prophylaxis (review). *Cochrane Lib* 2007:1–47.

De Simone R, et al. Migraine and epilepsy: Clinical and pathophysiological relations. *Neurol Sci* 2007;28:S150–S155.

Devine J, et al. Effect of daily migraine prevention on health care utilization in an insured patient population. *J Headache Pain* 2007;8:105–113.

Diamond ML. Emergency department treatment of the headache patient. *Headache Quarterly* 1992;3[Suppl 1]:28–33.

Diamond ML. The role of concomitant headache types and non-headache co-morbidities in the underlying diagnosis of migraine. *Neurology* 2002;58[Suppl 6]:S3–S9.

Dodick DW, et al. Cluster headache. *Cephalalgia* 2000;20:787–803.

Ebersberger A, et al. Is there a correlation between spreading depression, neurogenic inflammation, and nociception that might cause migraine headache? *Ann Neurol* 2001;49:7–13.

Ekbom K, Hardebo JE. Cluster headache: Aetiology, diagnosis, and management. *Drugs* 2002;62:61–69.

Erdemoglu AK, Varlibas A. The long-term efficacy and safety of botulinum toxin in refractory chronic tension-type headache. *J Headache Pain* 2007;8:294–300.

Ferro JM, et al. Headache associated with transient ischemic attacks. *Headache* 1995;35:544–548.

Forsyth PA, Posner JB. Headaches in patients with brain tumors: A study of 111 patients. *Neurology* 1993;43:1678–1683.

Frediani F, Villani V. Migraine and depression. *Neurol Sci* 2007;28:S161–S165.

Freeman M. Reconsidering the effects of monosodium glutamate: A literature review. *J Am Acad Nurse Pract* 2006;18:482–486.

Gardner KL. Genetics of migraine: An update. *Headache* 2006;46[Suppl 1]:S19–S24.

Geraud G, Keywood C, Senard JM. Migraine headache recurrence: Relationship to clinical, pharmacological, and pharmacokinetic properties of triptans. *Headache* 2003;43:376–388.

Goldstein J, et al. Acetaminophen, aspirin, and caffeine in combination versus ibuprofen for acute migraine: Results from a multicenter, double-blind, randomized, parallel-group, single-dose, placebo-controlled study. *Headache* 2006;46:444–453.

Goldstein J, et al. Acetaminophen, aspirin, and caffeine versus sumatriptan succinate in the early treatment of migraine: Results from the ASSET trial. *Headache* 2005;45:973–982.

Hardebo JE, Dahlof C. Sumatriptan nasal spray (20 mg/dose) in the acute treatment of cluster headaches. *Cephalalgia* 1998;18:487–489.

Jensen RM, et al. Burden of cluster headache 2007;27:535–541.

Jørgensen HS, et al. Headache in stroke: The Copenhagen Stroke Study. *Neurology* 1994;44:1793–1797.

Kaniecki RG. Migraine and tension-type headache. *Neurology* 2002;58[Suppl 6]:S15–S20.

Lipton RB, Bigal ME. Ten lessons in the epidemiology of migraine. *Headache* 2007;47[Suppl 1]:S2–S9.

Lipton RB, Dodick D, Sadovsky R, et al. A self-administered screener for migraine in primary care: The ID Migraine™ validation study. *Neurology* 2003;61:375–382.

Lygberg AC, et al. Incidence of primary headache: A Danish epidemiologic follow-up study. *Am J Epidemiol* 2005;161:1066–1073.

Mannix LK, et al. Efficacy and tolerability of naratriptan for short-term prevention of menstrually related migraine: Data from two randomized, double-blind, placebo-controlled studies. *Headache* 2007;47:1037–1049.

Mathew NT. Chronic refractory headache. *Neurology* 1993;43[Suppl 3]:S27–S33.

May A, Leone M. Update on cluster headache. *Curr Opin Neurol* 2003;16:333–340.

Merikangas KR, et al. Diagnostic criteria for migraine: A validity study. *Neurology* 1994;44[Suppl 4]:S11–S16.

Newman LC, et al. Episodic paroxysmal hemicrania: Two new cases and a literature review. *Neurology* 1992;42:964–966.

Obermann M, et al. Efficacy of pregabalin in the treatment of trigeminal neuralgia. *Cephalalgia* 2007;28:174–181.

Olesen J, Rasmussen BK. Management of acute nonvascular headache: The Danish experience. *Headache* 1990;30[Suppl 2]:541–544.

Primavera JP, Kaiser RS. Non-pharmacological treatment of headache: Is less more? *Headache* 1992;32:393–395.

Pringsheim T. Cluster headache: Evidence for a disorder of circadian rhythm and hypothalamic function. *Can J Neurol Sci* 2002;29:33–40.

Rapoport AM, et al. Zolmitriptan nasal spray in the acute treatment of cluster headache: A double-blind study. *Neurology* 2007;69:821–826.

Raskin NH, Green MW. Headache. In: Rowland LP, ed. *Merritt's Neurology*, 11th ed. Philadelphia: Lippincott Williams & Wilkins;2005:45–48.

Rhode AM, et al. Comorbidity of migraine and restless legs syndrome: A case-control study. *Cephalalgia* 2007;27:1255–1260.

Silberstein SD, et al. Menstrual migraine: Neuroendocrinology, pathophysiology, and management. *Headache* 2006; 46[Suppl 2]:S48–S68.

Silberstein SD, et al. Tramadol/acetaminophen for the treatment of acute migraine pain: Findings of a randomized, placebo-controlled trial. *Headache* 2005;45:1317–1327.

Silberstein SD. Intractable headache: Inpatient and outpatient treatment strategies. *Neurology* 1992;42[Suppl 2]:1–51.

Silberstein SD. Tension-type and chronic daily headache. *Neurology* 1993;43:1644–1649.

Silbert PL, Mokri B, Schievink WI. Headache and neck pain in spontaneous internal carotid and vertebral artery dissections. *Neurology* 1995;45:1517–1522.

Smith TR, et al. Sumatriptan and naproxen sodium for the acute treatment of migraine. *Headache* 2005;45:983–991.

Solomon S, Lipton RB, Newman LC. Clinical features of chronic daily headache. *Headache* 1992;32:325–329.

Stang PE, et al. Incidence of migraine headache: A population-based study in Olmsted County, Minnesota. *Neurology* 1992;42:1657–1662.

Stang PE, Osterhaus JT, Celentano DD. Migraine: Patterns of healthcare use. *Neurology* 1994;44[Suppl 4]:S47–S55.

Steward WF, et al. Prevalence of migraine in the United States. *JAMA* 1992;267:64–69.

Steward WF, Shecter A, Lipton RB. Migraine heterogeneity: Disability, pain intensity, and attack frequency and duration. *Neurology* 1994;44[Suppl 4]:S24–S39.

Stewart WF, et al. Population variation in migraine prevalence: A meta-analysis. *J Clin Epidemiol* 1995;48:269–280.

Stewart WF, et al. Prevalence of migraine headache in the United States. Relation to age, income, race, and other sociodemographic factors. *JAMA* 1992;267:64–69.

Stewart WF, Lipton RB. The impact of migraine. *Neurology* 1994;44[Suppl 4].

Tepper SJ, et al. The patent foramen ovale-migraine question. *Neurol Sci* 2007;28:S118–S123.

Warner JS, Fenichel GM. Chronic post-traumatic headache often a myth? *Neurology* 1995;46:915–916.

Welch, KMA. Relationship of stroke and migraine. *Neurology* 1994;44[Suppl 7]:S33–S36.

Wilmhurst P, Bryson P. Relationship between the clinical features of neurological decompression illness and its causes. *Clin Sci* 2000;99:65–75.

Wingerchuk DM, et al. Migraine with aura is a risk factor for cardiovascular and cerebrovascular disease: A critically appraised topic. *Neurologist* 2007;13:231–233.

Zissis NP, et al. A randomized, double-blind, placebo-controlled study of venlafaxine SR in out-patients with tension-type headache. *Cephalalgia* 2007;27:315–324.

Chapter 9

Balla J. Report to the Motor Accidents Board of Victoria on whiplash injuries. *Headache and Cervical Disorders* 1984; 10:256–269.

Britland S, Young R, Sharma A, Clarke B. Acute and remitting painful diabetic polyneuropathy: A comparison of peripheral nerve fiber pathology. *Pain* 1992;48:361–370.

Chelimsky TC, Low PA, Naessens JM, et al. The value of autonomic testing in reflex sympathetic dystrophy. *Mayo Clin Proc* 1995;70:1029–1040.

Cousins M, Phillips G. *Acute Pain Management.* Edinburgh: Churchill Livingstone, 1986.

Deyo R, Rainville J, Kent D. What can the history and physical examination tell us about low back pain? *JAMA* 1992;268:760–765.

Foley K. The treatment of cancer pain. *New Engl J Med* 1985;313:84–95.

Frymoyer J. Back pain and sciatica. *N Engl J Med* 1988;318:291–300.

Grushka M, Sessle B. Burning mouth syndrome. *Dent Clin North Am* 1991;35:171.

Huskisson E. Visual analogue scales. In: Melzack R, ed. *Pain Measurement and Assessment.* New York: Raven Press;1983:33–37.

Jannetta P. Microsurgical approach to the trigeminal nerve for tic douloureux. *Prog Neurol Surg* 1976;7:180–200.

Koes B, Scholten R, Mens J, Bouter L. Efficacy of epidural steroid injections for low-back pain and sciatica: A systematic review of randomized clinical trials. *Pain* 1995;63:279–288.

Kriegler J, Ashenberg Z. Management of chronic low back pain: A comprehensive approach. *Semin Neurol* 1987;7:303–312.

Kuslich SD, Ulstrom CL, Michael CJ. The tissue origin of low back pain and sciatica. *Orthop Clin North Am* 1991;22:181–187.

Max M, Lynch S, Muir J, et al. Effects of desipramine, amitriptyline and fluoxetine on pain in diabetic neuropathy. *N Eng J Med* 1992;326:1250–1256.

Melzack R. The McGill Pain Questionnaire: Major properties and scoring methods. *Pain* 1975;1:277–299.

Merskey H, Bogduk N. *Classification of Chronic Pain: Descriptions of Chronic Pain Syndromes and Definitions of Pain Terms.* Seattle: IASP Press, 1994.

Pearce J. Whiplash injury: A re-appraisal. *J Neurol Neurosurg Psychiatry* 1989;52:1329–1331.

Pfeifer M, Ross D, Schrage J, et al. A highly successful and novel model for treatment of chronic painful diabetic peripheral neuropathy. *Diabetes Care* 1993;16:1103–1115.

Portenoy R, Foley K. Chronic use of opioid analgesics in non-malignant pain: Report of 38 cases. *Pain* 1986;25:171–186.

Saal J, Saal J. Nonoperative treatment of herniated lumbar intervertebral disc with radiculopathy: An outcome study. *Spine* 1989;14:431–437.

Saarto T, Wiffen P. Antidepressants for neuropathic pain. *Cochrane Database Syst Rev* 2007;(4):CD005454.

Schwartzman R, Mclellan T. Reflex sympathetic dystrophy: A review. *Arch Neurol* 1987;44:555–561.

Spaccarelli K. Lumbar and caudal epidural corticosteroid injections. *Mayo Clin Proc* 1996;71:169–178.

Stanton-Hicks M, Jänig W, Hassenbusch S, et al. Reflex sympathetic dystrophy: Changing concepts and taxonomy. *Pain* 1995;63:127–133.

Sutherland J, Wesley R, Cole P, et al. Differences and similarities between patient and physician perceptions of patient pain. *Fam Med* 1988;20:343–346.

Watson C, Watt V, Chipman M, et al. The prognosis with post-herpetic neuralgia. *Pain* 1991;46:195–199.

Wiffen P, Collins S, McQuay H, et al. Anticonvulsant drugs for acute and chronic pain. *Cochrane Database Syst Rev* 2005;(3):CD001133.

Wiffen PJ, McQuay HJ, Edwards JE, et al. Gabapentin for acute and chronic pain. *Cochrane Database Syst Rev* 2005;(3): CD005452.

Wolfe F, Smythe H, Yunus M, et al. The American College of Rheumatology 1990 criteria for the classification of fibromyalgia: Report of the multicenter criteria committee. *Arthritis Rheum* 1990;33:160–192.

Woolf CJ, Doubell TP. The pathophysiology of chronic pain: Increased sensitivity to low threshold Ab-fibre inputs. *Curr Opin Neurobiol* 1994;4:525–534.

Zeppetella G, Ribeiro MD. Opioids for the management of breakthrough (episodic) pain in cancer patients. *Cochrane Database Syst Rev* 2006;(1):CD004311.

Chapter 10

Allen RP, Earley CJ. Restless legs syndrome: A review of clinical and pathophysiologic features. *J Clin Neurophysiol* 2001; 18:128–147.

Fletcher EC. Sympathetic overactivity in the etiology of hypertension of obstructive sleep apnea. *Sleep* 2003;26(1): 15–19.

Friedman M, Tanyeri H, La Rosa M, et al. Clinical predictors of obstructive sleep apnea. *Laryngoscope* 1999;109:1901–1907.

Gaus SE, Shiromani PJ, McCarley RW, et al. Ventrolateral preoptic nucleus contains sleep active, galaninergic neurons in multiple mammalian species. *Neuroscience* 2002;115:285–294.

Guilleminault C, Chowdhury S. Upper airway resistance syndrome is a distinct syndrome. *Am J Respir Crit Care Med* 2000;161:1412–1413.

Guilleminault C, Clerk A, Black J, et al. Nondrug treatment trials in psychophysiologic insomnia. *Arch Intern Med* 1995;155(8):838–844.

Hanly PJ. Mechanisms and management of central sleep apnea. *Lung* 1992;170:1.

Hauri P. *The Sleep Disorders*. Kalamazoo, Michigan: The Upjohn Company, 1982.

Hoffstein V. Is snoring dangerous to your health: Controversies in sleep medicine. *Sleep* 1996;19(6):506–516.

Jindal RD, Buysse DJ, Thase ME. Maintenance treatment of insomnia: What can we learn from the depression literature. *Am J Psychiatry* 2004;161(1):19–24.

Kovacevic-Ristanovic R, Dyonzak J. Sleep disorders associated with respiratory dysfunction. In: Goetz CG, Tanner CM, Aminoff MJ, eds. *Handbook of Clinical Neurology: Systemic Diseases*, Part I. New York: Elsevier Science, 1993;449–475.

Larzelere MM, Wiseman P. Anxiety, depression, and insomnia. *Prim Care* 2002;29(2):339–360.

Malhotra A, White DP. Obstructive sleep apnoea. *Lancet* 2002;360(9328):237–245.

Masand P, Popli AP, Weilburg JB. Sleepwalking. *Am Fam Physician* 1995;51(3):649–654.

Millman RP, Rosenberg CL, Kramer NR. Oral appliances in the treatment of snoring and sleep apnea. *Clin Chest Med* 1998;19(1):69–75.

Montplaisir J, Boucher S, Poirier G, et al. Clinical, polysomnographic, and genetic characteristics of restless legs syndrome: A study of 133 patients diagnosed with new standard criteria. *Mov Disord* 1997;12(1):61–65.

Morin CM, Hauri PJ, Espie CA, et al. Nonpharmacologic treatment of chronic insomnia. An American Academy of Sleep Medicine Review. *Sleep* 1999;22(8):1134–1156.

Neubauer DN. Pharmacologic approaches for the treatment of chronic insomnia. *Clin Cornerstone* 2003;5(3):16–27.

Roth T, Roehrs T. Insomnia: Epidemiology, characteristics, and consequences. *Clin Cornerstone* 2003;5(3):5–15.

Scammell TE. The neurobiology, diagnosis and treatment of narcolepsy. *Ann Neurol* 2003;53:154–166.

Schenck CH, Mahowald MW. REM sleep behavior disorder: Clinical, developmental, and neuroscience perspectives 16 years after its formal identification in sleep. *Sleep* 2002;(25):120–138.

Shahar E, Whitney CW, Redline S, et al. Sleep-disordered breathing and cardiovascular disease: Cross-sectional results of the Sleep Heart Health Study. *Am J Respir Crit Care Med* 2001;163:19–25.

Shamsuzzaman AS, Gersh BJ, Somers VK. Obstructive sleep apnea: Implications for cardiac and vascular disease. *JAMA* 2003;290(14):1906–1914.

Sher AE. Upper airway surgery for obstructive sleep apnea. *Sleep Med Rev* 2002;6(3):195–212.

Sherin JE, Shiromani PJ, McCauley RW, et al. Activation of ventrolateral preoptic neurons during sleep. *Science* 1996; 271:216–219.

Smith MT, Perlis ML, Park A, et al. Comparative meta-analysis of pharmacotherapy and behavior therapy for persistent insomnia. *Am J Psychiatry* 2002;159(1):5–11.

Spielman AJ, Caruso LS, Glovinsky PB. A behavioral perspective on insomnia treatment. *Psychiatr Clin North Am* 1987; 10(4):541–553.

Stradling JR, Davies RJ. Sleep. 1: Obstructive sleep apnoea/hypopnoea syndrome: Definitions, epidemiology and natural history. *Thorax* 2004;59(1):73–78.

Vgontzas AN, Chrousos GP. Sleep, the hypothalamic-pituitary-adrenal axis, and cytokines: Multiple interactions and disturbances in sleep disorders. *Endocrinol Metab Clin North Am* 2002;31(1):15–36.

Vgontzas AN, Zoumakis M, Papanicolau DA, et al. Chronic insomnia is associated with a shift of interleukin-6 and tumor necrosis factor secretion from nighttime to daytime. *Metabolism* 2002;51(7):887–892.

Winkelman JW. Clinical and polysomnographic features of sleep-related eating disorder. *J Clin Psychiatry* 1998;59(1): 14–19.

Yaggi H, Mohsenin V. Sleep-disordered breathing and stroke. *Clin Chest Med* 2003;24(2):223–237.

Chapter 11

Adams RD, Victor M. *Principles of Neurology*, 4th ed. New York: McGraw Hill, Inc., 1993.

Anthony JC, LeResche L, Niaz U, et al. Limits of the "mini-mental state" as a screening test for dementia and delirium among hospital patients. *Psychol Med* 1982;12:397–408.

Bedford PD. General medical aspects of confusional states in elderly people. *Br Med J* 1959;2:185–188.

Bruce AJ, Ritchie CW, Blizard R, et al. The incidence of delirium associated with orthopedic surgery: A meta-analytic review. *Int Psychogeriatr* 2007;19:197–214.

Cameron DJ, Thomas RI, Mulvihill M, Bronheim H. Delirium: A test of the Diagnostic and Statistical Manual III criteria on medical inpatients. *J Am Geriatr Soc* 1987;35:1007–1010.

Chèdru F, Geschwind N. Disorders of higher cortical functions in acute confusional states. *Cortex* 1972;8:395–411.

Devinsky O. *Behavioral Neurology: 100 Maxims.* St Louis: Mosby/Yearbook, 1992.

Devlin JW, Fong JJ, Fraser GL, Riker RR. Delirium assessment in the critically ill. *Intensive Care Med* 2007;33:929–940.

Devlin JW, Fong JJ, Schumaker G, et al. Use of a validated delirium assessment tool improves the ability of physicians to identify delirium in medical intensive care unit patients. *Crit Care Med* 2007;35:2721–2724.

Ebersoldt M, Sharshar T, Annane D. Sepsis-associated delirium. *Intensive Care Med* 2007;33:941–950.

Eidelman LA, Putterman D, Putterman C, Sprung CL. The spectrum of septic encephalopathy: Definitions, etiologies, and mortalities. *JAMA* 1996;275:470–473.

Fernandez F, Levy J, Mansell P. Management of delirium in terminally ill AIDS patients. *Int J Psychiatry Med* 1989;19(2):165–172.

Folstein MF, Folstein SE, McHugh PR. Mini-mental state: A practical method for grading the cognitive state of patients for the clinician. *J Psychiatry Res* 1975;12:189–198.

Francis J, Martin D, Kapoor WN. A prospective study of delirium in hospitalized elderly. *JAMA* 1990;263:1097–1101.

Garza-Treviño ES, Hollister LE, Overall JE, Alexander WF. Efficacy of combinations of intramuscular antipsychotics and sedative-hypnotics for control of psychotic agitation. *Am J Psychiatry* 1989;146:1598–1601.

Gustafson Y, Olsson T, Eriksson S, et al. Acute confusional states (delirium) in stroke patients. *Cerebrovasc Dis* 1991;1:257–264.

Harris D. Delirium in advanced disease. *Postgrad Med J* 2007;83:525–528.

Kirshner HS. Delirium: A focused review. *Curr Neurol Neurosci Rep* 2007;7:479–482.

Larson EB, Kukull WA, Buchner D, Reifler BV. Adverse drug reactions with global cognitive impairment in elderly persons. *Ann Intern Med* 1987;107:169–173.

Lipowski ZJ. Delirium (acute confusional states). *JAMA* 1987;258:17899–1792.

Lipowski ZJ. Delirium in the elderly patient. *N Engl J Med* 1989;320:578–582.

Liptzin B, Levkoff SE, Cleary PD, et al. An empirical study of diagnostic criteria for delirium. *Am J Psychiatry* 1991;148:454–457.

Lonergan E, Britton AM, Luxenberg J, Wyller T. Antipsychotics for delirium. *Cochrane Database Syst Rev* 2007;(2):CD005594.

Lundström M, Olofsson B, Stenvall M, et al. Postoperative delirium in old patients with femoral neck fracture: A randomized intervention study. *Aging Clin Exp Res* 2007;19:178–186.

Maneeton B, Maneeton N, Srisurapanont M. An open-label study of quetiapine for delirium. *J Med Assoc Thai* 2007;90:2158–2163.

Mesulam M-M. Attention, confusional states, and neglect. In: Mesulam M-M, ed. *Principles of Behavioral Neurology.* Philadelphia: FA Davis Co.;1985:125–168.

Michaud L, Büla C, Berney A, et al. Delirium Guidelines Development Group. Delirium: Guidelines for general hospitals. *J Psychosom Res* 2007;62:371–383.

Misra P. Hepatic encephalopathy. *Med Clin North Am* 1981;65(1):209–226.

Moraga AV, Rodriguez-Pascual C. Accurate diagnosis of delirium in elderly patients. *Curr Opin Psychiatry* 2007;20:262–267.

Prakanrattana U, Prapaitrakool S. Efficacy of risperidone for prevention of postoperative delirium in cardiac surgery. *Anaesth Intensive Care* 2007;35:714–719.

Pun BT, Ely EW. The importance of diagnosing and managing ICU delirium. *Chest* 2007;132:624–636.

Rabins PV, Folstein MF. Delirium and dementia: Diagnostic criteria and fatality rates. *Br J Psychiatry* 1982;140:149–153.

Rea RS, Battistone S, Fong JJ, Devlin JW. Atypical antipsychotics versus haloperidol for treatment of delirium in acutely ill patients. *Pharmacotherapy* 2007;27:588–594.

Romano J, Engel GL. Delirium. I: Electroencephalographic data. *Arch Neurol Psychiatry* 1944;51:356–377.

Rudolph JL, Jones RN, Rasmussen LS, et al. Independent vascular and cognitive risk factors for postoperative delirium. *Am J Med* 2007;120:807–813.

Sampson EL, Raven PR, Ndhlovu PN, et al. A randomized, double-blind, placebo-controlled trial of donepezil hydrochloride (Aricept) for reducing the incidence of postoperative delirium after elective total hip replacement. *Int J Geriatr Psychiatry* 2007;22:343–349.

Siddiqi N, Stockdale R, Britton AM, Holmes J. Interventions for preventing delirium in hospitalised patients. *Cochrane Database Syst Rev* 2007;(2):CD005563.

Sos J, Cassem NH. Managing postoperative agitation. *Drug Ther* 1980;10(3):103–106.

Steinhart MJ. The use of haloperidol in geriatric patients with organic mental disorder. *Curr Ther Res* 1983;333:132–143.

Strub RL, Black FW. *The Mental Status Examination in Neurology*, 3rd ed. Philadelphia: FA Davis Co., 1993.

Trzepacz PT, Baker RW. *The Psychiatric Mental Status Examination.* New York: Oxford University Press, 1993.

White C, McCann MA, Jackson N. First do no harm… Terminal restlessness or drug-induced delirium. *J Palliat Med* 2007;10:345–351.

Wilson LM. Intensive care delirium. *Arch Intern Med* 1972;130:225–226.

Wise MG, Brandt GT. Delirium. In: Yudofsky SC, Hales RE, eds. *The American Psychiatric Press Textbook of Neuropsychiatry*, 2nd ed. Washington, DC: American Psychiatric Press Inc.; 1992:291–309.

Young J, Inouye SK. Delirium in older people. *Br Med J* 2007;334:842–846.

Chapter 12

Alexopoulos GS, Streim J, Carpenter D, Docherty JP. Expert consensus panel for using antipsychotic drugs in older patients. Using antipsychotic agents in older patients. *J Clin Psychiatry* 2004;65[Suppl 2]:5–102.

American Psychiatric Association. *Diagnostic and Statistical Manual of Mental Disorders* (4th ed., text revision; DSM-IV-TR). Washington, DC: American Psychiatric Association; 2000:147–180.

American Psychiatric Association. Practice guidelines for the treatment of patients with Alzheimer's disease and other dementias of late life. *Am J Psychiatry* 1997;154:1–1539.

Anthony JC, LeResche L, Niaz U, et al. Limits of the "Mini-mental State" as a screening test for dementia and delirium among hospital patients. *Psychol Med* 1982;12:397–408.

Ballard C, Margallo-Lana M, Juszczak E, et al. Quetiapine and rivastigmine and cognitive decline in Alzheimer's disease: Randomized double blind placebo controlled trial. *BMJ* 2005;330:874–877.

Barry PP, Moskowitz MA. The diagnosis of reversible dementia in the elderly: A critical review. *Arch Intern Med* 1988;148: 1914–1918.

Belmin J, Expert Panel and Organisation Committee. Practical guidelines for the diagnosis and management of weight loss in Alzheimer's disease: A consensus from appropriateness ratings of a large expert panel. *J Nutr Health Aging* 2007;11:33–37.

Berg L. Clinical Dementia Rating (CDR). *Psychopharmacol Bull* 1988;24:637–639.

Besdine RW, Jarvik LF, Tangalos EG. Managing advanced Alzheimer's disease. *Patient Care* 1991;25:75–100.

Bleecker ML, Bolla-Wilson K, Kawas C, Agnew J. Age-specific norms for the Mini-Mental State Exam. *Neurology* 1988;38:1565–1568.

Briesacher BA, Limcangco MR, Simoni-Wastila L, et al. The quality of antipsychotic drug prescribing in nursing homes. *Arch Intern Med* 2005;165:1280–1285.

Brock DB, Foley DJ, Lanska DJ. Trends in dementia mortality from two National Mortality Followback Surveys. *Neurology* 2003;60:709–711.

Brodaty H, Ames D, Snowdon J, et al. A randomized placebo-controlled trial of risperidone for the treatment of aggression, agitation, and psychosis of dementia. *J Clin Psychiatry* 2003;64:134–143.

Brodaty H, Ames D, Snowdon J, et al. Risperidone for psychosis of Alzheimer's disease and mixed dementia: Results of a double-blind, placebo-controlled trial. *Int J Geriatr Psychiatry* 2005;20:1153–1157.

Caltagirone C, Bianchetti A, Di Luca M, et al. Guidelines for the treatment of Alzheimer's disease from the Italian Association of Psychogeriatrics. *Drugs Aging* 2005;22[Suppl 1]:1–26.

Canadian Task Force on the Periodic Health Examination. *Canadian Guide to Clinical Prevention Health Care.* Ottowa: Canada Communication Group;1994:902–909.

Casey DA. Pharmacological management of behavioral disturbance in dementia. *P&T* 2007;32:560–566.

Clarfield AM, Davis MB. Canadian consensus conference on the assessment of dementia, 5–6 October 1989. *CMAJ* 1990;144[Suppl]:1–38.

Clarfield AM, Foley JM. The American and Canadian consensus conferences on dementia: Is there consensus? *JAGS* 1993;41:883–886.

Clarfield AM, Larson EB. Should a major imaging procedure (CT or MRI) be required in the workup of dementia? An opposing view. *J Fam Pract* 1990;31:405–410.

Clarfield AM. The reversible dementias: Do they reverse? *Ann Intern Med* 1988;109:476–486.

Cohen-Mansfield J, Lipson S, Werner P, et al. Withdrawal of haloperidol, thioridazine, and lorazepam in the nursing home: A controlled, double-blind study. *Arch Intern Med* 1999;159:1733–1740.

Colenda CC, Wagenaar DB, Mickus M, et al. Comparing clinical practice with guideline recommendations for the treatment of depression in geriatric patients: Findings from the APA practice research network. *Am J Geriatr Psychiatry* 2003;11:448–457. (Erratum *Am J Geriatr Psychiatry* 2003; 11:604.)

Corey-Bloom J, Thal LJ, Galasko D, et al. Diagnosis and evaluation of dementia. *Neurology* 1995;45:211–218.

Cotter VT. The burden of dementia. *Am J Manag Care* 2007; 13:S193–S197.

Council on Scientific Affairs, American Medical Association. Dementia. *JAMA* 1986;256:2234–2238.

Crum RM, Anthony JC, Bassett SS, Folstein MF. Population-based norms for the Mini-Mental State Examination by age and education level. *JAMA* 1993;269:2386–2391.

De Deyn PP, Rabheru K, Rasmussen A, et al. A randomized trial of risperidone, placebo, and haloperidol for behavioral symptoms of dementia. *Neurology* 1999;53:946–955.

Dewa CS, Remington G, Herrmann N, et al. How much are atypical antipsychotic agents being used, and do they reach the populations who need them? A Canadian experience. *Clin Ther* 2002;24:1466–1476.

Erkinjuntti T, Wikström J, Palo J, Autio L. Dementia among medical inpatients: Evaluation of 2000 consecutive admissions. *Arch Intern Med* 1986;146:1923–1926.

Expert Consensus Panel for Dementia. The expert consensus guideline series. Treatment of dementia and its behavioral disturbances. *Postgrad Med* 2005:1–111.

Fillit H, Cummings J. Practice guidelines for the diagnosis and treatment of Alzheimer's disease in a managed care setting: Part II: Pharmacologic therapy. *Manag Care Interface* 2000;13:51–56.

Fillit HM, Doody RS, Binaso K, et al. Recommendations for best practices in the treatment of Alzheimer's disease in managed care. *Am J Geriatr Pharmacother* 2006;4[Suppl A]:S9–S24.

Fiske J, Frenkel H, Griffiths J, et al. Guidelines for the development of local standards of oral health care for people with dementia. *Gerodontology* 2006;23[Suppl 1]:5–32. Foley JM, Cassel K, Eastman P, et al. Differential diagnosis of dementing diseases. *JAMA* 1987;258:3411–3416.

Folstein MF, Folstein SE, McHugh PR. "Mini-mental state": A practical method for grading the mental state of patients for the clinician. *J Psychiatr Res* 1975;12:189–198.

Food and Drug Administration. FDA public health advisory: Deaths with antipsychotics in elderly patients with behavioral disturbances. At www.fda.gov/cder/drug/advisory/antipsychotics.htm. Accessed 12 Dec 2005.

Forette F, Henry JF, Orgogozo JM, et al. Reliability of clinical criteria for the diagnosis of dementia: A longitudinal multicenter study. *Arch Neurol* 1989;46:646–648.

Galasko D, Klauber MR, Hofstetter CR, et al. The Mini-Mental State Examination in the early diagnosis of Alzheimer's disease. *Arch Neurol* 1990;47:49–52.

Garcia CA, Reding MJ, Blass JP. Overdiagnosis of dementia. *JAGS* 1981;29:407–410.

Garrard J, Makris L, Dunham T, et al. Evaluation of neuroleptic drug use by nursing home elderly under proposed

Medicare and Medicaid regulations. *JAMA* 1991;265:463–467.

German PS, Shapiro S, Skinner EA, et al. Detection and management of mental health problems of older patients by primary care providers. *JAMA* 1987;257:489–493.

Giron MS, Forsell Y, Bernsten C, et al. Psychotropic drug use in elderly people with and without dementia. *Int J Geriatr Psychiatry* 2001;16:900–906.

Goldstein M, Gwyther LP, Lazaroff AE, Thal LJ. Managing early Alzheimer's disease. *Patient Care* 1991;25:44–76.

Gurland BJ, Dean LL, Copeland J, et al. Criteria for the diagnosis of dementia in the community elderly. *Gerontologist* 1982;22:180–186.

Gustafson L. Differential diagnosis with special reference to treatable dementias and pseudodementia conditions. *Dan Med Bull* 1985;32[Suppl 1]:55–60.

Hachinski V, Iadecola C, Petersen RC, et al. National Institute of Neurological Disorders and Stroke-Canadian Stroke Network vascular cognitive impairment harmonization standards. *Stroke* 2006;37:2220–2241. Epub 2006 Aug 17. (Erratum in *Stroke* 2007;38:1118.)

Henderson AS, Huppert FA. The problem of mild dementia. *Psychol Med* 1984;14:5–11.

Herr K, Coyne PJ, Key T, et al. Pain assessment in the nonverbal patient: Position statement with clinical practice recommendations. *Pain Manag Nurs* 2006;7:44–52.

Hoffman RS. Diagnostic errors in the evaluation of behavioral disorders. *JAMA* 1982;248:964–967.

Katz S. NIA Conference on Assessment. Assessing self-maintenance: Activities of daily living, mobility, and instrumental activities of daily living. *JAGS* 1983;31:721–727.

Katzman R. Should a major imaging procedure (CT or MRI) be required in the workup of dementia? An affirmative view. *J Fam Pract* 1990;31:401–405.

Kittner SJ, White LR, Farmer ME, et al. Methodological issues in screening for dementia: The problem of education adjustment. *J Chronic Dis* 1986;39:163–170.

Lanska DJ, for the Quality Standards Subcommittee, American Academy of Neurology. Practice parameters for diagnosis and evaluation of dementia (Summary statement). *Neurology* 1994;44:2203–2206.

Larson EB, Buchner DM, Uhlmann RF, Reifler BV. Caring for elderly patients with dementia. *Arch Intern Med* 1986;146:1909–1910.

Larson EB, Kukull WA, Buchner D, Reifler BV. Adverse drug reactions associated with global cognitive impairment in elderly persons. *Ann Intern Med* 1987;107:169–173.

Larson EB, Reifler BV, Featherstone HJ, English DR. Dementia in elderly outpatients: A prospective study. *Ann Intern Med* 1984;100:417–423.

Larson EB, Reifler BV, Sumi SM, et al. Diagnostic evaluation of 200 elderly outpatients with suspected dementia. *J Gerontology* 1985;40:536–543.

Lawlor BA. Behavioral and psychological symptoms in dementia: The role of atypical antipsychotics. *J Clin Psychiatry* 2004;65[Suppl 11]:5–10.

Lee PE, Gill SS, Freedman M, et al. Atypical antipsychotic drugs in the treatment of behavioral and psychological symptoms of dementia: Systematic review. *Br Med J* 2004;329:75–78.

Lyketsos CG, Colenda CC, Beck C, et al. Position statement of the American Association for Geriatric Psychiatry regarding principles of care for patients with dementia resulting from Alzheimer disease. *Am J Geriatr Psychiatry* 2006;14:561–572. (Erratum in: *Am J Geriatr Psychiatry* 2006;14:808.)

Marsden CD, Harrison MJ. Outcome of investigation of patients with presenile dementia. *Brit Med J* 1972;2:249–252.

McKeith IG, Dickson DW, Lowe J, et al. Diagnosis and management of dementia with Lewy bodies: Third report of the DLB Consortium. *Neurology* 2005;65:1863–1872. Epub 2005 Oct 19. (Erratum *Neurology* 2005;65:1992; summary for patients *Neurology* 2005;65:E26–E27.)

Mesulam M-M. Dementia: Its definition, differential diagnosis, and subtypes. *JAMA* 1985;253:2559–2561.

Miyasaki JM, Shannon K, Voon V, et al. Practice parameter: Evaluation and treatment of depression, psychosis, and dementia in Parkinson disease (an evidence-based review): Report of the Quality Standards Subcommittee of the American Academy of Neurology. *Neurology* 2006;66:996–1002.

Modi S, Moore C, Shah K, National Hospice Organization. Which late-stage Alzheimer's patients should be referred for hospice care? *J Fam Pract* 2005;54:984–986.

Musicco M, Caltagirone C, Sorbi S, et al. Italian Neurological Society guidelines for the diagnosis of dementia: Revision I. *Neurol Sci* 2004;25:154–182.

Nelson A, Fogel BS, Faust D. Bedside cognitive screening instruments: A critical assessment. *J Nerv Ment Dis* 1986;174:73–83.

Nelson JC. Increased risk of cerebrovascular adverse events and death in elderly demented patients treated with atypical antipsychotics: What's a clinician to do? *J Clin Psychiatry* 2005;66:1071.

Nott PN, Fleminger JJ. Presenile dementia: The difficulties of early diagnosis. *Acta Psychiat Scandinav* 1975;51:210–217.

O'Connor DW, Fertig A, Grande MJ, et al. Dementia in general practice: The practical consequences of a more positive approach to diagnosis. *Br J Gen Pract* 1993;43:185–188.

O'Connor DW, Pollitt PA, Hyde JB, et al. Do general practitioners miss dementia in elderly patients? *Br Med J* 1988;297:1107–1110.

Pinholt EM, Kroenke K, Hanley JF, et al. Functional assessment of the elderly: A comparison of standard instruments with clinical judgement. *Arch Intern Med* 1987;147:484–488.

Rabins PV, Lyketsos CG. Antipsychotic drugs in dementia: What should be made of the risks? *JAMA* 2005;294:1963–1965.

Reifler BV, Larson E, Hanley R. Coexistence of cognitive impairment and depression in geriatric outpatients. *Am J Psychiatry* 1982;139:623–626.

Reifler BV, Larson EB. Excess disability in demented elderly outpatients: The rule of halves. *JAGS* 1988;36:82–83.

Roca RP, Klein LE, Kirby SM, et al. Recognition of dementia among medical patients. *Arch Intern Med* 1984;144:73–75.

Rubenstein LZ, Scheirer C, Wieland GD, Kane R. Systematic biases in functional status of elderly adults: Effects of different data sources. *J Gerontology* 1984;39:686–691.

Santacruz KS, Swagerty D. Early diagnosis of dementia. *Am Fam Physician* 2001;63:703–713, 717–718. Retrieved February 5, 2008 from http://www.aafp.org/afp/20010215/703.html.

Schneider LS, Dagerman KS, Insel P. Risk of death with atypical antipsychotic drug treatment for dementia: Meta-analysis of randomized placebo-controlled trials. *JAMA* 2005; 294:1934–1943.

Shiroky JS, Schipper HM, Bergman H, Chertkow H. Can you have dementia with an MMSE score of 30? *Am J Alzheimers Dis Other Dem* 2007;22:406–415.

Singh S, Wooltorton E. Increased mortality among elderly patients with dementia using atypical antipsychotics. *Can Med Assoc J* 2005;173:252.

Sink KM, Holden KF, Yaffe K. Pharmacologic treatment of neuropsychiatric symptoms of dementia: A review of the evidence. *JAMA* 2005;293:596–608.

Small GW, Jarvik LF. The dementia syndrome. *Lancet 2* 1982; 1443–1446.

Smith JS, Kiloh IG. The investigation of dementia: Results in 200 consecutive admissions. *Lancet* 1981;1:824–827.

Task Force Sponsored by the National Institute on Aging. Senility reconsidered: Treatment possibilities for mental impairment in the elderly. *JAMA* 1980;244:259–263.

Teri L, Logsdon RG, Peskind E, et al. and Alzheimer's Disease Cooperative Study. Treatment of agitation in AD: A randomized, placebo-controlled clinical trial. *Neurology* 2000;55:1271–1278.

Teunisse S, Derix MM, van Crevel H. Assessing the severity of dementia: Patient and caregiver. *Arch Neurol* 1991;48:274–277.

Volkert D, Berner YN, Berry E, et al., and DGEM (German Society for Nutritional Medicine), ESPEN (European Society for Parenteral and Enteral Nutrition). ESPEN Guidelines on Enteral Nutrition. *Geriatrics Clin Nutr* 2006;25:330–360.

Waldemar G, Dubois B, Emre M, et al., and EFNS. Recommendations for the diagnosis and management of Alzheimer's disease and other disorders associated with dementia: EFNS guideline. *Eur J Neurol* 2007;14:e1–26.

Wang PS, Schneeweiss S, Avorn J, et al. Risk of death in elderly users of conventional vs. atypical antipsychotic medications. *N Engl J Med* 2005;353:2335–2341.

Whitehouse PJ (ed). *Dementia. Contemporary Neurology Series*, Vol. 40. Philadelphia: FA Davis Co., 1993;3–33.

World Health Organization. *International classification of impairments, disabilities, and handicaps: A manual of classification relating to the consequences of disease.* Geneva: Author, 1980.

Chapter 13

Brunko E, Zegers de Beyl D. Prognostic value of early cortical somatosensory evoked potentials after resuscitation from cardiac arrest. *Electroencephalogr Clin Neurophysiol* 1987;66:15–24.

Champion HR, et al. Alcohol intoxication and serum osmolality. *Lancet* 1975;1:1402–1404.

Childs NL, Mercer WN. Brief report: Late improvement in consciousness after post-traumatic vegetative state. *New Engl J Med* 1996;334(1):24–25.

Council on Scientific Affairs and Council on Ethical and Judicial Affairs. Persistent vegetative state and the decision to withdraw or withhold life support. Council report. *JAMA* 1990;263:426–430.

Cranford RE. The persistent vegetative state: The medical reality (getting the facts straight). *Hastings Ctr Report* 1988:27–32.

Fisher CM. The neurological evaluation of the comatose patient. *Acta Neurol Scand Suppl* 1969;36:45.

Jennett B, Bond M. Assessment of outcome after severe brain injury. *Lancet* 1975;1:480–484.

Jennett B, Teasdale G. Aspects of coma after severe head injury. *Lancet* 1971;1:878–881.

Jennett B. Severe head injuries in three countries. *J Neurol Neurosurg Psychiatry* 1977;40:291–298.

Leigh RJ, Shaw DA. Rapid regular respiration in unconscious patients. *Arch Neurol* 1976;33:356.

Levin HS, et al. Vegetative state after closed-head injury. A traumatic coma data bank report. *Arch Neurol* 1991;48:580–585.

Levy DE, et al. Prognosis in nontraumatic coma. *Ann Intern Med* 1981;94:293.

Levy DE, Knill-Jones P, Plum F. The vegetative state and its prognosis following nontraumatic coma. *Ann NY Acad Sci* 1978;315:293–304.

Lewis S. Topel J. Coma. In: Weiter W, Goetz C, eds. *Neurology for the Non-neurologist*. Philadelphia: JB Lippincott, 1994.

McQuillen MP. Can people who are unconscious or in the "vegetative state" perceive pain? *Issues Law Med* 1991;6(4):373–383.

Munsat TL, Stuart WH, Cranford RE. Guidelines of the vegetative state: Commentary on the American Academy of Neurology statement. *Neurology* 1989;39:123–124.

Sigsbee B, Plum F. The unresponsive patient: Diagnosis and management. *Med Clin North Am* 1979;63:813–834.

Susac JO, et al. Clinical spectrum of ocular bobbing. *J Neurol Neurosurg Psychiatry* 1970;33:771–775.

Wijdicks EF. Clinical scales for comatose patients: The Glasgow Coma Scale in historical context and the new FOUR score. *Rev Neurol Dis* 2006;3:109–117.

Chapter 14

Aktekin B, Dogan EA, Oguz Y, Senol Y. Withdrawal of antiepileptic drugs in adult patients free of seizures for 4 years: A prospective study. *Epilepsy Behav* 2006;8(3):616–619.

Beghi E. The management of a first seizure. *Epilepsia* 2008;49[Suppl 1]:1–61.

Ben-Menachem E. Strategy for utilization of new antiepileptic drugs. *Curr Opin Neurol* 2008;21:167–172.

Berkovic SF, Mulley JC, Scheffer IE, Petrou S. Human epilepsies: Interaction of genetic and acquired factors. *Trends Neurosci* 2006;29:391–397.

Blume WT, Lüders HO, Mizrahi E, et al. Glossary of descriptive terminology for ictal semiology: Report of the ILAE Task Force on Classification and Terminology. *Epilepsia* 2001;42:1212–1218.

Chadwick D. Starting and stopping treatment for seizures and epilepsy. *Epilepsia* 2006;47[Suppl 1]:58–61.

Chang BS, Lowenstein DH. Mechanisms of disease: Epilepsy. *N Engl J Med* 2003;349: 1257–1266.

Christensen J, Vestergaard M, Mortensen PB, et al. Epilepsy and risk of suicide: A population-based case-control study. *Lancet Neurol* 2007;6:693–698.

Costello DJ, Cole AJ. Treatment of acute seizures and status epilepticus. *J Intensive Care Med* 2007;22(6):319–347.

Crawford P. Best practice guidelines for the management of women with epilepsy. *Epilepsia* 2005;46[Suppl 9]:117–124.

Duncan JS, Sander JW, Sisodiya SM, Walker MC. Adult epilepsy. *Lancet* 2006;367:1087–1100.

Engel J, Jr.(Chair). Report of the ILAE Classification Core Group. *Epilepsia* 2006;47:1558–1568.

Falconer MA, Serafetinides EA, Corsellis JA. Etiology and pathogenesis of temporal lobe epilepsy. *Arch Neurol* 1964;10:233–248.

Fisher RS, van Emde Boas W, Blume W, et al. Epileptic seizures and epilepsy. Definitions proposed by the International League against Epilepsy (ILAE) and the International Bureau for Epilepsy (IBE). *Epilepsia* 2005;46:470–472.

French J, Smith M, Faught E, Brown L. Practice advisory: The use of felbamate in the treatment of patients with intractable epilepsy. Report of the Quality Standards Subcommittee of the American Academy of Neurology and the American Epilepsy Society. *Neurology* 1999;51:1540.

French JA, Kanner AM, Bautista J, et al. Efficacy and tolerability of the new antiepileptic drugs I: Treatment of new onset epilepsy. Report of the Therapeutics and Technology Assessment Subcommittee and Quality Standards Subcommittee of the American Academy of Neurology and the American Epilepsy Society. *Neurology* 2004;62:1252–1260.

French JA, Kanner AM, Bautista J, et al. Efficacy and tolerability of the new antiepileptic drugs II: Treatment of refractory epilepsy. Report of the Therapeutics and Technology Assessment Subcommittee and Quality Standards Subcommittee of the American Academy of Neurology and the American Epilepsy Society. *Neurology* 2004;62:1261–1273.

French JA, Williamson PD, Thadani VM, et al. Characteristics of medial temporal lobe epilepsy. I. Results of history and physical examination. *Ann Neurol* 1993;34:774–780.

Hauser WA, Kurland LT. The epidemiology of epilepsy in Rochester, Minnesota, 1935 through 1967. *Epilepsia* 1975; 16:1–66.

Hitiris N, Mohanraj R, Norrie J, Brodie MJ. Mortality in epilepsy. *Epilepsy Behav* 2007;10:363–376.

International League Against Epilepsy. Commission on Classification and Terminology of the International League Against Epilepsy Proposal for Revised Classification of Epilepsies and Epileptic Syndromes. *Epilepsia* 1989;30:389–399.

Jackson M. Epilepsy in women: A practical guide to management. *Pract Neurol* 2006;6:166–179.

Kotsopoulos IA, van Merode T, Kessels FG, et al. Systematic review and meta-analysis of incidence studies of epilepsy and unprovoked seizures. *Epilepsia* 2002;43:1402–1409.

Kwan P, Brodie MJ. Early identification of refractory epilepsy. *N Engl J Med* 2000;342:314–319.

Kwan P, Sander JW. The natural history of epilepsy: An epidemiological view. *J Neurol Neurosurg Psychiatry* 2004;75: 1376–1381.

Loddenkemper T, Kotagal P. Lateralizing signs during seizures in focal epilepsy. *Epilepsy Behav* 2005;7:1–17.

McGonigal A, Chauvel P. Frontal lobe epilepsy: Seizure semiology and presurgical evaluation. *Pract Neurol* 2004;4;260–273.

Mellers JDC. The approach to patients with "non-epileptic seizures." *Postgrad Med J* 2005;81:498–504.

Sheorajpanday RV, De Deyn PP. Epileptic fits and epilepsy in the elderly: General reflections, specific issues and therapeutic implications. *Clin Neurol Neurosurg* 2007;109:727–743.

Sheth RD, Binkley N, Hermann BP. Progressive bone deficit in epilepsy. *Neurology* 2008;70:170–176.

Siegel AM. Presurgical evaluation and surgical treatment of medically refractory epilepsy. *Neurosurg Rev* 2004;27:1–18.

Tecoma ES, Iragui VJ. Vagus nerve stimulation use and effect in epilepsy: What have we learned? *Epilepsy Behav* 2006; 8:127–136.

Téllez-Zenteno JF, Dhar R, Wiebe S. Long-term seizure outcomes following epilepsy surgery: A systematic review and meta-analysis. *Brain* 2005;128:1188–1198.

Wiebe S, Blume WT, Girvin JP, Eliasziw M. A randomized, controlled trial of surgery for temporal-lobe epilepsy. *N Engl J Med* 2001;345:311–318.

Williamson PD, French JA, Thadani VM, et al. Characteristics of medial temporal lobe epilepsy. II. Interictal and ictal scalp electroencephalography, neuropsychological testing, neuroimaging, surgical results, and pathology. *Ann Neurol* 1993;34:781–787.

Williamson PD, Spencer DD, Spencer SS, et. al. Complex partial seizures of frontal lobe origin. *Ann Neurol* 1985;18:497–504.

Zarrelli MM, Beghi E, Rocca WA, Hauser WA. Incidence of epileptic syndromes in Rochester, Minnesota: 1980–1984. *Epilepsia* 1999;40:1708–1714.

Chapter 15

Adams HP, Bendixen BH, Kappelle LJ, et al. Classification of subtype of acute ischemic stroke: Definitions for use in a multicenter clinical trial. *Stroke* 1993;24:35.

Adams RJ, Chimowitz MI, Alpert JS, et al. Coronary risk evaluation in patients with transient ischemic attack and ischemic stroke: A scientific statement for healthcare professionals from the Stroke Council and the Council on Clinical Cardiology of the American Heart Association/American Stroke Association. *Stroke* 2003;34:2310.

Albers GW, Amarenco P, Easton JD, et al. Antithrombotic and thrombolytic therapy for ischemic stroke. *Chest* 2004;126: S483.

Barnett HJM, et al. Benefit of carotid endarterectomy in patients with symptomatic moderate or severe stenosis. *New Engl J Med* 1998;339:1415.

Biller J, Mathews K, Love B. *Stroke in Children and Young Adults.* Boston: Butterworth-Heinemann, 1994.

Bogousslavsky J, Van Melle G, Regli F. The Lausanne Stroke Registry: Analysis of 1000 consecutive patients with first stroke. *Stroke* 1988;19:1083.

Brey RL, et al. Antiphospholipid antibodies and cerebral ischemia in young people. *Neurology* 1990;40:1190.

Broderick J, Connolly S, Feldmann E, et al. Guidelines for the management of spontaneous intracerebral hemorrhage in adults. 2007 update. A guideline from the American Heart Association, American Stroke Association Stroke Council, High Blood Pressure Research Council, and the Quality of Care and Outcomes in Research Interdisciplinary Working Group. *Stroke* 2007;38:2001.

Buehning L, et al. The utility of brain CT scanning in the management of acute stroke. *Stroke* 1989;20:150.

Come PC, Riley MF, Bivas NK. Roles of echocardiography and arrhythmia monitoring in the evaluation of patients with suspected systemic embolism. *Ann Neurol* 1983;13:527.

Coull BM, Goodnight SH. Antiphospholipid antibodies, prethrombotic states, and stroke. *Stroke* 1990;31:1370.

ECASS Study Group. Intravenous thrombolysis with recombinant tissue plasminogen activator for acute hemispheric stroke: The European Cooperative Acute Stroke Study (ECASS). *JAMA* 1995;274:1017.

European Heart Rhythm Association and the Heart Rhythm Society, et al. ACC/AHA/ESC 2006 Guidelines for the Management of Patients With Atrial Fibrillation: A Report of the American College of Cardiology/American Heart Association Task Force on Practice Guidelines and the European Society of Cardiology Committee for Practice Guidelines (Writing Committee to Revise the 2001 Guidelines for the Management of Patients With Atrial Fibrillation). *J Am Coll Cardiol* 2006;48:149.

Executive Committee for the Asymptomatic Carotid Atherosclerosis (ACAS) Study. Endarterectomy for asymptomatic carotid artery stenosis. *JAMA* 1995;273:1421.

Fisher CM. Lacunar strokes and infarcts: A review. *Neurology* 1982;32:871.

Fisher EA, Goldman ME. Transesophageal echocardiography: A new view of the heart. *Ann Intern Med* 1990;113:91.

Goldstein LB, Adams R, Alberts MJ, et al. Primary prevention of ischemic stroke: A guideline from the American Heart Association/American Stroke Association Stroke Council. *Stroke* 2006;37:1583.

Gordon DL, et al. Interphysician agreement in the diagnosis of subtypes of acute ischemic stroke: Implications for clinical trials. *Neurology* 1993;43:1021.

Johnston SC, Gress DR, Browner WS, Sidney S. Short-term prognosis after emergency department diagnosis of TIA. *JAMA* 2000;284:2901.

Hass WK, et al. Ticlopidine Aspirin Stroke Study Group: A randomized trial comparing ticlopidine hydrochloride with aspirin for the prevention of stroke in high-risk patients. *N Engl J Med* 1989;321:501.

Kay R, et al. Low-molecular-weight heparin for the treatment of acute ischemic stroke. *N Engl J Med* 1995;333:1588.

Leung DY, et al. Selection of patients for transesophageal echocardiography after stroke and systemic embolic events: Role of transthoracic echocardiography. *Stroke* 1995;26:1820.

Libman RB, et al. Conditions that mimic stroke in the emergency department: Implications for acute stroke trials. *Arch Neurol* 1995;52:1119.

Madden KP, et al. Accuracy of initial stroke subtype diagnosis in the TOAST study. *Neurology* 1995;45:1975.

Miller VT, et al. Ischemic stroke in patients with atrial fibrillation: Effect of aspirin according to stroke mechanism. *Neurology* 1993;43:32.

National Institute of Neurological Disorders and Stroke rt-PA Stroke Study Group. Tissue plasminogen activator for acute ischemic stroke. *N Engl J Med* 1995;333:1581.

North American Symptomatic Carotid Endarterectomy Trial (NASCET) Collaborators. Beneficial effect of carotid endarterectomy in symptomatic patients with high-grade carotid stenosis. *N Engl J Med* 1991;325:445.

Rem JA, et al. Value of cardiac monitoring and echocardiography in TIA and stroke patients. *Stroke* 1985;16:950.

Rorick MB, Nichols FT, Adams RF. Transcranial Doppler correlation with angiography in detection of intracranial stenosis. *Stroke* 1994;25:1931.

Rosamond W, Flegal K, Furie K, et al. Heart Disease and Stroke Statistics 2008 Update. A Report From the American Heart Association Statistics Committee and Stroke Statistics Subcommittee. *Circulation* 2007;117:E1.

Rothrock JF, Clark WM, Lyden PD. Spontaneous early improvement following ischemic stroke. *Stroke* 1995;26:1358.

Rothrock JF, et al. An analysis of ischemic stroke in an urban southern California population: The UCSD Stroke Data Bank. *Arch Intern Med* 1993;153:619.

Sacco RL, Adams R, Albers G et al. Guidelines for Prevention of Stroke in Patients With Ischemic Stroke or Transient Ischemic Attack: A Statement for Healthcare Professionals From the American Heart Association/American Stroke Association Council on Stroke: Co-Sponsored by the Council on Cardiovascular Radiology and Intervention. *Stroke* 2006;37:577.

Sacco RL, et al. Infarcts of undetermined cause: The NINCDS Stroke Data Bank. *Ann Neurol* 1989;25:382.

Siewert B, Patel MR, Warach S. Magnetic resonance angiography. *Neurologist* 1995;1:167.

The Stroke Prevention by Aggressive Reduction of Cholesterol Levels (SPARCL) Investigators. High-dose atorvastatin after stroke or transient ischemic attack. *New Engl J Med* 2006;355:549.

Toni D, et al. Clinical and prognostic correlates of stroke subtype misdiagnosis within 12 hours from onset. *Stroke* 1995;26:1837.

Toole JF, et al. Lowering homocysteine in patients with ischemic stroke to prevent recurrent stroke, myocardial infarction, and death: The Vitamin Intervention for Stroke Prevention (VISP) randomized controlled trial. *JAMA* 2004;291:565.

Chapter 16

Adams JH, Doyle D, Ford I, et al. Diffuse axonal injury in head injury: Definition, diagnosis, and grading. *Histopathology* 1989;15(1):49–59.

Anderson RW, Brown CJ, Blumbergs PC, et al. Impact mechanics and axonal injury in a sheep model. *J Neurotrauma* 2003;20(10):961–974.

Andrews BT. History, classification, and epidemiology of cranial trauma. In: Batjer HH, Loftus CM, eds. *Textbook of Neurological Surgery*. Philadelphia: Lippincott, Williams, &Wilkins;2003:2796–2798.

Blumbergs PC, Jones NR, North JB. Diffuse axonal injury in head trauma. *J Neurol Neurosurg Psychiatry* 1989;52(7):838–841.

Bracken MB, Shepard MJ, Collins WF, et al. A randomized, controlled trial of methylprednisolone or naloxone in the treatment of acute cervical cord injury: Results of the Second National Acute Spinal Cord Injury Study. *N Engl J Med* 1990;322:1405–1411.

Bracken MB, Shepard MJ, Holford TR, et al. Administration of methylprednisolone for 24 or 48 hours or tirilazad mesylate for 48 hours in the treatment of acute cord injury: Results of the Third National Acute Spinal Cord Injury Randomized Controlled Trial. National Acute Spinal Cord Injury Study. *JAMA* 1997;277:1597–1604.

Bricolo AP, Pasut LM. Extradural hematoma: Toward zero mortality. A prospective study. *Neurosurgery* 1984;14(1):8–12.

Bryant R. Disentangling mild traumatic brain injury and stress reactions. *N Engl J Med* 2008;358:525–527.

Bullock RM, Chestnutt RM, Clifton G, et al. Guidelines for the management of severe head injury. The Brain Trauma Foundation (New York), American Association of Neurological Surgeons (Park Ridge, Illinois), the joint section of neurotrauma and critical care, 1995.*Eur J Emerg Med* 1996;3(2): 109–127.

Collins JG. Types of injuries by selected characteristics: United States, 1985–1987. *Vital Health Stat* 1990;10:175.

Cushing H. *The Third Circulation in Studies in Intracranial Physiology and Surgery.* London: Oxford University Press; 1926:1–51.

Denis F. The three-column spine and its significance in the classification of acute thoracolumbar spinal injuries. *Spine* 1983;8:817–831.

Dickman CA, Hadley MN, Browner C, et al. Neurosurgical management of acute atlas-axis combination fractures. *J Neurosurg* 1989;70:45–49.

Eisenberg HM, Gary HE, Aldrich EF. Initial CT findings in 753 patients with severe head injury. A report from the NIH traumatic coma data bank. *J Neurosurg* 1990;73(5):688–698.

Evans RW. Mild traumatic brain injury. *Phys Med Rehab Clin North Am* 1992;3:427–439.

Geisler FH, Manson PN. Traumatic skull and facial fractures. In: Rengachary SS, Wilkins RH, eds. *Principles of Neurosurgery.* London: Wolfe;1994:18.1–18.32.

Gennarelli TA. Mechanisms of brain injury. *J Emerg Med* 1993; 1:5–11.

Greenberg MS. *Handbook of Neurosurgery.* New York: Thieme; 1997:660–663.

Greene KA, Marciano FF, Johnson BA, et al. Impact of traumatic subarachnoid hemorrhage on outcome in non-penetrating head injury. Part I: A proposed computerized tomography grading scale. *J Neurosurg* 1995;83(3):445–452.

Hadley MN. Injuries to the cervical spine. In: Rengachary SS, Wilkins RH, eds. *Principles of Neurosurgery.* London: Wolfe;1994:20.1–20.13.

Hadley MN, Dickman CA, Browner CM, et al. Acute traumatic atlas fractures: Management and long-term outcome. *Neurosurgery* 1988;23:31–35.

Hartl R, Froelic M. Mannitol and hypertonic saline: Going head to head. *Crit Care Med* 2008;36(3):1005–1006.

Hoge CW, McGurk D, et al. Mild traumatic brain injury in U.S. soldiers returning from Iraq. *N Engl J Med* 2008;358:453–463.

Jennett B, Teasdale G, Braakman R, et al. Prognosis of patients with severe head injury. *Neurosurgery* 1979;4:282–289.

Juul N, Morris GF, Marshall SB, et al. Intracranial hypertension and cerebral perfusion pressure: Influence on neurological deterioration and outcome in severe head injury. *J Neurosurg* 2000;92:1–6.

Jussen D, Papaioannou C, et al. Effects of hypertonic/hyperoncotic treatment and surgical evacuation after acute subdural hematoma in rats. *Crit Care Med* 2008;36(2):543–549.

Kraus JF. Epidemiology of head injury. In: Brown CL, Napora L, eds. *Head Injury.* Baltimore: Williams & Wilkins;1987:1–19.

Kraus FJ, Nourjah P. The epidemiology of mild, uncomplicated head injury. *J Trauma* 1988;28:1637–1643.

Lee JH, Martin NA, Alsina G, et al. Hemodynamically significant cerebral vasospasm and outcome after head injury: A prospective study. *J Neurosurg* 1997;87:221–233.

Levin HS, Mattis F, Ruff RM, et al. Neurobehavioral outcome following minor head injury. *J Neurosurg* 1987;66:234–243.

Lobato RD, Cordobes F, Rivas JJ. Outcome from severe head injury related to the type of intracranial lesion. A computerized tomography study. *J Neurosurg* 1983;59(5):762–774.

Manley G, Andrews BT. Complications of cranial trauma. In: Batjer HH, Loftus CM, eds. *Textbook of Neurological Surgery.* Philadelphia: Lippincott, Williams & Wilkins; 2003: 2889–2894.

Marion DW. Pathophysiology of cranial trauma. In: Batjer HH, Loftus CM, eds. *Textbook of Neurological Surgery.* Philadelphia: Lippincott, Williams, & Wilkins;2003:2800–2803.

McIntyr LA, Fergusson DA, Hebert PC, et al. Prolonged therapeutic hypothermia after traumatic brain injury in adults. A systematic review. *JAMA* 2003;289:2992–2999.

Narayan RK. Closed head injury. In: Rengachary SS, Wilkins RH, eds. *Principles of Neurosurgery.* London: Wolfe; 1994:16.1–16.20.

Obana WG, Andrews BT. The neurological examination and neurologic monitoring in the intensive care unit. In: Andrews BT, ed. *Neurosurgical Intensive Care.* New York: McGraw Hill Inc.;1993:31–42.

Palmer AM, Marion DW, Botscheller, et al. Traumatic brain injury-induced excitotoxicity assessed in a controlled cortical impact model. *J Neurochem* 1993;61:2015–2024.

Peterson K, Carson S, Carney N. Hypothermia treatment for traumatic brain injury: A systematic review and meta-analysis. *J Neurotrauma* 2008;25(1):62–71.

Raghopathi R, Margulies SS. Traumatic axonal injury after closed head injury in the neonatal pig. *J Neurotrauma* 2002;19(7):843–853.

Rimel RW, Giordani B, Barth JT, et al. Disability caused by minor head injury. *Neurosurgery* 1981;9:221–228.

Servadei F, Murray GD, Teasdale GM, et al. Traumatic subarachnoid hemorrhage: Demographic and clinical study of 750 patients from the European brain injury consortium survey of head injuries. *Neurosurgery* 2002;50(2):261–267.

Servadei F, Teasdale G, Merry G. Defining acute mild head injury in adults: A proposal based on prognostic factors, diagnosis, and management. *J Neurotrauma* 2001;18(7):657–664.

Smith DH, Nonaka M, Miller R, et al. Immediate coma following inertial brain injury dependent on axonal damage in the brainstem. *J Neurosurg* 2000;93(2):315–322.

Sonntag VKH, Hadley MN. Nonoperative management of cervical spine injuries. *Clin Neurosurg* 1988;34:630–649.

Stone JL, Lowe RJ, Jonasson O, et al. Acute subdural hematoma: Direct admission to a trauma center yields improved results. *J Trauma* 1986;26:445–450.

Taylor WR, Chen JW, Meltzer H, et al. Quantitative pupillometry, a new technology: Normative data and preliminary observations in patients with acute head injury. *J Neurosurg* 2003;98:205–213.

Temkin NR, Dikmen SS, Wilensky AJ, et al. A randomized, double-blind study of phenytoin for the prevention of post-traumatic seizures. *N Engl J Med* 1990;323(8):497–502.

Wilberger JE, Harris M, Diamond DL. Acute subdural hematoma: Morbidity, mortality, and operative timing. *J Neurosurgery* 1991;74:212–218.

Chapter 17

Blindauer K, Shoulson I, Kieburtz K, et al. A controlled trial of rotigotine monotherapy in early Parkinson's disease. *Arch Neurol* 2003;60:1721–1728.

Clarke CE, Guttman M. Dopamine agonist monotherapy in Parkinson's disease. *Lancet* 2002;360:1767–1769.

Crossman AR. Mechanisms of levodopa-induced dyskinesia. *Mov Disord* 1990;5:100–108.

Dauer W, Przedborski S. Parkinson's disease: Mechanisms and models. *Neuron* 2003;39:889–909.

Dekker MC, Bonifati V, van Duijn VN. Parkinson's disease: Piecing together a genetic jigsaw. *Brain* 2003;126:1722–1733.

Deuschl G, Schade-Brittinger C, Krack P, et al. A randomized trial of deep brain stimulation for Parkinson's disease. *N Engl J Med* 2006;355:896–908.

Dewey RB Jr., Hutton JT, Lewitt PA, Factor SA. A randomized, double-blind, placebo-controlled trial of subcutaneously injected apomorphine for parkinsonian off-state events. *Arch Neurol* 2001;58:1385–1392.

Gibb WRG, Luthert PJ, Marsden CD. Corticobasal degeneration. *Brain* 1989;112:1171–1192.

Gliadi N, McDermott MP, Fahn S, et al. Freezing of gait in PD: Prospective assessment in the DATATOP cohort. *Neurology* 2001;56:1712–1721.

Gill SS, Patel NK, Hotton GR, et al. Direct brain infusion of glial cell line-derived neurotrophic factor in Parkinson disease. *Nat Med* 2003;9:589–595.

Hughes AJ, et al. Accuracy of clinical diagnosis of idiopathic Parkinson's disease: A clinicopathological study of 100 cases. *J Neurol Neurosurg Psychiatry* 1992;55:181–184.

Jankovic J, Tolosa E. *Parkinson's Disease and Movement Disorders*, 4th ed. Philadelphia: Lippincott, Williams & Wilkins, 2002.

Koller WC, Hutton JT, Tolosa E, Capilldeo R. Immediate-release and controlled-release carbidopa/levodopa in PD: A 5-year randomized multicenter study. Carbidopa/Levodopa Study Group. *Neurology* 1999;53:1012–1019.

Krack P, Batir A, van Blercom N, et al. Five-year follow-up of bilateral stimulation of the subthalamic nucleus in advanced Parkinson's disease. *N Eng J Med* 2003;349:1925–1934.

Lang AE, Gill S, Patel NK, et al. Randomized controlled trial of intraputamenal glial cell line-derived neurotrophic factor infusion in Parkinson disease. *Ann Neurol* 2006;59:459–466.

Mancini F, Zangaglia R, Cristina S, et al. Double-blind, placebo-controlled study to evaluate the efficacy and safety of botulinum toxin type A in the treatment of drooling in parkinsonism. *Mov Disord* 2003;18:685–688.

Nutt JG, Burchiel KJ, Comella CL, et al. Randomized, double-blind trial of glial cell line-derived neurotrophic factor (GDNF) in PD. *Neurology* 2003;60:69–73.

Pahwa R, Wilkinson SB, Overman J, Lyons KE. Bilateral subthalamic stimulation in patients with Parkinson's disease: Long-term follow up. *J Neurosurg* 2003;99:71–77.

Parkinson Study Group. Effect of deprenyl on the progression of disability in early Parkinson's disease. *N Eng J Med* 1989;321:1364–1371.

Parkinson Study Group. Effects of tocopherol deprenyl on the progression of disability in early Parkinson's disease. *N Eng J Med* 1993;328:176–183.

Parkinson Study Group. Pramipexole vs levodopa as initial treatment for Parkinson disease: A randomized controlled trial. Parkinson Study Group. *JAMA* 2000;284:1931–1938.

Parkinson Study Group. Dopamine transporter brain imaging to assess the effects of pramipexole vs levodopa on Parkinson disease progression. *JAMA* 2002;287:1653–1661.

Parkinson Study Group. A controlled, randomized, delayed-start study of rasagiline in early Parkinson disease. *Arch Neurol* 2004;61:561–566.

Patel NK, Heywood P, O'Sullivan K, et al. Unilateral subthalamotomy in the treatment of Parkinson's disease. *Brain* 2003;126:1136–1145.

Rascol O, Brooks DJ, Korczyn AD, et al. A five-year study of the incidence of dyskinesia in patients with early Parkinson's disease who were treated with ropinirole or levodopa. 056 Study Group. *N Eng J Med* 2000;342:1484–1491.

Shoulson I, Oakes D, Fahn S, et al. Impact of sustained deprenyl (selegiline) in levodopa-treated Parkinson's disease: A randomized placebo-controlled extension of the deprenyl and tocopherol antioxidative therapy of parkinsonism trial. *Ann Neurol* 2002;51:604–612.

Shultz CW, Oakes D, Kieburtz K, et al. Effects of coenzyme Q10 in early Parkinson's disease: Evidence of slowing of the functional decline. *Arch Neurol* 2002;59:1541–1550.

Stacy M, Jankovic J. Differential diagnosis of Parkinson's disease and the parkinsonism plus syndromes. *Neurol Clin N Am* 1992;10:341–358.

Stacy M, Jankovic J. Advances in the treatment of Parkinson's disease. *Ann Rev Med* 1993;44:431–440.

Vitek JL, Bakay RA, Freeman A, et al. Randomized trial of pallidotomy versus medical therapy for Parkinson's disease. *Ann Neurol* 2003;53:558–569.

Whone AL, Watts RL, Stoessl AJ, et al. Slower progression of Parkinson's disease with ropinirole versus levodopa: The REAL-PET study. *Ann Neurol* 2003;54:93–101.

Chapter 18

Boerkoel CF, Takashima H, et al. Charcot-Marie-Tooth disease and related neuropathies: Mutation distribution and genotype-phenotype correlation. *Ann Neurol* 2002;51(2):190–201.

Brooks BR, Miller RG, et al. El Escorial revisited: Revised criteria for the diagnosis of amyotrophic lateral sclerosis. *Amyotroph Lateral Scler Other Motor Neuron Disord* 2000;1(5): 293–299.

Dalakas MC, Hohlfeld R. Polymyositis and dermatomyositis. *Lancet* 2003;362(9388):971–982.

Emery AE. The muscular dystrophies. *Lancet* 2002;359(9307): 687–695.

Hughes RA, Wijdicks EF, et al. Practice parameter: Immunotherapy for Guillain–Barré syndrome: Report of the Quality Standards Subcommittee of the American Academy of Neurology. *Neurology* 2003;61(6):736–740.

Keesey JC. Clinical evaluation and management of myasthenia gravis. *Muscle Nerve* 2004;29(4):484–505.

Lacomis D. Small-fiber neuropathy. *Muscle Nerve* 2002;26(2): 173–188.

Mathews KD. Muscular dystrophy overview: Genetics and diagnosis. *Neurol Clin* 2003;21(4):795–816.

Sieb JP, Gillessen T. Iatrogenic and toxic myopathies. *Muscle Nerve* 2003;27(2):142–156.

Singleton JR, Smith AG, et al. Increased prevalence of impaired glucose tolerance in patients with painful sensory neuropathy. *Diabetes Care* 2001;24(8):1448–1453.

Sumner CJ, Sheth S, et al. The spectrum of neuropathy in diabetes and impaired glucose tolerance. *Neurology* 2003;60(1): 108–111.

The Diabetes Control and Complications Trial Research Group. Effect of intensive diabetes treatment on nerve conduction in the Diabetes Control and Complications Trial. *Ann Neurol* 1995;38(6):869–880.

The Diabetes Control and Complications Trial Research Group. The effect of intensive treatment of diabetes on the development and progression of long-term complications in insulin-dependent diabetes mellitus. *N Engl J Med* 1993;329(14): 977–986.

The Diabetes Control and Complications Trial Research Group. The effect of intensive diabetes therapy on the development and progression of neuropathy. *Ann Intern Med* 1995; 122(8):561–568.

Zatz M, de Paula F, et al. The 10 autosomal recessive limb-girdle muscular dystrophies. *Neuromuscul Disord* 2003;13(7–8):532–544.

Chapter 19

Bal AM. Unusual clinical manifestations of leptospirosis. *Post Grad Med* 2005;51:179–183.

Centers for Disease Control and Prevention. Sexually transmitted diseases treatment guidelines 2006. *Morbidity and Mortality Weekly Report* 2006;55(RR11):1–94.

Centers for Disease Control and Prevention. Treating opportunistic infections among HIV-infected adults and adolescents. *Morbidity and Mortality Weekly Report* 2004;55(RR15):1–112.

Davis LE, DeBiasi R, Goade DE, et al. West Nile neuroinvasive disease. *Ann Neurol* 2006;60:286–300.

Dougan C, Ormerod I. A neurologist's approach to the immunosuppressed patient. *J Neurol Neurosurg Psychiatry* 2004;75(Suppl I):I43–I49.

Garcia HH, Del Brutto OH. Neurocysticercosis: Updated concepts about an old disease. *Lancet Neurol* 2005;4: 653–661.

Ginsberg L. Difficult and recurrent meningitis. *J Neurol Neurosurg Psychiatry* 2004;75:16–21.

Goonetilleke A, Harris JB. Clostridial neurotoxins. *J Neurol Neurosurg Psychiatry* 2004;75(Suppl III):III35–III39.

Halperin JJ, Shapiro E, Logigian A, et al. Practice parameter: Treatment of nervous system Lyme disease (an evidence-based review): Report of the quality of standards subcommittee of the American Academy of Neurology. *Neurology* 2007;69:91–102.

Johnson RT. Prion diseases. *Lancet Neurol* 2005;4:635–642.

Kennedy PG. Viral encephalitis. *J Neurol* 2005;252:268–272.

Laupland KB. Vascular and parameningeal infections of the head and neck. *Infect Dis Clin North Am* 2007;21:577–590.

McArthur JC, Brew BJ, Nath A. Neurological complications of HIV infection. *Lancet Neurol* 2005;4:543–555.

McAuley JH, Fearnley J, Laurence A, Ball JA. Diphtheritic polyneuropathy. *J Neurol Neurosurg Psychiatry* 1999;67: 825–826.

Perez-Velez CM, Anderson MS, Robinson CC, et al. Outbreak of neurologic enterovirus type 71 disease: A diagnostic challenge. *Clin Infect Dis* 2007;45:950–957.

Sendi P, Bregenzer T, Zimmerli W. Spinal epidural abscess in clinical practice. *Q J Med* 2008;101:1–12.

Shanley JD. The resurgence of mumps in young adults and adolescents. *Cleve Clin J Med* 2007;74:42–46.

Steiner I, Kennedy GE, Pachner AR. The neurotropic herpes viruses: Herpes simplex and varicella-zoster. *Lancet Neurol* 2007;6:1015–1028.

Thwaites GE, Hien TT. Tuberculous meningitis: Many questions, too few answers. *Lancet Neurol* 2005;4:160–170.

Torok ME. Human immunodeficiency virus associated central nervous system infections. *Pract Neurol* 2005;5:334–349.

Wormser GP, Dattwyler RJ, Shapiro ED, et al. The clinical assessment, treatment, and prevention of Lyme disease, human granulocytic anaplasmosis, and babesiosis: Clinical practice guidelines of the Infectious Disease Society of America. *Clin Infect Dis* 2006;43:1089–1134.

Chapter 20

Altrochi PH. Acute transverse myclopathy. *Arch Neurol* 1963;9:21–29.

Austin SG, et al. The role of magnetic resonance imaging in acute transverse myelitis. *Can J Neurol Sci* 1992;19:508–511.

Beck RW, et al. A randomized, controlled trial of corticosteroids in the treatment of acute optic neuritis. *N Engl J Med* 1992;326:581–588.

Beck RW, et al. Brain magnetic resonance imaging in acute optic neuritis: Experience of the Optic Neuritis Study Group. *Arch Neurol* 1993;50:841–846.

Beck RW, et al. The effect of corticosteroids for acute optic neuritis on the subsequent development of multiple sclerosis. *N Engl J Med* 1993;329:1764–1769.

Caldemeyer KS, et al. MRI in acute disseminated encephalomyelitis. *Neuroradiology* 1994;36:216–220.

Cree BA, et al. An open label study of the effects of rituximab in neuromyelitis optica. *Neurology* 2005;64(7):1270–1272.

Cree BA, et al. Neuromyelitis optica. *Semin Neurol* 2002; 22(2):105–122.

Cutler JR, et al. Evaluation of patients with multiple sclerosis by evoked potentials, and magnetic resonance imaging: A comparative study. *Ann Neurol* 1986;20:645–648.

Farlow MR, et al. Multiple sclerosis: Magnetic resonance imaging, evoked potentials, and spinal fluid electrophoresis. *Neurology* 1986;36:828–831.

Fazekas F, et al. Criteria for an increased specificity of MRI interpretation in elderly subjects with suspected multiple sclerosis. *Neurology* 1988;38:1822–1825.

Ford B, et al. Long-term follow-up of acute partial transverse myelopathy. *Neurology* 1992;42:250–252.

Giang DW, et al. Clinical diagnosis of multiple sclerosis: The impact of magnetic resonance imaging and ancillary testing. *Arch Neurol* 1994;51:61–66.

Goodkin DE, et al. Low-dose (7.5 mg) oral methotrexate reduces the rate of progression in chronic progressive multiple sclerosis. *Ann Neurol* 1995;37:30–40.

Goodkin DE, et al. The efficacy of azathioprine in relapsing-remitting multiple sclerosis. *Neurology* 1991;41:20–25.

Goodkin DE. Role of steroids and immunosuppression and effects of interferon beta-1b in multiple sclerosis. *West J Med* 1994;161:292–298.

Honig LS, Sheremata WA. Magnetic resonance imaging of spinal cord lesions in multiple sclerosis. *J Neurol Neurosurg Psychiatry* 1989;52:459–466.

Jacobs L, et al. Advances in specific therapy for multiple sclerosis. *Curr Opin Neurol* 1994;7:250–254.

Jacobs LD, et al. Intramuscular interferon beta-1a for disease progression in relapsing multiple sclerosis. *Ann Neurol* 1996;39:285–294.

Kanter DS, et al. Plasmapheresis in fulminant acute disseminated encephalomyelitis. *Neurology* 1995;45:824–827.

Kappos L, Polman CH, Freedman MS, et al. For the BENEFIT Study Group. Treatment with interferon beta-1b delays conversion to clinically definite and McDonald multiple sclerosis in patients with clinically isolated syndromes. *Neurology* 2006;67:1242–1249.

Kesselring J, et al. Acute disseminated encephalomyelitis: MRI findings and the distinction from multiple sclerosis. *Brain* 1990;113:291–302.

Kleinschmidt-Demasters BK, Tyler KL. Progressive multifocal leukoencephalopathy complicating treatment with natalizumab and interferon beta-1a for multiple sclerosis. *N Engl J Med* 2005;353(4):369–374.

Langer-Gould A, et al. Progressive multifocal leukoencephalopathy in a patient treated with natalizumab. *N Engl J Med* 2005;353(4):375–381.

Lee KH, et al. Magnetic resonance imaging of the head in the diagnosis of multiple sclerosis: A prospective 2-year follow-up with comparison of clinical evaluation, evoked potentials, oligoclonal banding, and CT. *Neurology* 1991;41:657–660.

Lefvert AK, Link H. IgG production within the central nervous system: A critical review of proposed formulae. *Ann Neurol* 1985;17:13–20.

Lennon VA, et al. A serum autoantibody marker of neuromyelitis optica: Distinction from multiple sclerosis. *Lancet* 2004;364(9451):2106–2112.

Lynch SG, Rose JW. Multiple sclerosis. *Dis Mon* 1996;42:1–55.

Lyons PR, et al. Methylprednisolone therapy in multiple sclerosis: A profile of adverse effects. *J Neurol Neurosurg Psychiatry* 1988;51:285–287.

Mandler RN, et al. Devic's neuromyelitis optica: A prospective study of seven patients treated with prednisone and azathioprine. *Neurology* 1998;51(4):1219–1220.

Miller DH, et al. Acute disseminated encephalomyelitis presenting as a solitary brainstem mass. *J Neurol Neurosurg Psychiatry* 1993;56:920–922.

Miller DH, et al. Detection of optic nerve lesions in optic neuritis with magnetic resonance imaging. *Lancet* 1986;1:1490–1491.

Miller DH, et al. Magnetic resonance imaging in isolated noncompressive spinal cord syndromes. *Ann Neurol* 1987;22:714–723.

Miller JR, et al. Occurrence of oligoclonal bands in multiple sclerosis and other CNS diseases. *Ann Neurol* 1983;13:53–58.

Milligan NM, et al. A double-blind controlled trial of high dose methylprednisolone in patients with multiple sclerosis. 1. Clinical effects. *J Neurol Neurosurg Psychiatry* 1987;50:511–516.

Ormerod IEC, et al. Disseminated lesions at presentation in patients with optic neuritis. *J Neurol Neurosurg Psychiatry* 1986;49:124–127.

Polman CH, et al. AFFIRM Investigators: A randomized, placebo-controlled trial of natalizumab for relapsing multiple sclerosis. *N Engl J Med* 2006;354(9):899–910.

Rizzo JF 3rd, Lessell S. Risk of developing multiple sclerosis after uncomplicated optic neuritis: A long-term prospective study. *Neurology* 1988;38:185–190.

Ropper AH, Poskanzer DC. The prognosis of acute and subacute transverse myelopathy based on early signs and symptoms. *Ann Neurol* 1978;4:51–59.

Sandberg-Wollheim M, et al. A long-term prospective study of optic neuritis: Evaluation of risk factors. *Ann Neurol* 1990;27:386–393.

Sanders KA, et al. Gadolinium-MRI in acute transverse myelopathy. *Neurology* 1990;40:1614–1616.

Smith AS, et al. High-signal periventricular lesions in patients with sarcoidosis: Neurosarcoidosis or multiple sclerosis? *AJR Am J Roentgenol* 1989;153:147–152.

Soges LJ, et al. Migraine: Evaluation by MR. *AJNR Am J Neuroradiol* 1988;9:425–429.

The IFNB Multiple Sclerosis Study Group. Interferon beta-1b is effective in relapsing-remitting multiple sclerosis: Clinical results of a multicenter, randomized, double-blind, placebo controlled trial. *Neurology* 1993;43:655–661.

The International MS Genetics Consortium. Risk alleles for multiple sclerosis identified by a genomewide study. *N Engl J Med* 2007;357(9):851–862.

The Optic Neuritis Study Group. The clinical profile of optic neuritis: Experience of the Optic Neuritis Treatment Trial. *Arch Ophthalmol* 1991;109:1673–1678.

Thompson AJ, et al. Relative efficacy of intravenous methylprednisolone and ACTH in the treatment of acute relapse in MS. *Neurology* 1989;39:969–971.

Tourtellotte WW, et al. Multiple sclerosis: Measurement and validation of central nervous system IgG synthesis rate. *Neurology* 1980;30:240–244.

Van Assche G, et al. Progressive multifocal leukoencephalopathy after natalizumab therapy for Crohn's disease. *New Engl J Med* 2005;353(4):362–368.

Weinstock-Guttman B, et al. Study of mitoxantrone for the treatment of recurrent neuromyelitis optica (Devic disease). *Arch Neurol* 2006;63(7):957–963.

Yousry TA, Major EO, Rhyschkewitsch C, et al. Evaluation of patients treated with natalizumab for progressive multifocal leukoencephalopathy. *New Engl J Med* 2006;354(9):924–933.

Chapter 21

Afra D, Baron B, Bonadonna G, et al. (GMT) Group: Chemotherapy in adult high-grade glioma: A systematic review and meta-analysis of individual patient data from 12 randomized trials. *Lancet* 2002;359:1011–1018.

Bent M, Chinot O-L, Cairncross G. Recent developments in the molecular characterization and treatment of oligodendroglial tumors. *Neuro Oncol* 2003;5(2):128–138.

Bindal AK, Bindal RK, Hess KR, et al. Surgery versus radiosurgery in the treatment of brain metastasis. *J Neurosurg* 1996;84:748–754.

Cairncross JG, Kim JH, Posner JB. Radiation therapy for brain metastases. *Ann Neurol* 1980;7(6):529–541.

Chamberlain MC, Kormanik P. Prognostic significance of 111Indium-DTPA CSF flow studies. *Neurology* 1996;46(6):1674–1677.

Chamberlain MC. Malignant meningiomas: Adjuvant combined modality therapy. *J Neurosurg* 1996;84:733–736.

Chamberlain, MC, Abitbol JJ, Garfin S. Epidural spinal cord compression: Treatment options. *Semin Spine Surg* 1990;2:203–209.

Clouston PD, DeAngelis LM, Posner JB. The spectrum of neurological disease in patients with systemic cancer. *Ann Neurol* 1992;31:268–273.

Dalmau J, Posner JB. Neurologic paraneoplastic antibodies (anti-Yo; anti-Hu; anti-Ri): The case for a nomenclature based on antibody and antigen specificity. *Neurology* 1994;44:2241–2246.

Davey P. Brain metastases: Treatment options to improve outcomes. *CNS Drugs* 2002;16(5):325–338.

Fadul C, Wood J, Thaler H, et al. Morbidity and mortality of craniotomy for excision of supratentorial gliomas. *Neurology* 1988;38:1374–1379.

Faul CM, Flickinger JC. The use of radiation in the management of spinal metastases. *Neuro Oncol* 1995;23:149–161.

Forsyth PA, Posner B. Headaches in patients with brain tumors: A study of 111 patients. *Neurology* 1993;43:1678–1683.

Freilich RJ, Kroll G, DeAngelis LM. Neuroimaging and cerebrospinal fluid cytology in the diagnosis of leptomeningeal metastasis. *Ann Neurol* 1995;38:51–57.

Glantz M, Jaeckle KA, Chamberlain MC, et al. A randomized trial of a slow-release formulation of cytarabine for the treatment of lymphomatous meningitis. *J Clin Oncol* 1999;17:3110–3116.

Goldsmith BJ, Wara WM, Wilson CB, Larson DA. Postoperative irradiation for subtotally resected meningiomas. *J Neurosurg* 1994;80:195–201.

Grant R, Liang BC, Page MA, et al. Age influences chemotherapy response in astrocytomas. *Neurology* 1995;45:929–933.

Grant R, Naylor B, Greenberg HS, Junck L. Clinical outcome in aggressively treated meningeal carcinomatosis. *Arch Neurol* 1994;51:457–461.

Grigsby PW, Simpson JR, Emami BN, et al. Prognostic factors and results of surgery and postoperative irradiation in the management of pituitary adenomas. *Int J Radiat Oncol Biol Phys* 1989;16(6):1411–1417.

Horwich MS, Cho L, Porro RS, Posner JB. Subacute sensory neuropathy: A remote effect of carcinoma. *Ann Neurol* 1977;2:7–19.

Laws ER, Parney IF, Huang W, et al. Survival following surgery and prognostic factors for recently diagnosed malignant glioma: Data from the Glioma Outcomes Project. *J Neurosurg* 2003;99:467–473.

Lennon VA, Kryzer TJ, Griesmann GE, et al. Calcium-channel antibodies in the Lambert-Eaton syndrome and other paraneoplastic syndromes. *New Engl J Med* 1995;332(22):1467–1474.

Lennon VA. Paraneoplastic autoantibodies: The case for a descriptive generic nomenclature. *Neurology* 1994;44:2236–2240.

McCormick PC, Bello JA, Post KD. Trigeminal schwannoma. *J Neurosurg* 1988;69:850–860.

Mehta MP, Rodrigus P, Terhaard CHJ, et al. Survival and neurologic outcomes in a randomized trial of motexafin gadolinium and whole-brain radiation therapy in brain metastases. *J Clin Oncol* 2003;21(13):2529–2536.

Moll JWB, Antoine JC, Brashear HR, et al. Guidelines on the detection of paraneoplastic anti-neuronal-specific antibodies. Report from the workshop to the fourth meeting of the Inter-national Society of Neuro-Immunology on paraneoplastic neurological disease, held October 22–23, 1994, in Rotterdam, The Netherlands. *Neurology* 1995;45:1937–1941.

Newton H, Slivka MA, Stevens C. Hydroxyurea chemotherapy for unresectable meningioma. *Neuro Oncol* 2000;49(2):165–170.

O'Neill BP, Buckner JC, Coffey RJ, et al. Brain metastatic lesions. *Mayo Clin Proc* 1994;69:1062–1068.

O'Neill JH, Murray NMF, Newsom-Davis J. HE Lambert-Eaton myasthenic syndrome. A review of 50 cases. *Brain* 1988;3:577–594.

Peterson K, Rosenblum MK, Kotanides H, Posner JB. Paraneoplastic cerebellar degeneration. I. A clinical analysis of 55 anti-Yo antibody-positive patients. *Neurology* 1992;42:1931–1937.

Pollack IF, Sekhar LN, Jannetta PJ, Janecka IP. Neurilemomas of the trigeminal nerve. *J Neurosurg* 1989;70:737–745.

Posner JB. Surgery for metastases to the brain. *New Engl J Med* 1990;322(8):544–545.

Prados MD, Scott C, Curran WJ, et al. Procarbazine, lomustine, and vincristine (PCV) chemotherapy for anaplastic astrocytoma: A retrospective review of radiation therapy oncology group protocols comparing survival with carmustine or PCV adjuvant chemotherapy. *J Clin Oncol* 1999;17(11):3389–3395.

Riggs JE. Rising primary malignant brain tumor mortality in the elderly. *Arch Neurol* 1995;52:571–575.

Roche PH, Regis J, Dufour H, et al. Gamma knife radiosurgery in the management of cavernous sinus meningiomas. *J Neurosurg* 2000;93(3):68–73.

Rohringer M, Sutherland GR, Louw DF, Sima AAF. Incidence and clinico-pathological features of meningioma. *J Neurosurg* 1989;71:665–672.

Ross DA, Wilson CB. Results of transsphenoidal microsurgery for growth hormone-secreting pituitary adenoma in a series of 214 patients. *J Neurosurg* 1988;68:854–867.

Ruff RL, Lanska DJ. Epidural metastases in prospectively evaluated veterans with cancer and back pain. *Cancer* 1989;63:2234–2241.

Samil M, Migliori MM, Tatagiba M, Babu R. Surgical treatment of trigeminal schwannomas. *J Neurosurg* 1995;82: 711–718.

Sawaya R, Ligon BL, Bindal AK, et al. Surgical treatment of metastatic brain tumors. *Neuro Oncol* 1996;27:269–277.

Schiff D, Shaw EG, Cascino TL. Outcome after spinal reirradiation for malignant epidural spinal cord compression. *Ann Neurol* 1995;37:583–589.

Schold SC, Cho ES, Somasundaram M, Posner JB. Subacute motor neuropathy: A remote effect of lymphoma. *Ann Neurol* 1979;5:271–287.

Shapiro WR, Green SB, Burger PC, et al. Randomized trial of three chemotherapy regimens and two radiotherapy regimens in postoperative treatment of malignant glioma. *J Neurosurg* 1989;71:1–9.

Siegal T, Lossos A, Pfeffer MR. Leptomeningeal metastases: Analysis of 31 patients with sustained off-therapy response following combined-modality therapy. *Neurology* 1994;44: 1463–1469.

Smalley SR, Laws ER, O'Fallon JR, et al. Resection for solitary brain metastasis. *J Neurosurg* 1992;77:531–540.

Sneed PK, Suh JH, Goetsch SJ, et al. A multi-institutional review of radiosurgery alone vs. radiosurgery with whole brain radiotherapy as the initial management of brain metastases. *Int J Radiat Oncol Biol Phys* 2002;53(3):519–526.

Sorensen PS, Borgesen SE, Rasmusson B, et al. Metastatic epidural spinal cord compression. Results of treatment and survival. *Cancer* 1990;65:1502–1508.

Stupp R, Mason WP, van den Bent M, et al. Radiotherapy plus concomitant and adjuvant temozolomide for glioblastoma. *N Eng J Med* 2005;352:987–996.

Taha JM, Tew JM Jr., van Loveren HR, et al. Comparison of conventional and skull base surgical approaches for the excision of trigeminal neurinomas. *J Neurosurg* 1995;82:719–725.

Thomas D, Brada M, Stening S, et al. Randomized trial of procarbazine, lomustine, and vincristine in the adjuvant treatment of high-grade astrocytoma: A Medical Research Council Trial. *J Clin Oncol* 2001;19(2):509–518.

Vecht CJ, Haaxma-Reiche H, Noordijk EM, et al. Treatment of single brain metastasis: Radiotherapy alone or combined with neurosurgery? *Ann Neurol* 1993;33:583–590.

Younis GA, Sawaya R, DeMonte F, et al. Aggressive meningeal tumors: Review of a series. *J Neurosurg* 1995;82:17–27.

Chapter 22

American Psychiatric Association. *Diagnostic and Statistical Manual of Mental Disorders*, 3rd ed. Revised. Washington, DC: American Psychiatric Association, 1987.

Antinori A, Arendt G, Becker JT, et al. Updated research nosology for HIV-associated neurocognitive disorders. *Neurology* 2007;69(18):1789–1799.

Brew BJ. AIDS dementia complex. *Neurol Clin* 1999;17(4):861–881.

Consensus recommendations for the postmortem diagnosis of Alzheimer's disease. The National Institute on Aging, and Reagan Institute Working Group on Diagnostic Criteria for the Neuropathological Assessment of Alzheimer's Disease. *Neurobiol Aging* 1997;18(Suppl 4):S1–S2.

Consensus report of the Working Group on 'Molecular and biochemical markers of Alzheimer's disease.' The Ronald and Nancy Reagan Research Institute of the Alzheimer's Association and the National Institute on Aging Working Group. *Neurobiol Aging* 1998;19:109–116.

Corder EH, Saunders AM, Strittmatter WJ, et al. Gene dose of apolipoprotein E type 4 allele and the risk of Alzheimer's disease in late onset families. *Science* 1993;261:921–923.

Corey-Bloom J. Alzheimer's disease. *Continuum* 2004;10:29–56.

Erkinjuntti T, Rockwood K. Vascular dementia. *Semin Clin Neuropsychiatry* 2003;8(1):37–45.

Evans DA, Funkenstein HH, Albert MS, et al. Prevalence of Alzheimer's disease in a community population of older persons. Higher than previously reported. *JAMA* 1989;262: 2551–2556.

Folstein MF, Folstein SE, McHugh PR. Mini-Mental State: A practical method for grading the cognitive state of patients for the clinician. *J Psychiatr Res* 1975;12:189–198.

Graff-Radford NR, Woodruff BK. Frontotemporal dementia. *Semin Neurol* 2007;27(1):48–57.

Growdon JH. Biomarkers of Alzheimer disease. *Arch Neurol* 1999;56:281–283.

Hachinski VC. The decline and resurgence of vascular dementia. *CMAJ* 1990;142(2):107–111.

Hansen L, Salmon D, Galasko D, et al. The Lewy body variant of Alzheimer's disease: A clinical and pathologic entity. *Neurology* 1990;40:1–8.

Hobson M. Medications in older patients. *West J Med* 1992; 157:539–543.

Hou CE, Carlin D, Miller BL. Non-Alzheimer's disease dementias: Anatomic, clinical, and molecular correlates. *Can J Psychiatry* 2004;49(3):164–171.

Hughes AJ, Daniel SE, Blankson S, Lees AJ. A clinicopathologic study of 100 cases of Parkinson's disease. *Arch Neurol* 1993;50:140–148.

Josephs KA. Frontotemporal lobar degeneration. *Neurol Clin* 2007;25:683–696.

Kertesz, A. Pick complex: An integrative approach to frontotemporal dementia: Primary progressive aphasia, corticobasal degeneration, and progressive supranuclear palsy. *Neurologist* 2003;9(6):311–317.

Knight RSG, Will RG. Prion diseases. *J Neurol Neurosurg Psychiatry* 2004;75:I36.

Knopman DS. Vascular dementia. *Continuum* 2004;10:113–134.

Kokmen E, Whisnant JP, O'Fallon WM, et al. Dementia after ischemic stroke. *Neurology* 1996;19:154–159.

Letendre S, Marquie-Beck J, Capparelli E, et al. Validation of the CNS Penetration-Effectiveness rank for quantifying antiretroviral penetration into the central nervous system. *Arch Neurol* 2008;65(1):65–70.

Letendre SL, McCutchan JA, Childers ME, et al. Enhancing antiretroviral therapy for human immunodeficiency virus cognitive disorders. *Ann Neurol* 2004;56(3):416–423.

Lopez OL, Larumbe MR, Becker JT, et al. Reliability of NINDS-AIREN clinical criteria for the diagnosis of vascular dementia. *Neurology* 1994;44:1240–1245.

Mace NL, Rabins PV. *The 36-Hour Day: A Family Guide to Caring for Persons with Alzheimer's Disease.* Baltimore, MD: The Johns Hopkins University Press, 1981.

Mariani E, et al. Mild cognitive impairment: A systematic review. *J Alzheimers Dis* 2007;12(1):23–35.

May S, Letendre S, Haubrich R, et al. Meeting practical challenges of a trial involving a multitude of treatment regimens: An example of a multi-center randomized controlled clinical trial in neuroAIDS. *J Neuroimmune Pharmacol* 2007;2(1):97–104.

Mayeux R, Denaro J, Hemenegildo N, et al. A population-based investigation of Parkinson's disease with and without dementia. Relationship to age and gender. *Arch Neurol* 1992;49:492–497.

Mayeux R, Saunders AM, Shea S, et al. Utility of the apolipoprotein E genotype in the diagnosis of Alzheimer's disease. Alzheimer's Disease Consortium on Apolipoprotein E and Alzheimer's Disease. *N Engl J Med* 1998;338:506–511.

McArthur JC, Haughey N, Gartner S, et al. Human immunodeficiency virus associated dementia: An evolving disease. *J Neurovirol* 2003;9:205–221.

McKeith I, Mintzer J, Aarsland D, et al. International Psychogeriatric Association Expert Meeting on DLB. Dementia with Lewy bodies. *Lancet Neurol* 2004;3(1):19–28.

McKeith IG, Dickson DW, Lowe J, et al. Diagnosis and management of dementia with Lewy bodies: Third report of the DLB Consortium. *Neurology* 2005;65(12):1863–1872.

McKhann G, Drachmann D, Folstein M, et al. Clinical diagnosis of Alzheimer's disease. *Neurology* 1984;34:939–944.

Mirra SS, Heyman A, McKee D, et al. The consortium to establish a registry for Alzheimer's disease (CERAD). Part II: Standardization of the neuropathological assessment of Alzheimer's disease. *Neurology* 1991;41:479–486.

Neary D, Snowden J, Mann D. Frontotemporal dementia. *Lancet Neurol* 2005;4(11):771–780.

Reisberg B, Doody R, Stoffler A, et al. Memantine Study Group. Memantine in moderate-to-severe Alzheimer's disease. *N Engl J Med* 2003;348:1333–1341.

Robinson A, Spencer B, White L. *Understanding Difficult Behaviors: Some Practical Suggestions for Coping with Alzheimer's Disease and Related Illnesses.* Ypsilanti, MI: Eastern Michigan University Press, 1992.

Tatemichi TK, Foulkes MA, Mohr JP, et al. Dementia in stroke survivors in the Stroke Data Bank cohort. Prevalence, incidence, risk factors, and computed tomographic findings. *Stroke* 1990;21:858–866.

Vanneste J, Augustijn P, Dirven C, et al. Shunting normal-pressure hydrocephalus: Do the benefits outweigh the risks? A multicenter study and literature review. *Neurology* 1992; 42:54–59.

Chapter 23

Austin S, Cohen H, Losseff N. Haematology and neurology. *J Neurol Neurosurg Psychiatry* 2007;78(4):334–341.

Averbuch-Heller L, Steiner I, Abramsky O. Neurologic manifestations of progressive systemic sclerosis. *Arch Neurol* 1992;49(12):1292–1295.

Chong JY, Rowland LP, Utiger RD. Hashimoto encephalopathy: Syndrome or myth? *Arch Neurol* 2003;60(2):164–171.

Crane R, Kerr LD, Spiera H. Clinical analysis of isolated angiitis of the central nervous system. *Arch Intern Med* 1991;151(11):2290–2294.

Fine EJ, Soria E, Paroski MW, et al. The neurophysiological profile of vitamin B12 deficiency. *Muscle Nerve* 1990;13(2):158–164.

Fraser CL, Arieff AI. Nervous system complications in uremia. *Ann Intern Med* 1988;109(2):143–153.

Guarino M, Benito-Leon J, Decruyenaere J, et al. EFNS guidelines on management of neurological problems in liver transplantation. *Eur J Neurol* 2006;13(1):2–9.

Kirkham FJ. Therapy insight: Stroke risk and its management in patients with sickle cell disease. *Nat Clin Pract Neurol* 2007;3(5):264–278.

Kissel JT, Rammohan KW. Pathogenesis and therapy of nervous system vasculitis. *Clin Neuropharmacol* 1991;14(1):28–48.

Lewis M, Howdle PD. The neurology of liver failure. *Q J Med* 2003;96(9):623–633.

Lewis MB, Howdle PD. Neurologic complications of liver transplantation in adults. *Neurology* 2003;61(9):1174–1178.

Mach JR, Korchik WP, Mahowald MW. Dialysis dementia. *Clin Geriatr Med* 1988;4(4):853–867.

Mitsias P, Levine SR. Large cerebral vessel occlusive disease in systemic lupus erythematosus. *Neurology* 1994;44(3 Pt 1):385–393.

Myers L, Hays J. Myxedema coma. *Crit Care Clin* 1991;7(1):43–56.

Neiman J, Haapaniemi HM, Hillbom M. Neurological complications of drug abuse: Pathophysiological mechanisms. *Eur J Neurol* 2000;7(6):595–606.

Owczarek J, Jasinkska M, Orszulak-Michalak D. Drug-induced myopathies: An overview of the possible mechanisms. *Pharmacol Rep* 2005;57(1):23–34.

Riordan SM, Williams R. Treatment of hepatic encephalopathy. *N Engl J Med* 1997;337(7):473–479.

Ruff RL, Weissmann J. Endocrine myopathies. *Neurol Clin* 1988;6(3):575–592.

Yarranton H, Machin SJ. An update on the pathogenesis and management of acquired thrombotic thrombocytopenic purpura. *Curr Opin Neurol* 2003;16(3):367–373.

Zandi MS, Coles AJ. Notes on the kidney and its diseases for the neurologist. *J Neurol Neurosurg Psychiatry* 2007;78(5):444–449.

Index